Pierson and Fairchild's

PRINCIPLES & TECHNIQUES OF
Patient Care

FIFTH EDITION

Pierson and Fairchild's

PRINCIPLES & TECHNIQUES OF

Patient Care

Sheryl L. Fairchild, BS, PT

Consultant
Stoneham, Massachusetts

ELSEVIER

ELSEVIER
SAUNDERS

3251 Riverport Lane
St. Louis, Missouri 63043

Executive Content Strategist: Kathy Falk
Senior Content Development Specialist: Megan Fennell
Publishing Services Manager: Patricia Tannian
Project Manager: Carrie Stetz
Design Direction: Margaret Reid

Printed in Canada

Last digit is the print number: 9 8 7 6 5 4 3

This fifth edition is dedicated to Frank M. Pierson
(August 27, 1930 – June 8, 2010).
He was sole author of the first two editions
of Principles & Techniques of Patient Care *and Director*
of the Allied Medical Professions Department
of Physical Therapy at The Ohio State University
from 1977 until his retirement in 1991.
Frank was an excellent teacher,
loving husband and father to Sally and his three children,
and, most of all,
a friend to all who knew him.
He is greatly missed.

Preface

The first edition of *Principles & Techniques of Patient Care* was written to clearly explain and depict many concepts, procedures, and techniques of patient care that were used clinically by health care professionals. The continued use of this book by students, educators, and clinicians prompted an update of the information in this fifth edition. I was fortunate to receive excellent suggestions and recommendations for revisions to this edition, many of which have been included, from former users and reviewers of the book.

I am especially grateful to the individuals who formally reviewed and provided a critique of the fourth edition and to reviewers of certain chapters in the fifth edition; the feedback received from them was extremely valuable. Every chapter has been revised to ensure that the material reflects acceptable principles and techniques of current clinical practice. Revisions or additions of one type or another occurred in almost every chapter. Several new photographs have been added. Many of the boxes, procedures, and tables have been updated, and new ones have been added. New charts related to the treatment of ICU patients and rehabilitation for amputees are included in Chapters 10 and 11, respectively. The principles associated with topics such as differential diagnosis, the IFC model, HIPAA, The Joint Commission standards, and examples of electronic documentation have been added to this edition. The concepts of preventive long-term positioning, lung auscultation, kinesiology taping, and updates to pressure ulcer staging and emergency management recommended by the American Heart Association are now found in this text. The Bibliography has been expanded, and video references for several techniques have been added. Efforts have been made to ensure that the content of this text is accurate, relevant, and current at the time of manuscript preparation.

I believe that the revisions and additions to the text and figures contained in this edition have improved the book's educational and clinical usefulness. Some individuals may not agree with all the techniques or procedures presented and may use other preferred approaches in their patient interventions. However, the information and interventions in this edition should provide safe, effective, and acceptable methods for caregivers to use in a variety of settings.

I encourage the reader to review the Acknowledgments page, which details the individuals who were involved with the development and preparation of this new edition. I sincerely appreciate and extend my gratitude to them for their contributions of ideas, suggestions, time, and effort. Without their assistance and support, it would not have been possible to prepare and complete this project. Any future success in the acceptance and use of this book is, in large measure, attributable to their participation.

Sheryl L. Fairchild

Acknowledgments

The manuscript and photographs for this edition could not have been prepared and obtained without the assistance and support of many individuals, health care institutions, and private organizations. I am grateful to the photographers of the fourth edition: Chuck Thompson of Thompson Photography, Humble, Texas; Kim Ranney of Ranney Photography Studio, Canal Winchester, Ohio; and PatientKeeper, Inc., Newton, Massachusetts. Kim Dunleavy, Wayne State University, and the students of the Rehab Institute of Michigan are to be commended for their preparation of the videos that accompany this fifth edition.

Thanks to Melissa Danoff Roberto, DPT, MS, ATC, for her contribution of the revision information on differential diagnosis and to Barbara H. Bjornson, MD, Winchester Hospital, Winchester, Massachusetts, for her review of many of the medical sections in this book.

Numerous persons volunteered to be subjects for the photographs that greatly enhance the written material. Sharli Mathis and James Craig Middleton assisted us in the ambulation and transfer photographs in the previous edition. Others in Houston, Texas, who were photo subjects for the previous edition include Jana Lowe, MPT; Joan Pepper, PTA; Len Sobel, OTR; Elizabeth Gibson, PTA; Cindy Danielson; Poonam Shukla, PTA; Harold Engle, RN; Maritza Kennedy, RN; Terry Buchanan, RN; Anna Carmona, MPT; Don Clayton; Cathy Daniels, RN; Jeff Danielson; Larry Garrett; Grace Gibson, PTA; Maria Honaski, MPT; Rachael Jordan, RN; Yvonne Lanning, LVN; Susan Lasiter, CNA; Sheryl Lenzmeier; Carla Maslakowski; Adrienne Muller, RN; Stacie Reed; Dennis Rowe; Jessica Tevepaugh, CNA; Susan Noe, PT; Ranga Nathan, MD; Barbara Evans, RN; Joshua Cano; Darryl Crawford; Justin Duke; Sid Holcombe; Gary Kinliel; Arfincie Nichols; Jack and Kathy Simmons; Chuck Thompson; and Cheryl Wood. Subjects in Columbus, Ohio, included Nicole Baltich, RN; Tony Cooper, PTA; Victor Davis; James Estep; Angela Hosking; Bonnie Robinson; Shenae Russell Lipsky, PT; Sally Pierson; Charlotte Snyder; and Robert Vanecko, PT.

The photographic subjects for this fifth edition include Eddie G. Morris, Luther Inkley, Paco Emeanuru, Helene Lamp, Dylan Fischbach, Jadon Nafziger, Robert Scheetz, and Joseph Wingens. Several members of the staff of Melrose Wakefield Hospital, Melrose, Massachusetts, were also photo subjects for the fifth edition, including Brian Clifford, DPT; Diane Dewhirst, PT; Kerry Fagan, DPT; Melissa Roberto, DPT, MS, ATC; and Nicole Szwanke, DPT.

I would be remiss if I did not recognize the many contributions that Megan Fennell provided in her role as Developmental Editor. She provided excellent guidance, suggestions, and assistance throughout the project. The preparation of the final manuscript was greatly improved due to her excellent editorial skills, careful review of the material, and supportive comments. I was very fortunate to have Megan assist me with this fifth edition.

Many thanks to the other individuals at Elsevier, especially Kathy Falk, Executive Editor, who provided support and assistance throughout the completion of the project. In addition, I appreciate and recognize the work of persons in the Production, Marketing, and Sales departments.

I extend my gratitude to friends and family members, especially Helene Lamp, who allowed me to spend the time that was necessary to plan, write, organize photo shoots, and prepare for the submission of the manuscript.

Sheryl L. Fairchild

Contents

Chapter 9 **Assistive Devices, Patterns,
and Activities, 212**

Chapter 10 **Special Equipment
and Patient Care
Environments, 264**

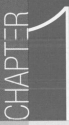

CHAPTER 1

Preparation for Patient Care Activities

objectives *After studying this chapter, the reader will be able to:*

- Describe a process for the examination and evaluation of a patient.
- Describe a health care directive and the need for such a directive.
- List the four components of a problem-oriented status note.
- Identify information that would be classified as "subjective" or "objective."
- Describe how subjective and objective information could be obtained through an evaluation.
- Discuss the importance of examining and evaluating each patient before establishing a plan of care.
- Describe the major components or categories of the patient management process.
- Describe evidence-based practice.
- List five barriers to communications and describe how they can be overcome.
- Describe five guidelines to use when communicating with a person who has an impairment.
- Describe the major components of a written home program.

key terms

Assessment   The measurement or quantification of a variable or the placement of a value on something (note that assessment should not be confused with examination or evaluation).

Caregiver   The person who is treating or working with the patient; examples are the therapist, therapist assistant, aide, or family member.

Communication   The exchange of information through verbal (oral), written, or nonverbal (visual) means.

Documentation   Written or printed matter conveying authoritative information, records, or evidence.

Electrodiagnostic tests   The use of an electrical current to assist with the diagnosis of a patient's condition.

Evaluation   A dynamic process in which the practitioner makes clinical judgments based on data gathered during the examination and identifies problems pertinent to patient/client management.

Examination   The process of obtaining a history, performing relevant systems reviews, and selecting and administering specific tests and measures.

Goniometry   The measurement of the range of motion of a joint of the body.

Health Insurance Portability and Accountability Act of 1996 (HIPAA)   A federal law enacted to protect health care–related information.

Kinesthesia   The sense by which position, weight, and movement are perceived.

Orthosis   An orthopedic appliance used to support, align, prevent, or correct deformities or to replace the function of parts of the body (e.g., a brace or splint).

Outcome measure   A quantifiable or objective means to determine the effectiveness of treatment or performance that is usually expressed in functional terms.

Problem-oriented medical record (POMR)   A system developed to organize a medical record that uses a common list of patient problems as its base.

Proprioception   Perception mediated by proprioceptors or proprioceptive testing; sensation and awareness about the movements and position of body parts or the body.

Prosthesis   The artificial replacement of an absent body part (e.g., an artificial limb).

Radiograph An image or a record produced on exposed or processed film through radiography; a roentgenogram.

SOAP An acronym, the letters of which identify each section of a patient's status: S, subjective; O, objective; A, assessment; P, plan.

Stereognosis The ability to recognize the form (shape) of an object by touch.

The Joint Commission A private, nonprofit organization whose purpose is to encourage the attainment of uniformly high standards of institutional medical care.

Two-point discrimination The ability to recognize or differentiate two blunt points when they are simultaneously applied to the skin.

INTRODUCTION

This book has been prepared to assist persons who are responsible for and involved with patient care to provide safe and effective care. The term "caregiver" (rather than therapist, nurse, health care practitioner, therapist assistant, technologist, technician, aide, or family member) is used to designate the person who is treating or working with the patient or client. Sometimes the term "client" is more appropriate to describe a person who receives treatment. Furthermore, the term "consumer" may be used to describe the person who receives care. However, for the sake of consistency, the term "patient" is used throughout this book to describe the person who receives treatment. Similarly, in some situations the term "intervention" may be used rather than the term "treatment," but for the sake of consistency, the term "treatment" is used in this book. The procedures and techniques contained in the book can be applied or adapted for use with a variety of patients to help them fulfill their functional needs or goals. The knowledgeable and experienced practitioner will realize that alternative techniques or procedures exist that provide safe and effective ways to perform many of the patient activities described in this book.

It is anticipated and expected that the health care practitioner or caregiver will modify or adjust any technique or procedure to benefit the patient or better suit a specific situation or environment. The safety of the patient and the persons involved with providing care must be maintained at all times. The patient should be encouraged to perform maximally whenever his or her active participation is desired.

The caregiver will need to guide, direct, and instruct each patient. For many patients, a brief demonstration of an activity or the use of equipment by the caregiver or another patient will enable the person to understand his or her role better. Verbal, written, and nonverbal communication (NVC) among the caregiver, the patient, and family members will be necessary. The purpose of each activity, its expected outcome, and the method of performance should be explained to the patient.

No activity should be attempted unless sufficient personnel and equipment are available to accomplish the task safely. All persons who assist with the patient's care must be trained and competent; the equipment must function properly and be safe and stable; and the patient must be evaluated to determine the capacity to assist with or perform a particular activity.

Patient examination and evaluation, patient safety, and communication between the caregiver and the patient are required to promote quality patient care. Lack of attention to any one of these areas usually will adversely affect the quality of care the patient receives.

INTERPROFESSIONAL COLLABORATION

Many organizations use a team of caregivers from different professions who review a patient's condition, determine the problems amenable to treatment, discuss potential treatment solutions, and make decisions to resolve problems. This interprofessional collaboration approach is particularly useful for patients with complex medical, social, economic, or other problems. To be successful, interprofessional collaboration requires the team members to meet collectively and periodically to solve problems and reach decisions about management of the patient. Collaboration, coordination, and communication are important factors used by the team to help the patient effectively fulfill goals or needs.

Interprofessional team members must be competent professionals who are willing to function interdependently to provide maximum benefit to the patient. Team members must be prepared to recognize and accept the value of other members' professional knowledge, skills, and expertise; work through role conflicts that may develop as a result of overlapping roles of the members; understand the basic components of each member's profession; communicate effectively with each other; and participate in leadership. The interprofessional team approach must be patient centered rather than profession centered; team members must therefore be able to provide advice, counsel, and recommendations, based on each member's knowledge and expertise, that will lead to the best outcome for the patient.

Group members need to be adept in the application of group process skills; thus it is recommended that a portion

Table **1-1** Interprofessional Collaboration

Rationale for Client/Patient	Rationale for Professional	Rationale Against Client/Patient	Rationale Against Professional
Comprehensive approach	Opportunity for members to better understand the skills, expertise, and roles of other professionals; better treatment planning and patient outcomes	Process may overwhelm the patient	May have personal and professional identity reduced, may lose professional autonomy
Reduction in duplication or fragmentation of professional services and activities	Opportunity for members to become more aware of and effective in their own professional expertise and knowledge	May not produce better quality care	Reduces personal decision making
Team is better able to address complex problems	Enhances ability and provides opportunity to network and refer to other professionals	May not result in best decisions because of professional role conflicts	Takes time away from other patients; is a time-consuming process
Team decision making is better because of input from different professionals	Broadens interaction with other professionals; leads to professional development	Likely to be more costly (e.g., time, money, and effort)	Causes separation from professionals, peers, and colleagues
Results in interventions for complex problems that exceed what an individual could accomplish	Creates a learning opportunity	May reduce the one-on-one relationship between the patient and individual professionals	Interprofessional collaboration may not be a value of the profession; professional becomes reluctant to participate

of their formal education be devoted to an introduction to and practice of techniques, skills, and activities associated with group interaction. Furthermore, the opportunity to collaborate with students from various professional programs (e.g., medicine, social work, nursing, law, theology, and allied health professions) to discuss and resolve complex case study patient scenarios would be beneficial to prepare for future interprofessional team collaboration. Table 1-1 presents rationales for the support of and opposition to the use of interprofessional collaboration from the perspective of the patient and the participating professional.

PROFESSIONAL COLLABORATION

Another concept used in patient care is professional teamwork or, more specifically, cotreatment. This method of treatment is particularly important for professions that have levels or types of caregivers. Examples are a physician and physician's assistant in the medical profession; a registered nurse and licensed practical nurse or nurse's aide in the nursing profession; an occupational therapist and occupational therapy assistant in the occupational therapy profession; and a physical therapist (PT) and PT assistant or aide in the physical therapy profession. In these professions, the assistant functions with direction, guidance, and, in some situations, direct supervision by the more responsible or primary caregiver in accordance with statutory, professional, or ethical requirements. In addition, the patient's limitations, condition, needs, response to treatment, and the

environment where the treatment is provided may influence or affect the relationship between the two caregivers.

An ideal relationship exists when the two caregivers cotreat the patient. In such a relationship, the two persons cooperatively establish the roles and activities each will perform. The primary caregiver evaluates the patient, provides a plan of care, determines the therapeutic interventions to be used, assigns tasks and responsibilities for the assistant to follow, establishes the goals or desired outcomes of treatment, and periodically evaluates the results of the treatment and the patient's responses to the treatment. The assistant performs the treatment activities for which he or she is qualified and communicates frequently, verbally and in writing, with the primary caregiver. Changes in the patient's condition, outcomes of the therapeutic procedures used, and observations by the assistant help the primary caregiver alter or adjust the plan of care. The primary caregiver eventually performs the activities necessary to terminate the treatment and discharge the patient from services.

It is imperative that the primary caregiver be aware of the activities of the assistant and that the assistant understand the rationale for the treatment and inform the primary caregiver of the patient's response. Furthermore, the cotreatment approach to patient care depends on the cooperation, collaboration, and coordination of the activities performed by the two caregivers to maximize the effectiveness of patient care.

ORIENTATION

Before seeing the patient, the therapist should perform a comprehensive review of the patient's medical record, including the physician's notes on the medical history, current history, physical findings, and diagnosis; test results; the physician request for treatment; nursing notes; medications prescribed; and any consultations to other medical/surgical specialties.

Before providing any form of treatment, including an examination and evaluation, the caregiver initially must orient the patient. This orientation consists of a personal introduction; informing the patient of the treatment goals, desired outcome, and potential risks; interviewing the patient (as part of the examination and evaluation) to obtain information; and instructing the patient regarding participation.

In a treatment setting, the caregiver should greet and identify the patient and state clearly his or her own name and professional or technical status. The patient should be informed why he or she has been referred to the service unit, the type of treatment to be received, and any serious risks or adverse effects associated with the proposed treatment. At this time the patient should have the opportunity to ask questions, obtain additional information, participate in the plan of care, and agree to or decline treatment. During the interview, the caregiver should confirm the patient's name and medical diagnosis and then progress to the assessment, examination, and evaluation of the patient. Next, the caregiver should instruct the patient more specifically about the treatment and the patient's role or expected level of performance. After the plan of care and objectives have been discussed with the patient, treatment can commence. During subsequent treatment sessions, several of the steps can be eliminated or modified as the patient becomes more familiar with the treatment process. However, the caregiver should always discuss each treatment activity with the patient and instruct or guide the patient's performance (Procedure 1-1).

AWARENESS OF CULTURAL DIVERSITY

Today, a caregiver is more likely to treat a person whose cultural or religious foundations vary greatly from what is often considered to be "mainstream" or "traditional." In preparation, the caregiver should be aware of his or her own personal biases, prejudices, attitudes, and values to better understand the effect these beliefs may exert on a patient if they are applied injudiciously. The caregiver should learn about or research the cultural norms and traditions associated with different ethnic or religious groups before treatment to be able to exhibit desirable behavior toward those individuals and their family members. Differences in language (both verbal and nonverbal), cultural or religious norms or traditions, and personal bias or prejudice can create problems between the caregiver and the patient (Box 1-1).

PROCEDURE 1-1

Patient Orientation

- Introduce yourself by name and title or professional designation.
- Verify the patient you are treating, using at least two patient identifiers such as patient name, medical record number, date of birth, or driver's license.
- Verify or confirm patient information you have received such as name, diagnosis, purpose of treatment, and referral source.
- Interview the patient to obtain relevant information; be alert for culturally different norms or traditions.
- Perform assessment, examination, and evaluation activities to establish the patient's capabilities, condition, problems, needs, goals, and a clinical diagnosis.
- Establish treatment goals and functional outcomes with patient input.
- Inform the patient of the treatment plan and techniques selected to fulfill outcome goals; include information about risks or adverse effects associated with the treatment.
- Encourage the patient to ask questions to enable the person to consent to or decline treatment.
- Request that the patient sign an informed consent document or record the oral consent in the medical record.

Understanding the cultural norms of a patient can help the caregiver enhance the effectiveness of the treatment by improving communication and developing respect between the two individuals. A judgment by the caregiver about a patient based on cultural or religious bias may affect the patient's care if the caregiver believes that the patient's behavior is "unusual" when compared with the caregiver's concept of "normal" behavior. The caregiver will want to become familiar with the basic cultural and/or religious expectations and traditions of each patient to understand fully the patient's needs and to develop a specific plan of care.

Because of their cultural or religious norms and traditions, some patients may rely on spiritual healing, family remedies, "folk" or "faith" healers, or supernatural power of healing more than traditional health care treatment. Herbal medicines, medicinal amulets, poultices, acupuncture, magnetic forces, and prayer vigils may be forms of alternative treatment used by persons from certain cultures and should be recognized by the caregiver as treatment adjuncts.

Furthermore, cultural norms may explain why some patients arrive late for an appointment, why some may not appear at all, or why some discontinue treatment early. The caregiver should be aware that gestures used by one culture may have a derogatory or offensive meaning or a meaning different from the one intended when a person of a different culture views or uses them. It is important to clarify the

Box **1-1** **Glossary of Terms Related to Cultural Diversity**

Culture
- The shared values, norms, traditions, customs, art, history, folklore, and institutions of a group of people

Cultural Competence
- A set of academic and interpersonal skills that allow individuals to increase their understanding and appreciation of cultural differences and similarities within, among, and between groups; this requires a willingness and ability to draw on knowledgeable persons of and from the community in developing focused interventions, communications, and other supports

Cultural Diversity
- Differences in race, ethnicity, language, nationality, or religion among various groups within a community, organization, or nation; a city is said to be culturally diverse if its residents include members of different groups

Cultural Sensitivity
- An awareness of the nuances of one's own and other cultures

Culturally Appropriate
- Demonstrating both sensitivity to cultural differences and similarities as well as effectiveness in using cultural symbols to communicate

Ethnic
- Belonging to a common group often linked by race, nationality, and language with a common cultural heritage or derivation

Race
- A socially defined population that is derived from distinguishable physical characteristics that are genetically transmitted

meaning or intent of the gesture when it is initially used. At times an interpreter may be needed so communication can be meaningful and appropriate relationships can be established. In some situations the interpreter may be a family member or friend; at other times a professional translator may be needed. A family member may insist on observing the treatment or remaining with the patient throughout the treatment session. (Note: Some institutions may have policies or procedures that restrict the use of a family member for interpretation unless a waiver is signed. If a family member is not present or refuses to sign a waiver, a professional interpreter may be hired.)

The intent of this section is to encourage the caregiver to become more knowledgeable about cultural and religious differences among patients and to be prepared to adapt to those differences when necessary to promote quality care. The words used and the actions exhibited should convey respect for differences in the age, gender, race or ethnicity, abilities, and sexual orientation of each person. Only a few examples of cultural or religious norms or traditions have

been presented. Many cultural rights are protected by the U.S. Department of Justice's Americans with Disabilities Act of 1990 and the Civil Rights Act of 1964. In addition, these or similar rights may be contained in institutional personnel policies, patient rights statements, and governmental documents.

HEALTH INSURANCE PORTABILITY AND ACCOUNTABILITY ACT

The Health Insurance Portability and Accountability Act of 1996 (HIPAA), which can be found at the U.S. Department of Health & Human Services Web site (www.hhs.gov), is a federal law enacted to protect health care–related information. The HIPAA Privacy Rule protects all "individually identifiable health information" held or transmitted by a covered entity or its business associate, in any form or media, whether electronic, oral, or on paper. The Privacy Rule calls this information "protected health information," as found at the U.S. Department of Health and Human Services Web site under Summary of the HIPPA Privacy Rule.

The Privacy Rule allows patients access to their individual health care–related information and control over the use of that information. HIPAA sets standards for the maintenance and transmission of patient information among health care organizations and facilities. According to the Office for Civil Rights Privacy Brief of the U.S. Department of Health and Human Services, individually identifiable information includes (1) demographic data that relates to the individual's past, present, or future physical or mental health condition; (2) the provision of health care to the individual; or (3) the past, present, or future payment for the provision of health care to the individual. Individually identifiable health information includes many common identifiers such as name, address, date of birth, and Social Security number. Care must be taken to avoid leaving paperwork that includes patient identifiers in a public area and to avoid open discussion of patients in a public area. Privacy screens should be added to computers that are in public patient treatment areas.

Violations of the Privacy Rule include sharing or discussing protected health information with other health care workers who are not involved in the care of the patient; accessing patient information when not involved in the patient's care, such as looking up information in the chart of a coworker, friend, or family member; and not providing a patient with access to his or her medical record within 30 days of the patient's request for such information. These violations are all case examples taken from the health information privacy section of the U.S. Department of Health and Human Services Web site. More information on HIPAA can be obtained at this Web site.

ADVANCE HEALTH CARE DIRECTIVES

An Advance Health Care Directive, also known as a "living will," is a set of instructions to give an appointed individual the right to make decisions concerning the health care actions to be taken when a person is no longer able to make decisions because of illness or incapacity. A standard advance directive form provides room to state additional wishes and instructions regarding organ donations.

A living will, which only becomes effective under the circumstances delineated in the document, is one form of advance directive that provides instructions for treatment. It is the oldest form of advance directive and was first proposed by an Illinois attorney, Luis Kutner, in the *Indiana Law Journal* in 1969. Kutner devised a way for persons to state their health care desires when they were no longer able to convey their wishes. Because this form of will was to be used while an individual was still living but unable to make decisions, it was called a "living will."

A living will generally provides specific instructions about the treatment to be followed by health care providers. It also can express wishes about withholding the food and water necessary to sustain life. A living will is used only when an individual is unable to give informed consent or refusal because of incapability. A living will can be general or specific.

Typically, before a living will is implemented, two physicians must verify that the patient is incapable of making medical decisions and that his or her condition is in compliance with the state's living will law. If a person's condition changes such that he or she regains the ability to make decisions, the living will is no longer in effect.

Appointing a power of attorney or health care proxy is another form of advance directive. A power of attorney or health care proxy is a person appointed by a patient to make decisions on behalf of the patient in the event that the patient is physically unable to make the decision. Before a medical power of attorney goes into effect, a person's physician must conclude that he or she is unable to make his or her own medical decisions. The appointed health care proxy has the same rights to request or refuse treatment that the individual would have. The primary benefit of the power of attorney is that the appointed agent can make real-time decisions in actual ongoing circumstances, as opposed to those recorded in a living will.

Advance directives are legally valid throughout the United States. The services of a lawyer are not needed to fill out an advance directive; the advance directive becomes legally valid as soon as it is signed in front of the required witnesses. Because advance directives vary by state, as does the nomenclature, it is important that a signed advance directive comply with the law of the state in which the person resides. Advance directives for many states can be found in the Bibliography under "Caring Connections."

INFORMED CONSENT

When obtaining informed consent, the more information provided by a caregiver about benefits of therapy, the alternatives, anticipated time frames, cost, and risks, the less likely it is that the caregiver will be held liable if a patient claims that the caregiver failed to provide adequate information.

As John J. Bennett wrote in the December 2007 issue of *PT Magazine*, states vary on what is determined concerning informed consent, but some states have informed consent statutes that apply to PTs. Two examples are Arkansas Code Annotated § 16-114-206(b), which applies to claims against PTs and contains specific provisions regarding what a plaintiff must prove to show lack of informed consent, and Utah Code Annotated § 78-14-3 (definition of health care provider) and § 78-14-5 (informed consent).

Before the initial treatment of a patient, the caregiver is responsible for informing the person about the proposed treatment, alternative treatments that are available, and associated primary known risks. The patient then has the right to consent to or reject the proposed treatment. This process is the process of informed consent.

To ensure that the patient is properly informed, the caregiver must provide sufficient information about the proposed treatment and any alternative treatment appropriate for the person's condition to permit the person to arrive at an intelligent and knowledgeable decision. The patient must be able to understand the information. Therefore it must be presented using terms and language that are comprehensible. A translator or an interpreter may be required for persons who do not speak or comprehend English. If a family member agrees to interpret for the patient, this accommodation should be documented in the medical record. Many health care facilities use an interpreter telephone service to meet the needs of patients who do not speak or understand English. This service is becoming more necessary in the United States as the number of patients whose first language is not English increases.

Known or potential primary risks associated with the treatment should be explained, and the person should have an opportunity to ask questions and receive responses to their questions regarding any aspect of the proposed treatment. Caregivers should provide responses within their level of knowledge, training, and competence based on expected or anticipated results or outcomes. The caregiver should not state or imply certain results or outcomes will occur, nor should the caregiver offer any indication to guarantee specific results or outcomes.

For patients who have not reached the legal age of consent and for those judged to be mentally confused or incompetent to participate in the informed consent decision-making process, it may be necessary to obtain consent from a legally qualified surrogate, such as a parent, guardian, family member, or court-appointed advocate.

The caregiver should document that the process of informed consent was performed in accordance with pre-established written policies and procedures of the service unit (e.g., department, rehabilitation unit, or office) or agency with which the caregiver is associated (e.g., a hospital department, school system, home health agency, outpatient facility, skilled nursing facility, or subacute care facility). In some situations, it may be prudent to have the patient or a surrogate sign a document to indicate the person has been informed of the proposed treatment and that consent to the treatment is authorized. The caregiver must use judgment and follow the recommendations of the facility or agency, risk manager, or legal counsel to determine whether each patient should be required to sign an informed consent authorization for treatment. If signed documents are not used, policies and procedures of the facility or agency must be specific and clearly indicate the process that each caregiver is to use when discussing informed consent decisions with the patient. Failure by the caregiver to fully inform a patient about the proposed treatment before the initiation of treatment, and to obtain his or her consent to receive treatment, may constitute professional negligence. Because informed consent is a right to which every patient is entitled, the caregiver is obligated to inform the patient of the proposed treatment, its alternatives, and its foreseeable risks before initiating that treatment (Box 1-2). (Note: If the patient refuses treatment, the refusal should be entered in the medical record and accompanied by the reason given for the refusal. The action taken by the caregiver also should be entered.)

PRINCIPLES OF DOCUMENTATION

The documentation of patient care is an important component of the written record maintained for each patient. Physicians, nurses, therapists, social workers, and many other persons involved with providing patient care perform documentation, which assists in better treatment planning and improved communication among disciplines. Documentation is closely scrutinized by funding sources to determine payment or denial of services. The American Physical Therapy Association Guidelines on Physical Therapy Documentation of Patient/Client Management uses these main documentation elements: initial examination/evaluation, visit/encounter, reexamination, and discharge or discontinuation summary (see the Bibliography). The following areas also should be considered for therapy documentation:

1. The patient's primary and treatment diagnosis
2. Physician's orders
3. The patient's barriers to treatment and their resolution
4. The patient's consent to treatment
5. The plan of care, which includes goals, interventions, proposed frequency and duration, and discharge
6. Short-term and long-term goals
7. Risk or benefit of treatment

Many health care settings use an electronic system for entering documentation into the medical record. This paperless system requires input from all medical disciplines to ensure that the necessary documentation is built into the

---

| Box **1-2** | Elements of the Informed Consent Process |

- Description of the patient's condition, diagnosis, or evaluative data and information
- Description or outline of the proposed, recommended treatment plan, techniques, or procedures
- Primary, known, anticipated, or potential risks, complications, and precautions associated with the proposed treatment
- Expected prognosis or outcome of the proposed treatment without a stated or implied guarantee of results (e.g., decrease or absence of pain, specific functional improvement, or specific flexibility or strength gain)
- Alternative forms of treatment appropriate for the person's condition with potential risks, complications, and precautions and the expected prognosis of the alternative treatment
- Questions from the patient and responses from the caregiver that are thorough and honest; if you are unsure of or do not know the response to a question, inform the patient and attempt to locate the information or refer the patient to a qualified resource (e.g., nurse, physician, social worker, pharmacist)
- Explain the potential or possible consequence of no treatment if the patient refuses treatment
- Document that you provided an opportunity for informed consent before initiation of treatment and the patient's decision to consent to or refuse treatment

---

system to satisfy the requirements of Medicare and other insurance payers. One advantage to an electronic medical record system is that necessary information can be built into a "check-off" format in which answers to questions such as "Does the patient consent to treatment?" would be checked off as "yes," "no," or "unable to respond." If "unable to respond" is checked, an explanation must be given before moving on to the next area in the record. Other advantages are that all patient information is readily available from other disciplines, including laboratory results, x-ray examinations, and so on and that interdepartmental communication is facilitated by improved readability and the ability of multiple users to access information simultaneously. Disadvantages are that the length of time to document is not much shorter than handwritten documentation, initial and ongoing staff training in the use of the computer program is required, and the software and hardware may be inadequate or may malfunction. Fig. 1-1 shows a health care worker using a mobile electronic documentation system. Refer to Appendixes 7, 8, and 9 at the end of the book for examples of electronic documentation.

Problem-Oriented Medical Record Description

Lawrence Weed developed the concept of the problem-oriented medical record (POMR) in the 1960s. This system

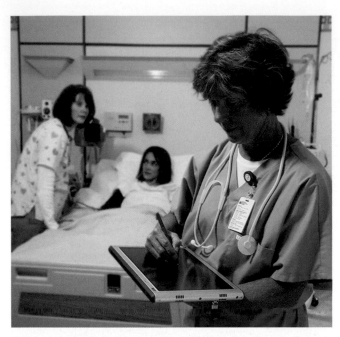

Fig. 1-1   A health care worker uses a handheld computer for electronic documentation. (Courtesy PatientKeeper, Newton, MA.)

is used by many health care facilities throughout the United States, some of which have developed their own variations. This system is based on a list of patient problems, a database, and a series of status (progress) notes designated as the "initial," "interim or ongoing," and "discharge" notes. When all departments or service units of a facility use POMR record keeping, a higher quality of patient care may be anticipated, better communication among the caregivers is more likely to occur, and better decisions about the patient's treatment can be made. Information about the patient and the plan of care is contained in the status notes, which are written in the SOAP format: *s*ubjective, *o*bjective, *a*ssessment, and *p*lan. The POMR has four phases:

1. Formation of a database (current and past information about the patient)
2. Development of a specific, current problem list (problems to be treated by various practitioners)
3. Identification of a specific treatment plan (developed by each caregiver)
4. Assessment of treatment plan effectiveness

When the POMR system is used, each practitioner adds evaluations, treatment planning, treatment decision-making information, and data to the patient's database and problem list.

SOAP notes should contain important, relevant information about the patient. They should indicate and clearly reflect the patient's condition and subsequent changes in condition, and they should be written frequently so that information is reported promptly and regularly. The method used to gather the information and the development of the examination and evaluation and planning phases is described in the section related to the patient management process. The relationship of the SOAP notes to the decision-making process and the purpose of documentation are described in several articles and textbooks. Excellent resources for information about the POMR and SOAP notes are listed in the Bibliography.

Guidelines for documentation and suggestions for improving the quality and meaningfulness of documentation are provided in Box 1-3.

Entry Corrections Occasionally it may be necessary to correct an entry. Careful and proper correction of an entry will help avoid accusations of tampering, changes to the entry for self-serving reasons or intent, or capricious alteration of the medical record, especially if litigation is involved or being considered. The following standard procedures should be followed when correcting a note in a handwritten medical record:

- Draw a single line through the inaccurate information, but be certain the material remains legible.
- Date and initial the correction, and add a note in the margin stating why the correction was necessary.
- Enter the corrected statement in the chronologic sequence of the record, and be certain it is clear which entry the correction replaces.
- Use black ink for all corrections and entries.

In some situations it may be beneficial to have the corrected statement witnessed by a colleague. Avoid alterations that create the appearance of tampering (e.g., erasing or writing over a word or phrase to improve legibility). Never attempt to obliterate material in the record by using a marker, correction fluid, a typewriter overstrike, or an eraser. Improper alteration of an entry can create many problems for the practitioner if the entry is questioned or used as evidence during litigation. The practitioner's credibility, honesty, and intent will be challenged, which may lead to charges of incompetence, negligent behavior, or poor judgment. Many errors of judgment are not negligent acts, but any attempt to hide them can create serious problem. Never enter a note or sign an entry for someone else, and do not ask someone else to perform such acts for you.

Many companies provide software programs for electronic documentation, including some used only for rehabilitation. These systems have guidelines explaining how an entry can be altered (e.g., "correction," "late entry," "entered in error," "addition," and/or "deletion"). The program will indicate when an entry has been altered and identify the person responsible. At least one system permits only the person who entered the original note to alter it.

During litigation or when questions arise about the patient's care, the medical record is the primary source of information about the care a patient received and his or her response to treatment. Accurate, timely, and proper documentation is therefore important. Failure to maintain proper documentation and records can delay or cause denial of

Box 1-3 Principles of Documentation

- Document every encounter/visit.
- Documentation must comply with regulatory requirements.
- Documentation must include identification of the patient/client and the PT or the PT assistant (or student where permitted by state and/or facility regulations).
- The patient's/client's full name and identification number (if applicable) must be included on all official documents.
- Documentation should indicate the referral source (physician or other practitioner, self-referral/direct access).
- All entries must be dated and signed with the PT's full name and title.
- Avoid general statements and provide specific, concise, clarifying information. Instead of stating "The patient is uncooperative," state "The patient refused to perform active assistive exercise."
- Use objective statements; instead of stating "Patient ambulates," state "Patient ambulates 25 feet in 1 minute using bilateral axillary crutches on a level surface, with assistance, using a 3-point pattern for 3 repetitions, with a 5-minute rest period between ambulations." Functional outcome measure statements more accurately describe the patient's condition and assist with obtaining reimbursement.
- Be complete with your statements; record the significant or important information about the patient's condition, progress, or response to treatment. (Remember: If an activity is not documented, it may be considered as not having occurred. If an unusual activity or procedure is used, document why it was selected and used. Unusual incidents, the action taken afterwards, and an objective description of the patient's condition or reaction should be recorded, dated, and timed. An incident report should be filed with the risk manager or similar individual, and it may be necessary to document that it was prepared and filed.)
- Provide continuity with your status (i.e., progress) notes. Be certain to indicate why or how you reached a particular decision about the care or treatment you provided, especially if it deviated from the acceptable care or treatment.
- Programs or treatment plans designed for the patient to follow at home should be well documented and include precautions. Your documentation should indicate how you determined (or the steps taken to ensure) the patient or family member understood and could comply with the instructions.
- Identify that you informed the patient of the treatment to be provided and its risks or hazards, the information was understood by the patient, and consent to treatment was given. If a consent form is used by the service unit, a copy signed by the patient should be in the medical record.
- Be prompt and timely with your entries, and write legibly. Be certain the information is accurate and consistent between entries. Investigate and clarify contradictory information; for example, is it the right hip or the left hip that requires treatment?
- Only use abbreviations that have been standardized or accepted and approved by the facility or the profession.
- Be certain there are no empty or open lines between entries and there are no open spaces within the notes. Use the format approved by the human information systems department or used by the facility or profession.
- Outline the major elements of the notes in your mind or on paper before you enter them in the record to avoid having to make a correction or a change in the notes. Avoid omissions, such as the date of initial or subsequent treatments, a change in treatment, or a discharge summary.
- Properly countersign the entries of other persons according to state statutes and facility requirements. Read the entry before countersigning it; it is prudent to review the proposed entry to ensure that it is accurate and complete before it is placed in the record.

reimbursement, lead to dismissal or disciplinary action against the practitioner, affect the accreditation status of the facility, weaken the defense of the defendant during litigation, or cause improper or poor-quality treatment to be delivered. The following basic principle should be followed: Maintain the record so that, if all the persons originally treating a patient were to disappear, the next group of practitioners could immediately continue to provide the best quality treatment by using only the information from the record.

Rationale Documentation is becoming more important as a means to assess or measure the quality of care received by the patient so the caregiver or facility will be more likely to receive payment from a third-party payer (e.g., Medicare or an insurance company). Persons who review claims and make reimbursement and treatment-related decisions focus on indicators of functional outcomes of treatment contained in the caregiver's documentation. Therefore the caregiver must be aware of the need to provide accurate, current, function-oriented documentation. In addition, the use of function-oriented, objective, and measurable data in the documentation process will result in the greatest likelihood of obtaining a favorable reimbursement response to submitted claims and gaining approval to continue treatment from the third-party payer. It seems reasonable to anticipate that a patient will have more motivation to accomplish a functional goal or task that is meaningful to the person than to strive to attain a given strength or range-of-motion value. In addition, well-organized, accurate, relevant, and prompt documentation improves communication among all persons providing care.

When a caregiver documents the treatment that has been provided or supervised, it is necessary to indicate the functional outcome or outcomes attained by the patient. The documentation must report the extent of change in the patient's condition that resulted from the treatment by using objective and measurable terms, language, or data. The results of initial and repeated muscle strength tests, goniometry measurements, and vital signs data are examples of objective, measurable information. However, it is also necessary to provide objective information that indicates the patient's ability or capacity to perform functional activities related to the activities in the home, workplace, or community and during recreation. Strength and range-of-motion data could be linked to the person's functional ability to perform dressing, feeding, and personal hygiene tasks at home; to reach, lift, and carry objects or use office equipment at work; to transfer and perform mobility activities in the community; and to participate in various sport or recreational activities. The caregiver should be certain that the functional outcomes directly relate to the preestablished treatment goals or outcome measures stated in the treatment plan.

PRINCIPLES OF PATIENT MANAGEMENT

Differential Diagnosis

When a patient exhibits symptoms that are associated with two or more illnesses or conditions, it becomes necessary to determine which of the illnesses or conditions the patient actually has. By using a systematic process, it can be possible to compare and contrast the symptoms and distinguish one illness or condition from another. The trained caregiver integrates knowledge gained from educational and clinical experiences and the evidence gained from information and data gathered from evaluation activities. The caregiver then can use reasoning to differentiate the symptoms and arrive at an initial diagnosis. An accurate diagnosis is the basis for better treatment decisions, plans, and outcomes and for the reduction of medical errors, and it limits the possibility of inappropriate treatment. Physicians have traditionally had the legal right to make a diagnosis, but recently certain types of nurses and therapists, especially PTs, have been given the legal right to make a diagnosis within the scope of their practice and as determined by state or federal statutes or policies.

Components of a Differential Diagnosis

The caregiver applies knowledge, evidence, and reasoning as the basis for a process to differentiate symptoms and reach an initial diagnosis. Two primary methods are used to gather information and data: (1) observation and interviews and (2) specific tests and measures. An examination should

provide information about the patient's current and previous medical, surgical, family, and social histories (see Table 1-3). If the caregiver is not a physician, certain symptoms or findings may indicate the need to refer the patient to a physician or other practitioner. For example, a referral should be made when the caregiver feels unqualified to provide treatment or when a patient exhibits chest pain at rest with diaphoresis, dyspnea, radiating chest or arm pain, increased pain with exertion, bowel and bladder incontinence of unknown origin, respiratory distress at rest, acute abdominal pain at rest or with pressure, changes in mental status (e.g., decreased alertness, cognition, memory, or consciousness), or increased agitation or seizure.

The components of the history reviews are listed in Box 1-4. During the interview of the patient or family members, open-ended questions should initially be used, followed by more specific questions. "Why are you here?" "What brings you here today?" and "What is bothering you today?" are questions that relate to the patient's primary symptoms. The request to "Tell me about your previous major illnesses and surgical procedures" will help identify previous medical and surgical events and treatment. Other possible approaches include the following questions: "Describe how you feel when you first wake up, later in the day, and when you go to bed." "What makes you feel better or worse?" "What can't you do because of your condition that you could do before you became ill?" To gain the most from the patient's response, use active listening skills to determine what the patient has actually told you. At the same time, look for nonverbal signs of discomfort (e.g., grimaces, frowns, and position changes), respiratory difficulties (e.g., rapid breathing, shallow breaths, and accessory muscle use), and decreased mental function (e.g., slow response, lack of eye contact, "flat" affect, and drowsiness).

While information is being gathered, determine whether a particular symptom is related to the body as a whole (i.e., a systemic symptom) or to a specific body system (e.g., musculoskeletal, neuromuscular, integumentary, or cardiovascular/pulmonary). The information gathered from various tests and measures is integrated with the interview and observational information to further aid in determinating the diagnosis. Examination and evaluation activities are

---

Box **1-4**   Components: Patient Medical History

- Primary complaint
- Current illness
- Previous medical history
- Previous surgical history
- Current medications
- Family history
- Social history
- Review of body systems

continued throughout the course of the patient's treatment to support the diagnosis, treatment plan, and outcome goals.

The information in this section introduces the process of "differential diagnosis"; it is not intended to be a complete explanation or a thorough presentation of this process. Refer to the Bibliography for additional information regarding this important activity.

Before initial treatment, the caregiver must develop and follow a process of gathering information and data so a quality plan of care can be developed and implemented. Major components of the process include assessment, examination, evaluation of the examination information and data, postulation of a diagnosis and prognosis, development of a plan of care, and the selection of intervention activities and techniques best suited to alter or change the patient's condition to attain desired functional outcomes (Procedure 1-2). The plan of care and the interventions should be derived from the diagnosis and prognosis. The caregiver should focus the plan of care so it will lead to the desired outcomes, usually expressed as short-term or long-term objectives and functional goals. Inherent in the process is the frequent reevaluation of the patient's condition and the response to treatment, which may result in a change in the interventions used or the modification of the functional goals. To complete the process—that is, planning and preparing for the termination of treatment (which could occur as early as the first or second treatment session)—a reevaluation must be performed. Refer to the Appendixes for examples of forms used to document patient care.

It is important to understand that the examination establishes a baseline of data and information that describes the patient's current condition and level of function and can be used to measure the patient's progress and response to treatment. Barriers to treatment (e.g., receptive aphasia or a mental, psychological, or social impairment) should be determined by the examination and documented in the medical record. The evaluation helps establish a functional diagnosis and prognosis for the patient, set outcome goals, and develop the plan of care.

The plan of care developed from decisions that the caregiver makes in accordance with the diagnosis and prognosis should contain treatment procedures, techniques, and activities that will be most effective in fulfilling the established goals and anticipated outcomes. The sequence and frequency of the program, the need for equipment, and the level of assistance required by the patient must be determined. At this time, consideration should be given to planning for the termination of treatment. Because of the cost containment requirements of most third-party payers, many patients will receive only a few treatment sessions from a qualified caregiver. Therefore the caregiver must plan and prepare a program of treatment activities to be performed at home or at another site after the patient's formal treatment program is terminated. Equipment needs, financial assistance, family education and training, referral proce-

---

PROCEDURE 1-2

Patient Management Process

- Examine the patient's medical record, including physician's orders, history and physical, special diagnostic tests, and nursing notes.
- Examine the patient, gather subjective and objective information and data, and perform tests and measures to determine the patient's current condition and functional abilities.
- Evaluate the information and data to make clinical judgments and decisions.
- Postulate a clinical diagnosis and prognosis based on the results of the evaluation.
- Form a plan of care based on the prognosis.
- Identify and select the intervention activities and techniques projected to be most effective to attain functional outcomes.
- Establish the sequence, frequency, and duration of the plan.
- Consider termination of treatment, including the development of a home treatment program if it becomes necessary.
- Implement the plan.
- Apply techniques, activities, or procedures selected to accomplish functional outcomes.
- Revise or modify the plan depending on the patient's response or progress.
- Evaluate and document the patient's response frequently; determine progress toward functional outcomes.
- Terminate the plan.
- Evaluate the patient's functional activities to determine the need for further treatment elsewhere.
- If appropriate, instruct family members or home caregiver and provide time for them to practice.
- Provide a written home program and place a copy in the patient's medical record; document the patient's functional outcomes; and document the date and time for reevaluation, if necessary.

---

dures, and follow-up or extended care may need to be considered as alternate treatment plans are developed.

Implementation of the procedures, techniques, and activities selected by the caregiver should be performed using the sequence and frequency previously determined. The caregiver must frequently and consistently reevaluate and measure the patient's progress and response to treatment. The extent to which the patient fulfills the short-term and long-term goals and accomplishes the functional outcomes must be measured and documented. For example, it is not sufficient to document that a patient's active range of motion of shoulder flexion has increased from 90 to 120 degrees. A functional outcome, such as the independent application and removal of clothing over the head, should be a component of the documentation. The caregiver must be prepared to continue, revise, or modify the treatment plan or the components of the treatment program based on the patient's progress and response to the treatment. Attention to the plan and program for treatment at home will be necessary. Education and training of the patient and a family member should be provided as well as the opportunity to practice the activities to be performed at home.

When the treatment program is to be terminated, the caregiver should evaluate and measure the patient's functional outcomes and compare them with the expected outcomes, and the home treatment program should be reviewed and finalized. The written or printed program should be given to the patient or family member, and a copy should be placed in the medical record or maintained in a separate file.

A summary of the patient's condition, the functional outcomes and goals that were accomplished, future treatment plans, and any reevaluation or follow-up care appointments should be documented in the medical record. Additional information about the patient management process can be found in several of the resources listed in the Bibliography.

Evidence-Based Practice

The use of the most current and valid research should be the basis of sound clinical decision making. The application of research to determine and guide a patient's course of treatment is referred to as evidence-based practice (EBP). Based on the caregiver's evaluation and diagnosis, the creation of an individualized and comprehensive treatment plan that is validated by evidence will assist the caregiver in delivering high-quality patient care safely and efficiently. With readily available access to the Internet, research has become much more prevalent for caregivers who seek to gain knowledge for their patients' outcomes. Sources that have been in the forefront of EBP are the American Physical Therapy Association, an organization that initiated a grassroots effort to develop a database containing current research evidence on the effectiveness of physical therapy interventions, and the American Occupational Therapy Association, which has links to online research through its Web site. Both of these professional sites require membership to access online research.

The use of EBP helps determine the effectiveness of the caregiver's interventions or outcome measures. Outcome measures help determine the difference the treatment has made to the patient's functional status, if any. Measurement of a patient's outcome helps validate the treatment the patient received for that particular diagnosis and may lead to future research and EBP.

A universal language is needed to measure outcomes and discuss health and impairment. Disablement models have been used since the 1960s with the development of the Nagi Disablement Model. Nagi's model describes how an active pathology can lead to impairments, functional limitations, and disability. The most current disablement model has

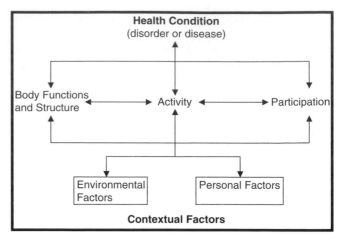

Fig. 1-2 The International Classification of Functioning, Disability and Health. (From International Classification of Functioning, Disability and Health: *ICF,* Geneva, Switzerland, 2001, World Health Organization; with permission of the World Health Organization.)

been created and edited by the World Health Organization (Fig. 1-2). The International Classification of Functioning, Disability and Health (ICF) takes into consideration the biologic, personal, and social domains when discussing health and impairment. Table 1-2 provides a comparison of the ICF and Nagi models. Fig. 1-3 illustrates an actual client condition using the ICF model. A patient's health status can be affected not only by the biologic processes occurring in the body, but also by environmental factors. By addressing all the domains of a patient's impairment, the caregiver is able to treat the cause and impact the impairment has created. The ICF common language can be used for the continuum of care from functional assessments, goal setting, treatment planning, and clinical outcome measures. When they are used correctly, disablement models promote value-driven patient care and clinical outcome measures that can be used for the development of EBP.

PRINCIPLES OF PATIENT EXAMINATION AND EVALUATION

The patient's emotional response or reaction to the condition, family unit interactions, the support system available, the potential for improvement or regression of the condition, and the goals or expectations that the person has for the treatment program also should be considered. The patient should be informed of the findings or results of the examination and evaluation and should be consulted and asked to assist with the development of the goals and outcomes of the treatment.

Goals of treatment should be established cooperatively between the patient and the caregiver. These goals usually are designated as interim (or short term) and terminal (or long term). Short-term goals are usually a specific component or lead-in activity for a long-term goal. An example of a short-term goal is "The patient will be able to perform

Table **1-2**	Disablement Models: Components and Comparison					

Model	Origin	Organ	Person Level	Societal Level	Other Domains
Nagi, 1965	Pathology	Impairment	*Functional limitations*	*Disability*	
World Health Organization International Classification of Functioning, 2001	Health condition	Body structure and function	*Activity*	*Participation*	*Environmental and personal factors*

Italics indicate dimensions that address health-related quality of life.

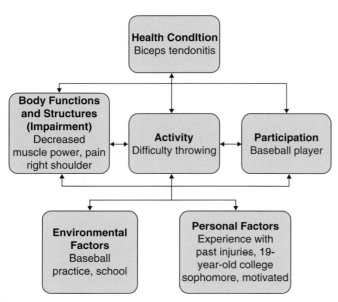

Fig. 1-3   Example of an International Classification of Functioning, Disability and Health client model.

a sitting push-up in a wheelchair 10 times in 1 minute within 2 weeks." This goal would lead to the following long-term goal: "The patient will be able to perform an independent sitting transfer from the bed to a wheelchair within 2 minutes and return to the bed within 2 minutes in no more than 3 weeks." Goals must be stated in objective, measurable terms and should indicate who will perform the activity, by what means the goal will be accomplished, the need for equipment or assistance, the time frame in which to accomplish the goal, and the functional outcome expected. Goals should be modified or revised depending on the patient's performance and progress. Finally, goals and outcomes should be realistic and attainable for each patient.

Table 1-3 is a guide to the areas that could be considered during the examination. Not all the activities will be necessary or appropriate for each patient, and the selection of the proper tests or procedures is the responsibility of the caregiver. However, for many patients, specific tests and measures will be required to obtain the data needed to develop the best plan of care. The purpose of the examination and evaluation is to identify the patient's abilities, the problems

to be treated, and the person's needs and goals so that outcomes can be established. The plan of care should result from the clinical diagnosis and prognosis determined by the caregiver and should include the intervention activities and techniques best suited to fulfill the goals and outcomes of the prognosis. The sequence, frequency, and duration of the plan of care must be established. Implementation of the plan of care, using preselected intervention procedures and techniques, provides the means to fulfill the treatment objectives, goals, and outcomes (Box 1-5).

The caregiver must be vigilant and conscientiously reexamine and reevaluate the patient frequently to maintain quality care. Failure to revise or adjust the treatment program based on the patient's response may delay the patient's recovery or limit the extent of improvement of functional skills and independence.

In summary, it is necessary to examine and evaluate the findings of the examination to form a basis for the development and implementation of the plan of care. Frequent examinations and evaluations must be performed to measure the patient's progress toward the treatment objectives, goals, and outcomes.

PATIENT AND FAMILY EDUCATION

The public continues to demonstrate an interest in and desire to become better informed about medical and health

Table 1-3 Guidelines for Patient Examination

Task	Guidelines
Gather subjective and objective information and data	Patient history: Interview the patient, family members, relatives, and other caregivers; review the medical record; observe the patient; perform/review tests and measures
	Identify the primary complaint or problem and its effect on function; identify prior function
	Obtain a history of the current illness or condition, including progression or regression of symptoms; pain factors (location, onset, duration, severity, description); factors that exacerbate or relieve symptoms; previous and current treatment, medications, modalities, activity
	Obtain history of previous medical/surgical interventions, particularly related to major body systems
	Obtain history of major family medical and surgical events, such as evidence of cancer, hypertension, coronary artery disease, other heart-related conditions, arthritis, and diabetes
	Obtain a history of social health/habits (current and past), employment or work, living environment, and lifestyle, such as use of tobacco, alcohol, controlled substances, and sexual activities
	Review information about four major body systems: musculoskeletal (gross range of motion, gross symmetry, gross strength, weight and height); neuromuscular (gross coordinated movement; motor control; motor learning; communication ability; consciousness; expected behavioral responses; orientation to place, time, and person; educational needs and barriers); integumentary (texture, skin color, presence of scar formation and integrity); and cardiovascular/pulmonary (blood pressure, edema, heart rate and respiratory rate)
Observe the patient	General appearance: body build, deformities, absence of body part
	Skin appearance: color, lesions, scars, texture
	Posture: Look for deviations while sitting and standing
	Ambulation: Consider mobility patterns, use of aids (e.g., wheelchair, crutches, walker, cane, other), level of independence, and ability to manage stairs, inclines, and uneven surfaces
	Balance, stability, coordination, equilibrium, motor control, and flexibility when standing, ambulating, sitting, and performing functional tasks
	Application of assistive devices such as a prosthesis, orthosis, splint, or bandage
Palpate patient areas	Skin and subcutaneous tissue to determine texture, temperature, color, laxity, firmness, pliability, edema, presence of scar formation, and nodules
	Muscles, tendons, ligaments to determine tone, pain, bulk, composition, stability, and laxity
	Joints to determine swelling, shape, response to movement, joint space, crepitus, stability, and presence of pain
	Bony structures to locate landmarks and to determine alignment, response to pressure, and presence of pain
	Arterial pulses to determine presence or absence, rate, rhythm, and force
	Respiratory rate
Test and measures	Muscle strength and endurance using manual or mechanical methods
	Joint motion and range using a goniometer; measured actively and passively
	Joint integrity; test actively and passively using manual or mechanical methods
	Sensory functions
	Protective reactions to pain, temperature, and pressure
	Discriminatory reactions such as kinesthesia, proprioception, stereognosis, two-point discrimination, touch, and feel (e.g., temperature, shape, and texture)
	Reflex responses related to tissue stretch, posture, and gross and fine motor skills
	Automatic reactions such as righting, equilibrium, and synergies
Cardiovascular/ pulmonary functions	Vital signs, respiratory capacity and rate, responses to exercise
	Review results of special cardiac and pulmonary function tests
Functional abilities and performance of daily tasks	Bed mobility, positional changes, and transfers
	Personal care and hygiene
	Application, removal, adjustment, and use of assistive devices or equipment
	Ambulation and mobility activities with and without the use of assistive devices or equipment
Mental and cognitive function	Problem solving, planning, decision making, comprehension, response to instructions, and communication skills (verbal and written)
Review other reports and tests when available	Radiograph films, scans, other imaging reports
	Laboratory reports such as blood chemistry, liver function, urinalysis, general chemistry, and arterial blood gases
	Electrodiagnostic tests such as electrocardiogram, electromyography, and electroencephalogram
	Biopsy reports
	Speech, hearing, language, and vision tests and reports
	Psychological evaluations

care in general and about the specific medical and health care that individuals receive. Patients and family members expect to be consulted and informed about the care they receive. Questions related to the need for, efficacy of, and expected results or outcome of treatment are routinely asked. The practitioner must be prepared to provide appropriate and accurate responses without expressing or implying a guarantee or promise that a specific outcome or result will be achieved. The patient must be informed, with language and terminology that is understandable, about the treatment to be received so an informed decision about its value and safety can be made.

The caregiver has the responsibility to educate the patient and family about the treatment program and activities, but patient confidentiality must be respected and the patient's permission must be obtained before sharing information with the family. Goals of treatment should be established cooperatively by the patient and caregiver once the patient has been informed of the various possibilities for his or her care. These goals should be stated in objective, measurable terms, which should include a time frame, how or by what means the goals will be accomplished, the need for equipment or assistive aids, and an indication of the expected functional outcome.

Interim (or short-term) goals and terminal (or long-term) goals must be developed and agreed upon. After the goals have been established, the caregiver can provide an overview or explanation of techniques or procedures that will be used to accomplish the goals. The effectiveness of the treatment program is measured by the accomplishment of the goals and subsequent patient outcomes. Goals can be revised when it is apparent the goal was an underestimate or overestimate of the patient's ability or progress (Table 1-4).

Another component of patient and family education is instruction for a home program. Some patients will require assistance from others to perform exercises and other activities in the environment of a home, health club, school, or other nonmedical facility. Ideally, the home program should be performed by the patient before termination of treatment, with a family member present and under the direction of the caregiver. The family member must be instructed about the responsibilities and level of assistance required. The patient and family member should practice the specific activities included in the home program while the caregiver observes and corrects improper performance. The home program should be printed or written and given to the patient for future reference (see Appendix 5 for an example). A copy is maintained with the patient's medical record or documentation materials at the treatment facility.

Instructions should include an outline of the exercises or activities, frequency of performance of the program, number of repetitions for each exercise, precautions or contraindications for each exercise, required equipment or supplies, specific instructions and diagrams to guide and direct the

Table **1-4**	Goal Statements
Goal Statement	**Guidelines**
General concepts	Objective terms are used
	Measurable outcomes are stated
	Realistic, attainable outcomes are identified
	Statements are oriented to the person involved, performance expected, time frame anticipated, functional outcome expected, and equipment or assistive aids needed
Short-term (interim) goals	Preparatory component of long-term goal
	Lead-in activity for long-term goal
	Sequential activities that produce cumulative effect
	Support and promote functional outcome
Long-term (terminal) goal	Evolves from short-term goals
	Describes maximal performance or desired outcome
	Describes functional outcome as a necessary component
	Should be revised or modified based on the patient's progress and performance

patient, caregiver's name and telephone number, and any scheduled reevaluation or reappointment sessions (Procedure 1-3). Finally, information about when or whether to terminate the program should be provided.

Information about the health care delivery system or resources in the community may need to be provided to assist the patient or family member to contact a particular agency or to obtain available benefits.

Education can be performed through direct contact between the patient and family members and the caregiver or through printed materials, DVDs or videotapes, and demonstrations. The specific instructional methods selected should coincide with the social, economic, mental, and physical factors manifested by or available to the patient and family members.

COMMUNICATION

Communication among persons is a primary function of life. For the caregiver, communication with patients, family members, other practitioners, and coworkers is a necessity. The caregiver should recognize that different forms of communication, such as verbal communication, NVC, and attentive listening, may be required depending on the purpose or situation related to the communication. Various barriers to communication should be recognized, documented, and avoided whenever possible. Patient-caregiver rapport can quickly be established by effective communication or delayed by the lack of it. The information in this chapter provides guidelines or reminders for the

PROCEDURE 1-3

Creating a Home Program

- Determine the need or value for the patient to continue treatment after the formal treatment concludes.
- Determine the environment and assistance available at home (family member), health club (health care practitioner), school (friend), or other.
- Prepare the program before termination of the scheduled treatment sessions.
- Instruct and supervise the patient and the assistant as they practice the program activities before termination of scheduled treatment sessions.
- Provide a typed or printed program with specific instructions, individualized for each patient.
- Outline and describe the activities, exercises, and positions to be used; provide diagrams as necessary.
- State goals and expected results, as necessary.
- Provide objective indicators of performance (i.e., repetitions, distance, and time) and the frequency and duration of the program.
- Provide indicators of successful completion, fulfillment, or accomplishment of goals, functional outcomes, or activities.
- Indicate equipment and supplies that will be needed.
- Indicate precautions or contraindications associated with the exercises or activities.
- Provide the date, time, and location of a scheduled reevaluation or appointment, if appropriate or necessary.
- Inform the patient when or whether to terminate the program.
- Provide caregiver's name, telephone number, and address.
- Document the preparation and assignment of the home program, and maintain a copy in the medical record or patient's file; contact the patient periodically to learn about problems, progress, or change in condition.

caregiver and should not be considered all-encompassing or complete.

Instructions and information can be presented to the patient verbally or nonverbally and with various audiovisual methods. Verbal communication is the most prevalent style used. When verbal communication is used, terms and concepts should be presented in language that the listener understands. Lay language is the most useful for most patients and family members. For example, "bend" is better than "flex," "turn" or "twist" is better than "rotate," and "straighten" is better than "extend" when instructing the patient or family. Directions should guide the patient to perform or act and should be brief and concise. Functional terms or phrases such as "push," "stand," "sit," "turn toward me," and "reach to the left" are more effective than nonfunctional phrases such as "Now, the first thing I want you to do is…" or "The next thing I want you to do is…" However, it is necessary to provide some transitional terms

and phrases, such as "Push with your hands on the armrests," "Straighten your hips and knees," or "Move your right crutch and left leg forward." The patient should be given time to process the message. The time required for processing will vary from person to person.

The tone, volume, and inflection of your voice can detract from or add to your message. You can either stimulate or calm a patient with your voice and behavior. For example, consider the mixed message you may give to a patient if you scowl or grimace while telling the patient that he or she performed well. When you want to encourage or stimulate a patient to act quickly, use a louder than normal volume and a sharper tone to your voice as you say, "Stand up, now!" and simultaneously clap your hands. For a nervous or apprehensive patient, you can use a lower than normal volume and a softer tone as you speak. It also may help assure the patient if you sit next to him or her or rest a hand on his or her shoulder while you talk. Think of other examples of how the volume, tone, and inflection of your voice, along with your nonverbal cues, can add to or detract from your message.

Observation of the patient's reaction to the message will help you determine whether the person understands it, has questions, or is puzzled. Maintaining eye contact with the patient allows both of you to relate to nonverbal cues and maintain better interaction. For example, when you are working with a patient's foot and ankle and he or she is supine or sitting, be certain to look at the patient's face, rather than at the foot, as you give your instructions.

It is helpful to provide an overview or a description of the total activity and its components before giving specific instructions or directions. The specific responsibilities or activities expected of the patient can be presented and emphasized later. Many caregivers find it helpful to have patients repeat the instructions to determine their ability to comprehend and retain the information and to estimate preparedness to perform. It is not sufficient to ask, "Do you understand what you are to do?" or "Do you understand the instructions?" because many patients will respond affirmatively even when they do not understand. Listen for the appropriate sequence and completeness of the repeated instructions. You may request the patient to demonstrate certain activities, such as prepositioning an extremity or the body or performing wheelchair tasks such as locking or unlocking the wheels, swinging away the front rigging, or positioning other equipment. These activities, when performed properly, help the caregiver assess the patient's level of comprehension and readiness to function.

NVC makes up the majority of human communication and may be even more effective than verbal communication. It is done through facial expressions, posture, gestures, body movements, and changes in body responses. Some forms of NVC are planned, whereas other forms are spontaneous, uncontrollable, or involuntary (Table 1-5). Most of us have been in embarrassing or stressful situations and

Table 1-5 Forms of Nonverbal Communication

Form	Examples
Appearance	Dress, grooming, cleanliness
Body movements	Abrupt, slow, threatening, caring
Body positions	Sitting, standing, walking, kneeling
Facial expressions	Smiling, frowning, grimacing
Gestures	Using hands and arms to guide or direct
Pantomime	Demonstrating the activity
Posture	Erect, slouched, rigid
Spontaneous response to stress	Blushing, perspiring, trembling
Touch	Therapeutic, caring, directive, guiding

have sensed a change in the color or temperature of our skin or experienced an increase in perspiration. These are examples of spontaneous, uncontrolled, or involuntary NVC. Facial expressions tend to be spontaneous, but at times they are planned for a specific effect. A frown or smile will indicate a negative or positive response to a patient's performance. When we use specific hand gestures or pantomime or demonstrate activities, we are using planned NVC. The skilled caregiver knows when and how to best use these various forms of NVC.

The caregiver also should observe the patient to identify how NVC is used. Often, more information and a more accurate estimation of the patient's response or reaction to instructions can be obtained through NVC.

The use of touch by the caregiver is another form of NVC. A brief hug, a hand squeeze, or a pat on the back can convey a message to a patient that cannot be sent as effectively with words. However, touch must be used in a therapeutic, caring way, and the caregiver must avoid any suggestion of sexual implications. Examples of improper and unacceptable forms of touch include patting, slapping, or stroking a patient's buttocks; squeezing the thigh; or stroking various body parts, except during a therapeutic massage or exercise activity. You must demonstrate care when you grasp, handle, or touch the patient, especially during massage and exercise when sensitive body areas are touched. The perineum and buttocks of all patients and the breasts of women and sometimes men should be draped, as described in Chapter 5. When it is therapeutically necessary to massage, grasp, hold, or touch a potentially sensitive area, it may be prudent to state the reason the area is being touched or handled. In some situations, it may be wise to have another person observe or assist as you perform a particular treatment to protect yourself and to demonstrate your concern for the patient. Because touch may be construed as having a sexual implication by any patient,

regardless of how careful the caregiver has been, any indication of impropriety must be avoided.

Written communication should follow guidelines similar to those listed for verbal communication. It should be brief, concise, and specific and use language the reader will be most likely to understand. The guidelines previously given for the development of home programs are applicable here. Typed or printed instructions are more easily read than handwritten ones. Diagrams, drawings, or photographs are extremely useful to show specific positions or the sequence of movements. DVDs and videotapes are other forms of communication that can be useful to educate or instruct a patient or the family.

The use of consistent language and the manner in which oral or written instructions or directions are given to a patient should enhance the patient's level of understanding and capacity to learn. This concept is particularly important when complex activities are being taught and when a patient's mental capacities have been altered. Repetition and practice of activities that require motor control or coordination will usually enhance the patient's skill and ensure a safer performance. A complex activity should be consistently performed in the same or a very similar manner, regardless of who is assisting or guiding the patient.

Many barriers can adversely affect verbal communication and NVC between a caregiver and the patient. A noisy treatment area, an excessive distance between the two persons, distractions in the treatment area, the language used by the caregiver (e.g., technical language instead of lay language), the position of furniture or equipment in relation to the persons who are communicating, the time available to communicate, and the individual values or biases of each person are some examples of deterrents and potential barriers to verbal communication and NVC. The astute caregiver is aware of and is able to identify these factors and avoids, eliminates, or reduces them. This awareness and the subsequent action to overcome these conditions or factors are important keys to effective communication (Box 1-6).

Attentive listening is another communication skill the caregiver should develop. Evaluating the patient's tone of voice, observing nonverbal cues, listening for the main theme of the message, focusing on the content of the message rather than on the way the message is communicated, and providing verbal feedback to clarify understanding of the message are examples of being an attentive listener. This aspect of communication may be overlooked by the caregiver, and the result may be a loss of information.

Communicating with a Person with an Impairment

Caregivers must be aware of their responsibility to communicate appropriately with a person with an impairment. You should first and foremost maintain the person's self-esteem by considering the person first in your words and

Box **1-6** Barriers to Effective Communication

- Distance between the sender and receiver (excessive distance decreases effectiveness)
- Noise and environmental confusion interfere with and may distort the message
- Inability of the receiver to comprehend the message
- Inability of the receiver to interpret or understand technical, medical, and professional terms, language, or abbreviations
- Inadequate amount of feedback between the receiver and sender
- Complex messages may be difficult to interpret and comprehend
- The sender and receiver may interpret the message differently
- Cultural, gender, or age differences between the sender and receiver may affect the interpretation or comprehension of the message
- Illegible writing affects the accuracy and comprehension of the message

Box **1-7** Guidelines for Communicating with Persons with Disabilities

- Interact directly with the person with the impairment.
- Greet the person with respect as you would a person without an impairment; shake hands or forearm, or use your left hand as appropriate.
- Identify yourself and other persons in a group to the person who is visually impaired.
- Stoop or squat to communicate with a person in a wheelchair; position yourself in front and at eye level.
- Avoid leaning or sitting on a person's wheelchair; use care when handling assistive aids.
- Avoid statements, gestures, or actions that patronize; interact as you would with persons who do not have an impairment.
- Tactilely or visually cue the person who is hearing impaired to indicate your presence.
- Be patient and listen carefully when interacting with a person who has difficulty speaking; use questions that require brief responses.
- Determine whether the person desires assistance before assisting him or her; wait for instructions.

thoughts. The person's health condition should be described accurately if it needs to be included in the message, but it is more important to emphasize the person's abilities rather than his or her impairment. For example, the statement "John, who has a spinal cord injury, uses a wheelchair for mobility" is more appropriate than "Because he has a broken back, John is confined to a wheelchair." The use of the term "person with an impairment" is preferable to the term "disabled person" to promote the person's self-esteem and recognition as a person first.

Some suggestions to improve communications with persons with disabilities are provided in Box 1-7. The caregiver should speak and interact directly with the person rather than with a companion and be prepared to shake hands. In some instances you may need to grasp the person's forearm or use your left hand rather than your right hand as you meet or greet the person. (Note: Some cultures may not permit the use of a handshake as a means of greeting, and some cultures may use variations of the traditional handshake as their form of greeting.)

Persons who are visually impaired appreciate knowing who is speaking, so you should identify yourself, similar to the way in which you identify yourself when using a telephone. It will be necessary to identify each individual in a group, and each individual should identify himself or herself when speaking. It is not necessary to increase the volume of your voice when speaking with a person who is visually impaired. When speaking with a person who is seated, stoop or squat and position yourself in front of the person and at his or her eye level.

A person who is hearing impaired may need to have tactile (touch, tap) or visual (hand wave, gesture) cueing from you before you begin speaking. If the person is able to

lip read, you should stand so that he or she can see your lips clearly; you also should speak slowly and enunciate carefully. Some persons who are hearing impaired may communicate by sign language (Fig. 1-4). Again, increasing the volume of your voice is unnecessary in most communication situations.

When you communicate with a person who has difficulty speaking, intensify your listening skills and provide feedback to the individual to indicate your understanding of the message. Avoid correcting, interrupting, anticipating what the person will say, or speaking for him or her. Be patient during the conversation, and wait for confirmation of your feedback before continuing. The use of questions that require brief responses or that can be answered by a head nod or shake may assist this person. At times you may sense that a person with an activity limitation may require assistance to perform a task or activity. When this occurs, you should ask the person whether assistance is desired and, if it is desired, ask for specific instructions or directions.

Occasionally, even the experienced caregiver may feel awkward or embarrassed when communicating with a person with a health condition, especially if an expression related to the impairment is used during the conversation. Examples are, "I'm looking forward to *seeing* you again," "I'll *see* you later," "Did you *hear* about the big fire?" and "Let's go over the plan one *step* at time." In most instances the person with an impairment will recognize these statements as expressions and components of the usual communication pattern, so there is no need to apologize or bring attention to the statement, but you may want to consider how you can limit the use of these expressions and others in the future. You should avoid the use of terms such as "victim,"

| Handshape **A to Z** | | | |

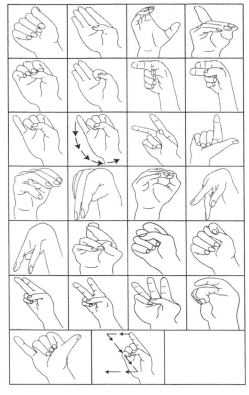

Fig. 1-4   American hand alphabet for the deaf. (Courtesy the Deaf Services Center, Worthington, OH, 2001.)

Box **1-8** Common Hospital Emergency Codes

- Code red = fire
- Code blue = heart or respiratory arrest
- Code orange = hazardous material spill or release
- Code gray = combative person
- Code silver = person with weapon/hostage situation
- Amber alert = infant and child abduction
- External triage = external disaster
- Internal triage = internal emergency
- Rapid response team = rapid response team
- Code name clear = to clear a code

"stricken," and "afflicted" because they tend to indicate an unhealthy status.

Being aware of and applying these suggestions will enable you to communicate appropriately with persons with an impairment, to maintain their self-esteem, and to recognize them as persons with abilities rather than stereotype them as being "disabled."

Communication between the caregiver and the patient is a critical aspect of patient care. The caregiver will be challenged to be aware of the importance of communication and to make every effort to communicate effectively. This goal can be accomplished through proper use of verbal, nonverbal, visual, and written communication.

SAFETY CONSIDERATIONS

Hospital Emergency Codes

In hospitals worldwide, a list of emergency codes is used to alert staff to various emergency situations. The use of codes is intended to convey crucial information quickly and with a minimum of misunderstanding to staff, while preventing panic or stress among visitors to the hospital. These codes may be printed on staff identification badges for ready reference or posted on placards throughout the hospital. A person calling a code should give the location of the emergency. Hospital emergency codes are commonly coded by color, and the color codes denote different events at different hospitals (Box 1-8). To date, emergency codes are not universal. For example, "code brown," which is used in some Texas hospitals, indicates that a severe weather warning has been issued for the area, but this particular code is not used in all regions of the United States.

Medical Errors

Patient safety should be the primary goal and focus of each person, facility, and service area involved with patient care. This goal and focus mean that no harm or injury should occur to the patient during, or as a result of, the care provided. Unfortunately, medical errors still occur with some frequency and have resulted in thousands of injuries or deaths. Medical errors occur when a planned treatment intervention does not work as it was intended or when an improper intervention is used. A 1999 study published by the Institute of Medicine indicated that more people die annually in hospitals as a result of medical errors than from motor vehicle accidents, breast cancer, or acquired immunodeficiency syndrome. Data from the same study showed that 1 in every 25 patients in hospitals sustained an injury as a result of a medical error.

Errors can occur at any location where treatment is provided, including the patient's home. Physicians and nurses are the persons most frequently associated with hospital-based or clinic-based patient care, but medical errors can be introduced by any caregiver, including therapists, pharmacists, laboratory and diagnostic technicians, administrators, or support personnel. Although it is important to realize that accidents related to patient treatment can and do occur, it is more important to determine how or why an event occurred and how a similar incident can be prevented. The Institute of Medicine, the Agency for Health Research and Quality, and The Joint Commission have been working cooperatively to develop strategies and standards designed to reduce medical errors in hospitals. Those lessons may be equally useful in the nonhospital setting.

Types of Errors Medical errors fall into two of four categories: sentinel (adverse) or potential adverse, and active

Table 1-6 Types of Medical Errors		
Sentinel vs. Potential Adverse Events	**SENTINEL EVENT** An injury is caused as a result of the medical management process rather than the condition or diagnosis of the patient	**POTENTIAL ADVERSE EVENT** No harm occurs either as a result of an intervention by an individual or because of chance; often referred to as a "close call" or "near miss"
Active vs. Latent Errors	**ACTIVE ERROR** Usually caused by an individual Effects of an active error becomes apparent quickly	**LATENT ERROR** Usually caused by a third party Causes may include faulty equipment (installation, maintenance, or irregularities), flaws in the care system, or organizational design Effects of a latent error may not become apparent quickly; they may only emerge after the fact

Data from the United States Department of Health & Human Services, Agency for Healthcare Research and Quality, PSNet, Patient Safety Network.

or latent (Table 1-6). In the hospital setting, an example of faulty equipment installation is when a piece of equipment, such as a patient lift, is attached to the ceiling or a wall but is not secured to a solid support such as a wall stud or ceiling rafter. Incorrect installation of equipment may be dangerous to patients and staff, which would make the improperly installed equipment both a latent error and a potential adverse event.

Medication Errors The primary types of medical errors result from errors in medication prescriptions or regimens, surgical procedures, diagnostic or laboratory report inaccuracies, and practice mistakes. Caregivers other than the physician and nurse who provide patient care should realize that the potential always exists for a medication error to occur. A medication error is one of the most common types of error and is a primary concern for the person who prescribes (physician), dispenses (pharmacist), and administers (nurse or therapist) the medication.

An adverse drug error is an example of a medication error. According to the U.S. National Library of Medicine, the three most common errors in nursing medication administration are wrong time, wrong rate, and wrong dose. To help reduce the number of medication errors, all caregivers should be aware of the five "rights" nurses use when they administer drugs (Box 1-9). Furthermore, it is important that each caregiver be aware of the potential adverse effects of the medications administered to each patient and how their action may be affected by the patient's physical activity, weight gain or loss, muscle gain or loss, and treatment activities.

Preventing Medical Errors In an effort to develop a more safety-conscious culture for health care providers, The Joint Commission requires that a root cause analysis be performed whenever a sentinel event is reported. The root cause analysis is designed to determine what happened, why

Box 1-9 Five "Rights" to Administering Medication
1. Right patient 2. Right drug 3. Right time 4. Right route 5. Right dose

or how it happened, and what could be done to prevent a recurrence of the event.

Several factors may be at play in medical errors:
- The complexity of the health care delivery system
- The number of caregivers involved in the patient's care
- Improper or faulty installation and maintenance of equipment
- Flaws in the design of systems, equipment, or organizational structure

The caregiver bears primary responsibility for the safety of each patient, regardless of the treatment provided and, in some situations, who provides it. Patient transfers, changes in position, exercise activities, and the transport of equipment or patients have the potential to cause injury; the caregiver must therefore maintain a safe environment and equipment that functions properly. Family members must be taught how to assist the patient safely and should be informed of any specific precautions related to the patient's care.

The patient also must assume some responsibility in maintaining his or her personal safety. Proper hygiene, skin care, changes in position, proper handling techniques, bowel and bladder management procedures, and transfer patterns may need to be performed or directed by the patient. The patient frequently knows the best approach, and the caregiver should listen and follow the patient's suggestions if they are reasonable and safe. Patients must be informed that they share responsibility for their health and safety within the limitations of their condition and abilities.

Incidents leading to patient injuries can be linked to the use of improperly functioning or poorly maintained equipment, a physical setting with hazardous obstacles or congested space, an excessive number of patients in the treatment area in relation to the personnel available to treat them, and the limited availability of personnel (as in the early morning, late afternoon, or during lunch). In addition, information about the various products used for treatment and equipment maintenance should be maintained in a notebook or manual (e.g., a Material Safety Data Sheet manual for easy reference and review).

The caregiver should be especially alert when treating a patient who is elderly, debilitated, or mentally disoriented; who is very young or has decreased mental capacity or a decreased physiologic status (e.g., open burns or wounds, a spinal cord injury, diabetes, or cardiopulmonary deficits); or who is emotionally disturbed. An elderly patient may experience physiologic changes that could adversely affect tolerance and ability to perform various tasks or activities. Some common changes of the aging process are listed in Table 1-7. It should be noted that, except for changes in vision, auditory acuity, mental capacity, and tactile sense, physiologic changes also may occur in younger persons who have been immobilized for a prolonged period.

During the examination and evaluation process, the caregiver should determine which of these changes have occurred and what effect they could have on the patient's ability to function and tolerate treatment. Activities that place the patient at risk, such as transfers, ambulation, bed positioning, and many types of exercise, should be performed cautiously. Decreased bone density can be a precursor for a fracture during transfers and ambulation, and decreased skin integrity may lead to skin tears during transfers, bed positioning, or exercise. The patient may need to be taught to use visual cues to compensate for the loss of proprioception, or kinesthetic sense. The reader is encouraged to consider other problems that may arise for the elderly patient who exhibits any of the changes presented. Furthermore, protective, preventive, or compensatory actions that could be taken to reduce the possibility of injury to the patient should be considered and performed. A patient with one or more of these conditions may have difficulty tolerating the treatment or may be more easily injured than other patients. The prudent caregiver will consider all the information related to the patient and will modify or revise the patient's treatment to reduce the likelihood of injury. The caregiver also should be aware of the need for safety and should follow established guidelines regarding body mechanics and personal health, as described in Chapter 4. Some recommendations for promoting safety are listed in Box 1-10.

Accidents and subsequent injuries tend to occur when health care personnel or family members are careless, inadequately trained, inattentive, or excessively busy. Additional information and suggestions regarding patient safety can be found in Chapters 2, 7, 8, 9, and 12.

Medical Errors in Allied Health Fields Several types of therapist errors were discussed by Anderson and Towell in the January 1, 2002, issue of the *Journal of Physical Therapy Education*. They are as follows:

Errors in diagnosis by the caregiver can occur when the examination is not thorough enough. An example would be when a patient with a medical diagnosis of stroke reports arm pain and the therapist must determine whether it is from musculoskeletal or neurologic causes. If the therapist determines an incorrect cause of the pain, therapy may not be effective and would lead to an unsatisfactory outcome. Another example would be a situation in which a patient reports pain from a headache and the therapist determines that it is a cervical musculoskeletal problem when actually it is a neurologic problem.

Table **1-7** Physiologic Changes Associated with Aging	
Physiologic Change	**Potential Problem or Deficit**
Decreased skin integrity	Skin tears; poor wound healing
Loss of bone density	Fractures, especially long bones and vertebrae
Decreased strength	Difficulty performing motor task
Decreased physical condition	Cardiopulmonary or cardiovascular systems may not respond adequately
Decreased muscle and connective tissue elasticity	Contractures; difficulty performing daily activities
Altered visual acuity	Falls; difficulty with tasks requiring visual input
Altered hearing acuity	Difficulty with tasks requiring auditory input
Decreased balance	Falls; difficulty maintaining safe sitting, standing, or walking activities
Altered proprioception	Falls; difficulty performing motor tasks, especially ambulation
Altered kinesthesia	Falls; difficulty performing motor tasks, especially ambulation
Altered mental capacity	Difficulty with comprehension of written, oral, or visual instructions
Decreased tactile sense	Burns; lacerations; difficulty differentiating objects or materials by touch

Box 1-10 Safety Recommendations

- Perform hand hygiene before and after treating each patient to reduce cross-contamination and transmission of disease; this is the single most important activity to prevent the spread of infection.
- Maintain sufficient space to maneuver equipment or perform a task; store equipment that is not in use so it will not interfere with patient care; position a patient to avoid the risk of being struck by passing personnel or equipment.
- Do not perform transfers or ambulation in an area where your view is obstructed, such as near a door or the corner of a hallway, or where space is inadequate or too congested for the activity.
- Routinely evaluate equipment to be certain it functions properly; establish a maintenance program for each item.
- Position equipment, furniture, and assistive aids so the items are stable, secure, and accessible when they are used; remove them when they are not in use so they do not interfere with patient and caregiver movements.
- Keep the floor clear of electrical cords, litter, loose rugs or floor mats, water, dirt, and other similar hazards.
- Do not leave patients unattended, especially if they are compromised physiologically or mentally.
- Protect the patient with safety straps, bed rails, or similar items when they are not closely attended, according to established agency, regulatory body, and state or federal restrictions and guidelines.
- Obtain the equipment and supplies needed, and prepare the treatment area before the patient arrives to avoid the need to leave the patient unattended.
- Be certain the personnel who provide patient care are trained, qualified, and competent in their assigned duties.
- Avoid storing potentially hazardous equipment or materials in a location where they are hidden from view or where there is a risk of a patient obtaining them; do not store chemicals or heavy objects on a shelf above shoulder level; clearly label the contents and weight of boxes or other containers.

Intervention errors occur when the chosen treatment is of no help or is even harmful to the patient. The therapist may choose a technique or modality that is incorrect for the injury; provide too little treatment with an inadequate patient response; provide excessive treatment, causing a physiologic response that is too intense and may cause further harm or increased pain; or apply the technique incorrectly.

Failure in communication can cause serious negative results in the patient's care. The patient's medical information must remain confidential; at the same time, the need to communicate important patient information with appropriate caregivers is crucial to the patient's care. Examples of communication errors include improper or inadequate documentation and not asking the correct questions of the patient. Lack of communication with PT assistants, physical therapy aides, or occupational therapy assistants also may result in a medical error.

Malpractice claims, judgments, and settlements are one indicator of the incidence of provider responsibility for medical error, as stated in an article by Robert Sandstrom in the *Journal of Allied Health*. The purpose of Sandstrom's study was to describe malpractice by PTs in the United States based on physical therapy malpractice reports in the National Practitioner Data Bank between January 1, 1991, and December 31, 2004. "Failure to monitor" (11.6%), "wrong procedure or treatment" (8.4%), "failure to supervise" (7.9%), and "improper management" (5%) were the top four reasons for a malpractice claim reported to the National Practitioner Data Bank. It was noted in this study that the overall risk of a malpractice payment for the actions of a PT is very low, with an estimated malpractice rate of 0.025% of PTs holding jobs in 2002.

Other physical therapy errors that have been mentioned in the mass media include dropping patients, sexual assault, leaving patients unattended on equipment, overextension of joints, failure to inform patients of risks, failure to supervise, and the use of broken equipment.

The Joint Commission Standards

The Joint Commission standards deal with organizational quality of care issues and the safety of the environment in which care is provided. The purpose of any survey is to evaluate an organization's compliance with nationally established Joint Commission standards. The Joint Commission changed the survey process in 2006 when it began unannounced surveys that focused on observations and interviews. The Joint Commission team currently surveys facilities by a "tracer methodology": a survey team enters a facility, selects a number of patients, and follows the patients' course throughout the facility. For example, the patient enters the facility through the emergency department, transfers to the intensive care unit, to an acute care floor, to diagnostic testing (e.g., magnetic resonance imaging, computed tomography scanning, or radiology), and to a rehabilitation floor if one exists. Record review and interviews may be conducted with any or all of the departmental personnel and/or the patient as addressed in the tracer. Through its tracer methodology, The Joint Commission surveys examine the following areas:

- Ethics, Rights, Responsibility, and Provision of Care
- Medication Management; Environment of Care
- Surveillance, Prevention, and Control of Infection; Leadership
- Improving Organizational Performance; Management of the Environment of Care
- Management of Human Resources; Management of Information

Box 1-11	The Joint Commission Hospital National Safety Goals for 2011

- Identify patients correctly
- Improve staff communication
- Use medicines safely
- Prevent infection
- Identify patient safety risks
- Prevent mistakes in surgery

Courtesy The Joint Commission.

- Medical Staff Co-Leaders; Nursing
- National Patient Safety Goals/Sentinel Events

The Joint Commission standards dictate that a health care organization must perform the following tasks to keep its patients safe from medical errors:

- Assess its own compliance with all applicable standards, national patient safety goals, and accreditation participation requirements
- Create plans of action to bring noncompliant standards into compliance and identify ways to measure the success of those plans
- Interact in a phone call with The Joint Commission staff to review and receive approval of plans of action and applicable measures of success
- Implement the plans to bring all standards and accreditation participation requirements into compliance
- Demonstrate a 12-month track record for all plans of action at the time of the triennial survey

Failure to comply with these standards may result in sanctions or lack of accreditation. The Joint Commission National Patient Safety Goals for 2011 can be found in Box 1-11.

SUMMARY

It is important to inform the patient of the planned treatment and his or her responsibilities and participation in the activity. The explanation should contain the anticipated or desired results or outcomes of the treatment and any potential adverse effects. The patient should have the opportunity to consent to or reject treatment based on the receipt of sufficient information to make an informed decision, and this decision should be documented. The presence of the patient in the treatment area should not be assumed to be an expression of consent for treatment.

A patient management process is necessary to examine and evaluate the patient, develop a clinical diagnosis and prognosis, establish a plan of care, and implement the plan. Before and after treating a patient, the caregiver should perform proper handwashing techniques to reduce the transmission of pathogens from one person to another. Documentation of the examination and evaluation information and data, plan of care, and treatment goals or outcomes is necessary to provide a written record of the treatment given and the results attained by the patient and to ensure reimbursement for the services rendered by the caregiver. For many patients, it may be necessary to educate the family or caregivers about further treatment or care, and a home program should be prepared.

Communication between the caregiver and each patient can be improved if the caregiver reduces or avoids certain communication barriers and develops the skills associated with being an attentive listener.

The safety of the patient must be the priority of all persons involved in all treatment activities performed. The responsibility for patient safety remains with the primary caregiver, even when the patient is treated by supportive personnel whom the caregiver supervises. An important activity related to patient safety is the use of proper and frequent hand hygiene techniques.

self-study ACTIVITIES

- Describe the possible short-term and long-term goals for a patient with left hemiparesis.
- Describe at least three reasons a patient's family members may need to be educated by a primary caregiver, and provide the rationale for each reason.
- Explain the types of communication you would use to instruct a patient to ambulate with crutches, instruct a patient to perform a standing assisted transfer, instruct a family member to guard a patient who uses crutches, and instruct a family member to perform active assistive exercise.
- List at least four factors you should consider related to the general aspects of patient safety.
- Explain why it is important and necessary to evaluate or assess each patient before beginning treatment or developing a treatment plan.
- What is the importance of evidence-based practice?
- Describe how each examination and evaluation component may help you make decisions or resolve clinical problems about the plan of care you develop with the patient.
- Explain why it is important to develop a treatment plan *with* the patient rather than *for* the patient.

problem SOLVING

1. You have a patient in the hospital who has just refused treatment from you. What documentation in the medical record should you consider?
2. You are the moderator in a meeting with three persons; one has a severe hearing deficit, another has a severe visual deficit, and the third is in a wheelchair. How will you seat each person, and what will you do to improve communications among the group members?
3. During a clinical education experience, you are treating four female patients with different cultural backgrounds: African American, Hispanic, Japanese, and Vietnamese. You are having difficulties interacting with each of them, and they are not responding to your instructions and suggestions. What may be the cause of the difficulties, and what will you do to improve the situation?

Approaches to Infection Control

objectives *After studying this chapter, the reader will be able to:*

- Define asepsis, medical asepsis, surgical asepsis, and contamination.
- Describe and perform proper techniques of hand hygiene for clean and sterile situations.
- Describe and demonstrate how to establish and maintain a sterile field.
- Describe and perform the proper application and removal of protective garments for clean and sterile situations.
- Explain the concept, use, and value of standard precautions and transmission-based precautions.

key terms

AIDS   Acronym for acquired immunodeficiency syndrome, which is caused by the human immunodeficiency virus (HIV).

Asepsis   Absence of microorganisms that produce disease; the prevention of infection by maintaining a sterile condition.

Contamination   When something is rendered unclean or nonsterile; an item, surface, or field is considered to be contaminated when it has come into contact with anything that is not sterile.

Decontamination   The use of physical or chemical means to remove, inactivate, or destroy bloodborne pathogens on a surface or item to the point at which they are no longer capable of transmitting infectious particles and the surface or item is rendered safe for handling, use, or disposal.

Disinfection   The destruction or removal of pathogenic organisms, but not necessarily their spores.

Health care–associated infection   Infections associated with health care delivery in any setting; previously known as nosocomial infection.

Hepatitis   Inflammation of the liver.

Infection   The production of a disease or harmful condition by the entrance of disease-producing germs into an organism.

Isolation   Separation from others.

Medical asepsis   Practices that help reduce the number and spread of microorganisms.

Microorganism   A tiny living animal or plant that can cause disease.

Nosocomial   Pertaining only to infections originating in a hospital.

Pathogen   A microorganism that produces disease.

Personal protective equipment (PPE)   Refers to a variety of barriers and respirators used alone or in combination to protect skin, mucous membranes, airways, and clothing from contact with infectious agents; includes gloves, respirators, masks, face shields, goggles, shoe covers, and gowns.

Respiratory hygiene   A new Centers for Disease Control and Prevention standard that applies to all persons entering a health care setting, including visitors, patients, and health care personnel; also known as "cough etiquette."

Sepsis   The presence of pathogenic microorganisms or their toxins in the blood or tissues.

Spore   A hard, thick-walled capsule formed by some bacteria that contains only the essential parts of the protoplasm of the bacterial cell.

Sterile   Containing no microorganisms; free from germs; aseptic.

Sterilization   A process by which all microorganisms, including spores, are destroyed.

Surgical asepsis   Practices that render and keep objects and areas free of all microorganisms.

Wound   A bodily injury caused by physical means, with disruption of the normal continuity of structures.

INTRODUCTION

According to the Centers for Disease Control and Prevention (CDC), health care–associated infections are estimated to affect 1 in every 20 patients in a hospital setting and are the fourth leading cause of death in the United States. Basic measures of prevention include frequent handwashing or hand rubs (before and after treatment of each patient) with use of proper hand hygiene techniques and the wearing of appropriate personal protective equipment (PPE) such as gloves, a gown, a cap, and a mask. Patients must be protected from health care–associated infections, which can be spread from patient to patient or to a given patient by a caregiver who is careless or does not follow accepted infection control measures. A caregiver may try to avoid one or more of these measures because of a perceived lack of time, poor access to the items, poor location of a sink or handwashing station, a lack of proper-sized apparel, dermatitis due to frequent handwashing, a reaction to the available soap or detergent, a reaction to latex gloves, a lack of understanding of the importance of using infection control methods for each patient, or poor motivation to comply with the policies and procedures for other reasons. Therefore it may be necessary for the employer or department supervisor to reduce as many of these factors as possible, whether real or perceived, to make it more convenient for the caregiver to comply with policies and procedures.

Many resources provide information about the prevention of disease transmission and the spread of pathogenic microorganisms. Much of the information is not new, but in recent years a greater emphasis has been placed on the concept that each patient should be treated as if he or she has a transmissible or infectious disease. The CDC's 2007 "Guideline for Isolation Precautions: Preventing Transmission of Infectious Agents in Healthcare Settings" updates and expands the 1996 "Guideline for Isolation Precautions in Hospitals." The emergence of new pathogens such as SARS-CoV (associated with severe acute respiratory syndrome), avian influenza in humans, community-associated methicillin-resistant *Staphylococcus aureus*, *Clostridium difficile*, and noroviruses, along with the development of new therapies (e.g., gene therapy) and a concern for the threat from bioweapons attacks, has brought about theses changes in isolation precautions. Because of the change in health care delivery systems from primarily hospitals to other settings such as long-term care, posthospital rehabilitation centers, home care, freestanding specialty sites, and ambulatory care centers, a need was created for guidelines that can be used in all health care settings. An important change is the recommendation to don the proper PPE (gowns, gloves, and mask) when entering the patient's room for those who require contact and/or droplet precautions because contaminated surfaces are important sources for transmission of pathogens, and interactions with the patient cannot be predicted with certainty. An additional recommendation for use of standard precautions pertains to respiratory hygiene and cough etiquette, which was designed to contain respiratory secretions.

The spread of and serious consequences associated with acquired immunodeficiency virus (AIDS), which is caused by the human immunodeficiency virus (HIV), and hepatitis, especially the type caused by the hepatitis B virus (HBV), have created a need for health care workers and others who may have close, personal contact with a person who has one of these two diseases to use caution during contact. Both diseases are life threatening. Hepatitis B is more easily contracted but can be prevented with a vaccine. Currently no vaccine is available to prevent or cure AIDS, but some drug regimens have demonstrated the ability to slow the disease process. Because these two life-threatening diseases are prevalent and are spread through contact with various body fluids, an emphasis continues to be placed on cleanliness and sterile techniques. According to a 2008 article in the *Journal of the American Medical Association*, the estimated number of new HIV infections in the United States in 2006 was 56,300, and the estimated incidence rate was 22.8 per 100,000 population. Forty-five percent of infections were among black individuals, and 53% were among men who have sex with men. From 1990 to 2002, the CDC reported that the incidence of acute hepatitis B declined 67%, from 8.5 per 100,000 population to 2.8 per 100,000 population. The CDC recommends the use of standard precautions to protect health care workers and reduce the transmission of these diseases.

According to the CDC, standard precautions are a group of infection prevention practices that apply to all patients, regardless of diagnosis. Standard precautions are a combination and expansion of universal precautions and body substance isolation. They are based on the principle that all blood, body fluids, excretions (except sweat), secretions, nonintact skin, and mucous membranes may contain transmissible infectious agents. For all patients in all health care settings, hand hygiene should be used after touching blood, excretions, secretions, body fluids, and contaminated items, as well as immediately after removing gloves and between patient contact. Nonsterile gloves should be used for touching blood, secretions, excretions, body fluids, contaminated items, mucous membranes, and nonintact skin. You should wear gloves and a gown during treatment procedures and patient care activities if your clothing or exposed skin might come in contact with blood/body fluids, excretions, and secretions. If splashes of blood, body fluids, or secretions are anticipated, a mask, goggles, and/or face shield should be worn, especially during patient suctioning and endotracheal intubations. Transmission-based precautions are used in addition to standard precautions if evidence exists for person-to-person transmission via droplet, contact, or airborne routes in both health care and non–health care settings and if patient factors increase the risk of transmission (e.g., diarrhea, diapered infants, and draining wounds). The rationale for this concept is explained in greater detail in the Infection Control and Isolation Precautions sections of this chapter.

Some excellent and basic sources of information about infection control are the CDC; Occupational Safety and Health Administration (OSHA); Environmental Protection Agency (EPA); city, county and state health departments; and the infection control department or similar department of a hospital. Furthermore, seminars and other types of continuing education programs, including hospital-based programs for employees regarding AIDS and hepatitis, are available to health care personnel. Many brochures, textbooks, pamphlets, newspapers, magazines, and visual aids contain information about these and other diseases; some of these sources are listed in the Bibliography.

Individual institutions and agencies have enacted policies and procedures to control the spread or transmission of infection and disease, the most important of which are those related to hand hygiene. The caregiver and all other persons who treat patients, handle soiled patient linen, remove wound dressings, or collect disposed items (e.g., needles and other sharps) that are used to treat patients must become familiar with and adhere to established policies and procedures and develop proper personal habits for maximal protection.

The caregiver may be required to interact with patients who require care of open wounds or whose condition requires the use of medical or surgical aseptic techniques. Remember that microorganisms are present on the skin, in the air, in patient wounds, and throughout the environment. Be aware of the process of contamination and infection so that you, the patient, and other persons or objects can be protected from pathogens or microorganisms. This protection can be enhanced by interrupting the cycle of infection.

PRINCIPLES AND CONCEPTS

Microorganisms and the Infection Cycle

Microorganisms move, or are transmitted, from place to place by various means in a cyclical manner (the cycle of infection). The interruption of this cycle means an interruption of the microorganism's ability to grow, spread, or cause disease.

The cycle of infection includes five elements:

- **Reservoir.** Microorganisms require a place where they can grow and reproduce (i.e., a host or reservoir); animals and human beings are both examples of microorganism hosts.
- **Exit.** Microorganisms also require a means by which they can leave the host (i.e., exit the reservoir). They can exit through a person's nose, mouth, throat, ear, eye, intestinal tract, urinary tract, body fluids (e.g., blood), or wounds.

- **Transmission.** Microorganisms must pass from one person to another to spread the infection. Transmission can occur through the air, droplets (from a cough or sneeze), or direct contact with items such as another person's skin, equipment, mat pads, instruments (e.g., needles, scalpels, and thermometers), eating utensils, linens, and body fluids such as blood, semen, saliva, and vaginal secretions.
- **Infection.** To infect another person, the microorganism must be able to enter that person (i.e., it must have a portal of entry). Examples of such portals are a break in the person's skin barrier, mucous membranes, the mouth, the nose, the ears, and the genitourinary tract.
- **Susception.** Finally, the person who receives the microorganisms must be susceptible to them (i.e., be a susceptible host). A person whose body systems cannot destroy, repel, remove, or ward off the microorganisms is a susceptible host (Box 2-1).

Some microorganisms are more difficult to destroy than others, and sometimes medications designed to kill or reduce the number of microorganisms (e.g., antibiotics) are necessary to augment the protective actions of the body's systems. Some pathogens are totally resistant to medications or actions taken to reduce their numbers or prevent their growth. For example, no effective treatment (medication or vaccine) has yet been found to destroy or effectively eliminate HIV, which is associated with AIDS.

Most microorganisms grow or proliferate best in a dark, warm, moist environment and are less likely to grow when they are exposed to a light, cool, dry, or extremely hot environment. Therefore steam, gas, ultraviolet rays, and dry heat frequently are used to sterilize contaminated objects.

| Box **2-1** | Cycle of Cross-Contamination and Infection |

- Reservoir for organism and host (e.g., a person with a staphylococcal infection)
  ↓
- Method of exit for the organism (e.g., a draining wound)
  ↓
- Method of transmission of the organism (e.g., soiled dressings, exudate from the wound, or soiled linen)
  ↓
- Method of entry of the organism into a new host (e.g., a cut, abrasion, cuticle tear, or any break in the skin)
  ↓
- Susceptible host (i.e., a person with low or limited systemic resistance to the organism)
  ↓
- Infection develops in the new host

  Barriers to interrupt the cycle include proper disposal of dressings and linen and use of standard precautions, protective clothing, gloves, and proper hand hygiene techniques.

Some microorganisms require oxygen to support their growth, whereas others do not, and some microorganisms produce cells called spores (e.g., anthrax, botulism, and histoplasmosis). Because of their thick, hard, protective walls, spores are very difficult to destroy, especially when they are located deep in a wound.

The caregiver is responsible for interrupting or establishing barriers to the infection cycle at any stage of the process. Some barriers to infection are the use of proper hand hygiene techniques, the wearing of gloves and other PPE, the proper removal and disposal of a contaminated dressing or bandage, and the use of isolation techniques when necessary. It may not be possible—nor is it the objective—to completely eliminate all pathogens from an area or object to create asepsis. However, it is usually possible to affect the number of pathogens in an area so their concentration, influence, or capacity to create an infection is reduced by a person's immune system or by the use of medications designed to kill the remaining pathogenic microorganisms.

Aseptic Technique

A caregiver may become involved in the management of wounds of patients who have a transmissible infection or may be required to care for patients who must be protected from the environment to avoid becoming infected. Therefore caregivers must understand how to protect themselves, the patient, and other persons from becoming contaminated or infected.

The primary purpose of the precautions is to protect persons or objects from becoming contaminated or infected by pathogenic microorganisms. It is important that the caregiver understand the three most common means of transmission—contact, droplet, and airborne—so quality care can be delivered and therapeutic procedures or activities can be applied safely.

Pathogens can be transmitted through body fluids, although the body uses several means to provide barriers to pathogens or to rid the body of these pathogens. The primary barrier is the skin when it is intact. The skin is relatively impermeable to the absorption of external substances and to the loss of certain body fluids, and cilia in the respiratory tract assist in filtering and trapping microorganisms to prevent them from entering the lungs. When these natural barriers are disrupted, protection is reduced, and the possibility of becoming infected is increased. Therefore when treating someone who has an infection or who is more likely to become infected, it is imperative to establish barriers in addition to the body's natural ones.

In the treatment area, general cleanliness of equipment, floors, and restrooms and proper control of heat, light, and air are important considerations. Proper disposal of soiled linen, PPE such as gowns, gloves, caps, and masks, and dressing material/bandages, plus other disposable items, is important.

Current standard precautions rely on the concepts of medical and surgical asepsis and how pathogens can be transmitted (Table 2-1). The use of appropriate techniques to maintain at least medical asepsis should be followed, especially hand hygiene activities. Each employee should understand and adhere to practices and procedures that can be used to protect a specific patient, other patients, and persons such as visitors or employees, as well as themselves, from infection or contamination.

Table 2-1   Comparison of Medical and Surgical Asepsis

Factor	Medical Asepsis	Surgical Asepsis
Objectives of the barrier	Confine pathologic organisms to the room, unit, or specified locale Reduce the number of organisms after they leave the body and prevents the spread to others Used in the care of the patient with infectious diseases to prevent reinfection of the patient	Prevent all microorganisms from reaching the patient or contaminating a sterile field and surgical wound
Equipment and supplies	Disinfect, sterilize, or dispose of after contact with the patient; use clean materials	Disinfect or sterilize before contact with the patient; all items must be sterile
Reservoir of infection	The patient	Other people and the environment
Caregiver instruction and PPE	Handwashing, gowning, face mask—must be clean PPE Follow facility policy regarding isolation procedures Discard PPE after contact with the patient Separate clean from contaminated materials	Must perform a surgical scrub; all PPE must be sterile to protect the patient, including the sterile gown, mask or face shield, gloves, special shoe coverings, and hair covering
Goal of action	Confine the organisms and prevent spread to others	Reduce the number of organisms and prevent the spread of infection to the patient

PPE, Personal protective equipment.

Medical Asepsis Techniques of medical asepsis are designed to keep pathogens confined to a specific area, object, or person. Medical asepsis may involve isolation of a patient to protect health care workers, other patients, and other persons from the pathogenic microorganisms associated with the patient. For example, patients with tuberculosis, hepatitis, a staphylococcal or streptococcal infection, or another communicable or transmissible disease may be isolated in a private room. Specific care must be taken by persons who have contact with the patient, including contact with soiled dressings or articles of clothing, to reduce the possibility of becoming infected. The use of PPE by the caregiver will be necessary to protect the caregiver from the patient. Extreme care must be used when removing PPE after treating a patient who is in isolation to reduce cross-contamination. This approach is referred to as a "clean approach."

Surgical Asepsis Surgical asepsis techniques are used to exclude all microorganisms before they can enter a surgical wound or contaminate a sterile field before or during surgery. All instruments, surgical and patient drapes, and any other inert object that may come in contact with the surgical site must be sterilized. All personnel who enter the sterile field must perform a surgical hand scrub with an antimicrobial agent and don sterile gloves and a sterile gown.

INFECTION CONTROL

According to a study by the CDC published in 2008, the volume of, incidence of, and hospitalizations for infections with resistant organisms in the United States have risen from 499,702 in 2000 to 947,393 in 2005. The CDC in 2007 revised its two-tiered approach to infection and isolation precautions termed "standard precautions" and "transmission-based precautions."

- Standard precautions are designed to protect health care workers and patients in a hospital and other health care settings regardless of their diagnosis or infection status; these precautions are considered to be the best means to control infections (Table 2-2).
  - These precautions apply to blood; all body fluids, secretions, and excretions (except sweat), regardless of whether they contain visible blood; nonintact skin; and mucous membranes.
  - Standard precautions synthesize the major components associated with universal precautions and apply to all bodily fluids, secretions, and excretions of any patient. Use of these precautions decreases the risk of transmission of pathogens from moist body substances and protects against the transmission of undiagnosed and diagnosed infections.
- Transmission-based precautions are designed to protect the caregiver from specialized patients with highly transmissible pathogens who are known or suspected to be infected by epidemiologically important pathogens that can be spread by direct contact with dry skin or contaminated surfaces, droplets of moisture, or airborne particles (Table 2-3).

The caregiver must follow proper infection control procedures, which include hand hygiene; using gloves or a gown when in contact with blood, body fluids, secretions, excretions, and a contaminated patient's skin or linen and personal items; and using a mask, eye protection, or shield when fluid sprays or splashes are anticipated.

Hand Hygiene

Hand hygiene is the most important activity that every caregiver and hospital visitor should perform before and after contact with a patient (Box 2-2). Consistent and proper use of recommended hand hygiene techniques will reduce the number of pathogenic microorganisms on one's hands and thus reduce cross-contamination. All newly hired employees who will touch, transport, or clean a patient's environment should receive information about proper hand hygiene techniques and participate in reeducation sessions annually.

Although it is believed that many microorganisms are not dangerous to a person whose immune system is fully functioning and whose other defenses to infection are normal, these same organisms may produce an infection in a patient whose immune system is compromised or whose ability to ward off an infectious process is diminished.

Pathogens can be transmitted through the following means:
- Direct contact
- Air currents
- Contaminated linen or clothing
- Inadequately cleansed eating utensils, instruments, or equipment
- Moisture droplets

Because the most common method of transmission is by direct contact, the habitual use of proper hand hygiene techniques is the single most effective way to protect the patient and the caregiver. Research studies have shown that routine hand hygiene reduces the spread of infection

---

Box **2-2** Criteria for Performing Hand Hygiene

Hand hygiene should be performed at the following times:
- Before and after patient contact
- Before and after contact with wounds, dressings, specimens, bed linen, and protective clothing
- After contact with secretions or excretions and when hands are soiled or considered contaminated
- Before and after toileting
- After sneezing, coughing, or nose blowing
- After removing gloves
- Before and after eating

Table **2-2** Standard Precautions

Topic	Precautions
Barriers	Gloves: for touching blood, secretions, excretions except sweat, body fluids, contaminated items, mucous membranes, and nonintact skin
	Protective clothing: during patient care activities and procedures when contact of clothing/exposed skin with blood or body fluids, excretions, and secretions is anticipated
	Mask, eye protection (goggles), or face shield*: during procedures and patient care activities likely to generate splashes or sprays of blood, secretions (especially suctioning), and body fluids (e.g., endotracheal intubation)
	Mouthpiece, intubation device, resuscitation bag, and other ventilation devices: during patient resuscitation (cardiopulmonary resuscitation) to prevent contact with mouth and oral secretions
Hand hygiene	Immediately after glove removal, wash hands after touching blood, excretions, secretions, body fluid, and contaminated items
	Avoid wearing artificial fingernails because they may separate from the real nail, producing a pocket for pathogen growth
	Avoid contact with the outer surface of the gloves when they are removed
	Wash your hands or use a hand rub before and after patient care
Sharps (needles, scalpel blades)	Do not bend, recap, break, or hand-manipulate used needles; use safety features when available and use a one-handed scoop technique only
	Dispose of all sharps in a puncture-proof container immediately after their use
	Do not uncap or expose needles until they are needed
	Use caution when you handle and dispose of the item to avoid wounding yourself
Soiled patient care equipment	Handle in a manner that prevents transfer of microorganisms to others and to the environment
Respiratory hygiene/ cough etiquette	Contain the source of infectious respiratory secretions in symptomatic patients beginning at the initial point of encounter (e.g., emergency departments, outpatient clinics, and physician offices)
	Instruct symptomatic persons to cover the nose and mouth when sneezing or coughing
	Use tissues and dispose in a no-touch receptacle
	Observe hand hygiene after soiling of hands from respiratory secretions
	Wear a surgical mask if tolerated or maintain spatial separation >3 feet if possible
Miscellaneous	Avoid eating, drinking, smoking, applying cosmetics or lip balm, and handling contact lenses in a patient care area
	Avoid hand contact with mucous membranes of your eyes, nose, mouth, or ears
	Handle all laundry and textiles carefully, especially linen soiled by a patient's body fluids or waste; dispose and transport it in the proper bag, hamper, or container
	Avoid unnecessary contact with a patient who places you at risk with contact of a body fluid or waste product, especially blood
	Report incidents of contact with a patient's body fluids or waste product on an unprotected area of your body and seek immediate assistance if a direct blood-to-blood contact occurs between you and a patient

Standard precautions are based on the concept that all blood, secretions, body fluids, excretions except sweat, nonintact skin, and mucous membranes may contain transmissible infectious agents. Standard precautions are used in all patient care environments.
*The Centers for Disease Control and Prevention state that during aerosol-generating procedures involving patients with suspected or proven infections transmitted by respiratory aerosols (e.g., severe acute respiratory syndrome), a fit-tested N-95 or higher respirator should be worn in addition to gloves, gown, and face/eye protection. The N-95 respirator should be worn if a patient has severe acute respiratory syndrome, measles, chickenpox, *Mycobacterium tuberculosis*, 2009 H1N1 virus, or avian or pandemic influenza.

significantly. The more likely it is that the patient has an infection or is contaminated, the more important it is to use hand hygiene. Furthermore, when wound care is performed, the proper application and removal of protective garments and adherence to established infection control procedures is required. One must be aware that many objects in a patient's room may harbor pathogens and that hands can become contaminated through contact with these objects.

In 2002 the CDC published guidelines for hand hygiene, which are available at their Web site (www.cdc.gov).

The two primary methods of hand hygiene are hand rubbing and handwashing.

Hand Rubbing Hand rubbing with an alcohol-based waterless antiseptic is the most effective technique to decontaminate hands when handwashing is not required. Fig. 2-1 shows a handwashing station with both hand soap and a waterless rinse for a hand rub. Hand rubs should be routinely performed before and after the treatment of each patient, even when gloves are worn to treat the patient.

Table 2-3 Transmission-Based Isolation Precautions

Category*	Description
Contact precautions	Used to prevent transmission of infectious agents, including epidemiologically important microorganisms that are spread by direct or indirect contact with the patient or the patient's environment Also used where the presence of excessive wound drainage, fecal incontinence, or other discharges from the body suggest an increased potential for risk of transmission and extensive environmental contamination; transmission-based isolation precautions are used in addition to standard precautions when a patient is in isolation Hands: wash thoroughly upon entering the room and wash with chlorhexidine gluconate antiseptic soap upon leaving the room Gloves: wear gloves upon entering the room Gown: wear a gown when having direct contact with the patient, environmental surfaces, or patient items; remove before leaving the room Room: Private or cohort, preferably >3 feet between beds Dedicated equipment: Patient care items (e.g., thermometer, stethoscope, and blood pressure cuff) should remain in the room; if any item must be removed, it must be disinfected or placed in a bag labeled "biohazard"
Droplet precautions	Used to prevent transmission of pathogens spread through mucous membranes or close respiratory contact with respiratory secretions Hands: wash thoroughly upon entering and leaving the room Mask: required when working in close contact with the patient Room: private Patient transport: place a surgical mask on the patient if possible and follow respiratory hygiene/cough etiquette
Airborne precautions	Used to prevent transmission of infectious agents that remain infectious over long distances when suspended in the air (e.g., varicella virus [chickenpox], rubeola virus [measles], *Mycobacterium tuberculosis*, and SARS-CoV) Hands: wash thoroughly upon entering and leaving the room Mask: an N-95 respirator (dust/mist respirator) or higher level must be worn before entering the room; it must be fit-tested prior to use; discard the mask upon leaving the room; whenever possible, nonimmune health care workers should not work with patients with vaccine-preventable airborne diseases (e.g., chickenpox, measles, and smallpox) Room: private, airborne infection isolation room; door must remain closed Patient transport: place a surgical mask on the patient if possible

*For each of these categories, visitors should report to the nurse's station before entering the room.

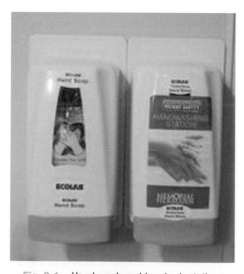

Fig. 2-1 Hand wash and hand rub station.

Hand rubbing, especially with alcohol-based rubs from a wall-mounted dispenser, has several advantages over handwashing:

• It requires less time to use
• It is more effective than soap and water
• It is more accessible than sinks
• It significantly reduces bacterial counts on hands
• It causes less damage to the skin than soap and water

Wall-mounted dispensers that contain antiseptic foam, gel, or spray are now found in many public facilities such as spas, restaurants, schools, restrooms, and workplaces. An alcohol-based hand rub product should contain 60% to 95% alcohol (e.g., isopropyl, ethanol, or n-propanol) and 1% to 3% skin conditioner (glycerol) as an emollient, which prevents skin irritation and dryness. Another method of decontamination is an antimicrobial/antiseptic hand wipe; however, the hand wipe is only as effective as handwashing as a decontaminant.

Table 2-4 Isolation Precautions

Isolation Type	Common Clinical Syndromes	Room Assignment	Mask	Gown	Gloves	Patient Transport/ Discontinuing Isolation
Contact	MRSA, VISA, VRE Aminoglycoside resistant Gram-negatives Uncontrolled diarrhea (*Clostridium difficile*), lice, scabies, impetigo	Private room or cohort patient with same infection Dedicated equipment in the room	No	Yes, with direct contact with patient, environmental surfaces, or items in the patient's room	Yes Use CHG soap for handwashing	Minimize transport as feasible Clearing the patient from MRSA or VRE isolation should not be attempted if receiving antibiotics (that treat that infection) See specifics below for D/C of isolation*
Droplet	Mumps (rubella) *Neisseria meningitidis*	Private room; does not require negative air flow	Yes, when working within 3 feet of patient	No	No	Minimize transport of patient Mask patient when transport is necessary†
	Streptococcus A			Contact precautions if skin lesions present—yes	Yes, if skin lesions are present	
Airborne	Measles (pulmonary) Tuberculosis	Private room with negative air flow; keep door closed (N-95 respirator)	Yes—dust/ mist mask	No	No	Minimize transport of patient Mask patient when transport is necessary‡
Airborne plus contact	Chickenpox, disseminated herpes zoster in immuno-compromised hosts, smallpox	Private room with negative air flow; keep door closed	Yes—dust/ mist mask (N-95 respirator)	Yes	Yes	Minimize transport of patient Mask patient when transport is necessary Continue for duration of illness

Data from the Clinical Epidemiology Department, The Ohio State University Medical Center, Columbus, OH, 2006. *CHG*, Chlorhexidine gluconate; *D/C*, discontinuation; *MRSA*, methicillin-resistant *Staphylococcus aureus*; *VISA*, vancomycin-intermediate *S. aureus*; *VRE*, vancomycin-resistant Enterococcus.

*VRE: Discontinuation at the admission of initial diagnosis is discouraged; outpatient is preferred; three paired negative perirectal screens plus original site (if present on inguinal, axillary, or umbilical areas); pairs should be obtained at least 7 days apart. MRSA: Three negative anterior nares screens plus original site (if present), obtained 24 hours apart.

†Isolation for *N. meningitidis* may be discontinued after 24 hours of appropriate antibiotic therapy.

‡Isolation must be continued for *Mycobacterium tuberculosis* until three negative acid-free bacillus smears are obtained.

PROCEDURE 2-1

Hand Rubbing

1. Remove jewelry from the hands and wrists.
2. Apply a cleansing agent (which may be in foam, gel, liquid, or spray form) from the dispenser to one palm.
3. Rub the hands vigorously using friction or rubbing motions to the following areas:
   - Palms together
   - Interlace fingers; rub web space and between and around each finger
   - Dorsum of each hand with the palm of the opposite hand
   - Fingertips of each hand in the opposite palm
   - Dorsal finger creases of each hand with the opposite palm
   - Each thumb while it is clasped by the opposite palm
   - Each wrist while it is clasped by the opposite palm
4. Rub for at least 15 seconds or until the hands are dry. Do not rinse the hands with water or dry them with a towel.

The basic steps for using a hand rub are as follows:
- Apply a small amount of the product to the palm of one hand; the amount delivered is usually premeasured by the manufacturer.
- Rub the product briskly over the hands, covering all surfaces of both hands as described for handwashing.
- Continue to rub until the hands are dry; do not rinse the hands with water. It may take 25 to 30 seconds for the hands to dry depending on the product.

Procedure 2-1 details these steps.

After several hand rubs have been performed, the hands may become sticky and handwashing should be performed to cleanse them. Some facilities may have a policy that recommends that a hand wash be performed after a specific number of hand rubs (e.g., after every 15 hand rubs or if the hands become soiled). However, the CDC does not list handwashing after a certain number of hand rubs as a requirement in its hand hygiene guidelines.

Handwashing Several techniques can be used to wash your hands; however, regardless of the method you use, it is important to cleanse your hands thoroughly. Avoid touching any potentially contaminated surface during or at the conclusion of the handwashing process. If gloves and other protective clothing are to be applied, they should be applied at the conclusion of the hand wash.

Although handwashing is not the most effective method of decontaminating hands, it is the preferred method when hands are visibly dirty, soiled, or considered to be contaminated. Handwashing for 15 to 30 seconds with ordinary soap and water will remove transient bacteria from the hands as a result of the mechanical action of the friction while rubbing and scrubbing during the wash (Procedure 2-2).

Hand washes frequently are required before entering an intensive care unit or operating suite. An antimicrobial or germicidal agent (e.g., 2% chlorhexidine gluconate) may be added to the cleansing medium to make it antiseptic (Procedure 2-3). This formula is sufficient for the wash used before entering most intensive care units, but 4% chlorhexidine gluconate is recommended for the wash before entering an operating suite. Furthermore, a hand wash is the better means of decontamination after treating a patient with a *C. difficile* infection.

Bar soap generally is not used in hospitals because it is considered contaminated. Pathogens can survive on a bar of soap, even if it has been rinsed before being replaced in a rack. Other objects that may contaminate hands during handwashing are the sink rims and basin, water that splashes from the sink, towel dispensers, faucet handles, and the operating lever of a dispenser of soap. Avoid contact with these items whenever possible, or at least recognize that they are contaminated. The safest way to access soap and water is through the use of knee-operated or foot-operated controls or automatic soap and water dispensers, or when the soap is contained in a one-time-use brush. Most health care facilities now provide wall-mounted dispensers that contain either non-antimicrobial soap or antimicrobial soap that is delivered in a premeasured amount.

Procedures for handwashing for medical asepsis can be found in Procedure 2-2; procedures for surgical asepsis are in listed in Procedure 2-3. Both procedures, however, follow these same basic principles:
- Before handwashing, remove jewelry from the hands and wrists, especially items with settings or irregular or rough surfaces, because they may harbor pathogens and cannot be cleansed effectively. Artificial fingernails and chipped nail polish should be avoided because they, too, may harbor pathogens.
- To reduce the collection of pathogens under the fingernails, nails should be trimmed to less than one-quarter inch so they are not visible when the hand is held in front of the face with the palm directed toward the face and the fingertips at eye level.
- Irritations, lesions, or breaks in the skin of the hands place the caregiver at a greater risk for self-contamination or infection. It is important that the caregiver take proper care of the hands and wear gloves if irritations, lesions, or breaks in the skin are present.
- Warm water should be used for comfort and to promote lather that will cleanse the hands more effectively and, when rinsed, carry pathogens away.
- After the skin is wet, apply soap and rub briskly, covering all surfaces of each limb with lather. Friction is an important component of handwashing to loosen dirt, dead skin cells, and pathogens from the skin.

PROCEDURE 2-2

Handwashing for Medical Asepsis

1. Remove jewelry from the hands and wrists; remember that the sink, soap dispenser, and towel container are considered to be contaminated.
2. Turn on the water and adjust it to a warm temperature so the soap will lather and there will be less irritation to the skin; avoid using cold or hot water.
3. Wet your wrists and hands, with the hands directed downward; avoid touching the sink rim or basin.
4. Apply soap (**A**); prepare to wash hands vigorously using friction or rubbing motions (**B**).
5. Wash for up to 30 seconds; wash longer if the hands have come in contact with body fluids, an infectious wound, or a contaminated patient.
   - Lather and scrub the palms together.
   - Interlace the fingers; scrub between and around each finger; wash the web space between each finger (**C**).
   - Scrub the dorsum of each hand with the opposite palm or brush (**D**).

- Scrub the fingertips and the dorsal finger creases of each hand with the opposite palm, or use a one-time, disposable brush or a pointed, disposable wood probe ("orange stick") to clean under each fingernail (**F**)
- Encircle each thumb and wrist with the opposite palm and scrub.

6. Rinse hands thoroughly from the wrist to the fingers; do not rinse the skin proximal to the area that has been washed; rinse the soap lather completely from all surfaces (**F**).
7. Dry the hands with a disposable paper towel; allow the water to flow while the hands are being dried.
8. Discard the towels used to dry the hands; use a clean, dry towel to turn off the faucet (**G**); discard all used towels in an appropriate container; avoid touching the container.

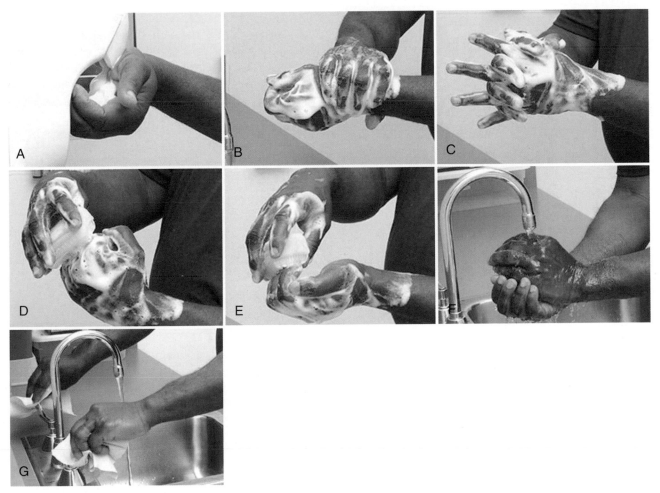

Fig. 2-2   Handwashing for medical asepsis.

PROCEDURE 2-3

Handwashing for Surgical Asepsis

1. Remove all jewelry from your hands, neck, and ears, and approach the wash area with your arms exposed to approximately 3 inches above the elbow. Avoid touching the sink and other nearby objects with your clothing or hands.
2. Turn on the water; adjust the water to a warm temperature.
3. Wet your hands and forearms; apply the soap or detergent according to the previous directions for medical asepsis.
4. Wash your hands as outlined for medical asepsis, except that you will need to wash your entire forearm to approximately 3 inches above your elbow. This process requires approximately 7 minutes (**A**).
5. Rinse your hands by holding them with your fingers upward so that the rinse water flows from a clean to an unclean area (i.e., from your fingers to your elbows). Do not allow your hands, forearms, or upper arms to contact the sink or your body.
6. Clean your fingernails, cuticles, and skin creases with a one-time-use brush using vigorous strokes; you may use a pointed, disposable wood probe ("orange stick") to clean under each fingernail. Discard the probe and brush after use.
7. Perform a final rinse with your hands directed upward (**B**).
8. Dry your hands, forearms, and the distal area of your upper arms thoroughly using a sterile towel or air dryer. Avoid contact between the towel and your clothing and between your washed skin and your clothing or other nonsterile areas. Wrap your hands and forearms in a dry, sterile towel before applying protective clothing or gloves; hold your hands above waist level and slightly away from your body until you begin your treatment or patient care activities.

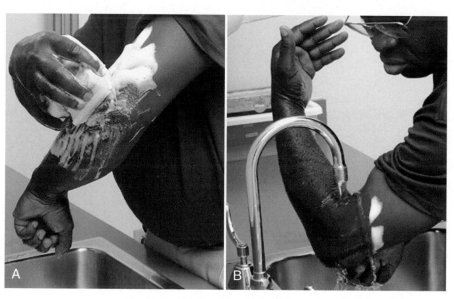

Fig. 2-3 Handwashing for surgical asepsis.

Isolation Precautions

Current isolation precaution guidelines are linked to the method by which pathogens are transmitted and hence are termed "transmission-based precautions" (see Table 2-3). This system relies on the concepts and principles associated with the cycle of infection, medical asepsis, and surgical asepsis to protect a person or object from becoming contaminated or infected by transmissible pathogens.

A patient may be isolated ("in isolation") from other patients and the hospital environment because of a disease or infection that is transmissible. The person may be placed in a private room or in a room with another patient with the same disease.

When a patient is in isolation, specific actions designed to interrupt the route of transmission of pathogens from the patient must be followed by any person who enters the patient's environment (Table 2-4). The use of proper hand hygiene techniques and the use of PPE (i.e., gloves, a gown, a mask, and eye protection or a face shield) are precautions that are usually required. The specific barriers used to interrupt the route of transmission of pathogens will depend on the type of disease or infection present and, most importantly, the mode of transmission of the pathogens associated with the disease or infection.

Three factors are involved with the use of transmission-based precautions (note the similarities between these factors and the stages in the previously discussed infection cycle):

1. A source (reservoir) of the infectious agent
2. A susceptible host with a portal of entry receptive to the agent
3. A mode of transmission for the agent

The CDC guidelines for isolation precautions are designed so that the routes of transmission of the microorganisms are interrupted or blocked within a health care facility. The disease-specific precautions are divided into three designations of precautions based on the route of transmission: contact (direct or indirect), droplet, and airborne.

- **Contact:** Microorganisms are transferred directly from one infected person to another or indirectly when the transfer of an infectious agent is through an object, medical equipment, furniture surface, or person. Some diseases that can be transmitted by contact are herpes simplex virus, *S. aureus*, vancomycin-resistant Enterococcus, and *C. difficile*.
- **Droplet:** Microorganisms are transferred by direct or indirect contact, but in contrast to contact transmission, respiratory droplets carrying infectious pathogens transmit infection when they travel a short distance directly from the respiratory tract of the infected individual to the mouth, conjunctivae, or nasal mucosa of the recipient. Droplet transmission necessitates that the caregiver wear a mask or face shield (Fig. 2-4). Respiratory droplets may be transmitted during a sneeze, cough, or talking. Some examples of diseases or conditions spread through droplet transmission are strep throat, meningitis, pneumonia, influenza, the common cold, pertussis (whooping cough), smallpox, and mumps.
- **Airborne:** Microorganisms are transferred by small infectious particles (infective over time and distance) in the respirable size range. Airborne transmission can occur with measles, varicella (chickenpox), and *Mycobacterium tuberculosis*. A fit-tested N-95 respirator (Fig. 2-5) or higher should be worn.

The modes of transmission vary by type of organism, and some infections can be transmitted by more than one route. Other transmission routes are considered environmental and include contaminated food, water, or medications.

Infections of the skin, gastrointestinal tract, and wounds are most likely to be spread by direct or indirect contact, especially when body fluids, secretions, excretions, or blood are involved. Box 2-3 presents the activities that caregivers, other personnel, and, at times, visitors must perform to reduce the spread of infection in a health care setting.

A cart containing protective garments, biohazard bags, and other materials along with appropriate directions for use should be located outside the patient's room so the items can be accessed before anyone enters the room. Containers for disposal of contaminated items should be located in the

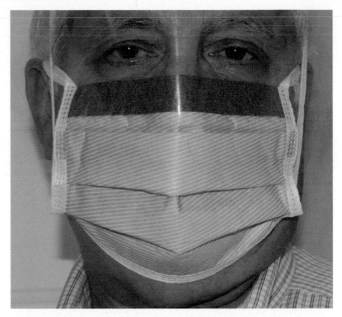

Fig. 2-4   A face shield.

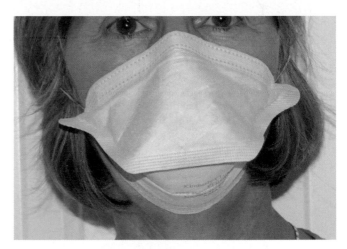

Fig. 2-5   A fit-tested N-95 respirator.

patient's room. The requirements for the amount and type of protection required for each category are listed on a color-coded card that is usually placed on the door or wall next to the patient's room (see Table 2-2). The medical record will indicate the isolation precautions in effect for the patient. Visitors of a patient who is in isolation must report to the nurse's station before entering the room.

The caregiver must be aware of the means of transmission of various diseases or infections to protect both the patient and the caregiver when working with the patient in an area other than the patient's room (e.g., the dialysis unit, rehabilitation unit or department, radiology unit, medical laboratory, or the patient's home). Consideration should be given to activities that may need to be performed before or after treatment (e.g., cleansing of treatment and transportation equipment, separation of the patient from other

- Proper hand hygiene techniques and wearing of gloves
- Use of masks, respiratory protection, eye protection, and face shields (especially when fluid splashes or sprays are anticipated)
- Use of gowns and protective apparel
- Handling and disposal of linen and protection of laundry personnel
- Cleaning or disposal of eating utensils and dishes
- Patient placement (i.e., in a private room or with a person who has the same disease)
- Protective transportation of an infected patient
- Use and care of patient care equipment and articles (e.g., disposal of sharps)
- Routine and terminal cleaning of the patient's environment (i.e., use of disinfectants and consistent housekeeping activities in the patient's room and treatment areas)

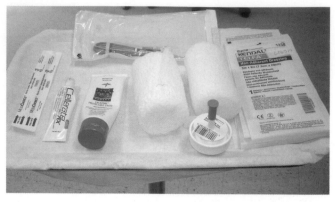

Fig. 2-6 Sterile packaging.

persons, and use of protective garments) when the patient is treated away from the room. These activities are especially important after treating a patient with a methicillin-resistant *S. aureus* infection, vancomycin-intermediate *S. aureus* infection, or vancomycin-resistant Enterococcus infection. Any equipment or treatment surface touched by the patient must be cleaned with a disinfectant wipe or solution. In addition, it is important that the caregiver know and understand the isolation system or precautions used in the facility so they are followed and the means of protection are used properly.

Occasionally, the term "protective isolation" may be used to designate a patient whose condition or disease causes a high risk of becoming infected through contact with another person. For example, patients with extensive open burns or wounds, a compromised immune system (i.e., a low white blood cell count), or a systemic infection (e.g., sepsis) may benefit from protective isolation. If this approach is used, it may be necessary for any person who enters the patient's room to apply protective items such as gloves and mask to reduce or prevent the transmission of pathogens to the patient. The sequence and method for applying the garments usually are more important than the method and sequence used to remove them when the patient is in protective isolation. The sequence and method of application are described later in this chapter.

The Sterile Field

As the term indicates, a sterile field is designed to maintain the sterility of objects contained within the field, such as dressings or bandages, and prevent contamination of objects that, in turn, could contaminate the patient. The sterile field is a form of surgical asepsis designed to keep the area

free from pathogens. Usually a nonabsorbent, sterile towel or the inside of the outer cover or wrapping of a package that contains sterile supplies is used as the base for the sterile field. Once the field has been established, additional sterile objects can be added to the field with care.

It is important to know and apply the following four rules of asepsis when you establish the field and when you use items that are part of the field:
1. Know which items are sterile
2. Know which items are not sterile
3. Separate sterile items from nonsterile items
4. If a sterile item becomes contaminated, remedy the situation immediately

Contamination occurs any time a sterile item physically contacts a nonsterile item. The remedy is to discard the contaminated item and reestablish the sterile field.

Only items that have been specifically sterilized or packaged and identified as sterile until the package is opened can be considered sterile. If an item has been autoclaved, be certain that black or green lines appear on the tape used to seal the package. These colored lines indicate that the item has been sterilized and is considered sterile. The outer packages of prepackaged sterile items should be checked to be certain that the items in the package were labeled as sterile when they were packaged and that they are still sterile and not outdated, and that the outer package is completely sealed and dry (Fig. 2-6).

Once the sterile field has been established (i.e., set up), care must be taken to maintain sterile conditions in the area and avoid contamination. Guidelines for maintaining the sterile field are presented in Box 2-4. In general, if the four rules of asepsis are followed, contamination of the field will be avoided. If you have any question about whether an item is nonsterile, consider it contaminated and do not use it. If the object has come in contact with other objects that are considered nonsterile, all the items should be discarded and only new items known to be sterile should be used.

It is imperative to maintain the sterile field once it has been established. The level of care provided by the caregiver

Box 2-4   Guidelines for Maintaining a Sterile Field

- Do not talk, sneeze, cough, or reach across a sterile field. The air currents or moisture droplets from your nose or mouth can convey pathogens onto the field.
- Do not turn your back to the field because contamination of the objects in the field can occur when you are not able to observe the field.
- Do not allow a nonsterile object to come in contact with a sterile object, and do not allow a sterile object to come in contact with a nonsterile object.
- Do not leave the field unattended, even if it is covered with a sterile towel or another sterile item. In your absence, the field can become contaminated.
- A 1-inch border along the edges of the field is considered to be nonsterile. Avoid placing any sterile item within 1 inch of the outer edge of the field, and do not touch this area with sterile gloves or other sterile objects.
- When you wear sterile protective clothing, the portions that are considered sterile (unless they come into contact with a nonsterile object or environment) are the gloves, the front of the gown above waist level, and both sleeves of the gown. The remainder of the gown is considered to be nonsterile.
- Remember that when forceps or other items that have been stored in a liquid disinfectant are used, they should be handled so the tip or end that has been in the disinfectant is held downward. If the tip or end of the object is held upward, the fluid will flow to a nonsterile area on the object. Then, when the tip or end is held downward again, the fluid will flow from the nonsterile area back to the sterile area and contaminate the object.
- The base and the area surrounding the field should be void of moisture because moisture is likely to contain microorganisms and can penetrate the field by direct contact, absorption, or the wicking property of any of the materials on the field. Moisture is considered to be a source of contamination, so the field must remain dry. If the base of the field or any of the sterile materials on the field becomes wet, they should be considered contaminated.
- To reduce or avoid movement over the field, position the items on the field so the items to be used first are nearest you.
- The area below the surface of the sterile field, which will usually be tabletop height or waist height, is considered nonsterile. Any item that falls to or is located below waist or tabletop level should be considered contaminated.
- General cleanliness of the treatment area, including the furniture, floor, walls, and lavatories, should be maintained to reduce the proliferation or deposition of microorganisms. Hand hygiene techniques and practices described previously should be used when a sterile field is required.

when a sterile technique is required may affect the healing process and possibly the patient's life. Procedures designed to protect the patient and the caregiver and to prevent wound contamination must be followed diligently and consistently.

PROTECTIVE GARMENTS

Protective clothing is recommended to safeguard the caregiver and the patient when it is necessary to reduce the transmission of pathogens from the caregiver to the patient, or vice versa. Gloves offer protection to the caregiver's hands to reduce the likelihood of becoming infected with microorganisms from an infected patient. Gloves also reduce the likelihood that the patient will receive microorganisms from the caregiver, and they reduce the possibility that a colony of microorganisms will develop on the caregiver's hands that could be transmitted to patients or to other personnel.

Protective clothing and apparel should be available to all caregivers and personnel who treat, transport, or handle items used for the patient whose condition requires the use of standard precautions. Items that should be available are gloves, gowns, masks, and protective eyewear such as eye shields or safety glasses. The necessary items should be applied before the patient is treated or before items associated with the patient are handled.

A gown, mask, and protective eyewear should be worn when spurting of blood is possible and in any other situation in which splashing of blood or other body fluids containing blood is anticipated or expected. Again, these examples are related to the patient for whom standard precautions are in effect. Several other reasons or patient conditions could require protective clothing to be worn. Specific institutional or agency policies and procedures regarding the use of protective clothing should be followed.

Gloves

Disposable gloves are usually sized small, medium, or large. They may be made of latex or nonlatex material and can be powdered or nonpowdered on the inside. These gloves can form an effective barrier between the caregiver's hands and the patient when they are applied and used properly. Regardless of the type of gloves you use, be careful when removing them to avoid any contact between the outside of the glove and your skin. Gloves should be worn routinely in situations in which it is necessary to control bleeding, perform a venipuncture, perform oral or nasal suctioning, perform endotracheal intubation, change a contaminated dressing, and handle or clean contaminated instruments or equipment. Wearing gloves to measure blood pressure or temperature usually is not necessary; however, if other reasons exist to wear gloves when performing these two procedures, they should be worn.

Gowns

A gown is used to protect the wearer's clothing from becoming contaminated or soiled by contact with a contaminant. A gown also provides a barrier to decrease the transmission of microorganisms from the caregiver's clothing to the patient or the environment. Techniques for the proper application, removal, and disposal of a gown are presented elsewhere in this chapter.

Masks

Masks are designed to reduce the spread of microorganisms that are transmitted through the air. They protect the wearer from the inhalation of particles or droplets that may contain pathogens. Masks also act as a filter to reduce the transmission of pathogens from the wearer to the patient. The proper techniques for application, positioning, removal, and disposal of a mask are presented elsewhere in this chapter.

Protective Eyewear

Protective eyewear, such as goggles, a facial shield, or eyewear with side shields, should be worn to prevent fluids from entering the eyes. It is especially important that protective eyewear be worn when blood splashes or spurts are likely to occur and when other body fluids are likely to be sprayed or splashed onto the face.

Application of Protective Garments

The caregiver may need to be protected from the patient, or the patient may need to be protected from the caregiver. In either situation, it is likely that protective clothing will be required. This section describes a method that can be used to apply clothing before treatment of a patient who has been placed in aseptic isolation (Procedure 2-4), along with a method that can be used to remove clothing after treatment of a patient who has been placed in isolation. When the patient is in protective isolation, the garment application sequence is extremely critical, but the garment removal sequence is less critical. When the caregiver is to be protected from the patient, the garment application sequence is less critical, but the garment removal sequence is extremely critical (Procedure 2-5).

Each health care facility or nursing unit has its own specific protocols related to the application and removal of protective clothing. The information in this chapter is sufficient to allow a caregiver to satisfactorily protect himself or herself or the patient, but it may not be as complete or specific as in many facility protocols. Therefore the caregiver should become familiar with the established protocols at the facility where patient care is provided.

After treating a patient in protective isolation, your gloves and clothing can be removed in any sequence because very little danger exists that you will become contaminated from a noninfectious patient. However, you should wash your hands or perform a hand rub after removing the gloves and clothing and avoid contact between your hands and your eyes, ears, nostrils, and mouth until you have washed your hands thoroughly.

Closed-Glove Technique for Asepsis   The closed-glove technique is used to reduce the possibility of glove contamination when the gloves are being applied. The exterior surface of the gloves is protected from contact with sources of contamination when this technique is performed properly (see Procedure 2-4).

Open-Glove Technique for Asepsis   In some situations the closed-glove technique is impractical or undesirable. The open-glove technique can be used in these situations, but it has a greater potential for glove contamination than the closed-glove technique unless you use extreme caution when you apply the gloves (Procedure 2-6).

Removal of Contaminated Protective Garments

You will frequently need to remove your contaminated protective garments without assistance after treatment of a patient for whom you had to use contact isolation precautions. When this situation occurs, you must avoid contaminating yourself while removing the garments. To protect yourself, do not touch any area of your body (e.g., your skin, eyes, ears, or hair) with your gloved hands. The sleeves and front of your gown will be the areas most likely to be contaminated, so do not touch those areas with your ungloved hands. You should remove your gloves without touching their outer surface with an ungloved hand. The paper type of gown can be removed similar to the way you would remove a cloth gown. You can release the neck and waist ties by tearing them rather than untying them (Procedure 2-7).

Because the furniture, sinks, linen, and other objects in the room may be contaminated, avoid touching them with any unprotected surface of your body. Remember to perform proper hand hygiene techniques before you apply and after you remove your protective clothing. Finally, do not wear protective clothing outside the patient's room or remove equipment from the room for use with patients in another area of the facility.

Some of the precautions you should follow when you treat a patient who is in protective isolation are as follows:

- Apply the protective clothing carefully, and follow the provided recommendations for their application.
- Avoid causing excessive air currents in the patient's room; move slowly and arrange linen or equipment carefully.
- Do not enter the patient's room with protective clothing or equipment that has been worn to treat patients in another area of the hospital—you may bring undesired microorganisms into the patient's environment.

Text continued on page 44

PROCEDURE 2-4

Clothing Application for Aseptic Isolation

1. Wash your hands as described previously for medical asepsis.
2. Apply a cap, but avoid touching your hair as much as possible. Include all your hair in the cap and, if possible, cover your ears (**A** and **B**).
3. Apply a mask, handling it by its ties or edges. Position the metal or plastic band of the mask over your nose, or center the dome type of mask over your nose and mouth. Gently open the mask so the bottom edge fits over your chin. Tie the upper ties snugly behind your head and above your ears; tie the lower ties snugly behind your neck. Avoid touching your neck or cap as you tie the mask (**C** and **D**). (Note: In some settings it may be preferred to apply the mask before the cap.)
4. Open the outer package of a sterile disposable gown and the sterile gloves, and place them on a table or counter in a sterile field at the approximate height of your waist. The inner cover of the gloves should remain closed (**E** to **G**).

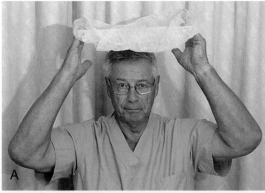

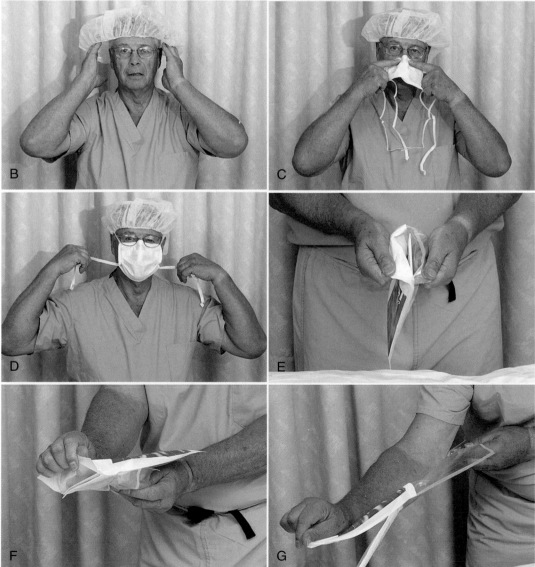

Fig. 2-7   Application of aseptic garments.

Continued

PROCEDURE **2-4**

Clothing Application for Aseptic Isolation—cont'd

5. Wash your hands as for surgical asepsis. (The medical asepsis technique may be acceptable for certain specific protocols.) Dry your hands thoroughly, and avoid touching your clothing or other objects with the washed areas of your skin.

6. Grasp the center of the gown with one hand, pick it up, and allow it to unfold without touching your body, clothing, or any other object. The gown will be folded inside out; avoid touching the outside of the gown (**H**).

7. Gently shake the gown so that it opens fully, and insert your left or right arm into the left or right sleeve. DO NOT ALLOW YOUR HAND TO EXTEND THROUGH THE GOWN CUFF; in this way a closed-glove technique can be used. Insert your other arm into the other sleeve, and keep that hand inside the cuff (**I** and **J**).

8. Ask another person to tie the neck and waist ties snugly. DO NOT ALLOW YOUR HANDS TO EXTEND THROUGH THE GOWN CUFFS when the gown is being tied (**K** and **L**). Note that the assistant should be gloved and wearing a cap.

9. When a disposable gown is applied with assistance from another person, care must be used to avoid contamination of the waist tie. **M** and **N** show proper handling of the tag of the tie so that the tie and gown remain sterile; the upper portion of the tag is sterile, and the bottom portion is not.

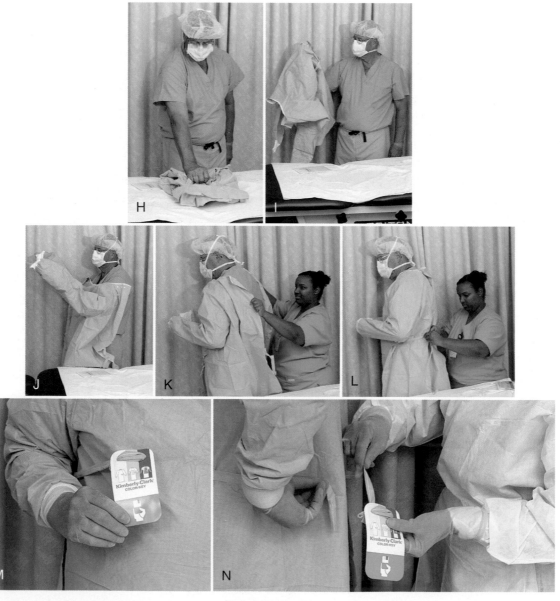

Fig. 2-7, cont'd

PROCEDURE 2-4

Clothing Application for Aseptic Isolation—cont'd

10. Carefully open the inner packet containing your gloves and pick up one glove with your hand, which is still inside the gown cuff. Place the glove palm down on its proper hand, so that the thumb of the glove rests on the thumb of your hand and the fingers of the glove are directed toward your elbow (**O** to **Q**).

11. Grasp the cuff of the glove through the cuff of the gown and peel the cuff over your hand to seal or enclose your hand within the glove cuff, and then gently maneuver your fingers and hand into the glove. Your other hand remains within the gown sleeve; do not extend it beyond the cuff (**R** to **T**).

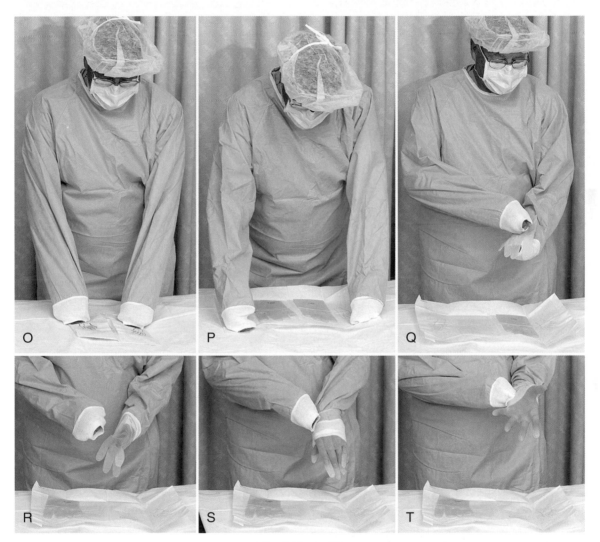

Fig. 2-7, cont'd

Continued

PROCEDURE 2-4

Clothing Application for Aseptic Isolation—cont'd

12. Repeat steps 10 and 11 to apply the other glove (**U** to **W**). Once both gloves have been applied completely, hold them above waist level and avoid touching your gown or other objects to maintain sterility (**X**). A sterile towel can be wrapped over your gloved hands to protect them until it is time to treat the patient.

13. The two-person method to apply sterile gloves is shown in **Y** and **Z**. All garments and gloves are sterile at this time; the glove is applied over the gown cuff.

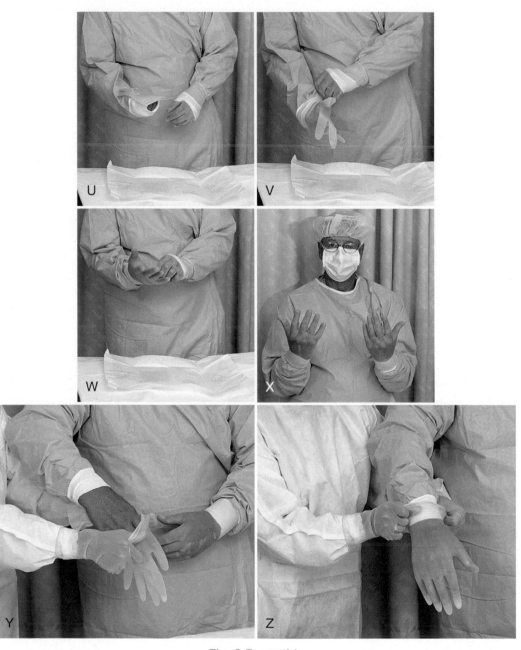

Fig. 2-7, cont'd

Clothing Removal for Isolation Precautions

1. Untie the waist tie of the gown and carefully untie the neck tie or unsnap at the neck. You should avoid touching your neck, cap, or the inner side of gown when untying/unsnapping the gown. Alternative method: the neck snaps can be pulled apart when grasping at the shoulders as described below (**A** and **B**).

2. Grasp the outer front shoulders of the gown by crossing the arms (i.e., your left hand grasps the right front shoulder, and your right hand grasps the left front shoulder). Gently remove the gown by pulling it over your arms with your arms extended in front of your body. Avoid touching the outer side of the gown with your bare arms or clothing. Gently roll the gown into a ball so that it will be turned inside out, and dispose of it. Avoid touching your skin or clothing with the gown or with your gloves (**B** to **F**).

3. The glove cuffs will have been turned down as the gown sleeves are removed from your arms. To remove the right glove, grasp the outside of it with your left hand and gently remove the glove so that it is inside out, and discard it. Use your ungloved right hand to grasp the inside of the left glove, and gently remove that glove so that it is inside out; discard it. Avoid touching the outside of the left glove with your ungloved hand or the ungloved skin with the left glove after the right glove has been removed (**G** to **K**).

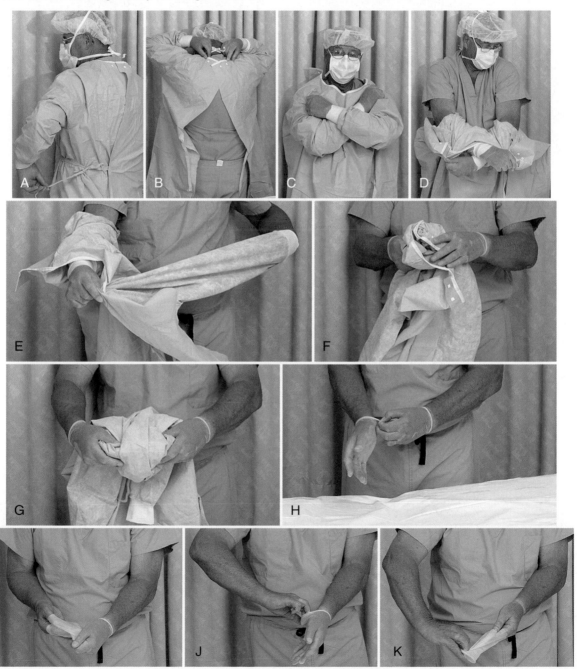

Fig. 2-8 Removal of protective clothing.

Continued

PROCEDURE 2-5

Clothing Removal for Isolation Precautions—cont'd

4. Wash your hands as described for medical asepsis.
5. Remove your mask by carefully untying each set of ties and handling it by the ties. Avoid touching the center of the mask with your hands, and dispose of it (**L** and **M**).

6. Remove the cap by handling it by its ties or by gently grasping the center at the top, and gently lift it from your head and dispose of it (**N** and **O**).
7. Wash your hands as described for medical asepsis.

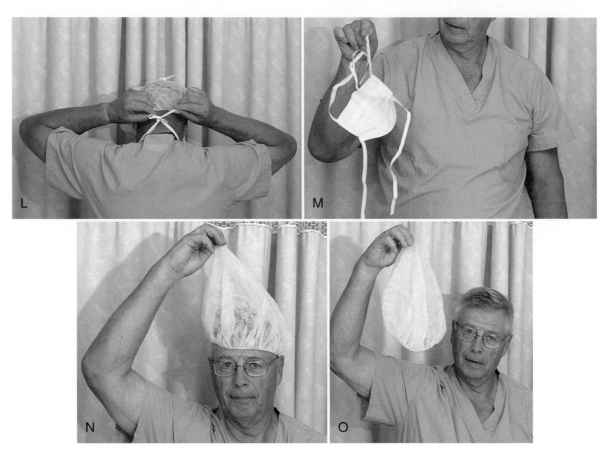

Fig. 2-8, cont'd

• Remember to perform proper handwashing before applying and after removing your protective clothing.

Adherence to these precautions will help protect both you and the patient from becoming infected.

DISPOSAL OF INSTRUMENTS AND CLOTHING

Instruments and equipment used to treat a patient should be cleaned or disposed of according to institutional or agency policies and procedures. Contaminated reusable equipment should be carefully placed in a container, labeled, and returned to the appropriate department for sterilization. Contaminated disposable items should be carefully placed in a container, labeled, and discarded according to institutional or agency policies and procedures.

Anyone who handles these instruments or equipment should wear gloves and wash or hand rub the hands before and after the gloves have been applied and removed. Needles, scalpels, and other sharp instruments should be placed in puncture-proof containers. No attempt should be made to recap, bend, or break the needle before it is discarded. The ear tips of a "community" or departmental stethoscope should be wiped with alcohol before and after each use. In some instances, it may be necessary to clean the diaphragm with alcohol. If the cuff of a sphygmomanometer becomes contaminated, it should be

PROCEDURE 2-6

Open-Glove Technique for Asepsis

1. Perform preparatory activities of handwashing.
2. Open the package containing the sterile gloves and place the gloves in the sterile field. Open the inner packet carefully, and arrange the gloves so that the cuffs are nearest you by touching only the inside of the folded cuffs with your hands. Avoid touching the outer surface of the gloves with your hands as you prepare to apply the first glove (**A**).
3. To apply the first glove, grasp the inner side or surface of the folded cuff of the glove. Caution: Do not touch the outside of either glove with an ungloved hand. Insert your hand and fingers into the glove and apply the glove as if you were applying a dress glove, but allow the cuff to remain folded; do not attempt to adjust the cuff or the fit of the glove at this time (**B** and **C**).

4. Using your gloved hand, lift the other glove by sliding your gloved fingers between the underside of the cuff and the outer side of the palm of the other glove. Caution: Do not touch the inside surface of the second glove or your ungloved hand with your gloved hand; to do so will contaminate them. Insert your hand and fingers into the glove, but do not allow the thumb of the hand you are using to apply the second glove to touch the inside of the cuff of that glove (**D** to **G**).
5. Pull the cuff of the second glove up by holding the outer surface of the cuff; avoid touching the skin of your hand with the outside of the first glove that was applied.
6. Once the cuff of the second glove is in place, slide your fingers under the cuff of the first glove and pull the cuff of that glove all the way up (**H**).

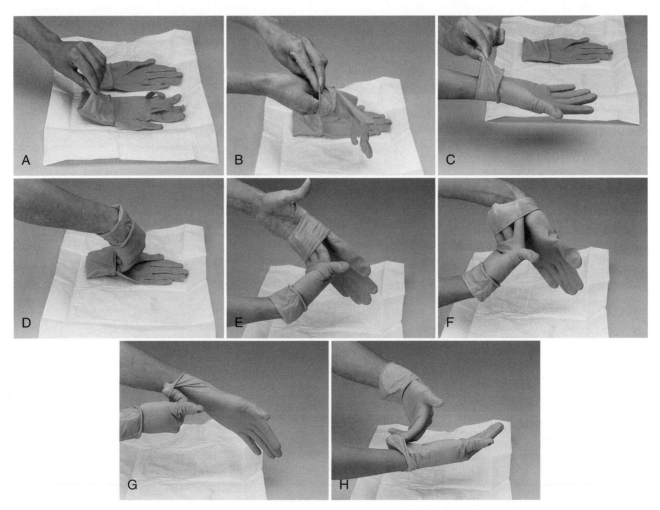

Fig. 2-9 Open-glove application technique. (From Young AP: *Kinn's the medical assistant: an applied learning approach*, ed 11, St Louis, 2011, Saunders.)

PROCEDURE 2-7

Independent Removal of Contaminated Protective Garments

1. Untie the waist tie and then carefully remove one glove by turning it inside out with the opposite hand. Caution: Do not touch the bare skin of your hand with the glove of your other hand as the glove is being removed. Dispose of the glove.
2. Untie the neck tie with your ungloved hand, but avoid touching the back of the gown, your neck, or your cap. Remove the gown, using your gloved hand to grasp the opposite outer anterior shoulder of the gown and using your ungloved hand to grasp the opposite inner anterior shoulder of the gown. Gently turn the gown inside out, and remove it from your arms. Avoid touching the outside of the sleeve or cuff with your ungloved hand; dispose of the gown. The remaining glove should roll down to expose the inside of the glove at your wrist.
3. Remove the remaining glove by grasping the inner surface of the glove at the cuff or by inserting one or two fingers at the base of your palm; peel the glove off by turning it inside out. Avoid touching your ungloved hand to the outside of the glove, and discard it.
4. Wash your hands as described previously.
5. Remove the mask and cap as described previously.
6. Wash your hands as described previously.

The following alternative method may be used:
1. Untie the waist tie and remove your cap, if it was applied after the mask, by grasping the top of it and lifting it from your head. Avoid touching your hair with your gloved hand. Dispose of the cap.
2. Grasp the outside of one glove at the cuff and fold it down to form a wide cuff; do the same to the opposite glove. Remove one glove by turning it inside out. Avoid touching your exposed hand with the outside of the other glove.
3. Remove the opposite glove by grasping the inside of the cuff of the glove and turning it inside out. Avoid touching the outside of the glove or the sleeve of the gown with your exposed hand. Dispose of the glove. Wash your hands, but avoid getting the cuffs of the gown wet.
4. Untie the mask, or grasp the inside of the mask with one hand and the elastic strap with the other hand; remove the mask carefully. Avoid touching the exposed skin of your hands or face with the outer side of the mask. Dispose of the mask.
5. Untie the tie at the neck of the gown and shrug the gown forward off your shoulders, or grasp the inside of the gown at the shoulders and pull it inside out over your extended arms. Roll the gown into a small ball by handling the inside of the gown. Avoid touching your clothing or exposed skin with the outside of the gown. Dispose of the gown.
6. Wash your hands as described previously.

disinfected in a manner similar to that used for clothing items.

Soiled linen should be handled as little as possible and with minimal movement to prevent contamination of the air and the persons who handle the linen. It should be disposed of and transported in bags that are leak proof and clearly designated as containing potentially contaminated linen. The bag can be color coded to indicate the type or condition of linen it contains. The risk of disease transmission from soiled linen contaminated with pathogenic microorganisms is negligible, but reasonable care should be taken when such linen is handled.

Protective clothing contaminated with blood or other body fluids subject to standard precautions should be disposed of and transported in bags or other containers that are nonporous and leak proof. Any person who is involved with the bagging, transporting, or laundering of contaminated clothing should wear gloves.

Contaminated dressings, bandages, materials, paper items, and other disposable items should be properly placed in a nonporous container or bag, labeled, and discarded according to institutional or agency policies and procedures.

Other contaminated items such as toys, magazines, personal hygiene articles, dishes, and eating utensils should be disposed of or disinfected and should not be used by others until they have been disinfected.

These precautions require greater emphasis when you are caring for patients whose susceptibility to infection is greatest. For example, patients who have open burns or wounds or a disease that compromises the immune system and patients who are receiving chemotherapy or body irradiation are more susceptible than other patients to transmitted pathogens. Protection of patients from pathogens is important, but it is particularly important for patients who have a reduced capacity to resist or overcome infection.

Sterilization

Sterilization is used to destroy all forms of microbial life, including high numbers of bacterial spores. An item can be sterilized by being subjected to steam under pressure (i.e., autoclaved), to ethylene oxide (a gas), or to a dry heat source, or it may be immersed in an EPA-approved chemical sterilant for 6 to 10 hours or according to the manufacturer's instructions. This last method should be used only for instruments or equipment that cannot be sterilized with heat, such as instruments or items that penetrate skin (e.g., needles or scalpel blades) or that come in contact with areas of the body that are not contaminated.

Disinfection

High-level disinfection destroys all forms of microbial life except high numbers of bacterial spores. Hot water pasteurization at 80° C to 100° C for 30 minutes or exposure to an EPA-approved sterilant chemical for 10 to 45 minutes or as directed by the manufacturer are the common methods used for this type of disinfection. This method can be used for reusable instruments or items that come into contact with mucous membranes (e.g., endotracheal tubes).

Intermediate-level disinfection destroys most viruses, most fungi, vegetative bacteria, and the tuberculosis bacterium, but it does not kill bacterial spores. The EPA-approved hospital disinfectant chemical germicides labeled for tuberculocidal activity and commercially available hard-surface germicides or solutions that contain at least 500 parts per million (ppm) of free available chlorine are the solutions most commonly used to accomplish this type of disinfection. Common household bleach in a solution of approximately one-quarter cup per gallon of water will produce an appropriate solution.

Low-level disinfection destroys most bacteria, some viruses, and some fungi, but it does not kill the tuberculosis bacterium or bacterial spores. The EPA-approved hospital disinfectants without a label claim for tuberculocidal activity are used for this type of disinfection. These types of agents are excellent cleaners and can be used for routine housekeeping or to remove soiling in the absence of visible blood contamination.

Environmental disinfection practices are used to clean and disinfect surfaces that have become soiled and are performed with any cleaner or disinfectant that is intended for environmental use. Environmental surfaces include floors, woodwork, mat or treatment table pads, countertops, walking aids, sliding or transfer boards, and sinks.

When liquids are used as cleaning agents, the person who uses them should protect the skin from repeated or prolonged contact with the agent by wearing gloves and other protective clothing as necessary.

Any item that is to be disinfected or sterilized should first be cleaned thoroughly to remove residual organic matter such as blood, excrement, or tissue. Different microorganisms will require different methods and levels of disinfection. The CDC, the local health department, or a hospital infection-control department can be contacted for current information regarding the best method to use and the level necessary to destroy or control various microorganisms.

The patient's room and the treatment area should be cleaned routinely by housekeeping personnel using EPA-approved cleansing products. It is unlikely the pathogenic microorganisms that are usually present on the walls, floors, carpet, furniture, and other objects in the area will be transmitted to persons or patients. Simple actions such as disposing of linen that drops onto the floor; avoiding shaking or rapidly moving linen, which could create air currents and lift microorganisms from the floor onto clothing; avoiding holding contaminated linen or protective clothing against your own clothing to reduce the transfer of microorganisms; and promptly discarding dressings and soiled linen according to institutional or agency policies and procedures will help reduce the transmission of microorganisms.

DECONTAMINATION

Several methods can be used to clean or decontaminate equipment or a surface area. By definition, decontamination is "to remove, inactivate, or destroy blood-borne pathogens on a surface or item to the point where they are no longer capable of transmitting infectious particles and the surface or item is rendered safe for handling, use, or disposal."*

Hands and other skin surfaces should be washed immediately and thoroughly after they have been contaminated by blood, wound drainage, or other body fluids to which standard precautions apply, even if gloves have been worn. The gloves should be removed carefully to avoid the external surface of the gloves coming in contact with your skin. The soiled gloves should be disposed of in a nonporous container; the same pair of gloves must not be worn to treat more than one patient.

Spills of body fluids should be removed as soon as possible, and the surface where the spill occurred should be cleansed with a solution of one part 5.25% sodium hypochlorite (bleach) diluted in 10 parts water or with an EPA-approved hospital disinfectant. Towels or linen used to clean up the spill must be disposed of properly, and the person involved in cleaning the spill should wear gloves and should consider wearing a gown. In general, it is better to be overprotected than underprotected when dealing with body fluids.

Infective waste products such as feces, urine, bulk blood, or suctioned fluid can be disposed of by carefully pouring them into a drain or toilet connected to a sanitary sewer, if this practice is permitted by institutional or local public health policies and procedures. In some instances, the waste product may need to be placed in a plastic bag that can be sealed so it can be transported. Individual bedpans and urinals, if not made of a disposable material, must be cleaned thoroughly and sterilized before use by another patient. Persons who are involved with the handling of these waste products should wear gloves, and a gown may be necessary if soiling of the handler's clothing is anticipated.

SUMMARY

Because a caregiver may need to treat a patient who has a transmissible pathogen or who requires protection from possible pathogens in the environment, the caregiver must know how to protect both the patient and himself or herself. The most effective method to reduce the transmission of pathogens is to routinely perform hand hygiene. Other methods include maintaining a barrier between the caregiver and the patient and disposing of dressings, sharps, and contaminated items properly. Most hospitals require that all employees adhere to the procedures established in

*Federal Register 56; 64175, December 6, 1991.

the CDC's standard precautions for blood-borne pathogens.

The caregiver should be able to apply and remove a dressing to protect the patient and himself or herself from contamination (see Chapter 11). The caregiver should know how to select the appropriate dressing and how to apply it to provide proper wound care.

Each institution has the responsibility to protect its employees from occupational exposure and transmission of pathogens, and the institution's employees have the responsibility to follow the institution's policies and procedures regarding infection control. Regulations established by OSHA are in effect for health care facilities and are designed to protect employees. The facility has the responsibility to provide its employees with information and instruction in techniques to protect themselves from infectious diseases, especially blood-borne diseases. Specifically, each health care facility must take the following steps:

- Educate employees on the methods of transmission and the prevention of HBV and HIV
- Provide safe and adequate protective equipment and teach employees where the equipment is located and how to use it
- Teach employees about work practices used to prevent occupational transmission of disease, including but not limited to standard precautions, proper handling of patient specimens and linens, proper cleaning of body fluid spills, and proper waste disposal
- Provide proper containers for the disposal of waste and sharp items and teach employees the color-coding system used to distinguish infectious waste
- Offer the HBV vaccine to employees who are at substantial risk of occupational exposure to HBV
- Provide education and follow-up care to employees who are exposed to a communicable disease

The following responsibilities of health care employees have been outlined by OSHA:

- Use protective equipment and clothing provided by the facility whenever the employee contacts, or anticipates contact, with body fluids
- Dispose of waste in proper containers, using knowledge and understanding of the handling of infectious waste and color-coded bags or containers
- Dispose of sharp instruments and needles into proper containers without attempting to recap, bend, break, or otherwise manipulate them before disposal

- Keep the work and patient care area clean
- Wash hands immediately after removing gloves and at all other times required by hospital or agency policy
- Immediately report any exposures, such as needle sticks or blood splashes, or any personal illnesses to a supervisor and receive instruction about any follow-up action

The desired outcome is to protect patients, visitors, and employees from contracting or transmitting pathogens. Information about the use of aseptic techniques and protective clothing, the proper handling of dressings and bandages, and methods to control the spread of disease in the hospital or a similar health care setting has been provided.

self-study ACTIVITIES

- Explain your duties or obligations when you treat a patient in isolation and when you treat a patient in protective isolation.
- Demonstrate the sequence you would use to apply and remove protective clothing when treating a patient in isolation and when treating a patient in protective isolation.
- Explain the concept and principles associated with standard precautions and describe the actions you would perform to comply with those principles when you provide patient care or treatment.

problem SOLVING

1. In your clinical setting, a 55-year-old male patient who is in isolation has a disease that is transmissible by air and has been referred to you for treatment. How will you prepare yourself to treat him in his room? In the course of his stay, he has progressed and is able to be treated in a site away from his room. What precautions would be required to transport and treat him in this area?

2. You have been selected to orient new employees about the techniques and procedures of hand hygiene. The employees represent nursing, physical and occupational therapy, and respiratory therapy. What teaching methods, equipment, and materials will you use? How will you determine that each participant has attained competence to perform all aspects of hand hygiene at the conclusion of the program?

3. You are the director of a patient care service unit in a health care facility. What actions or procedures would you recommend to your staff to prevent health care–associated infections in the unit?

Assessment of Vital Signs

objectives *After studying this chapter, the reader will be able to:*

- Provide the rationale for the need to measure, monitor, and record a patient's vital signs.
- Locate and palpate a patient's arterial pulse at various sites.
- Describe and define blood pressure.
- Accurately measure and record a patient's blood pressure, pulse and heart rates, respiration rate, and body temperature and determine a person's sense of pain.
- Describe the expected normal and abnormal changes in blood pressure, heart rate, and respiration rate resulting from exercise and other factors.
- Explain to a patient or family member the significance of measuring and monitoring vital signs.
- Describe pulmonary auscultation, breath sounds, and adventitious breath sounds.
- Describe the importance and methods of pain assessment.

key terms

Anoxia Absence of oxygen in the tissues.

Apical pulse The pulse that is found when a stethoscope is placed on the chest wall over the apex of the heart; also may be found by palpation.

Apnea The absence of breathing.

Arrhythmia Variation from the normal rhythm.

Auscultation Listening for sounds produced within the body by using the unaided ear or a stethoscope.

Bradycardia A slow heartbeat (i.e., pulse rate less than 60 beats/min); may be a normal finding in a well-conditioned person or an abnormal finding.

Cardiac output The amount of blood that is pumped from the heart during each contraction.

Diaphoresis Profuse perspiration.

Diastole The period when the least amount of pressure is exerted on the walls or the arteries during the heartbeat; usually indicates the resting phase of the heart.

Dyspnea Labored or difficult breathing.

Dysrhythmia Disturbance of rhythm.

Ectopic Arising or produced abnormally.

Expiration The passive phase of respiration when the person breathes out; also referred to as exhalation.

Fever Body temperature that is above the normal level; also referred to as pyrexia.

Hypertension Abnormally high blood pressure.

Hypotension Abnormally low blood pressure.

Inguinal Pertaining to the groin.

Inspiration The active phase of respiration when the person breathes in; also referred to as inhalation.

Intubation The insertion of a tube into the larynx to maintain an open airway.

Korotkoff's sounds Sounds heard during auscultatory determination of blood pressure; believed to be produced by the vibratory motion of the arterial wall as the artery suddenly distends when compressed by a pneumatic blood pressure cuff; the origin of the sound may be within the blood passing through the vessel or within the wall itself.

Occlude To fit close together; to close tight; to obstruct or close off.

Orthopnea A condition in which breathing is easier when the person is seated or standing.

Pulse A palpable wave of blood produced in the walls of the arteries with each heartbeat or contraction.

Pulse oximeter A medical device that measures levels of blood oxygen saturation, monitors pulse rate, and calculates heart rate.

Rale An abnormal, discontinuous, nonmusical sound heard on auscultation of the chest, primarily during inhalation; also called a crackle.

Rectal Pertaining to the rectum or the distal portion of the large intestine.

Respiration The act of breathing.

SOB Shortness of breath.

Sphygmomanometer An instrument used to measure blood pressure; it may use a mercury column or an enclosed air-pressure spring system.

Stethoscope An instrument used to convey sounds produced in the body of a person to the ears of the examiner; it is comprised of a diaphragm, tubing, and earpieces.

Stridor A shrill, harsh sound, especially the respiratory sound heard during inspiration in a person with a laryngeal obstruction.

Syncope A temporary suspension of consciousness caused by cerebral anemia; fainting.

Systole The period when the greatest amount of pressure is exerted on the walls of the arteries during heartbeat; usually indicates the contractile phase of the heartbeat.

Tachycardia An abnormally fast heartbeat (i.e., a pulse rate greater than 100 beats/min).

Vital signs Measurement of a person's body temperature, heart and respiration rates, and blood pressure; also referred to as cardinal signs.

INTRODUCTION

The patient's vital signs—that is, body temperature, heart rate (HR), pulse, blood pressure (BP), and respiration rate (RR)—are important because they are indicators of general health or physiologic status. In addition, the determination of a patient's sense or level of pain is frequently included with the measurement of vital signs. Normal values or ranges have been established for vital signs, and significant deviations from these norms may indicate an abnormal condition. It is important for the caregiver to know the normal values and determine the normal and abnormal changes that may occur as a result of illness, trauma, exercise, or physical condition.

For most patients, a baseline measurement of the vital signs at rest should be established so changes in the values caused by exercise or other activity can be determined. It is particularly important to establish baseline values for the following persons:

- Elderly patients (older than 65 years)
- Very young patients (younger than 2 years)
- Debilitated patients
- Patients who have performed limited aerobic activities for several weeks or months
- Patients with a previous or current history of cardiovascular problems
- Patients recovering from recent trauma, those with a condition or disease that affects the cardiopulmonary system (e.g., a spinal cord injury, a cerebrovascular injury, hypertension, peripheral vascular disease), or chronic obstructive pulmonary disease), or those recovering from recent major surgery

If abnormal values are found when the person is at rest, the cause of these values should be determined before the initiation of any activity that could affect the vital signs. Frequently a patient with abnormal resting values will be less able to tolerate physical activity or stress-producing events than a person with normal resting values.

Measurements of the patient's vital signs can be used to establish goals of treatment, assist with the development of a treatment plan, and assess a patient's response or treatment effectiveness.

General factors that frequently cause an increase or decrease in a person's vital signs are the level or amount of physical activity, the environmental temperature, the person's age, the emotional status of the person, and the physiologic status of the person (i.e., the existence of illness, disease, trauma, or use of medications).

Some possible adverse and potentially dangerous responses to activity are mental confusion, fatigue, exhaustion, lethargy, and slow reactions of movement or response to commands; decreased response to verbal and tactile stimuli; complaints of nausea, syncope, or vertigo; diaphoresis; a change in appearance (e.g., pallor or erythema); a decrease in BP; pupil constriction or dilation; and loss of consciousness. Many of these responses may be caused by anoxia. The caregiver should monitor the patient during and after treatment for any indication of these undesirable signs and symptoms. Prompt and appropriate care may need to be provided to reduce or relieve the symptoms, and modifications in the treatment program may be necessary to avoid them.

BODY TEMPERATURE

Body temperature is an indication of the intensity or degree of heat within the body. It represents a balance between the heat that is produced in the body and the heat that is lost. In humans, body temperature remains relatively constant regardless of the environmental temperature. However, some exceptions exist, such as when someone is exposed to extremes of heat or cold or when other factors such as humidity and physical exertion are involved.

Depending on the source, an accepted normal range for human oral core or body temperature is 96.8° F to 99.3° F (36° C to 37.3° C). The average temperature of 98.6° F (37° C) is the most generally accepted single value. The normal range for human rectal temperature is 97.8° F to 100.3° F (36.6° C to 38.1° C). Slight variations from these norms may occur in individuals; therefore it is important to establish a norm for each patient by repeated measurement of temperature. A person whose normal core temperature is 98.6° F or higher is considered to have a fever, or to be pyrexic, with a temperature higher than 100° F (38° C). A person is considered to be hyperpyrexic with a temperature higher than 106° F (41.1° C). Factors that affect body temperature are listed in Table 3-1.

Assessment of Body Temperature

It is suggested that a normal or baseline temperature be established for a person before the need arises to measure the temperature during an illness, especially when the patient is an infant or a toddler. Two or three serial measurements should be taken for infants younger than 3 months and for toddlers younger than 3 years when the presence or absence of a fever is a critical finding or when the operator is unfamiliar with the device used to measure temperature.

Although nursing personnel usually measure temperature, other health care personnel should be prepared to perform this task because treatment decisions may need to be made on the basis of the patient's body temperature or response to exercise. A person whose body temperature is elevated before treatment should not be asked to exercise. The cause of the abnormal temperature should be determined before exercise is begun.

The following points should be kept in mind:
- A person who has a normal body temperature before treatment can be monitored during or at the conclusion of the treatment to determine whether normal responses occur. If an excessive temperature value is measured or any signs or symptoms of excessive temperature are observed, the patient should have adequate periods of rest to allow the body temperature to become stabilized at the normal value.
- A person whose body temperature is lower than normal *before* treatment should be monitored to be certain the treatment is tolerated and to determine whether the temperature changes during or at the conclusion of the activity.
- A patient whose body temperature becomes lower than normal *during* treatment also may be demonstrating an abnormal response to the treatment.

In any of these abnormal situations, caution should be used if the treatment is continued, and it may be prudent to have the patient examined by an appropriate medical practitioner.

Sites used to assess a person's body temperature are the oral cavity, rectum, axilla, ear canal, forehead or temporal lobe, and occasionally the inguinal fold. The most common and convenient location to measure a person's temperature

Table 3-1	Factors Affecting Body Temperature
Factor	**Description**
Time of day	Body temperature is usually lower in the early morning and higher in the afternoon
Age	Body temperature tends to decrease slightly with age and is increased slightly in the very young
Environmental temperature	Body temperature may increase slightly in a hot environment and decrease slightly in a cold environment
Infection	Body temperature increases with a major or systemic infectious process
Physical activity	Body temperature usually increases slightly with physical activity but reaches a plateau as the person becomes better conditioned
Emotional status	Body temperature increases slightly during stressful or emotional periods (e.g., crying or anger)
Site of measurement	Body temperature values are slightly higher if measured rectally and slightly lower if measured in the axilla when compared with oral values
Menstrual cycle	Body temperature is slightly higher at the time of ovulation, and a pregnant woman's body temperature tends to be slightly higher than usual
Oral cavity temperature	Body temperature measurement may be inaccurate if measured orally within 14 to 30 minutes of ingestion of warm or cold substances or smoking; the body core temperature probably is not affected by these factors, but a false reading is obtained as a result of the temporary changes in the temperature of the oral cavity

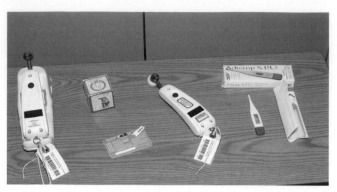

Fig. 3-1 Examples of temperature measurement devices.

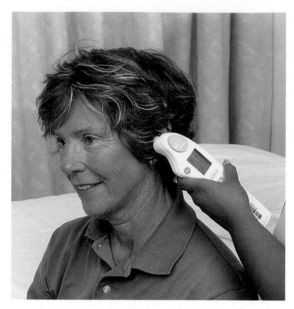

Fig. 3-2 Temperature measurement with an ear thermometer.

is the oral cavity, but the most accurate measurement of body temperature is obtained from the rectal cavity. Rectal, temporal lobe, or ear canal measurement can be used for infants or young children (i.e., preschool age) who are unable to maintain the thermometer/probe under the tongue or safely hold it between the lips. For unconscious patients or for patients who are unable to maintain the thermometer/probe in the mouth (e.g., a patient who is intubated), a rectal or ear canal measurement should be used. The axillary or inguinal folds are the least desirable sites because air currents may reduce the accuracy of the measurement. Therefore measurement at these sites should be used only when measurement at the other sites is neither possible nor safe. If the temperature is measured by the rectal, temporal ear, or axillary method, it should be so noted on the patient's record.

Equipment available to measure body temperature includes an oral thermometer with a probe; a chemical thermometer, which is discarded after one use; a temporal lobe scanner; or an infrared ear thermometer (Fig. 3-1).

Note: The use of an oral glass mercury thermometer is not included in this book because its use is prohibited by the Occupational Safety and Health Administration. This type of thermometer may still be used in the home, but it is no longer used in health care facilities. Two dangerous factors associated with this thermometer are the possibility of breakage and the toxicity of the mercury when it is released.

Ear Thermometer A thermometer that measures body temperature on the basis of heat generated by the ear canal and its surrounding tissue (Fig. 3-2) is especially useful for infants, toddlers, and older persons for whom it is difficult to use an oral thermometer probe. Most infrared ear thermometers require batteries as the power source, and disposable lens filters are used to protect the ear canal and lens cone. The lens filter should be cleaned thoroughly or discarded after each use to prevent cross-contamination or a false reading of the unit. The temperature value is obtained from a liquid crystal display in a window on one side of the

thermometer. According to a study by Craig and colleagues, the ear thermometer is not as accurate in taking body temperature as the rectal thermometer.

When a person has been lying on his or her ear, that ear should not be used for measurement until it has been exposed to the air for 2 to 3 minutes so the ear canal temperature can become stable. If the temperature of the ear canal is not permitted to acclimate, a falsely high reading may occur. A temperature differential may exist between the person's left and right ear, and so the same ear should be used for all measurements. When the results of the measurement are documented, the ear in which the thermometer cone was placed should be indicated.

Use of an ear thermometer is described in Procedure 3-1.

Oral Thermometer The oral thermometer has a probe connected to a unit containing a battery that measures a person's temperature and provides a digital reading. Use of the oral thermometer is described in Procedure 3-2.

PULSE

The pulse is an indirect measure of the contraction of the left ventricle of the heart and indicates the rate at which the heart is beating. It is defined as the movement of blood in an artery, which can be palpated at various sites of the body or measured through auscultation over the apex of the heart with a stethoscope. The rate or frequency of ventricular contractions of the heart is reported in beats per minute (beats/min).

Depending on the source used, the accepted normal range for the resting pulse is 60 to 100 beats/min in adults, 100 to 130 beats/min in newborns, and 80 to 120 beats/min in children aged 1 to 7 years. The normal resting pulse can

PROCEDURE 3-1

Measuring Body Temperature with an Ear Thermometer

- Wash your hands and obtain the ear thermometer, lens filter, recording form, and pen.
- Position the patient to expose one ear. An infant or a toddler may be held on your lap so the head can be stabilized; other persons may lie or sit.
- Apply a clean lens filter, and if the thermometer has an "oral" or "rectal" setting, select "rectal" for an infant or toddler and "oral" for an older child or adult. Regardless of the setting you select, the thermometer lens will be placed in the person's ear canal.
- Gently but firmly pull and hold the ear to straighten the ear canal. Pull straight back on an infant's ear and slightly downward; pull up and back on the ear of a person who is older than 1 year.
- Insert the thermometer lens cone, with a clean filter applied, into the ear opening. It may be necessary to

gently rock the lens cone back and forth to insert it far enough to seal the ear canal from the external air.
- Maintain the lens cone in the ear canal, and depress and hold the activation button for 1 second. After the beep, the temperature reading will appear in the liquid crystal display window; mentally record the value.
- Remove the lens cone from the person's ear and discard or thoroughly wash the lens filter if it is to be used again. Note: In the home it may be appropriate to wash and reuse a lens filter, but in other environments the used lens filter should be discarded. Wash your hands.
- Record the results using the value from the liquid crystal display reading; indicate whether the rectal or oral setting was used, and indicate which ear was used.
- Note: Do not attempt to take a temperature with an ear thermometer in an ear where an earache is suspected.

PROCEDURE 3-2

Measuring Body Temperature Orally

- Wash your hands and obtain a thermometer, probe cover, recording form, and pen.
- Position the patient and explain the procedure. Observe the patient and evaluate signs and symptoms related to body temperature: skin color, temperature (hot, warm, or cool), and condition (moist or dry).
- Turn on the unit and apply the disposable probe cover to the probe (**A**).
- Instruct the patient to open his or her mouth, position the probe under the tongue, hold the probe in place

with the lips, not with the teeth, and breathe through the nose (**B**).
- Leave the probe in place until the digital readout or alarm indicates that a constant temperature level has been reached; note the value.
- Remove the probe from the patient's mouth, discard the probe cover, turn off the unit, and wash your hands.
- Record the results, using even increments to report tenths of a degree.

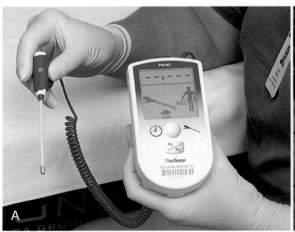 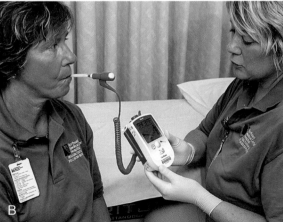

Fig. 3-3   Use of a thermometer for oral body temperature.

Table **3-2** Factors Affecting Pulse

Factor	Description
Age	Persons older than 65 years may exhibit a decreased pulse rate, whereas young persons (adolescents and younger) usually exhibit an increased rate
Gender	Male pulse rates are usually slightly lower than female rates
Environmental temperature	The pulse rate tends to increase with high temperature and decrease with low temperature
Infection	The pulse rate tends to increase with a major infectious process
Physical activity	Normally the pulse rate should rise rapidly in response to vigorous physical activity, plateau or stabilize as the intensity or severity of the exercise plateaus, and then decline as the intensity of the exercise declines; the pulse rate after exercise should revert to the person's resting pulse rate within 3 to 5 minutes after cessation of exercise; a person with a conditioned cardiopulmonary system will probably exhibit less change in the pulse rate, and the rate should return to its normal resting level in a shorter time than that required by an unconditioned or debilitated person
Emotional status	The pulse rate increases during episodes of high stress, anxiety, or emotion (e.g., anger or fear) and may decrease when the person is asleep or in a state of extreme calm
Medications	Various medications may cause the pulse rate to increase or decrease, depending on their effect on the cardiovascular system
Cardiopulmonary disease	Both the condition of the heart and the peripheral vascular system and their ability to function normally affect the pulse rate; for example, a patient with hypertension may exhibit a slower (lower) pulse rate, whereas a patient with hypotension may exhibit a faster (higher) pulse rate to compensate for the higher or lower blood pressure
Physical conditioning	Persons who perform frequent, sustained, vigorous aerobic exercise will exhibit a lower than normal pulse rate

Table **3-3** Pulse Measurement Sites

Artery	Site*
Temporal	Anterior and adjacent to the ear
Carotid	Inferior to the angle of the mandible and anterior to the sternocleidomastoid muscle
Brachial	Medial to the biceps in the antecubital fossa or on the medial aspect of the mid shaft of the humerus
Radial	At the wrist on the volar forearm medial to the stylus process of the radius
Femoral	At the femoral triangle slightly lateral and anterior to the inguinal crease
Popliteal	In the midline of the posterior knee crease between the tendons of the hamstring muscles
Dorsal pedal	Along the midline or slightly medial on the dorsum of the foot
Posterior tibial	On the medial aspect of the foot inferior to the medial malleolus

*These sites are accurate for most patients; however, for some patients it may be necessary to palpate the area surrounding a site to locate the pulse (see Fig. 3-4).

be established for each patient by repeated measurement of the pulse at the same site and under the same conditions. Wide variations in pulse rate are likely to be found among patients and may or may not be indicative of abnormalities. However, unusual or abnormal findings in a specific patient should be carefully evaluated to determine their potential cause and the potential effect the treatment may have on the patient. Factors that affect the pulse are listed in Table 3-2.

Assessment of Pulse

Sites used to measure pulse with the use of a stethoscope are the temporal, carotid, brachial, radial, femoral, popliteal, dorsal pedal, and posterior tibial arteries (Table 3-3; Fig. 3-4) and the apex of the heart. The most common sites used are the radial and carotid arteries because they are easily accessed. The temporal or carotid sites can be used when access to the radial site is restricted. The carotid or radial sites are usually preferred by persons when they are measuring their own pulse (Fig. 3-5). The apical pulse site is used when the peripheral sites are inaccessible or the pulse is difficult to palpate at those sites. The inguinal, popliteal, tibial, and pedal arterial sites are used to evaluate the pulse in the lower extremity. These measurements are important when patients with peripheral vascular disease or a disorder affecting peripheral blood flow are treated.

The pulse often is described subjectively according to its rate, rhythm, and volume. Examples of descriptive terms include the following:

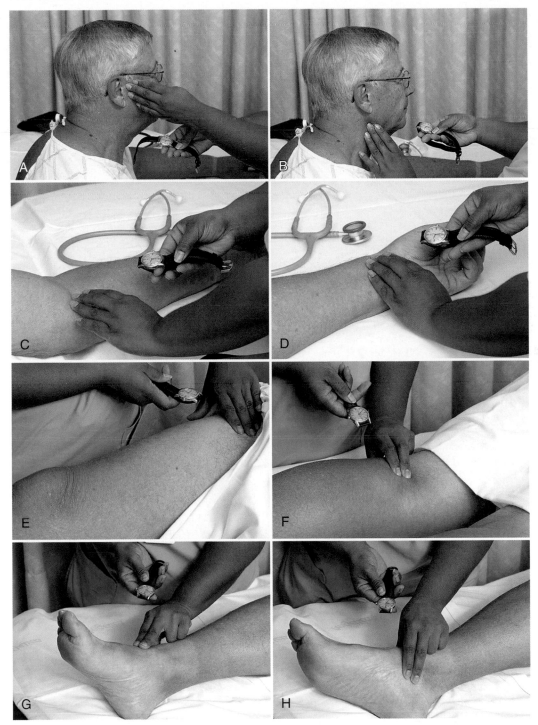

Fig. 3-4   Pulse measurement sites. **A,** Temporal. **B,** Carotid. **C,** Brachial. **D,** Radial. **E,** Femoral. **F,** Popliteal. **G,** Dorsal pedal. **H,** Posterior tibial.

- *Strong and regular* indicates even beats with a good force to each beat.
- *Weak and regular* indicates even beats with a poor force to each beat.
- *Irregular* indicates that both strong and weak beats occur during the period of measurement.

- *Thready* indicates a weak force to each beat and irregular beats.
- *Tachycardia* indicates a rapid HR (>100 beats/min).
- *Bradycardia* indicates a slow HR (<60 beats/min).
   A timepiece that allows the evaluator to easily count the pulse for 1 minute or part of a minute (e.g., 10, 15, 20, or

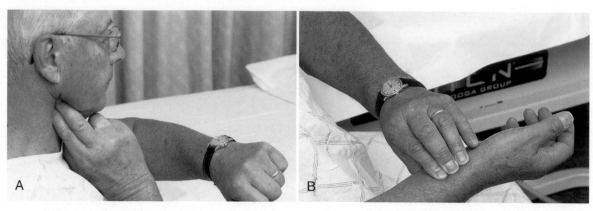

Fig. 3-5 Person measuring his own pulse at the carotid (**A**) and radial (**B**) sites.

PROCEDURE 3-3

Measuring the Pulse

- Wash your hands, obtain a timepiece that measures seconds, and explain the procedure to the patient. Observe the patient for signs or symptoms of stress, anxiety, or cardiovascular distress. The patient may be recumbent, sitting, or standing.
- Select an arterial site and firmly but gently place two or three fingertips over the artery. Avoid using your thumb, because you may perceive your own pulse rather than that of the patient and because the thumb's pad is less sensitive than that of the other fingers. Avoid applying excessive pressure, which may occlude the artery. An exception to light pressure is when you attempt to palpate the popliteal artery. Very firm, deep pressure may be required to locate that artery and palpate its pulse. When determining a patient's resting heart rate for the first time, allow the person to rest supine or seated for approximately 5 minutes before performing the measurement. Measure the pulse rate for a full minute to reduce the potential for error and improve the accuracy of the measurement.
- Mentally count each beat.
  - If you measure the rate for 10 seconds and multiply that value by 6, the margin of error is ±6 beats per minute (beats/min).
  - If you measure the rate for 15 seconds and multiply that value by 4, the margin of error is ±4 beats/min.
  - If you measure the rate for 30 seconds and multiply that value by 2, the margin of error is ±2 beats/min.
- Record the results in beats/min, indicate any variations in rhythm or volume, and identify the location you used to palpate and measure the pulse (such as 68 beats/min, regular, R brachial pulse; 86 beats/min, irregular [every fourth beat absent in 1 minute], L radial pulse, patient sitting).

- Measurement of the apical pulse usually requires a stethoscope, but manual palpation is possible. Wash your hands and explain the procedure to the patient. The patient must be positioned so the left anterior side of the chest is accessible.
  - Manual palpation: Place two or three fingertips on the patient's skin on the left lateral side of the base of the sternum in the intercostal space between the fourth and fifth or the fifth and sixth ribs; then count and record the pulse rate as previously described.
  - Auscultation: Clean the stethoscope's diaphragm and earpieces with an alcohol wipe. Position the earpieces in your ears with the earpieces directed forward. This position will be the most comfortable, and the earpieces will be in line with the auditory canal. Warm the diaphragm with your hand or by rubbing it with a cloth. Then place the diaphragm on the patient's skin in a location similar to the one described previously. In an adolescent or adult female patient, it may be necessary to position the diaphragm slightly medially or laterally and inferior to the left breast. Count and record the pulse rate as described previously. Remove the earpieces from your ears, and clean them and the diaphragm with an alcohol wipe. (Note: If the stethoscope is a personal one, only the diaphragm needs to be cleaned before and after use with a patient. If the stethoscope is loaned to other persons or belongs to the department, the earpieces should be cleaned using an alcohol wipe before and after use. This action will decrease the possibility of contamination of the earpieces and diaphragm and help prevent the spread of disease or infection from one person to another.)

30 seconds) is necessary to measure the pulse rate accurately. A stopwatch, clock, or wristwatch with a sweep second hand or a second digital readout is the most convenient and readily available timepiece. Materials to record the measured value and a stethoscope (if the apical pulse is to be measured) are other items that may be needed to measure the patient's pulse rate. Steps used to measure pulse are listed in Procedure 3-3.

In most persons, the apical and radial pulse rates will be equal. However, in patients with cardiac disease or

Abnormal Responses Exhibited by the Pulse

- The pulse rate slowly increases during active exercise.
- The pulse rate does not increase during active exercise.
- The pulse rate continues to increase or decreases as the intensity of exercise or activity plateaus.
- The pulse rate slowly declines as the intensity of the exercise or activity declines and terminates.
- The pulse rate does not decline as the intensity of the exercise or activity declines.
- The pulse rate declines during the exercise before the intensity of the exercise or activity declines.
- The increased pulse rate or the amount of the increase exceeds the level expected to occur during the exercise period.
- The rhythm of the pulse becomes irregular during or after exercise or activity (e.g., dysrhythmia, arrhythmia, or ectopic beats occur).

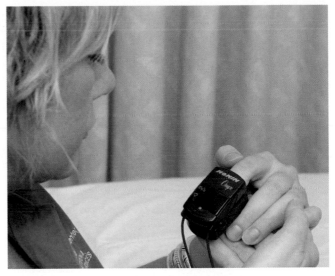

Fig. 3-6   A handheld pulse oximeter.

peripheral arterial disease, these two values may differ. Therefore the radial and apical pulse rates should be evaluated simultaneously during the initial evaluation of the patient. Two persons should monitor the two pulses simultaneously (i.e., one person monitors the radial pulse for 1 minute while the other person monitors the apical pulse for 1 minute), and the results are compared. Any difference in the two values is referred to as the "pulse deficit." Further evaluation of the patient is necessary to determine the cause of the difference between the two pulse rates. Both the left and the right radial pulses should be compared with the apical pulse. If a difference exists between the apical and radial pulse rates, only the apical pulse should be used to evaluate the patient. Such differences should be documented in the patient's medical record.

The expected normal responses of the pulse rate to exercise have been described (see Table 3-2). A patient with resting tachycardia or bradycardia should be carefully evaluated by an appropriate practitioner (e.g., a physician, nurse, cardiovascular exercise specialist) to determine the limitations or tolerance to exercise or treatment before treatment is initiated.

During the monitoring of the patient's pulse, the evaluator should be aware of abnormal pulse responses to exercise or other treatment activities. It may be necessary to modify or terminate treatment when these abnormalities are severe and/or persistent. Additional caution or consultation with other medical personnel may be necessary before treatment proceeds to protect the patient from harm or undue stress.

Abnormal responses of the pulse rate during or after exercise or physical activity are listed in Box 3-1.

Pulse Oximetry

A pulse oximeter measures the level of blood oxygen saturation, monitors pulse rate, and calculates HR. The pulse oximeter is placed over the fingertip of the forefinger or ring finger (or at times the earlobe). The normal blood oxygen saturation reading at or near sea level is between 95% and 100%. Hypoxemia is suspected if readings fall below 90%. Before applying the pulse oximeter, make sure the patient is not wearing fingernail polish. No blood samples need to be drawn because the oximeter performs a noninvasive examination. The primary use of a pulse oximeter is to measure blood oxygen levels among newborns, surgery patients, and patients with pulmonary disease.

Three types of pulse oximeters are available. A stationary digital pulse oximeter is used mainly in hospitals, in addition to patient monitoring devices, and has an alarm system that sounds when abnormal values are reached. Handheld oximeters consist of a fingertip probe and a handheld base unit that displays the results; they sometimes include a large memory bank that stores data, or the data can be downloaded onto a computer (Fig. 3-6). Finger pulse oximeters are compact units that usually operate with a single button. All finger probes should be cleaned after use by wiping the inner surface with isopropyl alcohol unless the unit is for single use only. External conditions such as altitude, temperature, and lighting can affect the readings. In general, oximeters accurately measure oxygen saturation between 70% and 100% regardless of the type of oximeter used.

BLOOD PRESSURE

Systemic arterial BP is a physiologic variable that reflects the effects of cardiac output, peripheral vascular resistance, and other hemodynamic factors. A sphygmomanometer (i.e., a BP cuff) measures BP and is an indirect measurement of the pressure inside an artery caused by blood flow through the artery. Specifically, it is the force exerted by the blood against any unit area of the vessel wall. BP is composed of the systolic and diastolic pressures:

Table **3-4**	Korotkoff's Sounds

Phase	Description
I	The first faint, clear tapping sounds are detected and gradually increase in their intensity; these sounds are the initial indication of systolic pressure in an adult, according to the American Heart Association
II	The sounds heard have a murmur or swishing quality to them
III	The sounds become crisp and louder than those previously heard
IV	There is a distinct and abrupt muffling of the sounds until a soft, blowing quality is heard; this phase is the initial indication of the diastolic pressure and is the best indicator of diastolic pressure in adults, according to the American Heart Association
V	The sounds essentially disappear totally; the phase is also referred to as the "second diastolic pressure phase"

Table **3-5**	Blood Pressure: Accepted Normal Values

Patient/Range	Systolic (mm Hg)	Diastolic (mm Hg)
Infants		
Birth to 3 mo	85-90	35-65
3 mo to 1 y	90-100	60-67
Children		
1-4 y	100-108	60
4-12 y	+2 per year to 100	60-70
Adolescents	100-120	65-75
Adults		
Normal	<120	<80
High normal	130-139	85-89
Elderly (≥65 y)	120-140	80-90
Hypertension ranges		
Prehypertension	120-139	80-89
Stage 1	140-159	90-99
Stage 2	160-179	100-109
Stage 3	180-209	110-119
Stage 4	>210	>120

- Systolic pressure is the BP at the time of contraction of the left ventricle (systole).
- Diastolic pressure is the BP at the time of the rest period of the heart (diastole).

Listening for Korotkoff's sounds with a stethoscope can identify the various phases of a person's BP. These sounds have been described as occurring in phases, as shown in Table 3-4. A large amount of practice and a quiet environment are necessary for the evaluator to differentiate these five phases. Phases I and V are the two most important phases to identify in most patients. However, in patients with a known or suspected cardiovascular condition, it may be important to identify most or all of the phases.

Depending on the source, accepted normal BP ranges in adults are systolic, 120 mm of mercury (mm Hg) or less, and diastolic, 80 mm Hg or less. A systolic/diastolic value of 120/80 mm Hg is frequently used as the normal value (Table 3-5).

When the resting systolic pressure is consistently found to measure more than 140 mm Hg or the resting diastolic pressure consistently measures more than 90 mm Hg, the person is usually considered to be stage 1 hypertensive. A consistent reading of 180/110 mm Hg is considered indicative of stage 3 hypertension. Factors associated with or that contribute to hypertension are obesity; physical inactivity; excessive use of nicotine, alcohol, or salt; arteriosclerosis; diabetes mellitus; oral contraceptives (in women); advanced age (i.e., middle age or older); kidney disease; race (i.e., greater incidence in those of African descent); and diet. In most persons, no signs or symptoms are associated with hypertension, and unless the person has his or her BP measured periodically, the condition often goes unrecognized

and undiagnosed. Persons with hypertension are more susceptible to coronary artery disease, cerebrovascular accident, peripheral vascular disease, and congestive heart failure. Therefore it is important that all persons have their BP evaluated several times a year. A new classification, "prehypertension," as designated by the American Heart Association, describes people with BPs between 120 and 139 mm Hg systolic or 80 and 89 mm Hg diastolic. This new prehypertension category focuses the attention of the physician, patient, and public on BP in these ranges in hopes that persons in this category will adopt health-promoting lifestyles. With lifestyle changes, it is believed that future high BP can be avoided.

Hypotension is defined as a systolic pressure that is consistently below 100 mm Hg. This condition is usually non-threatening, but some hypotensive patients may experience dizziness or syncope when abruptly standing from a previous lying, sitting, or squatting position.

Factors that affect BP are listed in Table 3-6.

Assessment of Blood Pressure

The most common site used to measure BP is the brachial artery. The femoral artery is occasionally used, particularly in patients with known or suspected lower extremity peripheral vascular diseases.

A stethoscope, sphygmomanometer, chair, support for the patient's upper extremity, alcohol wipes, and recording materials are necessary to measure and record the patient's BP. The cuff must be the proper size to obtain an accurate measurement. If the bladder in the cuff is too narrow in relation to the circumference of the patient's arm, the reading will be erroneously high; if the bladder is too wide,

Table **3-6** Factors Affecting Blood Pressure

Factor	Description
Age	Younger patients (adolescents and younger) exhibit lower systolic and diastolic values; elderly patients (≥65 years) may exhibit slightly higher systolic and slightly lower diastolic pressure
Physical activity	Systolic pressure should gradually increase with exercise, plateau as the exercise intensity plateaus, and then gradually decline as the exercise intensity declines; it should return to its normal resting value within 3 to 5 minutes after termination of the exercise
	Diastolic pressure should remain essentially unchanged throughout the exercise period, although an increase of approximately 10 to 15 mm Hg is usually not considered abnormal; an increase of more than 15 mm Hg constitutes abnormality
Emotional status	The BP will increase during episodes of high stress, anxiety, or emotion (e.g., anger or fear)
Medications	Various medications may cause BP to increase or decrease, depending on their effect on the cardiovascular system
	Medications frequently used to control hypertension may result in a temporary state of hypotension in some patients
Size and condition of arteries	Arteries that have a reduced lumen will produce an increased BP value, and arteries that have decreased elasticity will produce an increased systolic value and a decreased diastolic value; these two factors tend to account for the changes that occur in the BP values of the elderly
Arm position	When the person is seated or standing, the standard arm position is with the forearm maintained at the level of the fourth intercostal space and elbow extended; no adjustment in arm position is required when the person is supine because it is supported on the bed at the proper level; the BP may increase when the arm is lowered from the level previously described and may decrease when the arm is raised above that level
Muscle contraction	The patient should not maintain arm position by contraction of the upper extremity musculature because this contraction may produce an increase in the BP as a result of the increased resistance to blood flow
Blood volume	The BP decreases when a loss of blood occurs and increases with an increase in blood volume (i.e., after transfusion of whole blood or plasma)
Dehydration	A significant decrease of body fluids may cause low BP
Cardiac output	Systolic BP increases with increased cardiac output and decreases with decreased cardiac output
Site of measurement	The BP values are often higher in the left upper extremity than in the right upper extremity; if the thigh is used as the measurement site, the systolic pressure is usually higher than that found in the arm, partly because of the need to use a wider bladder in the cuff, but the diastolic pressure will be essentially the same as that found in the arm

BP, Blood pressure.

Table **3-7** Average Sphygmomanometer Bladder Measurements

Age	Measurement	
	Inches	Centimeters
Infant	1-1.5	2.5-4
Average-sized adult	3-6	7-15
Large adult		
Arm	6-8	15-20
Thigh	8-9	20-23

the reading will be erroneously low. The width of the bladder should be 40% of the circumference of the midpoint of the limb (Table 3-7). The length of the bladder is also important and should be approximately twice the width of the bladder, or 80% of the arm circumference.

Decisions regarding the size of the bladder should be based on the circumference of the patient's extremity, not on the patient's age or other personal factors. Steps to measure BP are shown in Procedure 3-4 (auscultation) and Procedure 3-5 (palpation).

If it is necessary to repeat the measurements, the cuff should be completely deflated and the patient should be allowed to sit quietly for 1 to 2 minutes before the measurements are retaken. This step allows any blood that may be trapped in the veins to be released and allows the circulatory system to return to normal. The caregiver should be alert to the potential sources of errors in measurement of BP so that they can be avoided or eliminated.

You will need to develop your hearing, vision, and manual dexterity so you can accurately hear phase I and V Korotkoff's sounds, read the value accurately, and properly operate the valve on the cuff-inflation bulb (i.e., close it, open it, control the rate of deflation) with your thumb and index finger.

Measuring Blood Pressure by Auscultation

- Wash your hands and obtain a stethoscope and sphygmomanometer (**A**). Explain the procedure and rationale for measurement to the patient. Observe the patient for signs or symptoms of stress or recent exercise. If the patient has exercised, ambulated, or experienced emotional stress, he or she should rest for 15 to 30 minutes before the blood pressure (BP) is measured. Position the patient sitting with the forearm supported on a firm object approximately at the level of the heart, with the thighs parallel to each other and the feet flat on floor. Position yourself so you are comfortable and can view the manometer gauge easily. If the patient is sitting or recumbent, you should sit facing the person. If the patient is standing, elevate the arm and support it between your arm and lateral area of the chest while you face the patient.

- Expose the antecubital space of the left or right arm; do not roll the shirt or blouse sleeve too tightly because it may partially occlude the artery. Palpate the brachial pulse so you will know where to place the diaphragm of the stethoscope.

- Apply the deflated cuff to the arm with the center of the bladder over the medial aspect of the arm so it will occlude the artery when it is inflated. The cuff should be applied approximately 2.5 cm above the antecubital space (about 1.5 fingerbreadths) with the manometer attached to the cuff or placed so that the needle and scale can be observed easily without being held in your hand (**B**).

- After cleaning the earpieces and diaphragm with an alcohol wipe, apply the stethoscope to your ears with the earpieces directed forward. Place the diaphragm on the skin where the brachial artery was palpated, but avoid

contact with the patient's clothing or the cuff. Apply firm but light pressure on the diaphragm to maintain contact with the skin (**C**).

- To initially determine the amount of pressure needed in the cuff to occlude the brachial artery, palpate the radial pulse and inflate the cuff by closing the valve on the inflation bulb and squeezing the bulb until the radial pulse is no longer palpable. This value can be used as a baseline for the cuff-pressure inflation level. Note this value and deflate the cuff. After waiting 30 to 60 seconds, reinflate the cuff to 15 to 20 mm Hg above the pressure that previously occluded the artery to ensure that the artery is fully occluded. (Note: Once the patient's systolic pressure has been determined several times and a normal systolic value has been established, the cuff can be inflated to approximately 15 to 20 mm Hg above that value each time the BP is measured.)

- To deflate the cuff, release the valve on the inflation bulb so that the needle drops at the rate of 2 to 3 mm Hq per second. Listen for normal Korotkoff's sounds, and mentally note the needle position (reading) when the initial sound is heard through the stethoscope. This reading is the systolic pressure value. Continue to deflate the cuff, listening for the absence of the sound of a pulse or beat, and mentally note the needle position. This reading is the diastolic pressure value. Allow the cuff to deflate completely, remove it from the patient, and remove the stethoscope from your ears. Record the values, including the patient position and extremity used (e.g., 130/70 right upper extremity [RUE], sitting; 140/80 left upper extremity [LUE], sitting). Clean the stethoscope earpieces and diaphragm with an alcohol wipe.

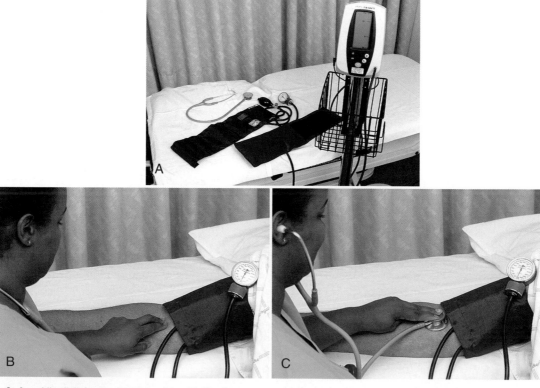

Fig. 3-7   **A,** A mobile digital sphygmomanometer. **B,** Blood pressure palpation method without use of a stethoscope. **C,** Use of a stethoscope and sphygmomanometer for measurement of blood pressure.

PROCEDURE 3-5

Measuring Blood Pressure by Palpation

- Perform steps 1 through 3 as outlined in Procedure 3-4.
- Palpate the brachial artery pulse in the antecubital space with two or three fingers, and maintain your fingers over the pulse (see Fig. 3-7, *B*).
- Inflate the cuff as described previously.
- Deflate the cuff as described previously and observe the manometer. Mentally note the needle position when the first pulse in the artery is palpated. This reading is the systolic pressure value.
- Continue to deflate the cuff while observing the manometer. Mentally note the needle position when the last distinct pulse is palpated. This reading is the diastolic pressure.
- Completely deflate the cuff and remove it from the patient.
- Record the values as described previously; indicate that the palpation method was used.

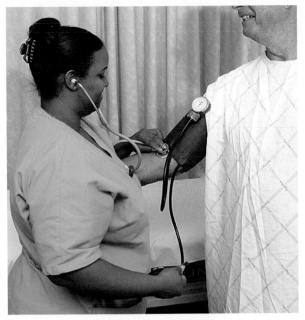

Fig. 3-8   Taking blood pressure for a standing patient.

You should develop the habit of reporting the values without "rounding" them to the nearest higher or lower value. For example, if you read the systolic pressure as 137 mm Hg, report it as 137 mm Hg; do not report it as 135 mm Hg.

Do not bias the findings by expecting a certain value rather than listening for it. Some patients will tell you what their usual values are before you actually take a measurement, or you may have read the values determined previously by another evaluator, or you may recall the values you measured during a previous treatment session. This information may bias you and lead you to predict or expect similar values rather than recording the values as you hear and measure them. When you eliminate, reduce, or avoid these potential sources of errors in the measurement of a patient's BP, you will increase the accuracy and precision of your measurement.

The patient may sit, stand, or lie for this procedure, but the upper extremity must be supported with the forearm and arm at the approximate level of the heart to reduce inaccurate measurements (see Procedure 3-4 and Fig. 3-8). If the extremity is positioned in a dependent (hanging) position, the hydrostatic pressure of the blood will be increased and such an increase may erroneously increase the value of the patient's BP. Do not allow the patient to position the upper extremity by contracting the muscles of the chest, shoulder, or arm. Isometric muscle contractions will partially occlude secondary blood vessels, and the patient's true BP may be distorted. In a normal subject, no significant difference in the BP should be found regardless of the person's position, as long as the upper extremity is properly positioned as described. Stimuli that may influence the BP should be controlled, eliminated, avoided, or accounted for (see Table 3-6).

An important factor to consider related to BP is the mean arterial pressure (MAP), the average pressure that occurs during a single cardiac cycle (contraction/relaxation). MAP is determined by using the following formula:

$$[\text{Systolic pressure} + (\text{Diastolic pressure} \times 2)]/3 = \text{MAP}$$

$$\text{Example: BP of } 130/80; [(130 + (80 \times 2)]/3 = 96.7 \text{ MAP}$$

An MAP of 60 mm Hg or higher is necessary to perfuse the body's major organs and vessels to maintain them. Therefore some facilities may have a policy that prohibits rehabilitation treatment of a patient whose MAP is less than 60 mm Hg.

The expected normal responses of BP during exercise have been described (see Table 3-6). A patient with a resting elevated BP (hypertension) or a resting depressed BP (hypotension) should be carefully evaluated by an appropriate practitioner to determine the limitations or anticipated tolerance to exercise or treatment before treatment is initiated.

During monitoring of the patient's BP, the caregiver should be aware of abnormal BP responses to exercise or other treatment activities (Box 3-2). It may be necessary to modify or terminate the patient's treatment if these abnormalities are serious or persistent. To ensure patient safety, additional caution or a consultation with medical personnel may be necessary before you proceed with treatment.

| Box **3-2** | Abnormal Responses Exhibited by Blood Pressure |

- Systolic pressure rapidly increases during active exercise.
- Systolic pressure does not increase during active exercise.
- Systolic pressure continues to increase or decreases as the intensity of the exercise or activity plateaus.
- Systolic pressure rapidly declines as the intensity of the exercise or activity declines and terminates.
- Systolic pressure does not decline as the intensity of the exercise or activity declines.
- Systolic pressure declines significantly below its resting level at the termination of the exercise or activity.
- Systolic pressure declines during exercise before the intensity of the exercise declines.
- The systolic pressure rate or the amount of systolic pressure increase is excessive during the exercise or activity period.
- Diastolic pressure increases more than 10 to 15 mm Hg during the exercise or activity period.

RESPIRATION (PULMONARY VENTILATION)

The physical components of respiration produce an inflow (inspiration) and outflow (expiration) of air between the environment and the lungs. Air moves into and is expelled from the lungs by muscle contraction and relaxation. One respiration comprises one inhalation and one exhalation.

Depending on the source used, the accepted normal range for respiration at rest is 12 to 18 respirations per minute (breaths/min) for adults and 30 to 50 breaths/min for infants. Resting values above 20 breaths/min or below 10 breaths/min are considered abnormal for adults.

Assessment of Respiration

Measurement of the rate, rhythm, depth, and character of respiration is performed by observation or touch. "Rate" refers to the number of breaths per minute, "rhythm" refers to the regularity of the pattern, "depth" refers to the amount of air exchanged with each respiration, and "character" refers to deviations from normal, resting, or quiet respiration. The evaluator observes or measures by touch the rate of movement of the patient's thorax, abdomen, or both. Patients who are extremely ill and in respiratory distress may have their respiration measured with a stethoscope. The amount of effort required and the sounds produced during resting respirations should be evaluated as part of the assessment.

Normal respiration requires minimal effort for inspiration and essentially no effort for expiration. A person may be classified as either an upper chest (thoracic) or abdominal breather. In an upper chest breather, the thorax elevates and expands during inspiration and the abdomen remains relatively motionless. During inspiration, an abdominal breather exhibits expansion of the abdomen and the thorax remains relatively motionless. During periods of respiratory distress, a person may exhibit both breathing patterns. Persons who have difficulty breathing while at rest experience dyspnea, or labored breathing. No sound should be heard during normal, resting respiration. Abnormal sounds include wheezing, rales, and stridor. Patients also may demonstrate orthopnea, or difficulty breathing, while recumbent. This condition is relieved when the patient sits or stands. Apnea, or absence of breathing, and shortness of breath also may be experienced by patients and may require the use of a ventilator if they persist.

A watch or clock that measures both seconds and minutes or a stopwatch and materials to record the results will be necessary for evaluation of a patient's respiratory rate (RR). Steps to measure RR are detailed in Procedure 3-6.

Factors affecting respiration are described in Table 3-8. A patient who exhibits problems or difficulty with breathing while at rest should be carefully evaluated by a qualified practitioner to determine the person's limitations or tolerance to exercise or treatment before treatment is initiated.

During monitoring of the patient's RR (see Fig. 3-9), the caregiver should be aware of abnormal respiration responses to exercise or other treatment activities. It may be necessary to modify or terminate treatment if these abnormalities impair function or are persistent. Additional caution or consultation with other medical personnel may be necessary before proceeding with treatment. Frequent monitoring of the patient's RR may be necessary during the initial treatment sessions to ensure the person is functioning within safe limits.

Factors that affect respiration are listed in Table 3-8. Abnormal responses to watch for while measuring respirations are listed in Box 3-3.

Pulmonary Auscultation Much practice is required to become competent in lung auscultation, that is, listening for breath sounds in the lungs, usually with the diaphragm of a stethoscope. During preparation of the patient and auscultation, the following factors must be remembered: the environment should be quiet; the patient should be sitting up or standing and not be leaning on anything (e.g., a wall or bed rails); the patient should be asked to breathe in and out through his or her mouth; you should warm the stethoscope with your hand; auscultation should only be performed over bare skin; care should be taken not to touch the stethoscope tube against bed rails or the patient's clothing; and to compare breath sounds, always auscultate one side and then the other, moving in a systematic direction. Fig. 3-10 illustrates the important areas of systematic auscultation.

PROCEDURE 3-6

Measuring Respiration Rate

- Wash your hands and obtain a timepiece that measures seconds. Observe the patient for signs or symptoms of abnormal respiration (e.g., gasping, panting, open-mouth breathing, and use of accessory neck muscles). The patient may be sitting, lying, or standing as long as the abdomen or thorax can be observed. To avoid voluntary control of respiration by the patient, do not explain the procedure.
- Simulate measurement of the radial pulse with the patient's forearm resting on the abdomen. Observe or tactilely measure the outward and inward movement of the patient's thorax or abdomen.
- Count either the inspirations or the expirations for 1 minute. (One inspiration and one expiration equal one respiration cycle.) The rate is reported in respirations per minute. Once the rate, rhythm, depth, and character of the person's respirations have been determined to be within normal parameters, the measurement period can be reduced to 30 seconds, but the number of inspirations or expirations must be multiplied by 2 to determine the rate for a full minute.
- Reposition the patient's clothing or bed linens if they were removed or adjusted to expose the patient's abdomen or thorax.
- Note and record the rate, depth, rhythm, and character of the person's respirations. Record the rate as respirations per minute and describe the depth, rhythm, and character of the pattern if they vary from normal.

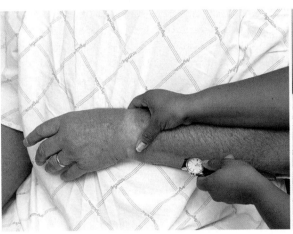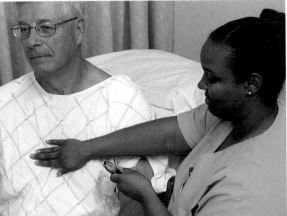

Fig. 3-9   Measuring a patient's respiration rate.

Table 3-8 Factors Affecting Respiration

Factor	Description
Age	Both very young patients (infant to 3 years) and elderly patients (≥65 years) tend to have higher respiration rates
Physical activity	The rate and depth of respiration increase during exercise
Emotional status	The rate and depth of respiration increase during episodes of high stress, anxiety, or emotion (e.g., anger or fear)
Air quality	Impurities in the atmosphere may cause the respiration rate to increase or decrease, depending on the effects of various components of the person's pulmonary system
Altitude	High altitudes cause the respiration rate to increase until a person is acclimated
Disease	Disease that affects various components of the pulmonary system usually increases the respiratory rate and also may affect the depth of respiration

Box 3-3 Abnormal Responses Exhibited by Respiration Rate

- The respiration rate slowly increases during exercise or activity.
- The respiration rate does not increase during exercise or activity.
- The respiration rate increases as the intensity of the exercise or activity plateaus.
- The respiration rate slowly declines as the intensity of the exercise or activity declines and terminates.
- The respiration rate does not decline as the intensity of the exercise or activity declines.
- The respiration rate declines during exercise or activity before the intensity of the exercise declines.
- The increase in the rate or the amount of increase in the patient's respiration rate is excessive during the exercise period.
- The rhythm of the respiration pattern becomes irregular during or after exercise or activity.

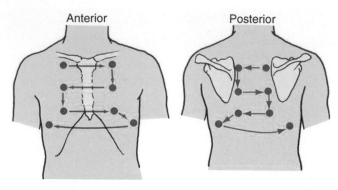

Anterior   Posterior

Fig. 3-10 Path of systematic auscultation. (From Des Jardins T: *Clinical manifestations and assessment of respiratory disease,* ed 6, St Louis, 2011, Mosby.)

Breath sounds occur during inspiration and expiration of air through the bronchial tree. These sounds are characterized by their pitch, qualities (harshness or loudness), intensity, and duration of the inspiratory and expiratory phases:

- Normal breath sounds are classified as tracheal, bronchial, bronchovesicular, or vesicular and depend on the area of the chest being examined.
- Tracheal breath sounds are best heard in the neck region and are high pitched, harsh, hollow, and loud.
- Bronchial breath sounds are loud, tubular, less-harsh sounds that are best heard over the manubrium of the sternum. These sounds are abnormal if heard in the peripheral lung fields and represent consolidation in a lobe.
- Bronchovesicular sounds are high pitched and soft and are best heard between the scapulae. These sounds come from the mainstem bronchi.
- Vesicular breath sounds are soft and low pitched and are heard over the periphery of both lung fields. The expiratory phase heard is shorter than the inspiratory phase.

Adventitious or abnormal breath sounds usually indicate disease and are superimposed upon normal breath sounds. They are classified as discontinuous, or nonmusical, and continuous, or musical, breath sounds. The discontinuous adventitious breath sounds are considered crackles (also known as rales) or pleural friction rubs and are sharp, discrete bursts of sound heard most commonly on inspiration. Crackles can be heard in persons with asthma, bronchitis, interstitial lung disease, bronchiectasis, and early congestive heart failure. Pleural rubs, which are heard during both inspiration and expiration, sound like brushing or creaking sounds and are found in patients with pneumothorax or a pleural effusion.

Wheezes, rhonchi, and stridor make up the continuous, musical abnormal breath sounds. Wheezes and rhonchi occur when air flows through a narrowed airway and are heard during expiration. Wheezes occur in patients with chronic obstructive pulmonary disease, asthma, chronic bronchitis, congestive heart failure, and pulmonary edema and can be heard anywhere in the lungs where obstruction exists. Rhonchi sound like snoring or gurgling and imply larger airway obstruction by secretions. Stridor is heard over the trachea and is an inspiratory musical wheeze that suggests obstruction of the trachea or larynx; it is considered a medical emergency.

PAIN

Pain is an unpleasant sensory and emotional experience associated with actual or potential tissue damage or described in terms of such damage. Response to pain is highly personal and subjective; it is whatever the patient says it is and exists wherever and whenever he or she says it does. Self-report of pain is considered the most reliable indicator of pain. Pain often is accompanied by emotional and/or spiritual responses, such as suffering or anguish, and effective management should include measures to address these responses. Each patient should be screened for pain upon admission and asked whether he or she has pain. A pain screen is a quantitative rating of the intensity of pain as reported by the patient using a standardized instrument that has demonstrated reliability and validity. If pain is reported, additional assessment data should be obtained. Pain assessment is an evaluation of the cause of the patient's pain, including, but not limited to, location, intensity, duration of pain (constant or intermittent), aggravating and relieving factors, effects of activities of daily living, sleep patterns, psychosocial aspects of the patient's life, and effectiveness of current strategies. Reassessment of pain will need to be performed several times per day to determine the effect of medications or other interventions designed to alleviate the pain. Written documentation of the patient's perception of pain is preferred rather than oral responses.

Pain management is the use of pharmacologic and nonpharmacologic interventions to control a patient's identified pain. Adverse effects of pharmacologic treatment (i.e., pain medication) may be respiratory depression, respiratory distress, change in mental status, myoclonus, uncontrolled nausea or vomiting, urinary retention, constipation, uncontrolled pruritus, and sensory/motor changes.

Application of nonpharmacologic measures should be considered based on patient preference and the degree of pain relief. Some nonpharmacologic measures are application of heat or cold; positioning; massage; distraction techniques such as music, videos, games, and reading materials; relaxation techniques such as imagery, meditation, and prayer; a quiet environment; self-hypnosis; or transcutaneous electrical nerve stimulation. Pain management extends beyond pain relief, encompassing the patient's quality of life and ability to work productively and to enjoy recreation.

The Joint Commission 2001 Pain Management Standards state that every patient has a right to have pain assessed and treated. The standard for the pain assessment, while stating that it is performed for all patients, has long been interpreted to mean "as appropriate to the reason the patient is presenting for care or services." In the 2004 Joint Commission standards, the element of performance states, "A comprehensive pain assessment is conducted as appropriate to the individual's condition and the scope of care, treatment, and services provided." As a requirement of the assessment design standard, the organization is expected to define in writing the scope of assessments, including the data gathered to assess patient needs. Criteria should be defined by the organization in respect to all services and settings.

Many patient pain assessment tools are available. These tools are largely focused on the adult population. Special considerations should be given to the very young and very old, known or suspected substance abusers, the cognitively impaired, and persons who do not speak or comprehend English. When developing a pain treatment plan, clinicians should be aware of the unique needs and circumstances of patients from various ethnic and cultural backgrounds.

Assessment of Pain

In many hospital environments, patient pain is considered the fifth vital sign. Some facilities have created comprehensive pain clinics or pain management teams, especially facilities that treat cancer patients or have a large population of orthopedic or neurologic patients. Pain management medical teams typically include some or all of the following individuals: a clergy member, a dentist/oral surgeon, a dietitian, an internist, a neurologist/neurosurgeon, a nurse, an occupational therapist, an oncologist, an orthopedist, a pharmacist, a physiatrist, a physical therapist, a radiologist, and a vocational counselor/social worker. Goals for an interdisciplinary pain team or for an individual clinician are to eliminate the source of pain when feasible; teach the patient to function within pain limitations; improve pain control through conservative physical and psychologic methods; relieve drug dependency; treat underlying depression and improve psychologic well-being; address areas of secondary gain; improve family and community support systems; provide access to occupational rehabilitation; provide patient education on pain, anatomy, physiology, posture, body mechanics, and medications; improve strength, flexibility, and general physical conditioning; and maximize the patient's functional level.

In the initial assessment of pain, the clinician should document the onset and temporal pattern of pain. Ask the patient to point to the exact location of pain on his or her body, on the clinician, or on a pain questionnaire, if available (Figs. 3-11 through 3-13 and Tables 3-9 and 3-10). Determine whether the pain radiates or spreads to other parts of the body. Ask the patient to describe the pain, because words can provide valuable clues to the cause. For example, patients who describe their pain as "burning" or "tingling" are likely to have a neuropathic cause of pain, particularly if associated with subjective numbness, loss of sensation, and weakness.

| Table 3-9 | Pain Descriptions and Related Structures |

Type of Pain	Structure
Cramping, dull, aching	Muscle
Sharp, shooting	Nerve root
Sharp, bright, lightning-like	Nerve
Burning, pressure-like, stinging, aching	Sympathetic nerve
Deep, nagging, dull	Bone
Sharp, severe, intolerable	Fracture
Throbbing, diffuse	Vasculature

From McGee DJ: *Orthopedic physical assessment*, ed 4, Philadelphia, 2005, Saunders Elsevier.

PROCEDURE 3-7

Assessment of Pain

In the initial assessment of pain, the clinician should determine and document the following elements:
- Pain onset
- Pattern of pain
- Exact location of pain
- Results of a pain questionnaire, if available
- Whether the pain radiates or spreads to other parts of the body
- Description of the pain; that is, when is it best and worst, whether it is constant or intermittent, what activities make the pain better and worse, and time of day when the pain is better or worse
- What work or social activity is affected by the pain
- Rate the pain from 1 to 10, with 1 being the least and 10 being the worst

An assessment of pain intensity should include an evaluation of the present pain intensity and when the pain is at its least and worst. Knowing factors that aggravate or relieve the pain helps clinicians design a better plan of care. The patient should describe the symptoms at onset, whether they are constant or intermittent, and which activities make the symptoms worse or better (e.g., bending, sitting, rising, standing, walking, or lying). Ask the patient if the symptoms are worse upon awakening, as the day progresses, or in the evening. Document whether the pain increases during a cough, sneeze, or strain and if bladder function is affected. The initial pain assessment should elicit information about changes in activities of daily living, including recreational and work activities, sleep patterns, sleeping postures and sleep surfaces, mobility, appetite, and mood (Procedure 3-7).

If the patient is cognitively impaired, the inability to communicate information concerning pain places them at high risk for insufficient pain control. Two common risk groups in palliative care include patients with underlying brain pathology such as dementia, stroke, Parkinson disease,

Initial Pain Assessment Tool

Date_____

Patient's name _____ Age _____ Room _____

Diagnosis_____ Physician_____

Nurse_____

I. Location: Patient or nurse marks drawing.

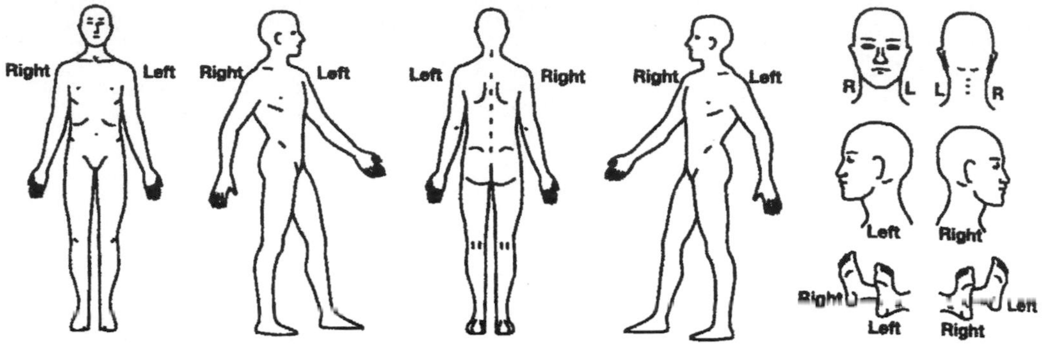

II. Intensity: Patient rates the pain. Scale used_____

Present:_____

Worst pain gets:_____

Best pain gets:_____

Acceptable level of pain:_____

III. Quality: (Use patient's own words, e.g., prick, ache, burn, throb, pull, sharp)

_____

IV. Onset, duration, variations, rhythms:_____

_____

V. Manner of expressing pain:_____

VI. What relieves the pain?_____

VII. What causes or increases the pain?_____

VIII. Effects of pain: (Note decreased function, decreased quality of life.)

Accompanying symptoms (e.g., nausea)_____

Sleep_____

Appetite_____

Physical activity_____

Relationship with others (e.g., irritability)_____

Emotions (e.g., anger, suicidal, crying)_____

Concentration_____

Other_____

IX. Other comments:_____

_____

X. Plan:_____

_____

Fig. 3-11   Initial Pain Assessment Tool. (From McCaffery M, Beebe A: *Pain: clinical manual for nursing practice,* St Louis, 1989, Mosby.)

Simple Descriptive Pain Distress Scale*

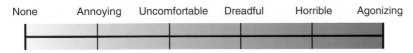

None   Annoying   Uncomfortable   Dreadful   Horrible   Agonizing

0-10 Numerical Pain Distress Scale*

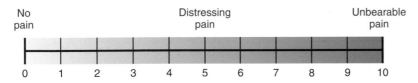

No pain   Distressing pain   Unbearable pain

0   1   2   3   4   5   6   7   8   9   10

Fig. 3-12   Pain Distress Scale. (From Jacox A, Carr DB, Payne R et al: *Management of cancer pain* [Clinical Practice Guideline No. 9, AHCPR Publication No. 94-0592], Rockville, MD, March 1994, Agency for Health Care Policy and Research, U.S. Department of Health and Human Services, Public Health Service.)

Visual Analog Scale (VAS)†

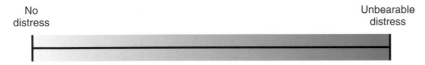

No distress   Unbearable distress

*If used as a graphic rating scale, a 10-cm baseline is recommended.
†A 10-cm baseline is recommended for VASs.

Instructions: Below is a thermometer with various grades of pain on it from "No pain at all" to "The pain is almost unbearable." Put an × by the words that describe your pain best. Mark how bad your pain is AT THIS MOMENT IN TIME.

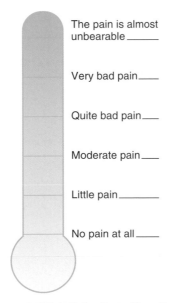

The pain is almost unbearable _____

Very bad pain _____

Quite bad pain _____

Moderate pain _____

Little pain _____

No pain at all _____

Fig. 3-13   "Thermometer" Pain Rating Scale. (From Brodie DJ, Burnett JV, Walker JM et al: Evaluation of low back pain by patient questionnaires and therapist assessment, *J Orthop Sports Phys Ther* 11:528, 1990.)

or developmental abnormalities and patients receiving sedating medications, such as intensive care unit patients who are given sedative/hypnotics to control the anxiety and agitation that can accompany mechanical ventilation. Assessing the pain of a cognitively impaired patient includes asking the patient, as some useful information may be attained; interviewing the family or caregivers for patient behaviors that may indicate pain (such as the patient placing a hand on his or her forehead to indicate a headache, restlessness, or loss of appetite); reviewing the medical record for known pain-inducing conditions such as a painful diabetic neuropathy or fracture that was present before the patient became cognitively impaired; and completing a physical assessment and checking the medical record for laboratory values that may indicate pain (e.g., a urinary tract infection). In addition, caregivers should use a validated pain rating system for cognitively impaired persons. Such rating systems focus on the following observational items: facial expression; body posture; vocalizations; interactivity; and appetite. Table 3-11 can be used as a reference tool for nonverbal pain indicators that may helpful in assessing pain in cognitively impaired persons, nonverbal patients, and patients with a language barrier. Other tools for pain assessment can be found in the Bibliography.

SUMMARY

It is important to monitor a patient's vital signs (i.e., body temperature, pulse, BP, RR, and pain) because they are

Table 3-10 Pain Rating Scales for Children

Pain Scale/Description	Instructions	Recommended Age/Comments
Faces Pain Rating Scale (Wong and Baker, 1988, 2000) Consists of six cartoon faces ranging from smiling face for "no pain" to tearful face for "worst pain"	**ORIGINAL INSTRUCTIONS** Explain to child that each face is for a person who feels happy because there is no pain (hurt) or sad because there is some or a lot of pain FACE 0 is very happy because there is no hurt FACE 1 hurts just a little bit FACE 2 hurts a little more FACE 3 hurts even more FACE 4 hurts a whole lot FACE 5 hurts as much as you can imagine, although you don't have to be crying to feel this bad Ask the child to choose the face that best describes his or her own pain assessment record **BRIEF WORD INSTRUCTIONS** Point to each face using the words to describe the pain intensity; ask the child to choose the face that best describes his or her own pain and record the appropriate number	For children as young as 3 y Using original instructions without affect words, such as happy or sad, or brief words resulted in same pain rating, probably reflecting the child's rating of pain intensity; for coding purposes, numbers 0, 2, 4, 6, 8, 10 can be substituted for 0-5 system to accommodate 0-10 system The FACES provide three scales in one: facial expressions, numbers, and words Use of brief word instructions is recommended
Oucher (Beyer et al., 1992) Consists of six photographs of a child's face representing "no hurt" to "biggest hurt you can ever have"; includes a vertical scale with numbers from 0-100; scales for children of Caucasian, African, and Hispanic descent have been developed (Villarruel and Denyes, 1991)	**NUMERIC SCALE** Point to each section of scale to explain variations in pain intensity: (0) No hurt (1-29) Little hurt (30-69) Middle hurt (70-99) Big hurt (100) Biggest hurt you could ever have Score is actual number stated by child **PHOTOGRAPHIC SCALE** Point to each photograph, starting from the bottom, on Oucher and explain variations in pain intensity using following language: First: no hurt Second: a little hurt Third: a middle hurt Fourth: even more hurt than that Fifth: pretty much or a lot of hurt Sixth: biggest hurt you could ever have Score pictures from 0-5, with the bottom picture scored as 0 **GENERAL** Practice using Oucher by recalling and rating previous pain experiences (e.g., falling off a bike) The child points to the number or photograph that describes the pain intensity associated with his or her experience Obtain a current pain score from child by asking, "How much hurt do you have right now?"	For children 3-13 y Use the numeric scale if the child can count to 100 by ones and identify larger of any two numbers, or by tens Determine whether the child has cognitive ability to use the photographic scale; the child should be able to seriate six geometrical shapes from largest to smallest Determine which ethnic version of Oucher to use; allow the child to select a version of Oucher, or use the version that most closely matches the physical characteristics of the child (Jordan-Marsh et al., 1994)

From Hockenberry MJ, Wilson D: *Wong's essentials of pediatric nursing,* ed 8, St Louis, 2009, Mosby.

indicators of the patient's general health or physiologic status. The caregiver should be able to differentiate between normal and abnormal findings and should have some knowledge of the possible causes of abnormal findings. It may be necessary to measure all or selected vital signs before, during, and after exercise or physical activity. The use of proper techniques during the measurement of vital signs will produce the most accurate findings.

In addition to measuring a patient's vital signs, a subjective determination of the response to exercise or aerobic

Table **3-11** Checklist of Nonverbal Pain Indicators*

Behavior	With Movement	At Rest
1. Vocal complaints: nonverbal (sighs, gasps, moans, groans, cries)		
2. Facial grimaces/winces (furrowed brow, narrowed eyes, clenched teeth, tightened lips, jaw drop, distorted expressions)		
3. Bracing (clutching or holding onto furniture, equipment, or affected area during movement)		
4. Restlessness (constant or intermittent shifting of position, rocking, intermittent or constant hand motions, inability to keep still)		
5. Rubbing (massaging affected area)		
6. Vocal complaints: verbal (words expressing discomfort or pain [e.g., "ouch," "that hurts"]; cursing during movement; exclamations of protest [e.g., "stop," "that's enough"])		
Subtotal scores		
Total score		

*Instructions: Observe the patient for the following behaviors both at rest and during movement.
Scoring: Score a 0 if the behavior was not observed. Score a 1 if the behavior occurred even briefly during activity or at rest. The total number of indicators is summed for the behaviors observed at rest, with movement, and overall. No clear cutoff scores exist to indicate severity of pain; instead, the presence of any of the behaviors may be indicative of pain, warranting further investigation, treatment, and monitoring by the practitioner.
Data from Feldt KS: The checklist of nonverbal pain indicators (CNPI), *Pain Manag Nurs* 1(1):13-21, 2000 and Horgas AL: Assessing pain in older adults with dementia. In Boltz M, series editor: *Try this: best practices in nursing care for hospitalized older adults with dementia* (serial online): http://consultgerirn.org/uploads/File/trythis/try_this_d2.pdf. Accessed October 31, 2011.

activity can be obtained with the use of a tool such as the Borg Scale of Perceived Exertion. The patient is asked to indicate the perceived level of exertion during exercise using a numerical scale (e.g., a 6 to 20 or a 0 to 10 range) or a descriptive scale. The scales progress from a minimum exertion of "none" (6) to a maximum exertion of "very, very hard" (18 to 20) or from "nothing" (0) to "very, very strong" or "maximum" (10). A printed copy of these scales can be displayed on the wall so the patient can report the exertion level to the caregiver during physical activity. This information could be used to evaluate the patient's response to the activity, to establish patient goals, to judge progress, or to establish parameters for aerobic conditioning. Adverse responses or reactions to exercise or activity should be reported to the patient's physician or to nursing personnel and documented by the caregiver. It may be necessary to adjust or modify the exercise or activity at future sessions to reduce or eliminate undesirable reactions. If it is apparent that the patient is in acute distress or the condition is life-threatening, emergency procedures should be implemented immediately. Contact skilled personnel using the 911 emergency exchange or an emergency number within the facility before you begin emergency care.

Pain assessment is an important part of every patient's medical history and record. Pain scales or pain questionnaires should be completed by the patient or the caregiver if the patient is unable to do so. The amount, type, location, and frequency of the pain a patient has should be reassessed throughout treatment.

self-study ACTIVITIES

• List the normal values for adult heart rate (HR), blood pressure (BP), and respiratory rate (RR).

• Explain the reactions a normal adult should exhibit to aerobic exercise or activity in terms of HR, BP, and RR.

• Discuss the factors that may affect a person's HR, BP, and RR; indicate why it is important for the caregiver to be knowledgeable about these factors.

• Describe three factors or procedures that can adversely affect the accuracy of BP values.

• List six specific sites at which a patient's HR (pulse) can be accurately palpated and measured.

• Describe the preparation of the patient and things to remember during pulmonary auscultation.

problem SOLVING

1. You have taken the blood pressure (BP) of a 34-year-old woman before treatment. She exercises on a bike for 20 minutes, and you are to reassess her BP 5 minutes after exercise. What would you expect her BP to be now in relation to her resting BP?

2. A 35-year-old man with a neck flexion-extension (whiplash) injury is treated in an outpatient setting 2 weeks after a motor vehicle accident. What questions would you ask concerning his pain?

3. You are completing a clinical education experience at a children's hospital and are treating a 6-year-old child with leukemia who reports frequent pain. One component of the treatment is to lessen the pain she experiences. What would you do to determine the location and severity of pain? How will you know whether your intervention is effective? Would you expect the child's BP to be higher while she is having pain?

CHAPTER 4

Body Mechanics

objectives *After studying this chapter, the reader will be able to:*

- Define the term "body mechanics."
- Describe the proper body mechanics to use to lift, reach, push, pull, and carry objects.
- Instruct or teach another person to use proper body mechanics.
- Explain specific precautions to use when lifting, reaching, pushing, pulling, and carrying objects.
- Provide basic information to educate another person about how to care for the back.
- Use proper body mechanics for lifting, reaching, pushing, pulling, and carrying objects.

key terms

Anterior   Situated at or directed toward the front of a body or object; the opposite of posterior.

Base of support (BOS)   The area on which an object rests and that provides support for the object.

Center of gravity (COG)   The point at which the mass of a body or object is centered.

Core stabilization   Relates to a group of muscles bounded by the abdominal wall, the pelvis, the diaphragm, and the lower back that are contracted to assist in posture, balance, and stability.

Dysfunction   Disturbance, impairment, or abnormality of the functioning of a body part.

Friction   The act of rubbing one object against another.

Gravity   The force that pulls toward the center of the Earth and affects all objects.

Isometric   Maintaining or pertaining to the same length.

Kyphosis   Abnormally increased convexity in the curvature of the thoracic spine as viewed from the side.

Lateral   Pertaining to a side; away from the midline of the body or a structure.

Lever arm   A component of a mechanical lever; it may be the force arm or the weight (resistance) arm; when the length of the force arm is increased or the length of the weight arm is decreased, a greater mechanical advantage is created for the lever system.

Lordosis   An increase in one of the forward convexities of the normal vertebral columns; a lumbar or cervical lordosis can occur.

Lumbar   Pertaining to the lower region of the back superior to the pelvis.

Medial   Pertaining to or situated toward the midline of the body or a structure.

Pelvic tilt (inclination)   Movement of the pelvis so the anterior superior iliac spine moves anteriorly or posteriorly to produce an anterior or a posterior tilt or inclination of the pelvis.

Posterior   Situated at or directed toward the back of a body or object; the opposite of anterior.

Recumbent   Lying down.

Sagittal plane   Anteroposterior plane or body section that is parallel to the median plane of the body.

Squat   To sit on the heels with the knees fully bent.

Stoop   To bend the body forward or downward by partially bending the knees.

Torque   The expression of the effectiveness of a force in turning a lever system; it is the product of a force multiplied by the perpendicular distance from its line of action to the axis of motion ($T = F \times D$).

Valsalva phenomenon or maneuver   Increased intrathoracic pressure caused by forcible exhalation against a closed glottis.

Vector   A quantity possessing magnitude and direction, such as a force or velocity.

Vertical gravity line (VGL)   An imaginary vertical line that passes through the center of gravity of an object.

INTRODUCTION

Good posture and proper body mechanics are essential to your health. Persons in the occupations of physical and occupational therapy are at high risk for injury, especially to the back. Any person required to lift, reach, push, pull, and carry objects should be instructed in proper body mechanics. This population includes our patients, family members or caregivers who are responsible for the care of the patient, and other health care workers who are responsible for the care of patients. Proper use of body mechanics and core stabilization will conserve energy, reduce stress and strain on body structures, reduce the possibility of personal injury, and produce safe movements of the spine.

According to Willson et al., the core of the body relates to the musculature and structures within the lumbo-pelvic-hip complex. Leetun and colleagues state that "core stability is instantaneous and relies heavily on muscular endurance and neuromuscular control." Kibler et al. conclude that "core stability provides a proper control of movement and positioning of the trunk over the pelvis and legs during activity thereby providing a stable base for limb movement and proficient absorption of forces transmitted through the extremities during complex multijoint activities." Tightening the core muscle group before a movement or a lifting task assists in stabilizing the body during movement. When the transversus abdominis contracts, it tightens the diaphragm, increasing intraabdominal pressure, which in turn provides stability to the spine. Different experts include different muscles in the core muscle group, but generally the core muscle group includes the muscles of the abdomen, torso, back, and pelvic floor. Most experts agree that the primary core deep stabilizing muscles are the transversus abdominis and the lumbar multifidus. Other muscles mentioned in the literature are the rectus abdominis, internal and external obliques, quadratus lumborum, psoas, gluteus maximus, latissimus dorsi, biceps femoris, erector spinae, and the diaphragm.

It is the action of the core muscle group contracting together that provides support to the spine and pelvis during movement and maintains neutral pelvic alignment. Core stability is essential for the maintenance of an upright posture and especially for movements and lifts that require extra effort, such as lifting a heavy patient from the supine position to sitting. Without core stability, the lower back is not supported from inside and can be injured by the strain caused by a heavy lift.

Body mechanics can be described as the use of one's body to produce motion that is safe, energy conserving, anatomically and physiologically efficient, and maintains body balance and control. Thus proper use of body mechanics will better protect the patient and the caregiver from injury. Stress and strain to many anatomical structures and body systems are reduced when proper body mechanics and good posture are used so that work and patient activities can be managed with greater safety. In addition, energy

Box 4-1   Value of Proper Body Mechanics

- It conserves energy
- It reduces stress and strain on muscles, joints, ligaments, and soft tissue
- It promotes effective, efficient, and safe movements
- It promotes and maintains proper body control and balance
- It promotes effective, efficient respiratory and cardiopulmonary function

expenditure can be reduced when habits of proper body mechanics are developed to encourage comfort and efficiency of movement (Box 4-1).

Patients should be taught to breathe normally when performing physical activity and avoid the potentially adverse effects of the Valsalva phenomenon or maneuver. This phenomenon can occur when the patient holds his or her breath and air is trapped in the thorax, which increases intrathoracic pressure. This increased pressure can affect the circulatory system by decreasing the return of venous blood to the right side of the heart, which decreases cardiac output and increases peripheral blood pressure. These events could result in the rupture of a cerebral vessel or a cerebrovascular accident, which could lead to death. This phenomenon is most likely to occur when the patient is performing heavy lifting, pushing, or pulling but can occur at any time during active or resistive exercise.

Body mechanics for the prevention of injury to a caregiver's hands while performing manual therapy will not be fully discussed in this text, but it is important to maintain your wrist and finger joints in mid range during any manual therapy procedure and to use products designed to assist in trigger point therapy to protect your finger joints (see Greene and Goggin in the Bibliography). An example of a tool to help protect the caregiver's hands during treatment is called the foot roller (Fig. 4-1), which can be used for the treatment of scars. Proper posture is of primary importance while performing any therapeutic procedure.

PRINCIPLES AND CONCEPTS OF PROPER BODY MECHANICS

Gravity and friction are forces that add resistance to many activities associated with lifting, reaching, pushing, pulling, and carrying an object. Therefore it is important to select and apply techniques that will, in some situations, reduce the adverse effects of gravity or friction and, in other situations, enhance the positive effects of these two forces to reduce expenditure of energy, avoid undue stress or strain on body systems, and maintain control of the body. You should review the concepts associated with mechanics as originally described by Sir Isaac Newton, especially the three laws of motion, which can be found in any basic physics or kinesiology textbook. Other forces involved with

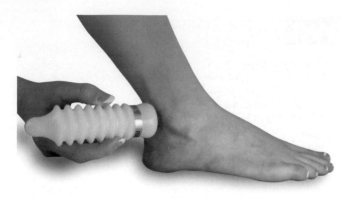

Fig. 4-1 A foot roller used for scar treatment helps protect the caregiver's hands. (Courtesy Core Products International, Inc.)

movement and body control are muscle forces and forms of external resistance.

Before you attempt to lift, pull, reach for, or carry an object, the following two actions are required to use proper body mechanics:

- Position yourself so your center of gravity (COG) and the object's COG are as close as possible.
- Increase your base of support (BOS).

An object's COG is located where the mass of an object is located; it is the heaviest area to move or the most difficult to adjust to a new position. The COG of a standing person is located approximately at the level of the second sacral segment in the center of the pelvis. Positioning your COG as close as possible to the object's COG will help reduce the torque required to move or carry the object, and your muscles will require less energy to contract, experience less strain, and function more efficiently. You should recognize that it may be easier to adjust the object's COG than to adjust your own. Raising or lowering a patient's bed to adjust the COG in relation to your COG before performing exercise is one example of this concept.

Positioning yourself close to the object's COG means that you also can use the changed body mechanics in your arms to aid in the lift. This proximity position will allow use of your upper extremities in a shortened position, like short lever arms. Your muscles will function more effectively and with less strain to the structures of your trunk because a lower torque is required by the muscles of the upper extremity when the object is held close to your body. When the upper extremity is positioned away from the body when attempting to lift, push, pull, reach, or carry, a larger torque is required by the muscles of the extremity to perform the task. This larger torque causes more energy to be expended and increases the strain placed on many body structures.

Stability is vital before attempting to lift, reach, push, pull, or carry an object. You can achieve stability by tightening your core stabilizers, increasing your BOS, lowering your COG, maintaining your vertical gravity line (VGL) within your BOS, and positioning your feet according to the

direction of movement you will use to perform the activity. When you place your feet farther apart in an anterior-posterior stance (i.e., one foot ahead of the other foot) or in a medial-lateral stance (i.e., with the feet farther apart in a sideward direction), you increase your BOS, and these positions will help maintain your VGL within your BOS to further increase your stability.

The VGL is an imaginary line that bisects your body in the sagittal plane beginning at your head and continuing through your pelvis and through your COG. It indicates the vertical positioning of your COG. The VGL must be within your BOS (i.e., between your feet) for balance and stability. Your VGL is affected by activities that alter your COG. For example, when you attempt to stand on one foot, initially you must shift your COG over that lower extremity and foot before you can lift the other foot. Failure to shift your body weight will result in a loss of balance because your COG will not be located within your BOS. A patient's BOS can be improved when walkers, crutches, or canes are provided to aid with ambulation or stability.

Another example of a change in the position of your COG is when you reach for an object. When reaching with your arms, the relative position of your COG is changed and you will need to adjust your BOS or use more muscles to maintain balance and stability. One way to increase your BOS is to widen your stance (preferably to shoulder width). Remember, the closer your feet are to each other, the more unstable you will be. When you squat, stoop, or kneel, you lower your COG, which increases your stability. Objects with a high COG tend to be unstable. Tall, columnar types of equipment (e.g., ultraviolet or infrared lamps and intravenous poles) frequently have a weighted BOS to lower the object's COG. In addition, the item is likely to have an enlarged base so its VGL is located within the BOS.

LIFTING PRINCIPLES AND TECHNIQUES

Through the years, several lifting methods or techniques have been described, proposed, and used. Each of the methods focuses on the posture or position of the lumbar spine and how it is maintained during lifting. The lumbar area of the spine is where most injuries due to lifting or associated activities (e.g., shoveling, raking, or reaching above the head) occur.

Stress to the lumbar spine can be caused by the posture a person uses to lift, the weight or size of the object lifted, the repetitiveness of the activity, the physical condition of the structures of the lumbar area, or the sustainment of a flexed lumbar spine. This stress can lead to discomfort, debilitating pain, or impairment. Pain-sensitive structures of the lumbar area include various ligaments, the lumbodorsal fascia, the anulus fibrosus of the intervertebral disk, the vertebral facets, the nerve roots, muscle tissue, and the vertebral body. Therefore persons who lift and reach excessively as part of their daily life should be advised to avoid

PROCEDURE 4-1

Principles of Proper Body Mechanics

- Mentally and physically plan the activity before attempting it.
- Position yourself close to the object to be moved so you can use short lever arms.
- Maintain your vertical gravity line within your base of support to maintain stability and balance.
- Position your center of gravity close to the object's center of gravity to improve control of the object.
- Tighten your "core" muscles before beginning the lift; use the major muscles of the extremities and trunk to perform movements or activities and maintain your normal lumbar lordosis.
- Roll, push, pull, or slide an object rather than lift it.
- Avoid simultaneous trunk flexion and rotation when lifting or reaching.
- Look straight ahead and do not twist or turn your body while lifting.
- Take your time and lift the item with a smooth motion; avoid jerking movements.
- Perform all activities within your physical capability.
- Do not lift an object immediately after a prolonged period of sitting, lying, or inactivity; gently stretch the back and lower extremities first.
- When performing a lift with two or more persons, instruct everyone how and when they are to assist; use a mechanical lift or other appropriate equipment if it is available.

Box 4-2 Common Causes of Back Problems or Discomfort

- Faulty posture
- Stressful living and work habits, such as being unable to relax or staying in a posture for a prolonged period
- Faulty, improper use of body mechanics
- Repetitive, sustained microtrauma to structures of the back and trunk
- Poor flexibility of muscles and ligaments of the back and trunk
- A decline in general physical fitness
- Use of improper techniques to lift, push, pull, reach, or carry
- Episodes of trauma that culminate in one specific or final event ("the final straw"); stress, strain, or tearing of a muscle or ligament; change in the shape of a disk that then impinges on nerve roots; irritation of vertebral joints

Box 4-3 Rationale for Lumbar Lordosis Posture

- Lordosis reduces mechanical stress to the lumbar ligaments and the intervertebral disk.
- When the back is in the lordosis posture, compression forces on the intervertebral disk are directed anteriorly rather than posteriorly, a direction that reduces the potential for a posterolateral rupture of the disk.
- Lumbar spine stability is increased as a result of the approximation of the vertebral facets.
- The function of the lumbopelvic force couple is maximized.
- The anterior and posterior lower trunk muscles and hip and thigh extensor muscles are positioned to function more effectively.

activities, postures, and positions that may lead to injury. Principles of proper body mechanics to follow when lifting and reaching are presented in Procedure 4-1. Injury resulting from lifting may be caused by the single act of lifting a heavy object, by lifting improperly, or by repetitive lifting. Most upper and lower back injuries are caused by cumulative episodes of microtrauma caused by repetitive lifting or overuse of the same muscles, even when light objects are involved (e.g., repetitive stress syndrome). To avoid injury and resultant dysfunction related to lifting, it is important that a person maintain general body strength and flexibility, proper nutrition, appropriate rest and sleeping habits, good posture, and the use of proper body mechanics. Box 4-2 describes some of the common causes of back discomfort that, if avoided, may prevent future discomfort or injury.

Lumbar belts, or "back belts," have been advocated as a preventive measure for use by persons whose job requires frequent or repetitive lifting. It has been hypothesized that such a belt, when applied properly, increases the intraabdominal pressure and serves as a reminder to the wearer to use proper body mechanics when lifting. Smith et al. and Cholecki et al. have shown that some evidence exists that the proper use of a lumbar belt can increase lumbar spine stability and slightly improve lifting ability. It is important

for the lifter to use proper body mechanics and follow lifting precautions.

The lumbar spine should be maintained in its normal or "neutral" position of lordosis when lifting is performed (Box 4-3). This position tends to reduce stress on the major structures of the lumbar area and, when combined with partial or full flexion of the hips and knees, will reduce the tendency to bend forward at the waist during the lift. Forward bending at the waist with the hips and knees straight and the lumbar spine in a flexed position when lifting or reaching produces excessive stress to many of the structures of the lumbar area. Flexion of the hips and knees allows the lifter to lower the COG closer to the COG of the object and provides an effective position for the muscles of the lower extremities to perform the lift. Contraction of the core stabilizing muscles at the beginning of the lift increases intraabdominal pressure to simulate a pneumatic cylinder that may provide additional stability and decrease the load to the lumbar spine. Caution: The lifter should avoid the Valsalva maneuver when contracting the abdominal muscles.

Persons whose occupation requires them to perform frequent or repetitive lifting or reaching overhead can develop faulty body mechanics or poor habits for these activities. If they have not sustained an injury or if they are recovering from an injury and are preparing to return to work, it will be important to teach them to lift or reach using proper body mechanics, core stabilizers, and good posture, as well as proper precautions. It may be worthwhile for the caregiver to observe the person at the work environment and to understand the requirements of the job. Although it is not possible to prevent all back injuries, patient education and practice using proper techniques have the potential to reduce injury and prevent loss of function.

Vladimir Janda introduced the terms "upper crossed syndromes" and "lower crossed syndromes" as they affect posture and body movement. He states, "Crossed syndromes are characterized by alternating sides of inhibition and facilitation in the upper quarter and lower quarter. Layer syndrome, essentially a combination of upper crossed syndrome and lower crossed syndrome, is characterized by alternating patterns of tightness and weakness, indicating long-standing muscle imbalance pathology." In the book *Assessment and Treatment of Muscle Imbalance, The Janda Approach*, Page et al. describe the theories of Janda's approach to muscle imbalance and how the sensorimotor system affects these syndromes and body movement. The theories on crossed syndromes are quite complex and beyond the scope of this text. See the Bibliography for references on the Janda Approach. Guidelines for lifting activities can be found in Box 4-4.

Lift Techniques

Before performing an activity, you should prepare yourself mentally and physically and plan for the series of events or movements that will be required to perform the activity. For example, before moving an object, estimate its approximate weight by attempting to slide, tilt or tip, or partially lift it. Look inside its container to determine its composition or read the information about the contents and its weight, which frequently is printed on the container. A patient's weight can be determined by asking the person or checking the medical record. The size, configuration, shape, and position of the object should be evaluated to determine whether the object can be moved or controlled safely and with relative ease. If the item cannot be moved easily, get help. The job may require two people, thereby splitting up the load, or it may require a hand truck, dolly, or lifting equipment.

Determine the best method for moving the object before you attempt to move it. For example, would it be easier and safer to roll or slide an object rather than lift it? The move itself should be planned so all obstacles are removed and a

---

Box 4-4 Guidelines for Lifting Activities

- Stoop or squat to lift any object below the level of your hips.
- Widen your feet to increase your base of support and improve your balance and stability.
- Move close to the object before you lift; keep the object close to your body as you lift or carry it.
- Maintain the lumbar curve in your lower back as you lift; do not flatten your lower back.
- Mentally plan the lift; be certain you can safely lift the object without assistance; have sufficient space to perform the lift, and test the weight of the object before you lift it.
- Tighten your core stabilizers before you perform the lift.
- Do not lift and twist your back simultaneously; instead, pivot when you need to turn.
- Do not lift quickly or with a jerky motion.
- Move the object by pushing, pulling, sliding, or rolling rather than by lifting when possible; push rather than pull.
- Avoid repetitive and sustained lifting; use equipment or assistance to lift heavy objects.
- Use care when removing groceries, tools, or other items from the trunk of a car; do not bend at the waist and lift; bend your hips and knees slightly, and move the object close to you before lifting it.

---

clear path from point A to point B is established. The distance of the move, the need for and availability of an assistant, or the use of equipment should be determined and the final location or placement of the object should be decided. Gravity and momentum can be useful adjuncts and should be used whenever possible. It may be helpful to rock an object back and forth to generate some momentum, or an incline or ramp may be used to lower a heavy object from one height to another. To conserve energy, you should roll, slide, push, or pull an object rather than lift it when any of those options are appropriate for the activity and the object (see Procedure 4-1).

Patients and persons who provide assistance must be instructed about their responsibilities and tasks before they perform the activity. They must be taught or trained what to do, how to do it, and when to do it. Asking them to repeat your instructions will help confirm their level of understanding and the level of comprehension of their roles and expected performance. In addition, ask them if they have any questions about their role or the expected outcome. If you are the primary caregiver, establish yourself as the leader or coordinator of the activity. Your instructions and directions should be brief, concise, and action oriented (e.g., "lift now," "push down," and "stand up"). You may find it helpful to lead into the action command by using phrases such as "ready"; "one, two, three"; "first, I want you to ..."; or "on the count of three, lift."

It is important that you give your full attention to the activity, which includes anticipating unusual or unexpected events. When you help a patient to transfer, be prepared to increase your assistance to a maximal effort at any time, even though the patient previously may have performed the transfer successfully with minimal assistance. You must guard and protect the patient until he or she is able to perform the activity safely and consistently.

Your safety and that of the patient will be enhanced by prepositioning and securing any equipment required for the activity. An evaluation of the patient to determine the need for assistance during a transfer also will improve safety. Using mechanical devices or equipment (e.g., a hoist, transfer board, wheeled stretcher, or cart) and performing other previously described actions (e.g., raising or lowering the object, decreasing the distance of the move, or using gravity or momentum) will make the transfer safer and easier to complete. Additional information about transfer activities is presented in Chapter 8. Obtain assistance before you begin any activity you cannot safely perform alone.

You should be aware of several precautions before lifting, reaching, pushing, pulling, or carrying. You must avoid simultaneous trunk flexion (bending) and rotation (twisting) when you lift or reach for an object. Prolonged trunk flexion causes stress and strain to muscles, ligaments, and articulations of the posterior area of the trunk, spine, and, at times, the lower extremities. Therefore when an object is below the level of your waist and must be lifted, you should stoop or squat or raise the object to avoid trunk flexion. A footstool or ladder should be used to reach an object located above the level of your head. Use caution if you elect to use a chair or other similar object that is not intended to provide support while standing. If you do use a chair, be certain to stand on the seat within the BOS of the legs of the chair. Finally, you must be fully aware of your personal abilities and the limits of your strength, stamina, and motor control as they relate to lifting, reaching, pulling, pushing, and carrying. You must perform within the known limits of your physical abilities to avoid injury to yourself or the patient. Therefore obtain human or mechanical assistance to lift or move a large, bulky, or heavy object.

Your primary goal is to perform any activity safely, efficiently, and with minimal stress or strain. Proper body mechanics, core stabilizers, good posture, clear and concise instructions to the patient or caregivers (family, friends, or other personnel), and adherence to the precautions contained in this chapter will benefit you and the patient.

All lifts should be initiated with co-contraction of your core stabilizers just prior to the lift.

Deep Squat Lift A deep squat is performed to position the hips below the level of the knees. The lifter's feet straddle the object, with the upper extremities parallel to each other. The lifter grasps the opposite sides, the handles, or the underside of the object. The lifter's trunk is maintained in a vertical position, and the lumbar spine remains in lordosis with an anterior pelvic tilt (inclination) (Fig. 4-2).

Power Lift In a power lift, only a half squat is performed so the hips remain above the level of the knees. The lifter's feet are parallel to each other and remain behind the object, with the upper extremities parallel to each other. The lifter grasps the opposite sides, the handles, or under the bottom of the object. The lifter's trunk is maintained in a more vertical than horizontal position, and the lumbar spine remains in lordosis with an anterior pelvic tilt (Fig. 4-3).

Straight Leg Lift In a straight leg lift, the lifter's knees are only slightly flexed or may be fully extended. The lower extremities are either parallel to each other or straddle the object, and the upper extremities are either parallel to each other or grasp the opposite sides of the object. The trunk may be positioned either vertically or horizontally, and the lumbar spine remains in lordosis (Fig. 4-4).

One-Leg Stance Lift ("Golfer's Lift") The one-leg stance lift can be used for light objects that can be lifted easily with one upper extremity. The lifter faces the object, with the body weight shifted onto the forward lower extremity. To pick up the object, the weight-bearing lower extremity is partially flexed at the hip and knee while the non–weight-bearing lower extremity is extended to counterbalance the forward movement of the trunk (Fig. 4-5). The lifter picks up the object in a manner similar to the way a golfer removes a golf ball from the cup and returns to an upright position.

Half-Kneeling Lift To perform the half-kneeling lift, the lifter aligns the body by kneeling on one knee positioned behind and on one side of the object and the opposite lower extremity to one side of the object with the foot flat and the hip and knee flexed approximately 90 degrees. The object is grasped and lifted by the upper extremities, placed on the thigh of the flexed lower extremity, and moved close to the body before the flexed lower extremity begins rising to standing. The opposite lower extremity assists with raising the body as the person continues to stand (Fig. 4-6). The lumbar spine is maintained in its normal lordosis throughout the lift. This lift allows the lifter to secure the object close to the body before standing. The half-kneeling lift is useful for persons of small stature, those with limited upper extremity strength, and for persons whose initial unilateral lower extremity strength and overall balance while rising to standing are exceptional. Caution: Persons with a knee condition that would be exacerbated

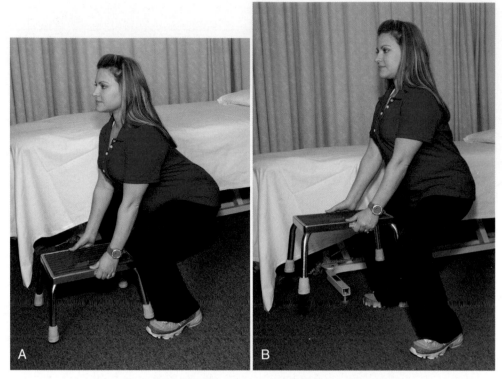

Fig. 4-2   Deep squat lift. **A,** Start position. **B,** Continuation of lift.

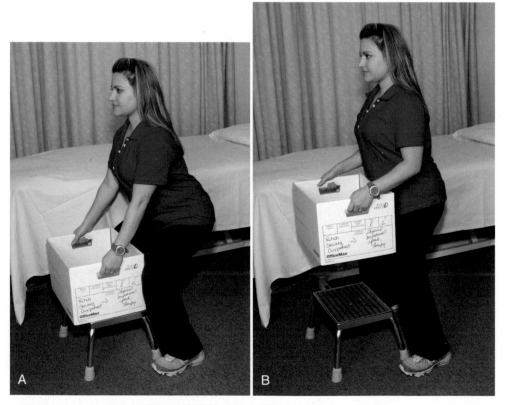

Fig. 4-3   Power lift. **A,** Start position. **B,** Midpoint of the lift.

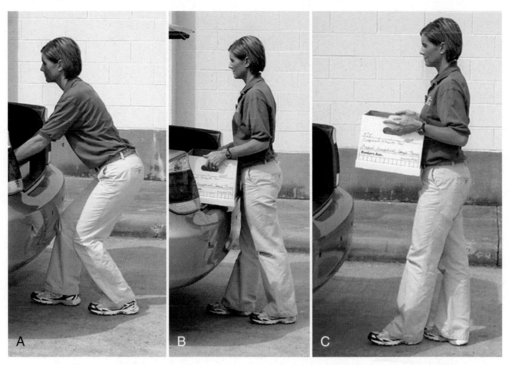

Fig. 4-4   Straight leg lift. **A,** Start position. **B,** Midposition of the lift. **C,** Completion of the lift.

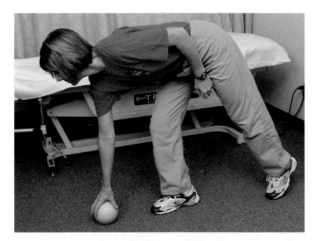

Fig. 4-5   One-leg stance lift ("golfer's lift").

by kneeling should avoid this lift, and rotating or twisting the trunk to position the object on the thigh should be avoided.

Traditional Lift To perform a traditional lift, the lifter faces the object with the feet anteroposterior on each side of the object and the lower extremities in a deep squat. This position provides a low COG and a wide BOS for the lifter. The person grasps the underside of the object with the upper extremities parallel or anteroposterior to each other. The

lift is begun by the flexor muscles of the upper extremities to partially lift the object, and then the lower extremities are used to raise the body with the object to an upright position as the hips and knees extend. The object should be held close to the body, and the lumbar spine should maintain its normal lordosis throughout the lift (see Box 4-3; Fig. 4-7). The lift provides stability and makes use of the large extensor muscles of the lower extremities to raise the body to full standing. Caution: This lift must be performed by the lower extremities, not by the back. To accomplish the lift with the lower extremities, elevation of the hips and pelvis before the body is raised by the lower extremities must be avoided, and normal lumbar lordosis must be maintained.

Stoop Lift When an object rests below the level of the waist but can be reached without squatting, the lifter can stoop to lift. The person partially flexes the hips and knees and maintains the lumbar spine in its normal lordosis. The lifter grasps the object and uses the lower extremities to raise the body and the object. To improve stability and balance, the feet are positioned at shoulder width and slightly anteroposterior to each other. When the object can be lifted by one upper extremity (e.g., a suitcase, briefcase, tool carrier, pail, or a shopping bag with handles), the other upper extremity can be used for support or balance (Fig. 4-8). This lift requires less energy expenditure than a lift that uses a deep or full squat.

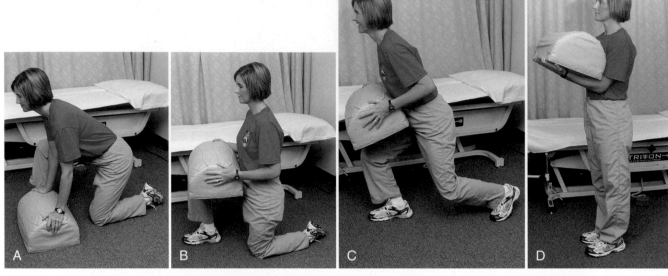

Fig. 4-6   Half-kneeling lift. **A,** Start position. **B,** Support position. **C,** Midpoint of the lift. **D,** Completion of the lift.

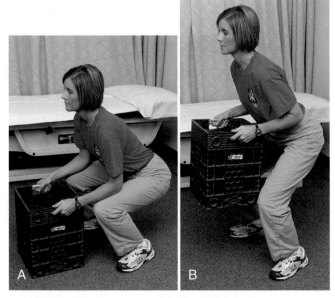

Fig. 4-7   Traditional lift. **A,** Start position. **B,** Continuation of the lift.

PUSHING, PULLING, REACHING, AND CARRYING

Many of the same principles described for lifting also apply to pushing and pulling activities. Use a crouched or semi-squat position to push or pull (Fig. 4-9). This position lowers your COG nearer to the object's COG, which increases stability, reduces energy expenditure, and improves control of the object. The force of the push or pull should be applied parallel to the surface over which the object is to be moved and in the line of the movement desired. This

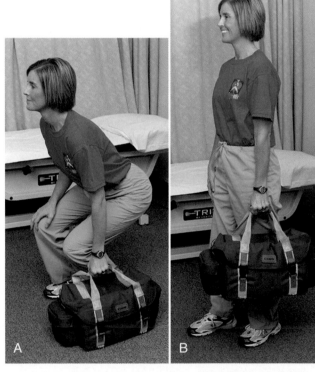

Fig. 4-8   Stoop lift. **A,** Start position. **B,** Continuation of the lift.

tactic reduces the effect of friction and moves the object in the proper direction. Initially, consideration should be given to how to overcome the effects of inertia and friction and the influence of vector forces. Inertia and friction are forces that impede the movement of an object. More force is required to start the movement of a stationary object than

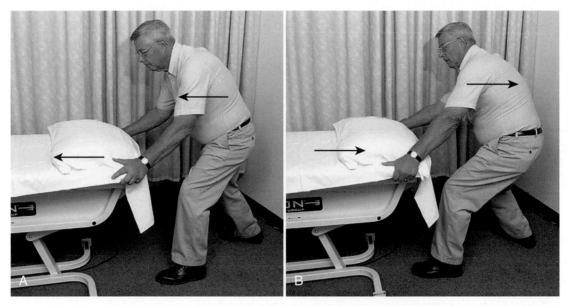

Fig. 4-9   **A,** Pushing an object. **B,** Pulling an object.

to continue its movement; therefore you should prepare yourself to exert greater effort when beginning to push or pull an object than you will need to continue to push or pull it. You may find that rocking the object to generate some motion helps to overcome its inertia; similarly, tipping or partially lifting the object to reduce contact between the object and the surface on which it rests reduces the friction between the object and the underlying surface. You can redirect the movement of the object with a force that alters the vectors of motion. Redirection can be accomplished by pushing harder with one upper extremity than the other, by pulling with one upper extremity and pushing with the other, or by positioning your body at one corner of the object and pushing or pulling at an angle to the line of forward motion. Remember, in most situations, energy will be conserved if an object is moved by sliding, rolling, or turning rather than by lifting or carrying.

Reaching for an object above your shoulder or head will be less strenuous if the object is lowered or if you raise your position by standing on a wide-based footstool or ladder (Fig. 4-10). These actions approximate the COG of the object and your COG, allow the use of shortened extremity lever arms, and decrease strain to back structures.

An object at arm's length should be brought closer to one's body before being lifted to reduce the torque produced by long lever arms. For example, move a patient from the center of the bed or mat to one edge of the bed or mat before performing exercises, or help a recumbent patient to move up or down or sit up to be nearer to you. When carrying an object, hold it close to your body, using your arms as short lever arms, and maintain its COG near your COG. Localize the COG of bulky objects by folding or otherwise positioning extended portions of the object toward its center. If you carry an object in a backpack or chest pack, be certain both

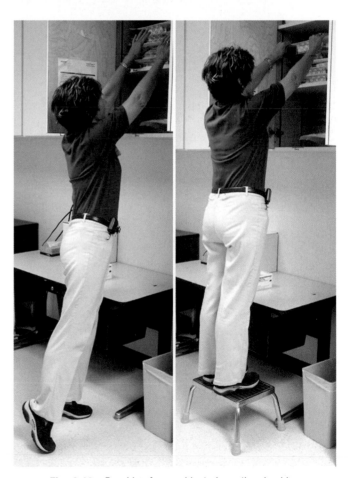

Fig. 4-10   Reaching for an object above the shoulder.

Box **4-5** Guidelines for Pushing, Pulling, Reaching, and Carrying Activities

PUSHING AND PULLING ACTIVITIES

Flex your knees and face the object squarely.

Use your arms and legs to push or pull; push with your arms partially flexed.

Push or pull in a straight line; your force should be parallel to the floor.

Be certain there are no objects in your path and doorways are wide enough for the object to pass through.

REACHING ACTIVITIES

Stand on a footstool or ladder to reach or place an object above your head.

Move the object close to you or move close to the object before grasping, lowering, or raising it; be certain you will be able to control the object safely.

Hold the object close to your body as you step down from or onto a footstool.

Do not simultaneously reach and twist your body.

CARRYING ACTIVITIES

When carrying an object, hold it close to your body; the best positions are in front of your body at the level of your waist or on your back.

If you carry an object in one hand (e.g., a suitcase or a briefcase), alternate carrying it in one hand and then the other; do not twist your back when moving the object from one hand to the other; stoop to lift it from the floor.

Balance the load whenever possible.

Some bulky or heavy objects can be carried on your shoulders, especially if you must carry them for a substantial distance.

Avoid carrying or balancing a small child on one hip; use an infant carrier, or hold the child close to your chest or on your back with use of an approved child carrier.

When a backpack is used, apply both shoulder straps.

---

shoulder straps are used and the weight is distributed in the pack with the weight close to your COG. You should avoid carrying the pack over one shoulder because that will affect your COG and require you to alter your posture, leading to increased strain of several structures (e.g., muscles, ligaments, tendons, and joint surfaces).

Guidelines for pushing, pulling, reaching, and carrying activities can be found in Box 4-5.

POSTURE AND BODY CONTROL

Good posture, strength, and flexibility are important factors in preventing back and neck problems. Core stability is essential for the maintenance of an upright posture and especially for movements and lifts that require extra effort. Chronic joint sprains and muscle strains often are caused by prolonged tension placed on muscles or joints because of poor posture. Poor physical condition leads to the loss of strength and endurance necessary to perform physical tasks without strain and is a predisposition to injury. Sustained posture, even if in good alignment, can cause fatigue. Reaching while holding heavy loads, sitting for long periods with the back unsupported, working with objects that are too low or far to reach, and even sleeping on an excessively firm or sagging mattress can cause back and neck pain and decreased range of motion.

As caregivers, it is our responsibility to observe a patient's posture while sitting, standing, and moving, regardless of the patient's diagnosis. Likewise, our posture should be correct when we are treating patients, even when we are

seated. Fig. 4-11 is an example of good posture when treating a patient while seated.

To test posture, the patient stands lateral to a plumb line. The ideal alignment requires that the line rests as follows: slightly anterior to the lateral malleolus; slightly anterior to a midline through the knee; through the greater trochanter; midway through the trunk (through the bodies of the lumbar vertebrae); through the shoulder joint; through the bodies of the cervical vertebrae; and through the lobe of the ear (Fig. 4-12). Persons with a history of low back pain or dysfunction and those whose lifestyle or occupation predisposes them to trauma to structures of the back (i.e., repetitive lifting) should be educated in ways to prevent further back injuries. Because sitting puts more stress on the back than lying, standing, or walking, it is important to instruct patients about proper sitting techniques when sustained sitting is necessary in their work (Fig. 4-13). The most important achievements in good sitting posture are a resting position for the upper extremities and correction of a forward head posture. Sustained standing or sitting with poor posture can cause kyphosis and postural fatigue throughout the musculoskeletal system. Fig. 4-14 shows where the plumb line would fall in a person with a posture of kyphosis-lordosis, swayback, and flat back and compares these postures to the ideal posture. Techniques for lessening this fatigue should be provided to the patient (Fig. 4-15; Boxes 4-6 and 4-7). Correcting faulty posture and guiding patients in healthy habits of good nutrition, physical fitness, stress management, rest, and the proper exercises will provide a healthier lifestyle.

An initial assessment or evaluation of the individual should be performed before starting patient education. Observe the individual's posture and review any previous history related to the present condition, the mechanisms of the current injury, the onset and type of symptoms, previous treatments, and current lifestyle and work activities, including the work environment (see Box 4-2).

Most patients, regardless of their condition or cause of injury, will benefit from basic education related to care of the structures of the back. This education often is performed through a formal program frequently referred to as a "back school." However, simple instructions and written home programs can provide the patient or family member with information about how to protect the back structures. In this book, only the most basic information is presented.

Initially the patient should receive verbal and written information about the basic anatomy of the body, especially the structures that affect the back. Instruction in the use

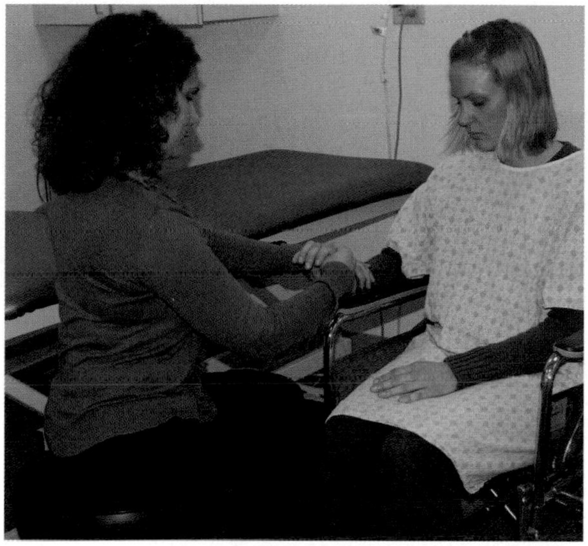

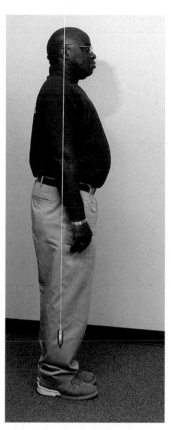

Fig. 4-11   Correct posture when seated without a back support.

Fig. 4-12   Assessing standing posture using a plumb line.

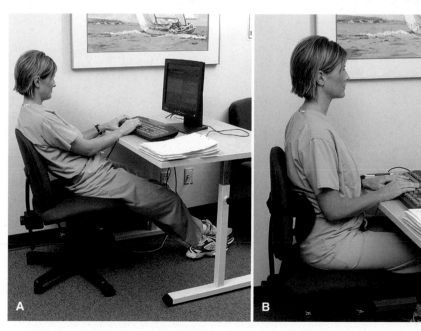

Fig. 4-13   Seated posture at a computer terminal. **A,** Improper seated posture. **B,** Proper seated posture. Notice use of a back support.

Box 4-6 Principles for Proper Posture

- Maintain the normal anterior and posterior curves of the spine for proper balance and alignment.
- Stand and sit with your body erect so the shoulders and pelvis (hips) are level; avoid slouching or "round back" positions.
- Stand with your ankles, knees, hips, and shoulders aligned; keep your head over your body, not in front of the shoulders.
- Stand with your abdominal wall flat, your head in neutral, your shoulders level, your chin parallel to the floor and slightly tucked, and your body weight evenly placed on each leg. Keep your knees slightly flexed and maintain lumbar lordosis.
- Sit with your head in a neutral position, your chin tucked or parallel to the floor, and your elbows, knees, and hips flexed to 90 degrees, with your feet flat on the floor or supported in a slightly inclined position. Your forearms and low back curve should be supported during prolonged sitting. Avoid slouching or a kyphotic posture.
- Avoid standing or sitting in one position for a prolonged time; occasionally alter your position. Move your head, neck, shoulders, back, hips, knees, and ankles periodically.
- When supine or partially lying on your side, flex your hips and knees. Use a pillow under or between the knees for support, and avoid lying prone. Use a small or medium-sized pillow to support your head, but do not position it under the shoulders. Use a bed mattress that is firm and provides support to the natural curves of the spine.

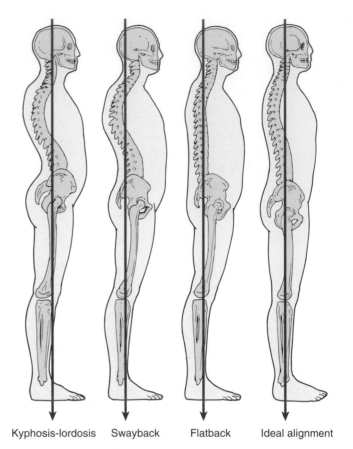

Kyphosis-lordosis   Swayback   Flatback   Ideal alignment

Fig. 4-14 A comparison of faulty postures of kyphosis-lordosis, sway-back, and flat back to the ideal posture.

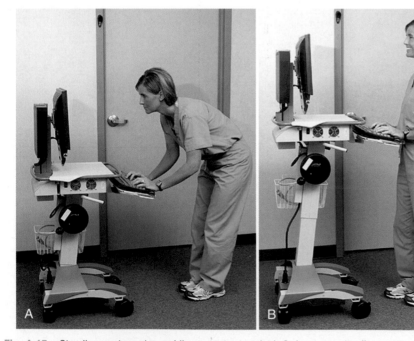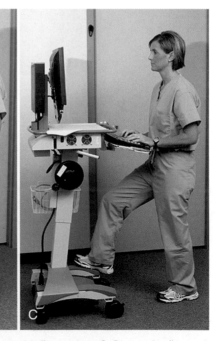

Fig. 4-15 Standing posture at a mobile computer terminal. **A,** Improper standing posture. **B,** Proper standing posture. **C,** Proper standing posture with the use of a support.

Box 4-7 Guidelines to Reduce Stress-Producing Positions or Activities

- Alter your posture or position frequently; avoid prolonged standing or sitting.
- Avoid bending at the waist while working, washing your face, brushing your teeth, or performing activities that are below your waist (e.g., bathing children in a bathtub or removing clothes from the washer or dryer); sit, stoop, or kneel instead of bending.
- For activities that require prolonged standing, use a cushioned mat and wear low-heeled shoes with good arch supports. Place one foot on a footstool or railing, and alternate feet occasionally for comfort (as when ironing or washing dishes). Perform a 30-second exercise routine every hour that includes low back flexion and extension, hip and knee flexion (knee to chest while standing), neck extension, lateral bending, and shoulder range of motion in all planes.
- When seated at a work station for prolonged periods, keep elbows, knees, and hips level and bent at 90 degrees; feet should be flat on the floor or supported at a slight incline; forearms should be supported by armrests, and the back should be supported by the chair back or a lumbar roll.
- When seated at a computer terminal, the vision display terminal should be directed about 10 degrees below horizontal. The chair used should encourage a supported lumbar lordosis with a seat pan that is tilted slightly forward. The keyboard should be pushed forward to permit the arms to rest in front of it, ideally, with the wrists supported on a padded surface. Performing a 1-minute exercise break every hour to include neck flexion, extension, and lateral bending stretching exercises, chin tucks, wrist flexion and extension stretches, shoulder pendulum exercises, tennis elbow stretch, and standing back bends is recommended.
- Enter and leave an automobile with a sideward rather than a twisting motion of the trunk. Adjust the car seat so your knees are at the same level as or slightly higher than your hips, tuck your chin and hold your head erect, and use a lumbar support. Stop frequently when driving long distances to walk or stretch your arms, legs, and back.

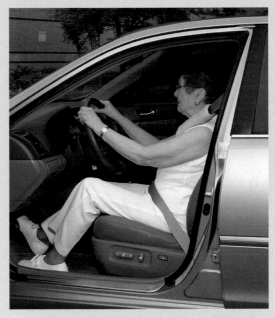

Fig. 4-16   Proper seated posture for driving.

of proper body mechanics, core stabilization, and how to correct faulty standing, sitting, or recumbent postures should be presented. Suggestions on ways to identify and correct improper work, recreational, or daily life habits will be beneficial. Simple exercises to promote a healthy back include shoulder blade retraction, chest stretches, the posterior pelvic tilt, knee to chest while supine, partial sit-ups, hamstring stretches, hip extension stretch, press-ups, wall slides, neck glide, core stability exercises, and neck stretches. Methods that can be used to protect or relieve back stress, such as the placement of one foot on a footstool while standing (Fig. 4-17) or the use of a lumbar cushion or roll while sitting (see Fig. 4-13, B), should be recommended (see Box 4-7). Information about the use of body mechanics should be given to the patient. Instructions in ways to maintain the proper condition and function of muscles, ligaments, and joint structures through the use of relaxation, flexibility, strengthening activities, and aerobic exercise are important components of patient education.

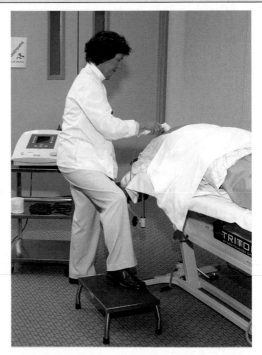

Fig. 4-17   Use of a footstool to relieve stress on the lumbar spine.

A person should be cautioned to balance work, recreational activities, and rest activities to avoid chronic overuse syndromes or the development of a specific dysfunction. Evaluating the person's work or home environment may be necessary so that specific suggestions related to those settings can be provided. The person should be advised to reduce, eliminate, or frequently change sustained or repetitive positions, postures, and activities that cause back stress, strain, or discomfort such as trunk flexion, prolonged sitting or standing, and combined lifting and twisting motions (see Box 4-7). The names and locations of qualified practitioners who can be contacted when professional advice or treatment is needed should be made available. Many booklets, brochures, posters, videotapes, and other educational materials are available, and most treatment units that care for patients with back dysfunction will have these materials.

The patient should be encouraged and motivated to develop a sense of individual responsibility for proper care of the back. The patient must realize that he or she is the only person who has direct control over his or her lifestyle, behavior, posture, and use of the body. Therefore the most appropriate person to assume responsibility for the care of the back is the individual, as long as sufficient information and guidance have been provided. Suggested guidelines for performing the activities in the chapter are presented in Boxes 4-4 to 4-7.

SUMMARY

The use of proper body mechanics helps the caregiver avoid excessive and unnecessary stress or strain to various body systems, reduces energy requirements, and enhances patient safety. For these reasons, persons and patients should be instructed in the use of proper body mechanics, core stabilization, and posture when they perform lifting, reaching, carrying, pushing, and pulling activities.

Effective body mechanics depends on the stability of a person's BOS, maintenance of the VGL within the BOS, foot and body positions in relation to an object, and the use of short lever arms when lifting, reaching, or carrying. Patients should be provided with information about ways to reduce stress-producing posture or to improve work position. Methods of stretching, strengthening, increasing flexibility, and relaxing body areas that are overused during work should be taught. Finally, a sense of personal responsibility for the proper care and use of one's body should be developed by each caregiver and patient.

self-study ACTIVITIES

- Define your concept of proper body mechanics.
- Describe at least four adverse effects that could occur if you use improper body mechanics to lift, push, pull, reach, or carry an object or transfer a patient.
- Outline a program and the instructions you would provide to a patient to promote proper back care.
- Describe different types of lifts and explain when you would use them.
- Outline and describe five suggestions you would provide to a person who wants information about the prevention of low back stress or injury.
- Describe the use of proper body mechanics when moving a recumbent person, lifting any object from the floor, pushing or pulling a piece of equipment, reaching and removing any object from a shelf above your head, and carrying an object with both upper extremities or one upper extremity.
- Explain core stabilization, exercises to strengthen the "core," and when to utilize your core during lifting activities.

problem SOLVING

1. You and another student are asked to educate a group of 10 nursing students in the most effective and safe use of body mechanics for lifting, pushing, pulling, and reaching. Before you meet with them, you must review your plan and teaching methods with your clinical instructor. Prepare a plan, including the teaching methods you will use and the equipment you will need.

2. You are treating a patient whose job requires him to transfer 5-lb boxes at a rate of five per minute from a waist-high conveyor belt to a pallet on the floor. The boxes contain fragile items and can be stacked only two boxes high. What suggestions or instructions would you give him or his employer to enable him to perform the task safely and effectively?

CHAPTER 5

Positioning and Draping

objectives *After studying this chapter, the reader will be able to:*

- Describe proper positioning of the trunk, head, and extremities with the patient supine, prone, side-lying, or sitting.
- Describe the use of patient restraints.
- Describe proper draping of the patient.
- Discuss precautions related to positioning a patient who is supine, prone, side-lying, or sitting.
- Present a rationale for the use and application of proper patient positioning.
- Present a rationale for the use and application of proper draping of a patient.

key terms

Abduction   Movement away from an axis or from the median plane of the body; movement of a body part away from the middle of the body.

Adduction   Movement toward an axis or toward the median plane of the body; movement of a body part toward the middle of the body.

Blanch   To become pale.

Comatose   Pertaining to or affected with coma; a state of unconsciousness.

Contracture   Shortening or tightening of the skin, muscle, fascia, or joint capsule that prevents normal movement or flexibility of the involved structure.

Extension   Movement that increases or straightens the angle between two adjoining body parts or bones.

External rotation (lateral)   Outward turning or pivoting around an axis.

Flexion   Movement that decreases the angle between two adjoining body parts or bones.

Hyperextension   Extension of a limb or part beyond the normal limit; overextension of a limb or part.

Internal rotation (medial)   Inward turning or pivoting around an axis.

Ischemia   Deficiency of blood in a part of the body from functional constriction or obstruction of a blood vessel.

Ischial tuberosity   The protuberance of the ischium; the inferior, distal portion of the pelvis.

Maceration   The softening of a solid by soaking.

Necrosis   Morphological changes indicative of cell death.

Occipital tuberosity   The protuberance of the occipital bone; the posterior area of the skull.

Perineum   The pelvic floor and associated structures occupying the pelvic outlet.

Prone   Lying face downward on the ventral (front) surface of the body; lying on the abdomen and chest.

Restraint (drug)   Medication used to control behavior or restrict the patient's freedom of movement that is not a standard treatment for the patient's medical or psychiatric condition.

Restraint (physical)   Any manual method, physical or mechanical device, material, or equipment that immobilizes or reduces the ability of a patient to move his or her arms, legs, body, or head freely.

Reverse T position   The position of the upper extremities when they are abducted to 90 degrees and externally rotated at the shoulders, with the elbows flexed to 90 degrees.

Seclusion   The involuntary confinement of a person in a room or area where the person is physically prevented from leaving.

Shear   An applied force that tends to cause an opposite, but parallel, sliding motion of the planes of an object; to subject to a shear force.

Spasticity   Continuous resistance to stretching by a muscle because of abnormally increased tension.

Supine   Lying with the face upward or on the dorsal (back) surface of the body; lying on the back.

T position   The position of the upper extremities when they are abducted to 90 degrees and internally rotated at the shoulders, with the elbows flexed to 90 degrees.

INTRODUCTION

Patient positioning must be considered before, during, and at the conclusion of treatment and when a patient is to be at rest for an extended period. It is important to teach other caregivers and family members the methods of proper positioning and the rationale behind positioning (i.e., prevention of pressure and contracture). Rehabilitation staff can play a significant role in both the prevention and treatment of skin breakdown. Physical and occupational therapists bring a unique set of skills to the multidisciplinary pressure ulcer prevention team. Although patient comfort is a consideration and constitutes one reason to position a patient, the caregiver must be aware that a position of comfort may be a position that could lead to the development of a soft-tissue contracture or a pressure ulcer. Therefore frequent changes in the dependent patient's position—at least every 2 hours—are necessary to prevent contractures and relieve pressure on the skin, subcutaneous tissue, and the circulatory, neural, respiratory, and lymphatic systems, as well as other structures. As an adjunct to long-term positioning, the use of compression stockings and/or lower extremity pneumatic devices to prevent deep vein thrombosis should be considered. Figure 5-1 demonstrates some of the preventive positions used for patients who are in bed for a prolonged time. The greatest pressure is placed on the tissues that cover bony prominences (Fig. 5-2). Table 5-1 provides an outline of the areas that receive the greatest pressure when the patient is in a specific position.

It is important to prevent an injury to the skin from friction and shearing forces during repositioning and transfer activities. The proper number of caregivers should be available to move patients when appropriate to decrease friction that may occur during the move. Assistive devices such as mechanical lifts, a trapeze, lift sheets, or transfer boards may be useful adjunctive devices to minimize tissue injury. Cornstarch can be used to reduce friction when necessary.

Intervention to reduce pressure over bony prominences is of foremost importance. Immobile patients need to be maintained in proper alignment. Attention must be focused on maintaining and/or enhancing functional ability. A turning schedule should be established for patients who are confined to bed. Data do not indicate how often patients should be turned to prevent ischemia of soft tissue, but 2 hours in a single position is the maximum duration recommended for patients with normal circulatory capacity. Most positions can be altered slightly (i.e., without a full position change) at the 1-hour mark, allowing for pressure relief.

The caregiver should use caution when positioning a patient who has decreased sensation to pressure, is unable to alter his or her position independently and safely, is immobile, is confused, is heavily medicated, has minimal soft-tissue protection over bony prominences, and is unable to express or communicate discomfort. The patient's trunk, head, and extremities should be supported and stabilized and proper alignment of the axial and appendicular skeletal segments should be maintained to provide a position that promotes efficient function of the patient's body systems. Flaccid or weak extremities should not be placed in a gravity-dependent position to alleviate the potential for dependent edema. The most distal part of the extremity should be higher than the heart; this position can be achieved with the use of pillows or bolsters. The patient should be positioned to enable the caregiver to administer treatment effectively, efficiently, and safely. Therefore caregivers should determine how the patient's position may affect his or her body mechanics and the application of the treatment program before initiating treatment.

PRINCIPLES AND CONCEPTS

The patient should be draped with clean linen and only the areas or body parts to be treated should be exposed, with the remainder of the patient's body covered to maintain modesty and warmth. Precautions must be taken to avoid unnecessary exposure of sensitive areas of the patient's body. For example, draping of the anterior chest (breasts) of female patients and the perineum (genitalia) of both male and female patients must be performed carefully and may need to be adjusted periodically to ensure that the drape is secure. Standards of modesty differ among individuals and cultures, and thus each patient should be draped to limit exposure of any body area that, when uncovered, is considered by the person to be immodest.

The linen used to drape each patient should be clean and unused before it is applied. Because the draping material may become soiled with perspiration, lubricants, or wound drainage, the patient's clothing should not be used as a drape. In many instances, undergarments and outer garments may need to be removed to prevent soiling and provide patient comfort. Before removing any garments, explain to the patient why they need to be removed and obtain the patient's permission to remove them. You may need to assure the patient that his or her modesty will be maintained throughout the treatment session or activity.

Folds or wrinkles in the linen beneath the patient should be removed or reduced to avoid increased pressure on the skin. Folded or wrinkled linen creates a thickness greater than that of the other areas of the linen and may cause localized pressure. Linen used to protect the patient's axilla, perineum, or gluteal cleft must be discarded as soon as it is removed from the patient because it is likely to be soiled. Previously used linen should never be reapplied to a patient or used for any other patient until it has been laundered.

Be certain to instruct or direct the patient about how to position and initially drape the body. A gown or other suitable item should be provided if removal of clothing or protection of sensitive areas is required. The treatment table or mat should be prepared with linen and pillows before the patient is positioned. The caregiver's instructions and directions should inform the patient exactly what to do, what position to assume, and how to apply the gown and drape.

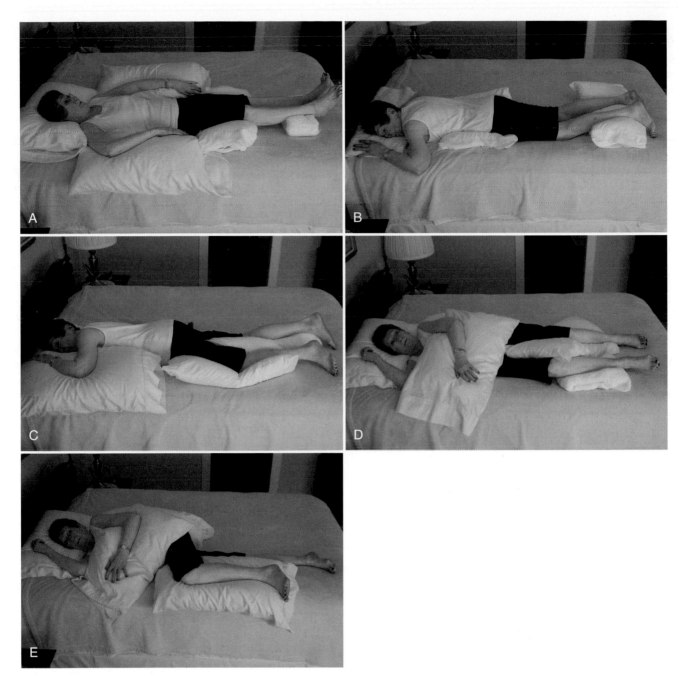

Fig. 5-1 Preventive positioning. **A,** Supine position. **B,** Prone position. (Note: The patient's arms may be placed at his or her sides if that position is more comfortable for the patient.) **C,** Three-quarters prone position. **D,** Three-quarters supine position. **E,** Side-lying position.

Pillows, rolled towels, or commercially available devices (e.g., bolsters and foam wedges) can be used to support or stabilize body segments to relieve strain to the patient's joints, ligaments, muscles, tendons, connective tissue, and nerves. A firm mattress usually enhances proper positioning, but the patient's condition and ability to alter a position should be considered when determining the type of surface on which the person will be placed (Procedure 5-1).

POSITIONING

The recommendations provided for short-term positioning should be appropriate for most patients. However, opinions differ about the use (or nonuse) and placement of pillows, towel rolls, bolsters, and similar items. Specific patient needs and the treatment to be provided will affect the position the caregiver selects. The positions described in this text should be modified based on criteria the caregiver determines to be necessary for each patient. Specific patient conditions, such as the loss of or decreased sensory awareness, paralysis, decreased skin integrity, poor nutrition, impaired circulation, and a predisposition to contracture development require special attention for positioning. For a patient with any of these conditions, it will be necessary to inspect the patient's skin, especially over bony prominences, before and immediately after the treatment session. Red areas indicate areas of pressure, and pale (or blanched) areas may indicate severe, dangerous pressure. Complaints of numbness or tingling are indicators of excessive pressure, as is localized edema or swelling.

Wheelchair-bound patients who sit for long periods need appropriate seating surfaces that safely reduce pressure while

still providing adequate support and stability. The following areas are at particularly high risk for a seated person:
- Ischial tuberosities
- Scapular and vertebral spinous processes
- Olecranon processes
- Medial epicondyles of the humerus if the patient is resting on a hard surface
- Back of the knees if the patient is resting against the seat
- The heels and feet

Use of donut cushions should be avoided because they can cause tissue ischemia. Selection of customized chair cushions may be needed for patients who are wheelchair bound for a long period.

For patients who are temporarily chair bound, consideration should be given to cushions that furnish maximum pressure reduction over the ischial tuberosities, adequate support, and comfort. Patients who are able to reposition themselves should be instructed to do so at 10- to 15-minute intervals. For patients who have a tendency to slide forward in their wheelchair, a wedged cushion can be placed so that the wider side of the cushion is to the front of the chair. Patients who have good upper body strength should be taught to do wheelchair push-ups to alleviate pressure on the ischial tuberosities. Leaning side to side to alleviate ischial tuberosity pressure is another option if the patient is unable to perform push-ups from the arm supports.

Proper body alignment is essential for chair-bound patients. Caution is necessary because pressure on a localized area of soft tissue, especially where an underlying bony prominence is located, produces local ischemia, which can lead to tissue necrosis over time. You must be particularly

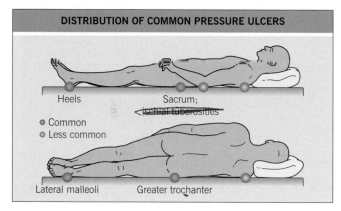

Fig. 5-2   Common bony pressure areas in the supine and side-lying positions. (Courtesy Bolognia JL, Jorizzo JL, Rapini RP: *Dermatology*, ed 2, St Louis, 2007, Mosby Elsevier.)

Table **5-1**   Bony Prominences that May Cause Pressure Injuries

Area	Supine Position	Prone Position	Side-Lying Position (Lowermost Extremity)	Side-Lying Position (Uppermost Extremity)	Sitting Position
Head and trunk	Occipital tuberosity Spine of scapula Inferior angle of scapula Vertebral spinous processes Posterioriliac crest Sacrum	Forehead Lateral ear Tip of acromion process Sternum Anterosuperior iliac spine	Lateral ear Lateral ribs Lateral acromion process	—	Ischial tuberosities Scapular and vertebral spinous processes (if leaning against back of chair); sacrum if the patient is slouched
Upper extremity	Medial epicondyle of humerus Olecranon process	Anterior head of humerus Clavicle	Lateral head of humerus Medial or lateral epicondyle of humerus	Medial epicondyle of humerus (if resting on a hard surface)	Medial epicondyle of humerus Olecranon process (if resting on a hard surface)
Lower extremity	Posterior calcaneus Greater trochanter, head of fibula, and lateral malleolus with excessive external rotation of the hip	Patella Ridge of tibia Dorsum of foot	Greater trochanter of femur Medial and lateral condyles of femur Malleolus of fibula and tibia Fifth metatarsal	Medial condyle of femur Malleolus of tibia	Greater trochanter Popliteal fossa Posterior calcaneus if resting against a hard surface

PROCEDURE 5-1

Guidelines for Positioning and Draping

- Introduce yourself to the patient by providing your name and title (e.g., physical therapist, physical therapist assistant, physical therapy student, aide, or technician). Confirm the patient's identity and current, relevant information (e.g., diagnosis, complaints, previous treatment and response, and name of the patient's physician).
- Inform the patient of the planned treatment, apply the principles of informed consent, and obtain consent for treatment.
- Specifically describe how the patient is to be positioned and provide assistance if required.
- If the patient is wearing street clothes, indicate the specific articles of clothing to be removed or request permission to remove them if assistance is necessary.
- Provide temporary clothing or linen to protect modesty and provide warmth.
- Ensure that sufficient linens, pillows, and equipment needed for the treatment are available in the cubicle or treatment area.
- Provide safe and secure storage for the patient's personal items.
- Specifically describe how you want the patient to apply linen items, a gown, a robe, or exercise clothing to cover (drape) the body; provide privacy while the patient is disrobing and dressing.
- Instruct the patient to inform you when he or she is positioned and draped, or confirm that the patient is clothed or draped before you enter the cubicle.
- At the end of treatment, take the following steps:
  - Instruct the patient to remove draping items and temporary clothing and put on his or her own clothing; provide assistance if required or provide privacy while the patient is dressing.
  - Provide linen so the patient can remove perspiration, massage lotion, electrotherapy gels, water, or other substances.
  - Return personal items to the patient.
  - Dispose of used linen in the proper container.
  - Prepare the cubicle or treatment area for future use or assign the task to another person.

Note: Depending on the gender of the caregiver and the patient and the area or areas of the patient to be exposed for treatment, it may be necessary for the caregiver to ask another person to help the patient with undressing, positioning, draping, and redressing to protect modesty.

Box 5-1   Rationale for Proper Positioning

Proper positioning is important for the following reasons:
- It prevents soft-tissue injury, pressure, and joint contracture.
- It provides patient comfort.
- It provides support and stability for the trunk and extremities.
- It provides access and exposure to areas to be treated.
- It promotes efficient function of patient's body systems.
- It relieves excessive, prolonged pressure on soft tissue, bony prominences, and circulatory and neurologic structures.

participate in activities without the risk of physical harm. Restraints are recommended for short-term use only and should not be used to hinder or restrain the patient for several hours. A patient who is comatose, experiences spasticity, has extensive paralysis, or is unable to mentally or physically maintain a safe position may require some form of temporary restraint or protective positioning. These protective measures are to be differentiated from the use of restraints for a prolonged period.

Unless a patient needs to be restrained for his or her own protection or to protect others from being harmed by the patient, physical or drug restraints are not to be used without the voluntary consent of the patient and a physician's ongoing order. Furthermore, a restraint should be used only when less restrictive interventions have been tried and found to be ineffective. Some examples of restraints are wrist or ankle belts or straps, a tightly wrapped bed sheet that constrains the patient's upper and lower extremities and trunk, a cloth body garment (e.g., a Posey vest or "straight jacket"), and, at times, bed rails when they are elevated. A drug can be a restraint when it is used to control behavior or restrict a patient's freedom of movement and when the drug is not a usual form of treatment for the patient's condition. According to The Joint Commission, the use of physical or drug-induced restraints, as well as seclusion, must be prescribed by a physician or other licensed independent practitioner who is responsible for the care of the patient and is authorized to order restraint or seclusion by hospital or facility policy in accordance with state law. The attending physician must be notified as soon as possible if he or she did not order the restraint or seclusion. These orders are good for not longer than 4 hours for adults, 2 hours for persons 9 to 17 years of age, and 1 hour for children younger than 9 years. The total time limit of an order is 24 hours, at which time a new order may be prescribed.

After a patient is placed in restraints or seclusion, he or she must be evaluated face-to-face within 1 hour by a physician or licensed independent practitioner or by a registered

aware of these possible consequences when you treat a patient whose condition involves the contributing factors previously described in this paragraph (Box 5-1).

Restraints

Restraints, or safety straps, may be used to protect the patient from falling out of bed or to permit the patient to nurse or physician assistant who has been trained according to the new requirements. The family should be notified of the method and reason for the restraint, if possible.

Some items not considered physical restraints are straps used for surgical or radiographic positioning, an arm board used to protect an intravenous infusion site, a protective helmet, surgical dressings or bandages, orthopedic appliances, table top chairs, and postural supports, as well as the therapeutic holding or comforting of children.

Rules, regulations, and guidelines related to the use of restraints and seclusion have been developed and are enforced by various state, local, and federal agencies and by accreditation organizations. Examples include local and state mental health agencies, the Department of Public Health, the Centers for Medicare and Medicaid Services, The Joint Commission, and the American Osteopathic Association. Facilities regulated or accredited by any of these agencies or organizations should have written policies and procedures for the application, use, and alternative actions associated with restraints and seclusion. Staff must be trained and able to demonstrate competency before performing restraint or seclusion, as part of orientation, and, subsequently, on a periodic basis.

Examples of alternative measures or actions include having a family member or health care personnel present with the patient, using a bed enclosure or Vail bed, having scheduled timing for toileting activities, using pain management techniques, using bowel and bladder function assessment and training activities, using cushions or pads for support, providing music or a television for distraction, providing frequent changes of scenery, offering frequent verbal instructions or directions, and rearranging furniture so the patient has better access to objects or controls.

Standards and rules related to the use of restraints and seclusion are contained in the Hospital Conditions of Participation: Patients' Rights (42 CFR Part 482) of the Medicare and Medicaid Programs, which was published in the *Federal Register* on December 8, 2006. The 1999 Health Care Financing Administration–based standards were derived from the concept that "patients have the right to be free from the use of seclusion or restraint, of any form, as a means of coercion, convenience, discipline or retaliation by staff." Compliance with these standards and the rules that accompany them are required for any facility that treats patients insured by Medicare or Medicaid as a Condition of Participation. The Joint Commission states that noncompliance with restraint/seclusion for hospitals will affect the accreditation decision.

The use of restraints and seclusion in the short-term and long-term care of patients is monitored closely by various local, state, and federal agencies and accreditation organizations. Two additional documents that support the intent of the Health Care Financing Administration standards are the Patient Rights and Organization Ethics standards established by The Joint Commission and the Patient's Bill of Rights contained in the Consumer Bill of Rights and Responsibilities developed by the Presidential Advisory Committee on Consumer Protection and Quality in the Health Care Industry. The caregiver is obligated to be knowledgeable about and trained in the application of restraints and to comply with the rules, regulations, and policies and procedures related to the appropriate use of restraints or seclusion of a patient. Settings covered by the rules are all hospitals, including short-term psychiatric rehabilitation facilities, long-term facilities, children's health care facilities, and alcohol/drug treatment facilities that receive Medicaid and Medicare funds. See the Bibliography for additional sources of information pertaining to the use of restraints or seclusion for patients.

Supine Position

A small pillow or a cervical roll may be placed under the patient's head, but excessive neck and upper back flexion or scapular abduction (round shoulders) should be avoided (Fig. 5-3). A small pillow, rolled towels, or a small bolster can be placed in the popliteal spaces (i.e., behind the knees) to relieve lumbar lordosis and promote comfort. Some patients may prefer to use a small lumbar roll or pillow. Because having an item behind the knees encourages hip and knee flexion and may contribute to lower extremity contractures of the iliopsoas (hip flexor) and hamstring (knee flexor) muscles, this position should not be maintained for a prolonged period. A small, rolled towel or small bolster may be placed under the patient's ankles to relieve pressure to the calcaneus (heel), but knee hyperextension should be avoided.

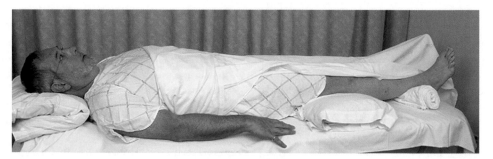

Fig. 5-3   Supine position.

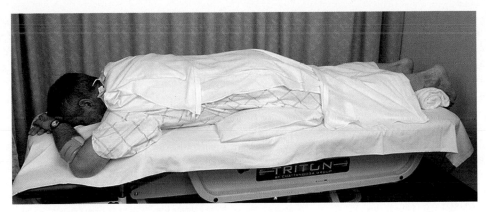

Fig. 5-4   Prone position.

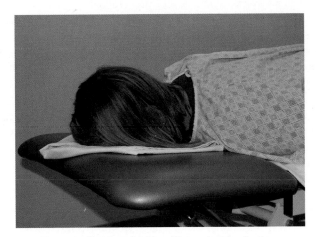

Fig. 5-5   Treatment table with a cutout for the face.

The patient's upper extremities may be elevated on pillows or positioned in whatever way the patient desires for comfort (such as by the patient's side, in a reverse T position, or folded on the chest). The patient's body and extremities should be totally supported on the mat or table. No part or portion of the body or extremities should project beyond the surface, because if the patient's hands or feet extend beyond the mat or treatment table, they could be struck and injured by a piece of equipment or another object. Therefore the patient should not be positioned so that his or her hands or feet project off the mat or treatment table, unless the patient is protected by a wall. This guideline is particularly important when the patient is screened by a cubicle curtain or sheet and parts of the patient's body might extend into an area where personnel move equipment or walk.

Remember that the areas of greatest pressure when the patient is supine are the occipital tuberosity, the spine and inferior angle of the scapula, the spinous processes of the vertebrae, the olecranon process, the posterior iliac crests, the sacrum, and the posterior calcaneus (see Table 5-1). Other possible pressure areas, depending on how the patient

is positioned, are the medial epicondyle of the humerus, the head of the fibula, the greater trochanter of the hip, and the lateral malleolus if excessive external rotation of the hip occurs. Elbows can be supported or protected, and if the patient has a flaccid extremity, the hand should be placed higher than the elbow to avoid dependent edema. A wedge, rolled towel, or sandbag can be used to maintain the hip in a neutral position. The hip should be moved toward internal rotation, and the wedge, towel, or sandbags should be placed against the lateral aspect of the soft tissue of the thigh and lower leg.

Prone Position

When a patient is in the prone position, place a small pillow or towel roll under the patient's head, or position the head to the left or right (Fig. 5-4). Some patients in the prone position may be more comfortable if they rest their forehead on a folded towel or a special headrest. A treatment table that has a cutout portion for the face and supports the head provides the most comfortable positioning (Fig. 5-5). This type of table usually maintains the neck in a neutral or a slightly flexed position. A pillow placed under the patient's lower abdomen will reduce lumbar lordosis. (For some patients, maintenance of the normal lumbar lordosis may be desired, and a pillow may be placed under the upper or middle chest or positioned lengthwise from the pelvis to the thorax to maintain lordosis.) A rolled towel should be placed under each anterior shoulder area to adduct the scapulae, reduce the stress to the interscapular muscles, and protect the head of the humerus. A treatment table with forearm rests can be used to alleviate stress to the interscapular muscles (see Fig. 5-5). The use of a pillow, towel roll, or small bolster under the anterior portion of the patient's ankles will relieve stress on the hamstring muscles and feet and will allow the pelvis and lower back to relax. However, placement of a pillow at the ankles causes knee flexion and may contribute to contracture of the hamstring (knee flexor) muscles. To avoid the development of a contracture, this position should not be maintained for a prolonged period. One alternative is to protect the patellae by placing towel rolls under the distal thigh areas, which lessens knee flexion.

The patient's upper extremities may be positioned for comfort (e.g., along the sides of the body, in a T position, or with the hands under the head).

Remember that the areas of greatest pressure when the patient is prone are the forehead or lateral ear, the tip of the acromion process, the anterior head of the humerus, the sternum, the anterior superior iliac crest, the patella, the crest of the tibia, and the dorsum of the foot (see Table 5-1).

Side-Lying Position

Initially a patient in a side-lying position should be positioned in the center of the bed, mat, or table with the head, trunk, and pelvis aligned (Fig. 5-6). Both of the patient's lower extremities should be flexed at the hip and knee. The uppermost lower extremity should be supported on one or two pillows and positioned slightly forward of the lowermost extremity. A small towel roll can be placed just proximal to the lowermost lateral malleolus to relieve pressure. The lowermost lower extremity provides stability to the patient's pelvis and lower trunk. One or two pillows should be used to support the patient's head. A folded pillow placed at the patient's chest is used to support the uppermost upper extremity and to prevent the patient from rolling forward. Placement of a folded pillow along the posterior area of the patient's trunk may be necessary to prevent the patient from rolling backward. To protect the lowermost greater trochanter, a rolled towel or pillow may be placed proximal to the trochanter, and if necessary, a pillow may be used under the thigh below the greater trochanter.

If you determine that the patient will not be able to maintain a side-lying position independently and safely, safety straps or a foam bolster should be applied. The lowermost upper extremity can be positioned to promote patient comfort and stability. If the lowermost greater trochanter requires protection, place a pillow distal to the trochanter under the lowermost lower extremity and a second pillow under the trunk proximal to the trochanter.

It is important that a patient whose condition predisposes him or her to the development of a pressure ulcer be positioned to avoid direct pressure to the lowermost trochanter and the lowermost shoulder. This position can be accomplished by placing the person in a slightly supine reclined position or a 30-degree lateral tilt position with use of a wedge or pillows to stabilize the patient.

Remember that the areas of greatest pressure for the lowermost portion of the body when the patient is in a side-lying position are the lateral ear, lateral ribs, lateral acromion process, lateral head of the humerus, medial or lateral epicondyles of the humerus, greater trochanter of the femur, lateral condyle of the femur, malleolus of the fibula, medial condyle of the femurs, and malleolus of the tibia (if the uppermost lower extremity is positioned directly over the lowermost lower extremity). The greatest areas of pressure for the uppermost portion of the body are the medial epicondyle of the humerus (if the patient is resting on a hard surface), the medial condyle of the femur, and the malleolus of the tibia.

Sitting Position

The patient should be seated in a chair with adequate support and stability for the trunk, which can be provided by pillows, belts, straps, or the back of the chair, or by leaning forward onto a treatment table. The patient's lower extremities should be supported with the feet on a footstool, on the footrests of a wheelchair, or on the floor. The distal, posterior thigh tissue and deeper structures should be free of excessive pressure from the edge of the chair or the wheelchair seat. When the patient receives treatment with the trunk leaning forward against the treatment table, one or more pillows should be used to support the anterior area of the trunk (Fig. 5-7). Use one or more pillows behind the patient when he or she is seated, with the trunk leaning back against the chair. The patient's upper extremities can be supported on pillows, the chair armrests, the treatment table, a lap board, or a pillow in the patient's lap. To improve access to the patient's back, he or she can sit in an armless chair with the chair back directed to the left or right.

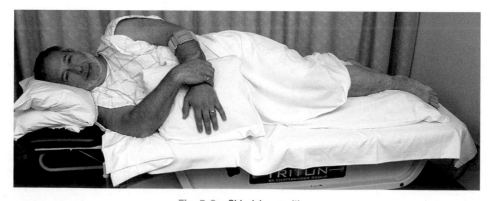

Fig. 5-6 Side-lying position.

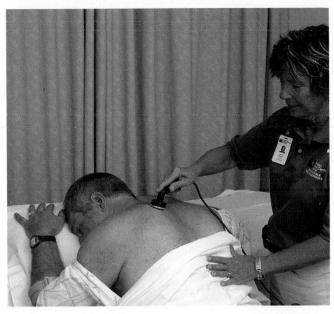

Fig. 5-7   A patient seated for treatment. Notice the use of pillows to support the trunk, head, and upper extremities; only the area to be treated is exposed.

| Box 5-2 | Common Soft-Tissue Contracture Sites Related to Prolonged Positioning |

Box 5-2	Common Soft-Tissue Contracture Sites Related to Prolonged Positioning
Supine	Hip and knee flexors
	Ankle plantar flexors
	Shoulder extensors, adductors, and internal rotators
	Hip external rotators
Prone	Ankle plantar flexors
	Shoulder extensors, adductors, and internal/external rotators
	Neck rotators, left or right
Lying on the side	Hip and knee flexors
	Hip adductors and internal rotators
	Shoulder adductors and internal rotators
Sitting	Hip and knee flexors
	Hip adductors and internal rotators
	Shoulder adductors, extensors, and internal rotators

Note: Forearm, elbow, wrist, and finger contractures can develop, depending on the position used.

Box 5-3	Precautions for Patient Positioning

- Avoid clothing or linen folds beneath the patient.
- Observe skin color over bony prominences before, during, and after treatment.
- Protect bony prominences from excessive and prolonged pressure.
- Avoid positioning the patient's extremities beyond the support surface.
- Avoid excessive, prolonged pressure on soft tissue, circulatory, and neurological structures.
- Use additional caution when positioning patients who are mentally incompetent or confused, comatose, very young or elderly, paralyzed, or lacking normal circulation or sensation.

Remember that the areas of greatest pressure when the patient is sitting are the ischial tuberosities and the posterior areas of the thigh. Other possible areas of pressure are the sacrum and the spinous processes of the vertebrae if the patient leans against the chair back and the medial epicondyle of the humerus and olecranon if the elbow rests on a hard surface such as a lap board.

Positioning Summary

In general, a patient who is inactive, has restricted mobility, or is unable to alter body positions should not be positioned for an extended period (more than 30 minutes) in any position that causes or produces the following:

- Excessive rotation or bending of the spine
- Bilateral or unilateral scapular abduction or a forward head position
- Compression of the thorax or chest
- Plantar flexion of the ankles and feet
- Hip or knee flexion; hyperextension of the knees
- Adduction and internal rotation of the glenohumeral joint
- Elbow, wrist, or finger flexion
- Hip adduction or internal/external rotation

These positions promote excessive stress or strain to various structures and may promote the development of a soft-tissue contracture or patient discomfort (Box 5-2). You must observe the areas of pressure on patients who are susceptible to skin irritation or breakdown (e.g., older adults, patients who have decreased subcutaneous tissue, patients with lack of sensation, and patients who are paralyzed). A reddened or blanched area that does not return to a normal appearance within an hour after the treatment session must be monitored. The use of the position that caused the problem should be avoided in the future. Various aids (e.g., elbow and heel protectors, footboards, seat cushions, lap boards, slings, splints, cones, or bolsters) can be helpful to reduce soft-tissue stress, support or stabilize a joint or segment, relieve pressure, or immobilize a segment. However, these items must be applied carefully and removed or adjusted periodically to avoid secondary problems. Straps on protective devices or splints may occlude peripheral circulation if applied too tightly; an unpadded lap board may cause excessive pressure to the medial humeral epicondyle; and bolsters, cushions, or cones may create a source for the development of perspiration, which may lead to skin maceration if not dissipated. Therefore cautious and judicious use of these aids is recommended (Box 5-3).

Be particularly careful when positioning a patient who is older, confused, mentally incompetent, very young, comatose, paralyzed, agitated, or known to have an impaired cardiopulmonary system. These persons may not tolerate remaining in one position for more than a few minutes. Their circulation or respiration may become impaired and their skin may develop a lesion more readily as a result of pressure or shear forces created by the position. These patients may have more difficulty complying with instructions to maintain a given position, they may lack the ability to sense the need to change their position, or they may be unable to alter their position without assistance. Such patients should be monitored frequently to avoid the adverse complications associated with improper positioning.

PREVENTIVE POSITIONING

It is recommended that a patient's position be altered frequently to avoid excessive or prolonged pressure, to reduce the development of contractures, to avoid postural malalignment, and to prevent other adverse effects. In addition, specific positions should be avoided for certain patients because their diagnosis or condition predisposes them to complications related to short-term or prolonged positioning. The functional ability or capacity of the patient may be compromised because of problems caused by improper positioning techniques, which may affect the patient's independence or quality of life. Some conditions in which selected positions should be avoided are discussed in the following sections.

Transfemoral Amputation

Prolonged hip flexion should be avoided for a patient with a transfemoral amputation. The residual limb (RL) should not be elevated on a pillow while the patient is supine for more than a few minutes of each hour. The amount and length of time the patient is permitted to sit should be limited to no more than 40 minutes of each hour. Having the residual limb elevated on a pillow while the patient is supine or sitting for more than 40 minutes promotes the development of a contracture of the patient's hip flexor muscles. If those muscles become contracted, the patient is likely to experience difficulty using a prosthesis for ambulation. In addition, it may not be possible to fit the patient with a prosthesis if contractures occur.

Hip abduction of the RL should be avoided to prevent a contracture of the hip abductor muscles. If this contracture develops, the patient will experience difficulty ambulating with a prosthesis. The patient should be encouraged to maintain the pelvis in a level position and to maintain the trunk in proper alignment while recumbent to avoid developing back discomfort and an abnormal posture. When the patient stands or is recumbent, the RL should be maintained in extension. Lying in the prone position periodically is recommended.

Transtibial Amputation

Prolonged hip and knee flexion should be avoided for the patient with a transtibial amputation. The RL should not be elevated on a pillow while the patient is supine for more than a few minutes of each hour. If the RL is elevated, the knee should be maintained in extension. The amount and length of time the patient is permitted to sit should be limited to no more than 40 minutes of each hour. Having the residual limb elevated on a pillow while the patient is supine and sitting with knee extended for longer than 40 minutes promotes the development of contracture of the patient's hip flexor muscles. Allowing the patient to sit in a chair for longer than 40 minutes promotes the development of contracture of the patient's knee flexor muscles. If these muscles become contracted, the patient will experience difficulty using a prosthesis for ambulation. In addition, it may not be possible to fit the patient with a prosthesis if contractures occur. When the patient sits, stands, or is recumbent, the hip and knee should be maintained in extension. Lying in the prone position periodically is recommended.

Hemiplegia

When the patient's upper extremity is involved, the following positions should be avoided: prolonged shoulder adduction and internal rotation; elbow flexion; forearm supination or pronation; wrist, finger, or thumb flexion; and finger and thumb adduction. These positions are most likely to lead to soft-tissue contractures caused by muscle spasticity, reduced function of the opposing muscles, and lack of active motion. The use of a sling to support the involved extremity places the shoulder in adduction and internal rotation, the elbow in flexion, and the forearm in pronation; in addition, the wrist and fingers may be flexed. This position is comfortable for many patients, but if contractures of the muscles of the upper extremity develop, the potential for functional use of the extremity will be reduced. Therefore the upper extremity should be positioned in varying amounts of shoulder abduction and external rotation, elbow extension, slight wrist extension, thumb abduction and extension, and finger extension and slight abduction.

When a patient's lower extremity is involved, prolonged hip and knee flexion, hip external rotation, and ankle plantar flexion and inversion should be avoided. These positions are the ones that are most likely to lead to soft-tissue contractures caused by muscle spasticity, reduced function of the opposing muscle, and lack of active motion. The potential for function of the lower extremity will be reduced if contractures develop; therefore the lower extremity should be positioned in varying amounts of hip and knee extension, hip abduction and internal rotation, and ankle dorsiflexion and eversion.

However, static positioning of the extremities may not be the most effective treatment technique depending on the patient's neurological condition and response to positioning. The extremities should be exercised several times per day and should not remain in a single position for a prolonged period.

The normal alignment of the patient's head and trunk should be maintained when the person is sitting or lying. Frequent adjustments of posture or position may be necessary to ensure proper alignment.

Rheumatoid Arthritis

Rheumatoid arthritis is a systemic disease, and one of the major systems involved by the disease is the musculoskeletal system, especially the joints. Prolonged immobilization of the affected extremity joints should be avoided, particularly if the joint is maintained in flexion. Bony prominences, especially the elbows and greater trochanters, should be protected for the person who is immobile in bed. Gentle, careful, and frequent active or passive movement of the involved joints should be performed several times per day unless the joints are in a state of acute inflammation. The uninvolved joints should be exercised actively.

Contractures may develop even when various therapeutic measures are used. Carefully applied exercise can benefit most patients, but each patient should be given a treatment plan specifically designed for him or her. The patient will need to assume a great deal of the responsibility to maintain the body at its maximal level of function after being instructed by the appropriate caregiver or practitioner.

Split-Thickness Burns and Grafted Burn Areas

Healing or regenerating skin is likely to develop scar tissue, and contractures are likely to occur. It is important to avoid prolonged positioning of the joints that have been affected by the burn or the graft used to repair the wound. It is particularly important to avoid positions of comfort. A position of comfort for the patient with a burn is the position that does not produce stress or tension to the wound or graft. Prolonged flexion or adduction of most peripheral joints should be avoided when the burn is located on the flexor or adductor surface of a joint. The patient should be encouraged to perform gentle, careful, and frequent movement of the involved joints and should exercise the uninvolved joints. When the patient is unable to perform active exercise, passive exercise should be performed. It is important for the caregiver to adhere to the physician's instructions when treating a recently grafted area.

Usually the patient should not be allowed to assume the position that provides the greatest comfort for an extended period because contractures are more likely to develop when the position of comfort is maintained. Once a contracture has developed, time, exercise, and perseverance by the patient and health care providers will be necessary to return the joint to a normal position and functional use. The patient is likely to experience a great deal of pain and discomfort during the process used to restore normal joint motion. Everyone involved with the care and management of the patient, including the patient, must understand that prevention of a contracture is far more desirable and less costly than the treatment required to overcome one.

These examples of patient conditions illustrate the need for proper positioning techniques for selected patients. Many other patient problems require thoughtfulness and planning to prevent the development of contractures or to maintain function. The general rule to remember is that prolonged immobilization and failure to change positions frequently are precursors to the development of contractures, pressure areas, and decreased function.

Orthopedic Surgical Conditions

For a patient who has had a total knee replacement, it is important to keep the affected knee in extension. This position is not comfortable for the patient initially, but it will enhance future restoration of motion. Many patients are treated with a continuous passive motion machine immediately after surgery, which enhances knee motion. When the patient is not undergoing treatment with a continuous passive motion machine, the knee should be placed in full extension (with no pillow) and in a neutral position at the hips. A rolled towel or wedge can be used at the hip or lower leg, if necessary, to maintain a neutral position. Active assisted exercises and active range of motion exercises, as well as getting the patient out of bed at the earliest possible time, will benefit the patient.

For a patient who has undergone a total hip replacement, motion of the affected limb must be restricted to avoid excessive hip adduction, rotation, and flexion. An adduction pillow can be used to prevent excessive adduction, and a wedge or rolled towel will assist in preventing excessive hip rotation. Prevention of hip flexion beyond 90 degrees is most important when getting the patient out of bed or placing him or her in a chair and is covered in another chapter of this book.

DRAPING

The primary reasons to appropriately drape or clothe a patient are to expose or free an area to be treated; address modesty concerns; maintain a comfortable body temperature; and protect the skin and clothing from becoming soiled or damaged (Box 5-4). The caregiver must be aware that each patient has his or her own concept of modesty. Some patients may be embarrassed or consider their body to be excessively exposed when only the upper or lower extremity is uncovered. Others may seem to have a disregard for their modesty and may expose themselves, to the embarrassment of other patients or the caregiver.

A patient's cultural, religious, or personal preferences may affect the caregiver's ability to drape the patient to expose sufficient areas of the skin or body parts for treatment. For example, a Muslim woman may not permit any area of her body to be exposed to a man, so it may be necessary for a woman to perform the treatment. A man of the same faith will need to be treated by a man. Similar limitations may exist for nuns or other devout religious persons who are members of a particular group or sect. Therefore before positioning and draping a patient, it will be important for the caregiver to determine whether the patient has specific cultural, religion-based, or personal requests or preferences that would affect the draping process. Each patient should be informed of the type of clothing to be worn for the treatment session, or the facility may provide suitable clothing. Before treatment, the caregiver should inform the patient that clothing may need to be removed and why this step is necessary. The patient should be told that the body will be protected by linen or substitute garments, except for the areas to be treated. In some instances the caregiver will need to inform the patient that clothing may become soiled even though clean linen is used as protection.

The area to be treated must be exposed and have freedom of motion so treatment can be performed effectively and observation or palpation of the area can occur. However, if the patient senses or experiences exposure of a sensitive area of the body (e.g., the perineum, gluteal region, or anterior chest area in female patients), it is doubtful that the treatment session will be effective.

Another person may need to help the patient remove or apply clothing or drape material in preparation for treatment. If it is necessary to undress the patient, request

permission to do so. To avoid or reduce the transference of disease or infection from one patient to another, clean and previously unused linen and garments must be used for each patient. Soiled linen and garments must be properly disposed of at the conclusion of each treatment session. If body fluids have soiled the items, wear gloves when you handle them and discard them in an appropriate container. If an undergarment is removed, it is imperative that the patient's modesty be preserved throughout the treatment session.

Remember that some patients may be reluctant to remove their clothing, even after you have indicated that their modesty will be preserved. You can help reduce their apprehension by providing sufficient and appropriate draping materials, giving them instructions about how to apply or use the items, ensuring that the treatment cubicle is shielded by a closed curtain or door, asking permission to enter the cubicle and ensuring that they are draped, and, if necessary, having a caregiver who is the same gender as the patient help the patient to undress and dress. Access to the treatment area should be permitted only for persons required to provide treatment. Whenever the caregiver leaves the treatment cubicle, the patient should be dressed or draped so the body is not unduly exposed in case another person enters or looks into the cubicle.

With the patient supine, the upper extremities can be exposed for treatment (Fig. 5-8). Either the caregiver or the patient should remove any restrictive clothing, splints, or other devices to expose the areas to be treated. It may be necessary to provide a gown for the patient and to be certain that any clothing that was not removed does not restrict movement or access to the extremity. A towel, gown, or sheet can be used to drape the patient's anterior chest and lower extremities. The drape should not restrict joint motion or access to the area to be treated. In some instances it may be necessary to apply the drape into the axilla to shield the anterior and lateral areas of the chest.

With the patient supine, the lower extremities also can be exposed for treatment (Fig. 5-9). Either the caregiver or the patient should remove any restrictive clothing, splints, or other devices to expose the areas to be treated. Clothing

---

Box 5-4   Rationale for Patient Draping

Draping is important for the following reasons:
- It provides modesty for the patient.
- It helps the patient maintain an appropriate body temperature.
- It provides access and exposure to areas to be treated while protecting other areas.
- It protects the patient's skin or clothing from being soiled or damaged.

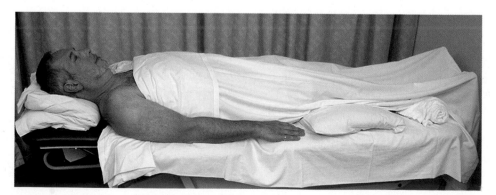

Fig. 5-8   Draping of a supine patient for treatment of the upper extremity.

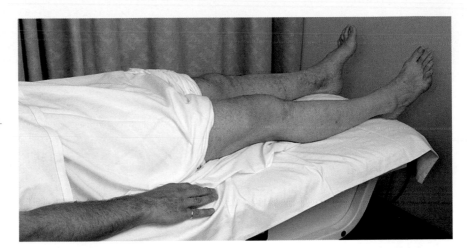

Fig. 5-9 Draping of a supine patient for treatment of the lower extremities.

not removed should not restrict motion or limit access to the area to be treated. A towel or sheet can be used to drape the patient's perineum (groin); the cover must be applied high in the groin and under the thigh to shield the perineum fully. Ascertain that the drape remains secure throughout the treatment and does not restrict joint motion of the hip or knee. If it is not to be treated, the patient's upper body and opposite lower extremity should be covered for warmth and to preserve modesty.

Draping material is frequently used to absorb perspiration, water, and various lubricants or to prevent these fluids from contacting the patient's clothing. It also is used to protect the patient's modesty and maintain body warmth. Therefore this material must not be used for another patient and must be disposed of at the termination of treatment. The patient should be instructed to dress or helped to dress at the end of the treatment. The caregiver should evaluate the patient's response to treatment at its conclusion. Specific draping techniques necessary for massage are beyond the scope of this book and are not presented; however, they are available in other textbooks.

SUMMARY

Use of proper techniques to position and drape a patient is important because these techniques protect the patient from injury, provide stabilization to an area, provide access while exposing only the specific area to be treated, maintain body temperature, and provide protection for unnecessary exposure of body areas, especially the breasts and perineum.

Prolonged use of any one position should be avoided to reduce the development of a soft-tissue contracture, soft-tissue pressure, or patient discomfort. Pillows, towel rolls, wedges, or similar devices can be used to promote comfort and stability, but they should be used with caution to avoid a position that may lead to a contracture. The caregiver should be aware of the body areas that will be affected most by pressure and by the positions selected so the areas can

be protected, the pressure can be relieved periodically, or the positions can be avoided.

self-study ACTIVITIES

- List at least three possible adverse effects of improper or prolonged positioning to the musculoskeletal, neuromuscular, and cardiopulmonary systems.
- Describe why proper patient positioning and draping are important for the practitioner.
- Explain why or how the patient positions presented in the text provide comfort for the patient.
- Outline the precautions you would use if it were necessary to position a patient who has decreased sensation, is elderly, is mentally confused, is unable to independently change position, has impaired respiration, or has impaired peripheral circulation.
- Explain how you would position and drape a patient for treatment to the right upper and lower extremities while supine and for treatment to the left upper and lower extremities while lying on the side.

problem SOLVING

1. A 55-year-old female inpatient with rheumatoid arthritis and acute inflammation of her left knee is to be examined and evaluated for exercise. Explain the procedures for draping, precautions to consider, and patient positioning.

2. A 65-year-old man with a left cerebral vascular accident has arrived in the department for treatment. The treatment plan includes passive, active assistive, and active exercise to the right upper and lower extremities. He wears a sling to support the right upper extremity and an ankle-foot orthosis on the right lower leg. Describe the procedures for assisting, draping, and patient positioning.

3. A female outpatient arrives for treatment of ultrasound and deep-tissue massage to the upper back, posterior neck, and shoulder areas. What instructions or directions would you give her before positioning her for treatment, and how would you position her for maximal comfort and exposure of the area to be treated?

CHAPTER 6

Basic Exercise: Passive and Active Range of Motion

objectives *After studying this chapter, the reader will be able to:*

- Differentiate among passive exercise, active assistive exercise, active exercise, and active resistive exercise.
- Provide a rationale for the use or objectives of each form of exercise.
- Discuss the principles of preparation for these forms of exercise.
- Discuss the principles of application of these forms of exercise.
- Demonstrate the application of passive, active assistive, and active resistive exercise.

key terms

Active assistive exercise Exercise performed by a person with manual or mechanical assistance; can be static or dynamic.

Active exercise Exercise performed by a person without any manual or mechanical assistance.

Active resistive exercise Exercise performed by a person against manual or mechanical resistance.

Adhesion A fibrous band of scar tissue that binds together anatomic structures that are normally separate.

Atrophy A decrease or reduction in the size of normally developed cells, tissues, organs, or body parts.

Capsular pattern A characteristic pattern for a given joint that limits joint motion and indicates that a problem exists within that joint.

Concentric contraction An overall shortening of a muscle as it develops tension and contracts; positive work is performed or movement is accelerated.

Contraction A drawing together or a shortening or shrinking (e.g., a muscle contracts).

Contracture A condition of shortening and hardening of muscles, tendons, or other tissue, often leading to deformity and rigidity of joints.

Dorsal Relating to the back or posterior of a structure (as opposed to the ventral, or front, of the structure). Some of the dorsal surfaces of the body are the back, buttocks, calves, and the knuckle side of the hand.

Eccentric contraction An overall lengthening of a muscle as it develops tension and contracts to control motion performed by an outside force; negative work is performed or movement is decelerated.

End feel The quality of the movement a person senses when pressure is applied passively to a joint at the end of its available range of motion.

Extrinsic Being, coming, or acting from the outside; not inherent.

Hypertrophy An increase in the cross-sectional size of a fiber or cell.

Isokinetic exercise A form of active resistive exercise; the speed of movement of the limb is controlled throughout the arc or range of motion, and the resistance offered is in direct proportion to the force offered by the patient throughout the range of motion of the exercise.

Isometric contraction A muscle contraction that develops tension but does not perform any mechanical work; no appreciable joint motion occurs, and the overall length of the muscle remains constant.

Isotonic contraction   A muscle contraction whereby tension is developed and movement of a joint or body part occurs; an eccentric or concentric contraction can occur, and the muscle may lengthen or shorten.

Joint play   The laxity or elasticity of a joint capsule that allows movement of the joint surfaces within the capsule.

Length-tension curve   The curve that accounts for the active and passive elements of muscle tension and dictates that optimal tension is developed at one point known as the resting length, the point in its range where peak torque is developed.

Passive exercise   Exercise performed on a person by manual or mechanical means; no voluntary muscle contraction occurs.

Phlebitis   Inflammation of a vein.

Pronation   The position of the forearm that places the palm downward; medial rotation of the forearm. The motion occurs in the forearm.

Proprioceptive neuromuscular facilitation (PNF)   A treatment technique that uses various stimuli to affect the muscle or joint proprioceptors to facilitate or alter movement responses.

Range of motion (ROM)   The normal extent of movement in a joint; the amount of motion allowed between two bony levers.

Resistance   A force external to the body that creates additional work for a muscle when it contracts.

Soft tissues   Tissues that lack bony or skeletal components; these tissues include muscle, ligament, joint capsule, tendon, skin, and fascia.

Stretching   Any therapeutic technique or procedure designed to lengthen or elongate shortened soft-tissue structures and to increase the range of motion.

Supination   The position of the forearm that places the palm upward; lateral rotation of the forearm. The motion occurs in the forearm.

Thrombophlebitis   Inflammation of a vein associated with the formation of a thrombus.

Thrombus   An aggregation of blood factors, primarily platelets and fibrin, with entrapment of cellular elements that frequently leads to a clot and obstruction of a blood vessel.

Volar   Pertaining to the palm; indicating the flexor surface of the forearm, wrist, or hand.

INTRODUCTION

Exercise is an important therapeutic intervention that is used to improve the functional capacity of patients. The general goals of exercise are to enhance the metabolic and physiological function or capacity of muscle, maintain or improve joint motion and range, and enhance efficiency of the cardiopulmonary system and independent function of the body. Exercise can affect strength, endurance, joint flexibility, coordination, and one's general sense of well-being.

The two basic types of exercise are active and passive. Each type has several benefits and limitations. In general terms, active exercise requires the patient to assist with or independently perform the exercise with the use of an active, voluntary contraction of muscle. In contrast, passive exercise is used for patients who are unable or not permitted to contract the muscles or who need to avoid undesired muscle contraction because of pain or adverse effects to the cardiopulmonary, musculoskeletal, or neuromuscular systems that may be associated with muscle contractions. When exercise is performed, the caregiver should consider the goals of providing exercise, the effect of gravity, the amount and type of stability and support necessary for the patient during the exercise, the purpose of the exercise, the ability of the patient to perform or participate in the activity, and the safety measures or protection required to avoid injury, an increase in the patient's symptoms, or worsening of the patient's condition.

Support should be provided to relieve stress to a joint or body area, control the weight of an extremity or body part, or compensate for the loss of muscle strength. The caregiver may need to use one or both hands to provide support to the segment or area. Support is used to promote motion or movement, whereas stabilization is used to avoid, limit, or prohibit movement. Use of stabilization is appropriate to protect the site of a healing fracture, areas of extensive soft-tissue trauma or damage, and the site of a recently injured, healing musculotendinous structure. Stabilization also may be used when movement of an uninvolved joint or body part is to be avoided. The caregiver will need to use both hands to stabilize the area by grasping above and below the site of the problem or securing one structure (e.g., the scapula) while moving or mobilizing another structure. In some instances, an external splint or bandage can be used as the stabilizing force provided it does not restrict or prevent the desired movement. The hand positions used by the caregiver may need to be revised as the exercise is performed to maintain proper control, support, or stability. The illustrations in this chapter will help you identify where to place your hands to provide support and stabilization. Future decisions about hand placement should be based on the individual patient's condition and the caregiver's knowledge, skill, experience, and competence.

The caregiver must integrate knowledge of the musculoskeletal, neuromuscular, and cardiopulmonary systems to properly determine and implement an exercise program. In addition, concepts and principles such as torque, force, force couples, levers, axis of motion, joint structures and components, muscle contractility and elasticity, stresses to skeletal and soft tissue, joint biomechanics, ligamentous and muscular attachments, sensation, neural innervation patterns, and muscle tone should be considered and applied by the caregiver. An explanation of these terms, concepts, and principles is beyond the scope of this textbook; see the Bibliography for appropriate resources.

The desired outcome of exercise must be determined and measured throughout the treatment program. Patient progression toward preestablished objectives or goals is the key determinant of the effectiveness of the treatment program and its procedures, techniques, or activities. The progression of the patient should be measured frequently and recorded in the patient's medical record.

Goniometric measurements (or measurements of joint range of motion with a goniometer) should be taken upon initial examination of the patient and throughout the treatment program. Practice of the art and science of goniometry is not covered in this book. The Centers for Disease Control and Prevention Joint Range of Motion Video (see the Bibliography) is an excellent goniometric measurement resource.

According to Wintz, "Manual Muscle Testing is a procedure for the evaluation of the function and strength of individual muscles and muscle groups based on effective performance of a movement in relation to the forces of gravity and manual resistance." Manual muscle testing of the patient must be performed initially and throughout the course of treatment. These measurements help establish short-term and long-term treatment goals and provide specific information to the patient and caregiver. Manual muscle testing will not be discussed further because it is beyond the scope of this book.

CARDINAL OR ANATOMIC PLANES OF MOTION

The cardinal planes of motion are associated with and described according to the anatomic position. A person who is standing upright is considered to be in the anatomic position when the upper extremities are relaxed along the sides of the trunk, the shoulders are externally rotated, the forearms are supinated, and the fingers are extended and adducted; the lower extremities are parallel and in neutral rotation, the heels are approximately 4 inches apart, and the toes are directed forward; and the face is directed forward with the head in neutral flexion-extension, rotation, and lateral bending.

The three cardinal planes are the sagittal, frontal or coronal, and transverse planes (Figure 6-1). The sagittal

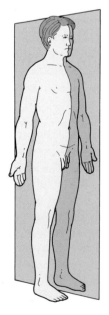
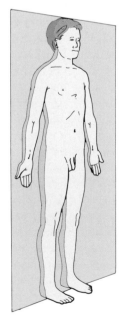
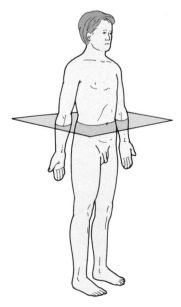

Sagittal plane   Frontal or coronal plane   Transverse plane

Fig. 6-1 Anatomic body planes. (From Cameron MH, Monroe LG: *Physical rehabilitation: evidence-based examination, evaluation, and intervention,* Philadelphia, 2007, Saunders Elsevier.)

plane is a vertical plane that divides the body into left and right components; flexion and extension occur in this plane. The frontal plane is a vertical plane that divides the body into front (anterior) and back (posterior) components; except in the thumb, abduction and adduction occur in this plane. The transverse plane is a horizontal plane that divides the body into upper and lower components; rotation occurs in this plane.

TYPES OF EXERCISE FOR RANGE OF MOTION

Passive range of motion (PROM) is the movement of a joint or body segment by a force external to the body within an unrestricted and normal ROM without active, voluntary muscle contraction by the patient. The external force may be applied in three ways: (1) manually by the patient or another person; (2) mechanically with the use of weights or pulleys, a continuous passive motion unit, or the passive mode on an isokinetic unit; or (3) by gravity. PROM differs from passive stretching. When PROM is used, no increase in joint range should be expected; rather, the goal or objective is to maintain the unrestricted joint range. When passive stretching is used, the goal or objective is to increase the restricted joint range to full joint range. Only PROM techniques are described in this book.

Active range of motion exercise (AROM) is the movement of a joint or body segment produced by active, voluntary muscle contractions by the patient within the unrestricted, normal ROM. No increase in joint range should be expected, but strength and endurance can be increased.

Active assistive ROM exercise is a form of active exercise whereby an external force is used to help the patient perform the exercise. The assistance may be applied manually, mechanically, or by gravity. The patient still must perform active, voluntary muscle contractions to the extent that he or she is able to do so. This technique may be used when muscular weakness, fatigue, or pain limit the patient's performance and when active, voluntary muscle contractions are desired.

Indications for Passive Range of Motion Exercise

In general, PROM is used when a patient is unable to perform any form of active exercise. Examples of indications for PROM are when paralysis is present, when the patient is comatose, when pain occurs if an active muscle contraction is attempted, and when recovery from trauma or a surgical procedure prohibits active muscle contraction. PROM also is used to avoid exercise of an unhealed fracture when healing of the fracture would be disrupted with active muscle contractions. PROM is used to counteract the negative aspects of immobilization, evaluate joint range and

Box **6-1** Benefits of Passive Exercise

- Preserves and maintains range of motion
- Minimizes contracture formation
- Minimizes adhesion formation
- Maintains mechanical elasticity of muscle
- Promotes and maintains local circulation
- Promotes awareness of joint motion (i.e., sensory awareness)
- Evaluates joint integrity and motion
- Enhances cartilage nutrition and stimulates movement of synovial fluid
- Inhibits or reduces pain

flexibility, provide sensory stimulation and awareness, and reduce stress on the cardiopulmonary system.

PROM is usually contraindicated when passive movement increases the patient's symptoms or intensifies the condition and when the person is capable of and would benefit from some type of active exercise.

Several benefits can result from PROM. It can assist in preserving and maintaining existing ROM; it can minimize the development of muscle shortening or the development of capsular, ligamentous, or tendinous adhesions resulting from immobilization; and it can assist in maintaining the mechanical elasticity of muscle. PROM also assists in maintaining local circulation and maintaining or developing a patient's awareness of joint motion by enhancing kinesthesia, proprioception, mental imaging, and sensory awareness. PROM can be used to evaluate joint ROM, stability, flexibility, and muscle tone. Cartilage nutrition and movement of the synovial fluid in the joint capsule are enhanced by PROM. The movement a patient is expected to perform with active exercise can be demonstrated passively to help the patient learn the desired movement. Finally, PROM may reduce or inhibit pain when proper support is given to a specific joint or body segment (Box 6-1).

The caregiver should be aware of the limitations of PROM. It cannot prevent muscle atrophy; maintain or increase muscle tone, strength, or contractile endurance; or reduce adipose tissue. Although PROM can assist in maintaining local circulation, it is not as effective as active exercise. The caregiver usually will find it difficult to apply PROM when the patient's muscles are fully innervated and the patient is conscious or when pain occurs with movement.

The best results can be expected when PROM is performed by a conscientious individual who integrates what is palpated, sensed, and observed during treatment. The progression to active assistive exercise, observation of changes in the joint range, and being alert to additional patient responses are the responsibilities of the primary caregiver, particularly if the exercise activities are assigned to supportive persons (e.g., family members, aides, or assistants).

Indications for Active Range of Motion Exercise

In general, AROM is used when a patient is able to voluntarily contract, control, and coordinate muscular movements with or without assistance, when no contraindications to its use exist, and when its established benefits are desirable to fulfill the goals of the patient's treatment.

AROM may be contraindicated in patients with cardiopulmonary dysfunction, an unhealed and unprotected fracture site, an unhealed and unprotected recent surgical site, or severe soft tissue trauma. Caution in the use of AROM is recommended when soft tissue or joint pain or joint swelling is apparent, which may occur with many conditions such as acute osteoarthritis, acute rheumatoid arthritis, or hemophilia. If active exercise increases the patient's symptoms or the condition intensifies, or when improper or substitutive movement patterns are used, active exercise may be contraindicated.

Benefits associated with AROM include maintaining the physiological elasticity, strength, and contractile endurance of muscle and increasing the local circulation. AROM also provides increased sensory awareness of joint motion, which is associated with proprioception, kinesthesia, and coordination. The cardiopulmonary functions of cardiac output, capillary efficiency, stroke volume, oxygen uptake, gas exchange in the lungs, and overall cardiac efficiency can be maintained or improved when multiple muscles contract simultaneously and the patient is in a deconditioned physiological state. Active exercise such as repetitive ankle dorsiflexion-plantar flexion ("ankle pumping") can be used to assist in preventing the development of a thrombus, thrombophlebitis, or phlebitis in the peripheral veins of the lower legs. The stimulus of stress that is produced by muscle contraction will help the tendon-bone interface maintain its structural integrity. Finally, AROM can improve muscle strength in a patient whose strength is measured at a grade of "fair" (50% or less of normal) on a manual muscle test. Muscles that initially are stronger than fair need to contract against external resistance, in addition to the weight of the segment, to increase the strength of the muscle (Box 6-2).

AROM will not develop strength in muscles when the initial strength is measured at a grade of "good" (75% or more) on a manual muscle test. Furthermore, cardiopulmonary efficiency in a normally conditioned or well-conditioned person may be maintained but will not be increased unless vigorous aerobic exercise is performed.

AROM is usually more beneficial than PROM for a patient, but the caregiver must determine which type of exercise should be used. A treatment program may begin with PROM, progress to active assistive ROM exercise and

---

Box **6-2** Benefits of Active Exercise

- Maintains physiological elasticity, strength, and contractile endurance of muscle
- Increases local circulation
- Increases awareness of joint motion and sensory awareness
- Maintains and improves cardiopulmonary functions, especially with aerobic exercise
- May help prevent thrombus formation in lower extremities when ankle flexion-extension movements are used (i.e., "ankle pumping")
- Maintains and promotes the structural integrity of the tendon-bone interface
- Improves muscle strength with the use of external resistance

---

then to active free exercise, and eventually lead to active resistive exercise, depending on the goals of treatment and the patient's physical abilities. This progression requires the skill and knowledge of the caregiver to determine when the exercise progression should occur. The patient should be encouraged to perform within his or her ability but at maximal effort levels whenever possible. Caregivers are cautioned to remind patients to breathe normally while performing active exercise to avoid the potential adverse effects of the Valsalva phenomenon, described in Chapter 4.

PROM and AROM can be performed in the traditional anatomic planes or in diagonal planes of motion using the patterns of proprioceptive neuromuscular facilitation (PNF). Motion also may be performed in specific arcs or planes of motion of any joint to better affect a given muscle or portion of the joint range. The caregiver will need to decide which motions to perform and whether to perform them through the full range or through only a portion of the range. The decisions should be based on evaluation and observation of the patient's responses to the exercise and the patient's condition.

PREPARATION FOR APPLICATION OF PASSIVE RANGE OF MOTION AND ACTIVE RANGE OF MOTION

Initially, you should examine and evaluate the patient and obtain information from the medical record or other reliable sources to assist in determining the goals of treatment and the type of exercise to be used. Introduce yourself to the patient and explain the rationale or purpose, the risks if any exist, and the desired outcome of treatment. Obtain the patient's consent to perform treatment before you begin. You should be prepared to respond to questions regarding the treatment before you start the exercise program.

PROCEDURE 6-1

Procedures for Basic Exercise Activities

- Examine and evaluate the patient to determine the exercise needs and establish appropriate outcome goals; discuss the exercise program with the patient.
- Develop a treatment plan designed to meet the patient's needs and outcome goals (i.e., frequency, duration, and sequence); obtain consent from the patient.
- Select the treatment activities, techniques, and procedures that will most likely fulfill the predetermined needs and outcome goals effectively and within an acceptable period.
- Be prepared to protect structures that are unstable or vulnerable to injury during exercise (e.g., hypermobile or flaccid joints, healing fracture or surgical sites, and muscle and ligamentous strains or sprains).
- Instruct the patient about performance responsibilities and maintaining a breathing pattern to avoid the Valsalva maneuver.
- Perform movements smoothly and slowly throughout the unrestricted range of motion; resistive exercises should be performed within the patient's physical limits.
- Proper precautions must be established; equipment must be secure and free from damage, and proper body mechanics should be used by the patient and caregiver.
- The caregiver should monitor the effects of the exercise, especially when cardiopulmonary dysfunction exists.
- The exercise plan, activities, techniques, or procedures should be revised or modified depending on the patient's response and progress toward the outcome goals; the program should be discontinued if adverse effects occur and persist for 24 hours or longer.

Box 6-3 Principles of Exercise Activities

- The patient should not be challenged to exceed maximal physical capabilities.
- The patient should be instructed to maintain a normal breathing pattern to avoid the Valsalva maneuver.
- Avoid applying excessive stress to the patient's skin, soft tissues, joints, and bones when manual or mechanical resistance is used.
- Protect structures that are unstable or vulnerable to injury, such as hypermobile joints, healing fracture sites, healing surgical sites, and muscle or ligamentous strains or sprains.
- Monitor the effect of exercise closely for patients who have a known history of cardiopulmonary dysfunction (e.g., monitor vital signs and observe for signs of exercise intolerance such as a flushed face or a frown or grimace).
- Evaluate the equipment being used to ensure that it is secure and stable and that it functions properly.
- The caregiver and patient should use proper body mechanics during exercise.

PRINCIPLES OF PASSIVE RANGE OF MOTION EXERCISE

PROM can be a beneficial treatment approach when a patient is unable to actively move a body segment; to avoid pain, undesired movements or patterns of motion, or development of undesired muscle tone; and to reduce stress to a localized site of poor integrity or to the cardiopulmonary system. The patient does not assist with the movements—instead, an external manual, mechanical, or gravitational force is used to provide motion of the segment. None of these external mechanical forces is described or depicted in this book, but sources of such information can be found in the Bibliography.

Manual PROM can be performed by the patient (self-performed ROM), by a family member, or by a trained professional. Gentle, firm support and stabilization through proper hand placement and control should be provided to avoid stress to the structures or segment being moved. Practice will help the caregiver determine the best hand placements (areas of grasp) to provide smooth, controlled, and complete motion with minimal adjustments. All planes of motion of the joint should be exercised, which may require moving the joint through a variety or combination of motions. Although it is possible to passively move several joints simultaneously, initially you should evaluate the range of each joint individually. This step will assist in determining whether a limitation exists in the range of one or more of the joints. If all joint ranges of the segment or extremity are similar, time can be saved by performing PROM to multiple joints simultaneously.

Position the patient to have access to the extremities, align and support the trunk and extremities, enhance your body mechanics, and provide patient comfort to the extent that it is compatible with the treatment. Restrictive clothing, orthoses, and linen should be removed or loosened. Be certain that sufficient space exists to perform the treatment, and drape the patient to protect modesty, maintain warmth, and expose the area or segment to be treated. Remember to use proper body mechanics when performing the exercises. Use of proper body mechanics can be facilitated by adjusting the height of the bed; adjusting the position of the patient on the bed, treatment table, or chair; and positioning yourself close to the patient. Obtain assistance in moving or positioning the patient when necessary (Procedure 6-1 and Box 6-3).

Table **6-1** End Feel: Normal and Abnormal

End Feel	Normal	Abnormal	Example
A "hard" unyielding painless sensation	Hard—bone to bone		Elbow extension
A yielding compression that halts further movement	Soft—soft tissue approximation		Knee or elbow flexion
A firm (springy) type of movement with a slight give; toward the end of the ROM, there is a feeling of elastic resistance	Firm—tissue stretch		Hip rotation, ankle dorsiflexion, finger extension
This end feel is invoked by movement, usually with pain; the end feel is sudden and hard; the muscle spasm occurs early in the ROM, almost as movement starts		Early muscle spasm	Acute protective spasm indicative of inflammation
This end feel occurs late in the ROM at or near the end of range; it is caused by instability and resulting irritability caused by movement		Late muscle spasm	Spasm caused by instability as in the apprehension test for shoulders
This end feel is similar to firm tissue stretch but does not occur where one would expect; the end feel has a thick feel to it and limitation comes abruptly after a smooth, frictionless movement		Hard capsule	Frozen shoulder, chronic conditions
This end feel is similar to "normal" but with a restricted ROM; often found in acute conditions, with stiffness early in the range and increasing until the end of range; it has a soft, boggy end feel		Soft capsule	Synovitis, soft tissue edema
This abnormal bone-to-bone end feel comes well before the normal end of ROM		Bone to bone	Osteophyte formation
This end feel occurs when considerable pain is produced by movement; the movement is stopped by pain with no mechanical resistance		Empty	Acute subacromial bursitis
This end feel is similar to a tissue stretch, but occurs unpredictably; it usually occurs in joints with a meniscus and there is a rebound effect, which usually indicates an internal derangement		Springy block	Meniscus tear

ROM, Range of motion.
From Watkinson A: *End feel.* Available at www.watkinson.co.n2\end_feel.htm.

PROM should be performed through the entire unrestricted, normal range of the joint and soft tissue. The caregiver must be aware of normal joint range parameters and must perceive or sense the resistance, or lack of resistance, from the soft tissue or joint capsule and other joint structures as the exercise is being performed. This is the concept of *end feel*, or the "feel" of the resistance of the tissue at the end or completion of the range. To determine that feel, an excess pressure known as "overpressure" is applied at the end of the range. End feels are described as "soft" when soft tissues are compressed or stretched (as in elbow or knee flexion), "firm" when joint capsules or ligaments are stretched (as in hip rotation), "hard" when a bony block or resistance is reached (as in elbow extension), or "empty" when no end feel is elicited because the patient does not permit full motion to occur, usually because of acute pain. An abnormal end feel may result from muscle guarding, a muscle spasm, muscle spasticity, or an intraarticular block such as a torn articular cartilage or

a loose body in the joint. The caregiver should evaluate the ROM in relation to these normal and abnormal end feels, or capsular patterns, and adjust the treatment as necessary. When assessing passive movements, the caregiver with a proper evaluation of end feel can assist in determining a prognosis for the condition and learn the severity of the problem. Table 6-1 explains normal and abnormal end feels as described by Alan Watkinson (see Bibliography).

Muscles that cross more than one joint (i.e., multijoint muscles) must be identified and given special consideration when PROM is performed. Some examples of multijoint muscles are the biceps and triceps, extrinsic finger flexors and extensors, the quadriceps (rectus femoris), the hamstrings, and the gastrocnemius. It is important to differentiate between the available or normal joint range and the muscle range when multijoint muscles are involved. To allow full joint motion to occur, multijoint muscles must be relaxed and must not be lengthened simultaneously over the joints they cross. Joint motion is important because it assists in maintaining proper capsular and ligamentous flexibility. Motion over the full muscle range is performed to assist in maintaining the length or flexibility of the muscles and tendons that cross a given joint. Multijoint muscles must be lengthened simultaneously over each joint they cross to maintain their functional length.

This concept is particularly important when you are applying PROM to the extrinsic flexors and extensors of the fingers. For example, to maintain the length of the extrinsic finger extensors, wrist flexion should be combined with finger flexion. Conversely, to maintain the length of the extrinsic finger flexors, wrist extension should be combined with finger extension. However, at least one patient condition exists for which full lengthening of the extrinsic finger flexors usually is contraindicated: a patient with a spinal cord injury that has spared the C6 nerve root may benefit from tightness or limited range of the extrinsic finger flexors. Limited range of the finger flexors, when combined with active wrist extension, can provide the person with a passive grasp. As the wrist is extended, the finger flexors, already limited in length, are elongated or stretched over the volar area of the wrist, which further shortens them. When this stretching occurs, a gross, passive grasp develops, known as a "tenodesis" (tendon fixation or suturing) grasp or movement. Relaxation of the wrist extensors allows the hand to lower and releases the passive tension on the finger flexors. This phenomenon is the opening phase of the grasp-and-release action.

Other persons with a spinal cord injury may benefit if their erector spinae muscles are not elongated by passive exercise because their trunk stability when they sit may be improved by the limited length or range of those muscles. Stability of a hypermobile joint may be enhanced if the muscles that cross or support the joint are not elongated fully, but a contracture of the joint should be avoided.

Another contraindication to be considered during ROM exercises is a total hip replacement. If the total hip replacement was done posteriorly, no hip adduction past neutral, no hip flexion past 90 degrees, and no internal hip rotation past neutral on the affected side should be performed.

Techniques for ROM exercise to be used with a hemiplegic patient vary somewhat from other diagnoses in that sensory stimulation, along with passive or active assistive movement, may assist the patient; therefore PNF patterns, as shown later in this chapter, may be of benefit. In an *eMedicine* article, Gould and Barnes state that PROM should be performed with a gentle, slow motion, a rhythmic stabilization, or a voluntary contraction followed by gentle stretching or relaxation. If the hemiplegic patient has flaccid musculature or hypermobility in the joints, ROM will need to be performed with the joints supported and stabilized. If the patient demonstrates hypertonicity in the musculature,

slower gradual movement during ROM will be necessary to avoid unwanted spasticity. The goals in ROM exercises for hemiplegic patients are to prevent contractures, maintain ROM, and provide protection from shoulder subluxation by proper positioning of the affected side.

Although most of the photographs in this book show patients in the supine or prone position when PROM is performed, other positions also may be used depending on the patient's condition. Many PROM activities can be performed with the patient sitting in a wheelchair or other type of chair, lying on his or her side, or standing. Mechanical devices such as pulleys or continuous passive motion units can be used as adjuncts to manual PROM techniques.

Research studies have not specifically determined the frequency or number of repetitions necessary for PROM to be effective. Many factors affect joint or muscle range, and no assurance exists that PROM will, in and of itself, maintain the free, unrestricted range of a given joint or muscles. The results of PROM activities are affected by the use of protective equipment, the positioning regimens that are utilized, the general medical and nursing care that is provided, and the patient's specific type of illness or trauma. The skill, knowledge, and judgment of the caregiver are required to reach decisions regarding the actual protocol that is applicable for each patient. Therefore the caregiver must evaluate the patient's response to treatment frequently and consistently and make adjustments to the plan of care for the patient as needed.

The caregiver also must understand and recognize which muscles or soft tissues are affected by the application of PROM. In general, a passive movement should be performed in the direction opposite to the movement the muscle would produce if it were to contract actively. For example, passive elbow extension is performed to lengthen the biceps, passive knee flexion is performed to lengthen the quadriceps, and passive ankle dorsiflexion is performed to lengthen the gastrocnemius-soleus muscle complex. This concept can be applied to movement of other muscles, soft tissues, and joints. A muscle or soft tissue that is limited in its ability to relax or lengthen will produce a contracture in the same direction as the movement the muscle would produce if it were to contract actively. Some muscles that can and often do produce contractures are the biceps, hamstrings, and gastrocnemius.

Before starting PROM, determine the purpose or goals of each exercise and discuss the goals with the patient. It is helpful to establish a sequence for the exercise program so you will be more likely to perform each motion and be less likely to omit a motion. For example, perform all shoulder movements, then exercise the elbow, and then exercise the forearm, wrist, and fingers. For the lower extremity (LE), perform all hip movements, then all knee movements, and then all ankle and foot movements. In some situations, it may be desirable or beneficial to perform two or more movements simultaneously; in other situations, it may be undesirable to combine movements. These situations are explained as they arise in the progression of the exercise program.

During the application of PROM, you must be alert in order to perceive and determine the patient's response to the exercises. Although these exercises are passive for the patient, the caregiver must be physically and mentally involved. Position yourself so you are able to observe the patient's face as you perform each exercise and as you exercise the extremity nearest to you. To reduce strain on your body, decrease the expenditure of energy, and ensure safety for the patient, avoid reaching across an extremity or the patient's trunk to exercise the more distant extremity.

All motions should be performed slowly, with a brief pause at the point of greatest joint range or elongation of a muscle. You should sense or perceive when the terminal, unrestricted joint range or muscle elongation has occurred and stop the exercise at that point. Remember that PROM exercise is different from stretching and that no increase in joint range or muscle length should be anticipated.

Proper support and stabilization of segments and joints must be incorporated into the exercise. The patient must develop trust and confidence that the caregiver will not cause further injury or pain during the performance of the exercises. This trust and confidence can be established by the manner in which the caregiver physically handles the patient and by explaining the intent or purpose of each exercise. After several exercise sessions have been completed, it should not be necessary to reexplain the intent or purpose of each exercise unless new exercises are initiated (Procedure 6-2).

Traditional Passive Range of Motion Movements

Upper Extremity Movements

Traditional Anatomic Planes. Position the properly draped patient supine on a firm surface and close to the near edge of the treatment table, mat table, or bed. Other positions can be used depending on the patient's condition and the caregiver's preference.

Elongation of Multijoint Muscles. Review the information presented earlier in this chapter with regard to the concepts related to joint range and the range of multijoint muscles. Initially, all motions should be performed individually so that the multijoint muscle is elongated over only one joint. This technique will assist in determining the muscle's free unrestricted range and will prevent excessive elongation of the muscle or excessive stress to the joint and its capsule.

Lower Extremity Movements

Traditional Anatomic Planes. The primary patient position is supine on a firm surface, properly draped, and

---

PROCEDURE 6-2

Application of Passive Exercise

- Position the patient for support, stability, and access to the area or segment to be exercised; drape the patient as necessary.
- Explain the purpose and goals of passive exercise and obtain consent for treatment.
- Position the patient to promote use of proper body mechanics by the patient and caregiver.
- Grasp the part to be treated to provide support, stability, and control. Refer to the photographs and instructions in this chapter for specific information about this step.
- Perform exercises through the complete, unrestricted range of motion.
- Perform the predetermined number of repetitions and frequency of exercises based on the patient's needs and goals.
- Perform the exercises smoothly and slowly; pause at the start and end positions of the exercise.
- At the conclusion of treatment, position the patient for proper alignment, support, and safety; drape or replace clothing for modesty and body temperature control.
- Evaluate the patient's response to treatment and document important findings.

---

positioned close to the near edge of the treatment table. Other positions can be used depending on the patient's condition and the caregiver's preference.

Elongation of Multijoint Muscles. For the hamstrings, start with the patient supine and the knee extended; perform hip flexion while maintaining the knee in extension. Terminate the motion when you sense maximal tension in the hamstring muscles or when the patient reports discomfort (see Fig. 6-27).

Trunk Movements

Traditional Anatomic Planes. You must use proper body mechanics when performing some of these motions to prevent unnecessary strain on the structures of your back and to protect the patient from discomfort and injury. Caution: Before applying PROM exercises to the cervical spine, the caregiver should use the vertebral artery occlusion test to evaluate the ability of the vertebral artery to maintain adequate blood flow to the brain (Procedure 6-3). Patient complaints of dizziness, lightheadedness, or visual problems (i.e., diplopia) indicate a compromise of the arterial blood flow. Further treatment should be withheld or performed cautiously until the results of additional medical tests are available. The physician should be notified about any abnormal vascular insufficiency observed during patient testing.

PROCEDURE 6-3

Vertebral Artery Occlusion Test

Position the person so he or she is supine and passively perform the following movements:
- Full head and neck extension
- Full head and neck rotation to the left and right with the head and neck in the neutral position
- Full head and neck rotation to the left and right with the head and neck in extension
- Simulated mobilization movements* and unilateral posteroanterior oscillation of C1-C2 facet joints with the head rotated left and right (prone lying)

Maintain each position for 10 to 15 seconds or until symptoms occur; wait 10 seconds between each test after returning the head and neck to a neutral position. Positive findings include complaints of dizziness, diplopia, light-headedness, or visual disturbances.

Data from Magee DJ: *Orthopedic physical assessment,* ed 4, Philadelphia, 2002, Saunders Elsevier.
*Simulated mobilization movement: passively position the cervical spine for each mobilization or manipulation without actually performing the mobilization.

Diagonal Patterns for Passive Range of Motion Movements Instead of using traditional anatomic planes of motion, diagonal patterns can be used. These patterns have the following stated and reported advantages:
- They incorporate rotation with all movements.
- The midline of the body is crossed with many of the movements.
- The movements tend to be more functional than traditional straight plane or anatomic plane movements.
- A combination of motions occurs within each pattern.
- Efficiency of treatment is achieved by exercising multiple joints with one motion.

The patterns were developed as components of the therapeutic approach known as PNF. The patterns can be performed actively by the patient, passively by a caregiver, or resistively against an external force. This book is not meant to be a complete resource for PNF patterning; more information can be found in *Proprioceptive Neuromuscular Facilitation* by Voss, Ionta, and Myers (see the Bibliography).

Two basic diagonal patterns are used for the upper and LE—diagonal 1 and diagonal 2—and each of them can be performed in flexion and extension, resulting in a total of four different movements. Thus the patterns are identified as "diagonal 1 flexion," "diagonal 2 flexion," "diagonal 1 extension," and "diagonal 2 extension." Furthermore, each pattern can be performed by the upper and lower extremity and thus is termed "diagonal 1 flexion upper extremity,"

"diagonal 1 flexion lower extremity," and so on. Common abbreviations of the patterns are D1 Fl UE (diagonal 1 flexion upper extremity), D2 Fl UE (diagonal 2 flexion upper extremity), D1 Ex UE (diagonal 1 extension upper extremity), D2 Ex UE (diagonal 2 extension upper extremity), D1 Fl LE (diagonal 1 flexion lower extremity), D2 Fl LE (diagonal 2 flexion lower extremity), D1 Ex LE (diagonal 1 extension lower extremity), and D2 Ex LE (diagonal 2 extension lower extremity).

The patterns are named according to the position of the proximal joint of the pattern (i.e., the shoulder or the hip) at the conclusion of the pattern. Thus the pattern is initiated with the proximal joint positioned opposite to its position at the conclusion of the pattern. Each pattern contains a flexion or extension component, an abduction or adduction component, and an internal or external rotation component for the proximal joint. All three motions must be performed, especially the rotation component. Other extremity joints or components also will have a final position, but the patterns are described according to the final position of the proximal joint. Refer to Table 6-2 for a description of each pattern.

The caregiver should be positioned so he or she is able to move in a diagonal direction as the patterns are performed. Pivoting on the feet is necessary to avoid improper and stress-producing body movements. Proper positioning and movement must be used consistently by the caregiver when diagonal patterns are performed passively to reduce stress and strain and to complete each pattern.

Remember that these patterns describe the positions of the proximal components at the completion of the pattern. To start a pattern, the proximal joint of the extremity is placed in the position that is the reciprocal of the completed pattern. For example, to initiate D1 Fl UE, the shoulder is positioned in D1 Ex UE. How would you position the extremity to initiate D1 Fl LE or D2 Fl UE? Note that when PNF patterns are used for any form of active exercise, the hand placement by the caregiver should provide a tactile contact and stimulus to the major muscles involved in producing the desired extremity movement. For those situations, the caregiver's grasp must contact the skin surface overlying the muscle or muscles that are to contract and avoid contact with the muscle or muscles that are to relax during the exercise. However, when diagonal patterns are used for PROM, hand placement is not as critical and may be altered to provide better support and stability to an extremity. Therefore the caregiver's hand placement in the photographs depicting the use of diagonal patterns for PROM may vary from the hand positions that would be used to tactilely stimulate the contracting muscles.

Upper Extremity

Flexion and Extension with the Elbow Extended. These four patterns can be performed with the elbow flexed. Hand

Text continued on page 125

UPPER EXTREMITY MOVEMENTS: TRADITIONAL ANATOMIC PLANES

Scapulothoracic

Movement: Scapular elevation and depression
Hand placement and motion: Cup the inferior angle with one hand while resting the other hand on the superior border of the scapula; move the scapula upward and downward.
Movement: Scapular protraction (abduction) and retraction (adduction)
Hand placement and motion: Rest one hand over the medial (vertebral) border while resting the other hand over the acromion process of the scapula; move the scapula toward and away from the spinous processes.

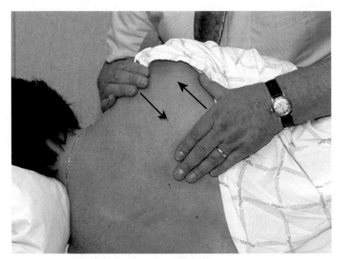

Fig. 6-2   Scapular elevation and depression.

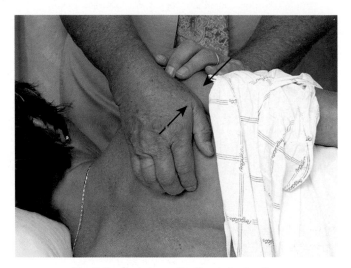

Fig. 6-3   Scapular protraction and retraction.

Movement: Scapular vertebral border lift ("winging")
Hand placement and motion: Slide the fingertips of one hand under the medial (vertebral) border of the scapula; gently lift the scapula from the ribs. It will be easier to grasp the vertebral border if the patient's UE is relaxed behind the trunk while in a side-lying position.

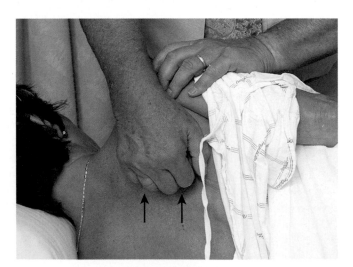

Fig. 6-4   Scapular vertebral border lift.

Glenohumeral

Movement: Shoulder flexion and extension

Hand placement and motion: For the right UE, grasp the right wrist and hand with your left hand and grasp the right elbow with your right hand; lift the extremity through the available range and return. Extension of the arm beyond the midline of the body produces hyperextension. You can accomplish this movement with the patient supine and the shoulder at the edge of the support surface or with the patient in a side-lying or prone position.

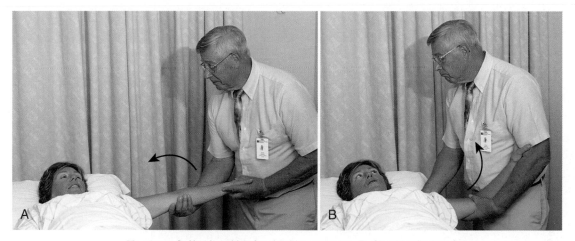

Fig. 6-5   **A,** Hand position for shoulder extension. **B,** Shoulder flexion.

Movement: Shoulder abduction and adduction

Hand placement and motion: Grasp the wrist and elbow; move the extremity away from the trunk and return it to its original position. The elbow may be extended or flexed, but avoid shoulder flexion and maintain the arm horizontal to the floor. It may be necessary to externally rotate the humerus to reduce impingement of the humeral head on the acromion process. In some instances it may be helpful to prevent excessive elevation of the scapula by placing one hand over its superior border. When the exercise is performed with the elbow extended, adjust your position by moving toward the patient's head.

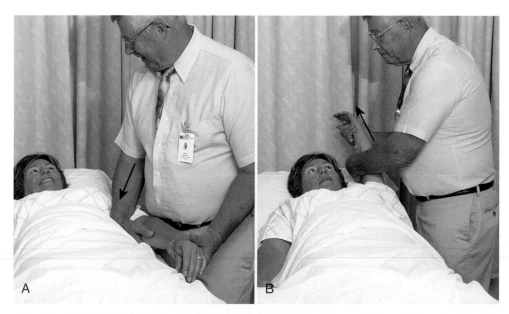

Fig. 6-6   **A,** Shoulder abduction with the elbow extended. **B,** Shoulder abduction with the elbow flexed.

Continued

Movement: Shoulder horizontal adduction and abduction

Hand placement and motion: Grasp the wrist and elbow; begin with the patient's shoulder abducted to 90 degrees and parallel to the floor. Lift the arm up and across the upper chest and return it to its original position. To attain full abduction, the patient's shoulder must be at the edge of the supporting surface to allow the humerus to clear the edge of the table. The elbow may be flexed or extended.

Movement: Shoulder internal (medial) rotation

Hand placement and motion: Abduct the shoulder to 90 degrees and flex the elbow to 90 degrees. Position yourself opposite the patient's elbow and face the patient. Grasp the patient's wrist with one hand and support the hand; rest the other hand on the acromion process or use it to support the distal end of the humerus (**A**). Move the forearm forward toward the floor, causing the humerus to rotate (**B**). Stop the motion when the acromion process tips forward, indicating that the head of the humerus has been blocked by the acromion.

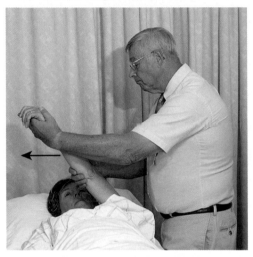

Fig. 6-7   Shoulder horizontal adduction.

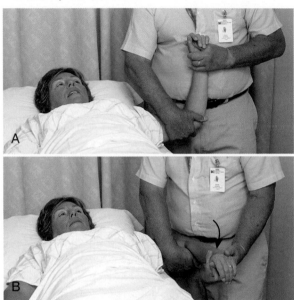

Fig. 6-8   **A,** Hand positions for shoulder rotation. **B,** Internal (medial) shoulder rotation.

Movement: Shoulder external (lateral) rotation

Hand placement and motion: Use the same hand placement described for internal rotation. Move the forearm backward toward the floor, causing the humerus to rotate. Stop the motion when the forearm is horizontal to the floor. (Note: Shoulder internal/external rotation can be performed with the elbow extended and the extremity positioned along the patient's side. To do so, grasp the humerus just above the epicondyles and grasp the forearm at the wrist; turn or roll the entire extremity inward and outward. As an alternative method, start with the humerus next to the trunk and the elbow flexed to 90 degrees. Grasp the distal end of the forearm, support the patient's hand, and move the forearm toward and away from the chest without abducting or adducting the shoulder. When this technique is used, internal rotation will be incomplete because the forearm will strike the chest before the complete range is attained.)

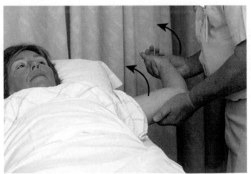

Fig. 6-9   External (lateral) shoulder rotation.

Humeral-Ulnar

Movement: Elbow flexion and extension

Hand placement and motion: For the right UE, grasp the patient's distal forearm and support the hand with your left hand; use your right hand to support and stabilize the distal end of the humerus. Flex and extend the elbow with the forearm neutral, pronated, and supinated, but avoid any shoulder motion.

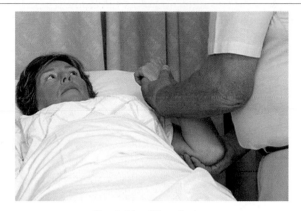

Fig. 6-10   Elbow flexion.

Radial-Ulnar

Movement: Forearm supination and pronation

Hand placement and motion: For the right forearm, grasp the distal end of the forearm and support the patient's hand with either your left or your right hand; use your other hand to support and stabilize the humerus. Supinate and pronate the forearm. This exercise can be performed with the elbow flexed or extended, but the motion must occur in the forearm. Avoid shoulder rotation and reduce stress to the wrist by grasping the distal end of the forearm. This motion can be combined with elbow flexion and extension.

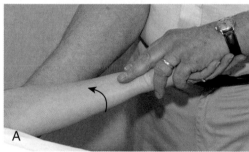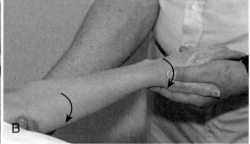

Fig. 6-11   **A,** Elbow extension with forearm supination. **B,** Forearm pronation.

Carpal-Radial-Ulnar

Movement: Wrist flexion and extension

Hand placement and motion: Grasp the patient's hand over its palmar and dorsal surfaces with one hand; use the other hand to support and stabilize the forearm. Move the palm toward the forearm, and move the dorsum toward the forearm. Allow the patient's fingers to relax, and do not stress the carpals. This motion can be performed with the elbow flexed or extended. After the range of the extrinsic finger flexors and extensors has been evaluated, you may want to combine wrist and finger flexion and wrist and finger extension. Review the information on multijoint muscles before combining wrist and finger motions.

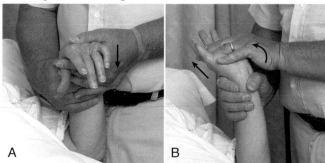

Fig. 6-12   **A,** Wrist flexion. **B,** Wrist extension.

Continued

Movement: Wrist radial and ulnar deviation

Hand placement and motion: Grasp the patient's hand as described for wrist flexion and extension; maintain the hand in neutral flexion-extension. Move the hand in a radial and ulnar direction, but avoid wrist flexion and extension.

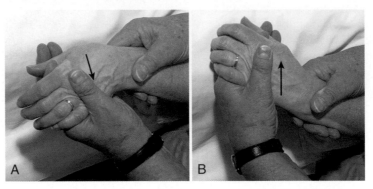

Fig. 6-13   **A,** Ulnar deviation of the wrist. **B,** Radial deviation of the wrist.

Metacarpal Head Joint Play

Movement: Elevation and depression of individual metacarpal heads

Hand placement and motion: Grasp the dorsal and palmar surfaces of the metacarpal of a finger just proximal to its head with the thumb and index finger of one hand; use your other hand to stabilize the adjacent metacarpal with a similar grasp. Using the first hand, move the head of one metacarpal upward and downward, but do not allow the adjacent metacarpal to move. Progress to the next metacarpal until all four distal metacarpals have been moved. Note: This technique should not be applied to the thumb.

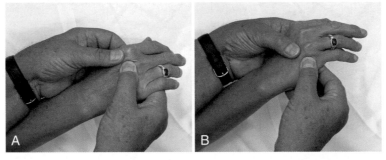

Fig. 6-14   Elevation (**A**) and depression (**B**) of individual metacarpal heads.

Metacarpophalangeal

Movement: Flexion and extension of the metacarpophalangeal (MCP) joint

Hand placement and motion: Grasp the dorsal and palmar surfaces of a metacarpal just proximal to the metacarpal head with the thumb and index finger of one hand, and use the thumb and finger of your other hand to grasp the dorsal and palmar surfaces of a proximal phalanx. Stabilize the metacarpal while you move the phalanx upward and downward. Perform the motion for each articulation on each hand; use the same techniques for the thumb.

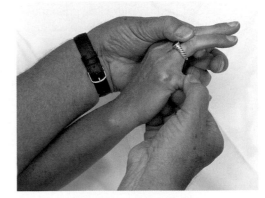

Fig. 6-15   Flexion of the metacarpophalangeal joint.

Distal and Proximal Interphalangeal

Movement: Flexion and extension of the distal interphalangeal (IP) joint

Hand placement and motion: Use the grasp described for MCP flexion and extension. Stabilize the more proximal phalanx, and move the more distal phalanx upward and downward. Perform the motion for each articulation on each hand, and use the same technique for the thumb.

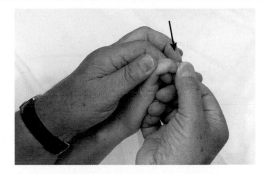

Fig. 6-16   Flexion of the distal interphalangeal joint.

Metacarpophalangeal and Interphalangeal (Combined Motions)

Movement: Finger flexion and extension of the MCP and IP joints

Hand placement and motion: Place one hand over the patient's extended fingers; use your other hand to support and stabilize the forearm. Gently fold the fingers into a fist, and return them to an extended position; use the same technique for the thumb by flexing the thumb into the palm and returning it to an extended position. Maintain the wrist in a neutral position. This motion can be performed with the elbow flexed or extended.

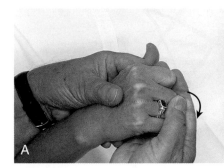 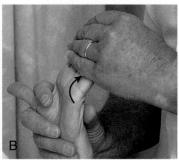

Fig. 6-17   **A,** Finger flexion. **B,** Finger extension.

Metacarpophalangeal

Movement: Abduction of the MCP joints

Hand placement and motion: Use one hand to grasp and stabilize the distal IP joints of the first, second, and third fingers; use your other hand to grasp the fourth finger. Keeping the MCP and IP joints extended, gently move the fourth finger away from the third finger; then stabilize the first and second fingers and move the third finger away from the second finger. Next, stabilize the second, third, and fourth fingers, and move the first finger away from the second finger. The second finger can be moved to the left and to the right independently and without stabilization of any of the other fingers. (Note that these motions are performed independently of the thumb and are used to maintain the web spaces between the four fingers.)

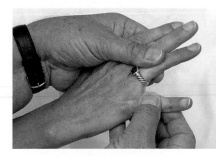 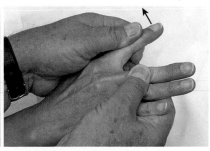

Fig. 6-18   Abduction of the metacarpophalangeal joints.

Continued

Thumb Metacarpal-Carpal and Metacarpophalangeal

Movement: Thumb opposition

Hand placement and motion: Grasp the patient's thumb with the thumb and fingers of one hand; use your other hand to grasp the fifth metacarpal and finger. Roll the thumb toward the fifth finger, maintaining the MCP and IP joints in extension. Return the thumb to a position of full extension to maintain its web space.

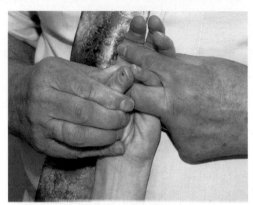

Fig. 6-19 Thumb opposition.

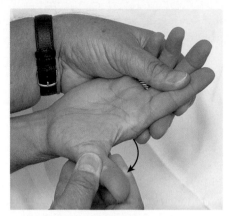

Fig. 6-20 Thumb abduction.

Metacarpal-Carpal of the Thumb

Movement: Thumb abduction and adduction

Hand placement and motion: Grasp the patient's thumb with the fingers and thumb of one hand; use the other hand to stabilize the second metacarpal. Lift the thumb away from the palm so it is perpendicular to the palm, but maintain the MCP and IP joints in extension. Return the thumb to the palm parallel to the second metacarpal.

Movement: Thumb extension and flexion

Hand placement and motion: Grasp the patient's thumb with the fingers and thumb of one hand; use the other hand to stabilize the second metacarpal. Move the thumb away from the index finger and horizontal to the palm; widen the web space to its maximum. Return the thumb so that it rests next to the side of the second metacarpal.

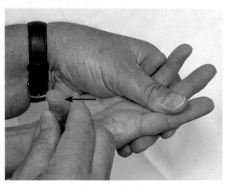

Fig. 6-21 Thumb extension.

Thumb Metacarpophalangeal and Interphalangeal

Movement: Thumb flexion and extension

Hand placement and motion: Grasp the patient's metacarpal with the thumb and fingers of one hand; use the thumb and index finger of the other hand to flex the distal joints of the thumb. Return the distal joints to extension.

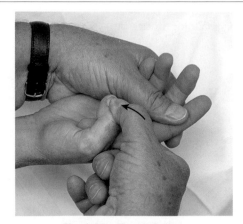

Fig. 6-22 Thumb flexion.

UPPER EXTREMITY MOVEMENTS: ELONGATION OF MULTIJOIONT MUSCLES

Biceps Brachii

Start with the patient supine and the shoulder at the edge of the support surface, with the elbow extended and the forearm pronated. Grasp the elbow with one hand; use the other hand to grasp the wrist. Lower the arm below the level of the support surface (i.e., hyperextend the shoulder) until you sense maximal tension in the muscle or the patient reports discomfort along the anterior (upper) aspect of the extremity.

Triceps Brachii (Long Head)

Start with the patient supine, lying on his or her side, or sitting. Grasp the wrist with one hand; use the other hand to support the distal end of the humerus. Flex the elbow maximally and simultaneously flex the shoulder. The patient must be lying on his or her side, sitting, or standing for maximal elongation to occur. Terminate the motion when you sense maximal tension in the muscle or when the patient reports discomfort along the posterior aspect of the arm.

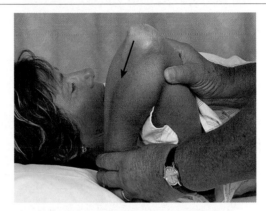

Fig. 6-23   Elongation of the triceps brachii.

Extensor Digitorum

Place one hand over the dorsum of all the fingers of the patient's hand; use your other hand to support and stabilize the forearm. Gently and sequentially flex the distal IP, proximal IP, and MCP joints, and carefully flex the wrist. Terminate the motion when you sense maximal tension in the muscle or when the patient reports discomfort along the dorsal surface of the wrist, hand, or fingers. This motion can be performed with the elbow flexed or extended.

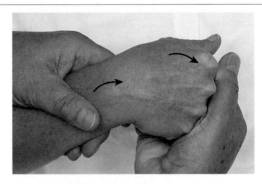

Fig. 6-24   Elongation of the extensor digitorum.

Flexor Digitorum Superficialis and Profundus

Place one hand over the palmar surface of all the fingers of the patient's hand; use your other hand to support and stabilize the forearm. Gently and sequentially extend the distal IP, proximal IP, and MCP joints and then carefully extend the wrist. Terminate the motion when you sense maximal tension in the muscles or when the patient reports discomfort along the palmar surface of the wrist, hand, or fingers. Avoid hyperextension of the MCP joints. This motion can be performed with the elbow flexed or extended.

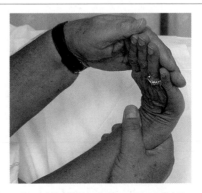

Fig. 6-25   Elongation of the flexor digitorum superficialis and profundus.

LOWER EXTREMITY MOVEMENTS: TRADITIONAL ANATOMIC PLANES

Acetabular-Femoral and Tibial-Femoral

Movement: Hip and knee flexion and extension

Hand placement and motion: Use one hand to cradle the patient's heel; place your other hand in the popliteal space. Lift the LE, allowing the hip and knee to flex. Slide your hand from under the knee to the lateral area of the thigh to prevent hip abduction as the hip and knee flex. Approximate the thigh to the chest and the leg to the posterior area of the thigh; return to the starting position. The patient will need to have the hip at the edge of the support surface to perform hip hyperextension by lowering the extremity toward the floor. Terminate the movement when the pelvis rotates anteriorly or when lumbar lordosis is increased. (Note: Hip hyperextension can be performed more easily when the patient is in a side-lying or prone position.)

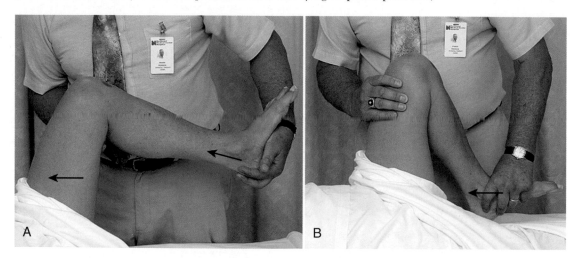

Fig. 6-26 **A,** Hip and knee flexion. **B,** Knee flexion.

Acetabular-Femoral

Movement: Hip flexion and extension with the knee extended (straight leg raising)

Hand placement and motion: Use one hand to support the distal end of the patient's leg; use your other hand to initially provide support in the popliteal space. Shift your hand from the popliteal space to the anterior area of the knee as the hip is flexed to maintain knee extension and to lift the entire LE to flex the hip. Terminate the motion when you sense maximal tension in the hamstring muscles or when the patient reports discomfort along the posterior area of the thigh or knee. Do not attempt to increase the range of the hamstrings by forcibly flexing the hip with the knee extended. It may be necessary to stabilize the knee of the opposite LE as you perform this motion. Some caregivers prefer to place the ankle of the exercised extremity on one shoulder and lift the LE by moving the body forward.

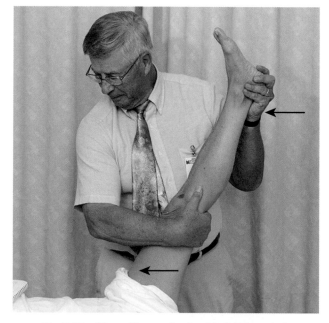

Fig. 6-27 Hip and knee extension (straight leg raise).

Movement: Hip abduction and adduction

Hand placement and motion: Use one hand to support the patient's distal leg; use your other hand to provide support in the poplitcal space and to maintain the knee in an extended position. Move the extremity away from the opposite LE, keeping it parallel to the floor and in a neutral internal-external rotation. Return the extremity to a position of adduction. To attain complete adduction of the exercised extremity, the opposite LE must be adducted. Some persons adduct the extremity by lifting it above the opposite extremity so that more adduction is attained.

Movement: Hip adduction—side-lying position

Hand placement and motion: With the patient in a side lying position and with the uppermost hip and knee extended and the lowermost extremity flexed, use one hand to support the knee or distal area of the thigh. With the other hand, grasp the ankle and lower the extremity toward the floor, keeping the knee extended.

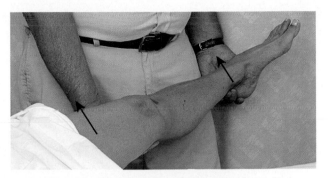

Fig. 6-28   Hip abduction.

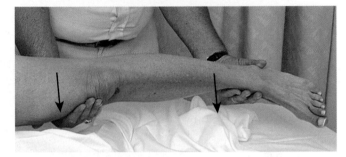

Fig. 6-29   Hip adduction in the side-lying position.

Movement: Hip internal and external rotation

Hand placement and motion: With the patient's hip and knee extended and resting on the treatment table, use one hand to grasp the distal area of the thigh proximal to the knee; use your other hand to grasp proximally to the ankle. Roll the extremity inward and outward, but do not abduct or adduct the hip. Be certain that motion occurs in the hip.

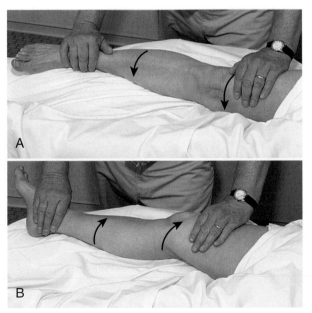

Fig. 6-30   **A,** Internal (medial) hip rotation. **B,** External hip rotation.

Continued

For an alternative technique, flex the hip and knee to 90 degrees. Use one hand to provide support under the patient's knee; use your other hand to grasp the ankle or cradle the leg. Move the leg inward and outward to cause the femur to rotate, but do not abduct or adduct the hip. Be cautious; avoid excessive stress to the medial or lateral aspects of the structures of the knee. Terminate the motion when you sense maximal tension in the muscle or joint or when the patient reports discomfort in the groin or lateral area of the hip.

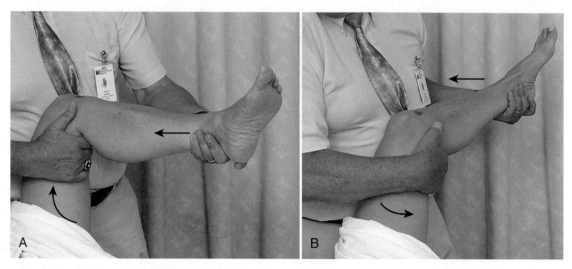

Fig. 6-31   **A,** External (lateral) hip rotation (alternative method). **B,** Internal (medial) hip rotation (alternative method).

Tibial-Femoral

Movement: Knee flexion with the hip extended

Hand placement and motion: With the patient supine and the thigh supported with the knee and leg at the edge of the support surface, use one hand to support the patient's ankle; use your other hand or a towel roll to protect the posterior area of the thigh. Lower the leg to flex the knee over the edge of the table. You will need to stoop to attain full range and to avoid unnecessary strain to the structures of your back.

You also may perform this motion with the patient prone. Use one hand to grasp the ankle; use your other hand to rest on the buttock. (Place a folded towel between your hand and the patient's buttock to preserve modesty.) Bend the knee by moving the heel toward the buttock. Terminate the motion when you sense maximal tension in the quadriceps muscle, when the patient reports discomfort along the anterior area of the thigh, or when hip flexion occurs. Hip flexion indicates that the rectus femoris has reached its fullest elongation and causes anterior pelvic rotation, resulting in hip flexion. To elongate the rectus femoris, the hip is extended simultaneously with knee flexion.

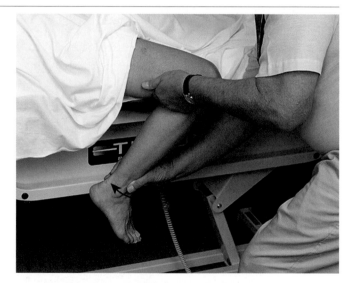

Fig. 6-32   Knee flexion with the hip extended.

Crural-Tibial

Movement: Ankle dorsiflexion and plantar flexion

Hand placement and motion: Dorsiflexion: Use one hand to grasp both sides of the calcaneus, place your forearm along the plantar surface of the foot, and use your other hand to stabilize the distal end of the tibia. Pull downward on the calcaneus while pushing upward with the forearm against the metatarsal heads. It is important that the calcaneus move, and you should avoid pushing only against the metatarsal heads or the forefoot. The knee can be extended or flexed slightly. When it is flexed, a more complete range of ankle motion will be possible because the gastrocnemius, a multijoint muscle, is partially relaxed. When the knee is extended, the gastrocnemius will be elongated more and will limit the range of ankle dorsiflexion.

Plantar flexion: Use one hand to grasp the dorsum of the foot; use your other hand to stabilize the distal end of the tibia. Press down on the foot to produce plantar flexion, but avoid pressure over the toes.

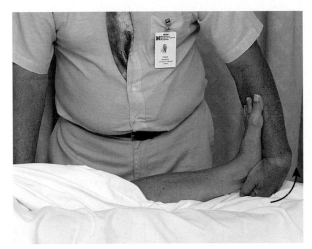

| Fig. 6-33   Ankle dorsiflexion. | Fig. 6-34   Plantar flexion. |

Talar-Crural

Movement: Ankle inversion and eversion

Hand placement and motion: Use one hand to grasp the dorsum of the foot; use your other hand to stabilize the distal end of the tibia. Turn the foot inward and outward, avoiding hip rotation. All motion should occur at the lower ankle joint.

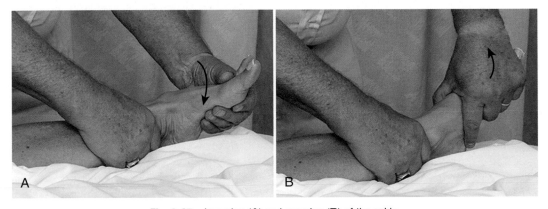

Fig. 6-35   Inversion (**A**) and eversion (**B**) of the ankle.

Continued

Metatarsophalangeal and Interphalangeal

Movement: Toe flexion and extension

Hand placement and motion: Use one hand to grasp and stabilize the foot or to stabilize each proximal area of the bone, similar to the technique described for the fingers. Use the thumb and index finger of your other hand to grasp the phalanx immediately distal to the metatarsal being stabilized; flex and extend the phalanx. All the metatarsophalangeal and IP joints may be moved simultaneously after the range of each joint has been evaluated. Avoid ankle dorsiflexion or plantar flexion by stabilizing the foot. The toes can be abducted using a technique similar to that described for the fingers.

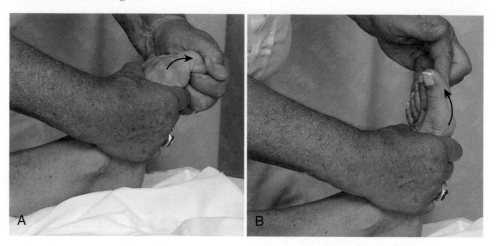

Fig. 6-36   Flexion (**A**) and extension (**B**) of the toes.

Metatarsal Head Joint Play

Movement: Elevation and depression of the metatarsal heads

Hand placement and motion: Use the thumb and index finger of one hand to stabilize one metatarsal; use the thumb and index finger of your other hand to grasp the adjacent metatarsal. The metatarsal that is not being stabilized is moved upward and downward. Avoid simultaneous movement of two metatarsals.

LOWER EXTREMITY MOVEMENTS: ELONGATION OF MULTIJOINT MUSCLES

Rectus femoris

Start with the patient prone and perform simultaneous knee flexion and hip extension. This motion also can be performed with the patient in a side-lying position, provided he or she is secure and you can stabilize the pelvis to prevent an anterior pelvic tilt. Terminate the motion when you sense maximum tension in the quadriceps muscle, when lumbar lordosis increases, or when the patient reports discomfort.

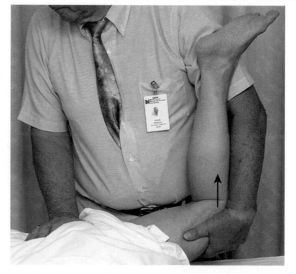

Fig. 6-37   Elongation of the rectus femoris.

Tensor fasciae latae (Iliotibial Band)

Start with the patient in a side-lying position and with the hip and knee of the uppermost extremity extended. Perform the motion described for hip adduction by lowering the uppermost extremity toward the floor or surface of the table. Terminate the motion when you sense maximum tension in the tensor fasciae latae or when the extremity ceases to move downward (see Fig. 6-29).

Gastrocnemius

Start with the patient supine and with the hip and knee extended. Perform the motion described for ankle dorsiflexion by moving the dorsum of the foot toward the shin; be certain that the calcaneus moves. This motion also can be combined with straight leg raising. Terminate the motion when maximal tension is sensed in the gastrocnemius or when the patient reports discomfort (see Fig. 6-33).

TRUNK MOVEMENTS: TRADITIONAL ANATOMIC PLANES

Cervical Spine

Stand at the patient's head and face the patient. With the patient's shoulders at the edge of the support surface, support the patient's head in your hands. Perform the motions slowly and cautiously.

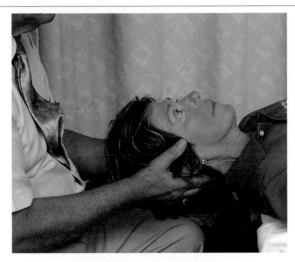

Fig. 6-38   Hand positions for mid position of the cervical spine.

Forward Bending (Flexion)

Support the patient's head with your hands placed firmly at the occiput. Lift the head so the chin moves toward the chest. Encourage the patient to relax the posterior neck muscles.

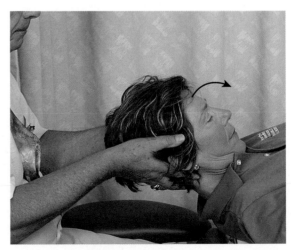

Fig. 6-39   Forward bending (flexion) of the cervical spine.

Continued

Backward Bending (Extension or Hyperextension)

Support the patient's head with your hands at the occiput. Lower the head so the occiput moves toward the floor. Encourage the patient to relax the anterior neck muscles.

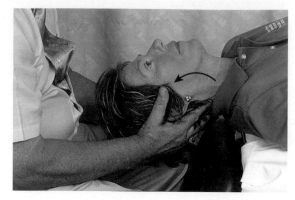

Fig. 6-40   Backward bending (extension or hyperextension) of the cervical spine.

Side Bending (Lateral Flexion)

Support the patient's head at the occiput and move the head so one ear moves toward the ipsilateral acromion. Maintain the cervical spine in neutral flexion-extension, and do not allow the scapula to elevate toward the ear. Encourage the patient to relax the lateral neck muscles on the side of the neck opposite to the direction in which you move the head.

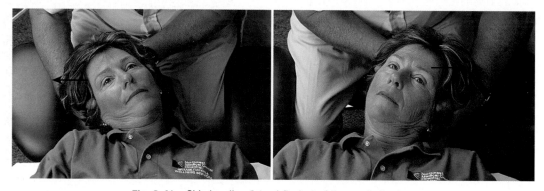

Fig. 6-41   Side bending (lateral flexion) of the cervical spine.

Rotation

Support the patient's head at the occiput, and turn the head to the left and to the right. Maintain the cervical spine in neutral flexion-extension. Perform this motion slowly to avoid vertigo. Encourage the patient to relax the muscles of the neck.

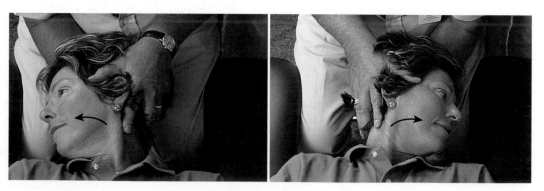

Fig. 6-42   Rotation of the cervical spine.

Lumbar Spine

Stand on one side of the patient at the level of the pelvis with the body close to the near edge of the support surface.

Lumbar Flexion

With the patient supine, lift both of the thighs toward the chest by performing hip and knee flexion (i.e., a bilateral knee-to-chest maneuver). Elevate the distal portion of the sacrum from the support surface to produce full posterior pelvic rotation. Caution: Do not attempt this maneuver when the patient's lower extremities are too heavy or too large for you to control and lift safely; be alert for indications of patient discomfort.

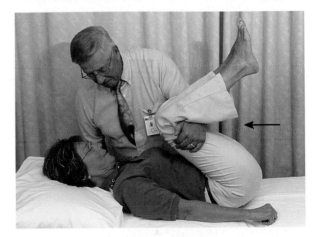

Fig. 6-43   Lumbar flexion.

Lumbar Extension

With the patient prone, flex both knees and lift both thighs to cause an anterior pelvic tilt and lumbar spine extension. Caution: Do not attempt this maneuver when the patient's lower extremities are too heavy or too large for you to control and lift safely; be alert for indications of patient discomfort. For small patients, the patient's chest can be lifted from the support surface by grasping the anterior surface of both shoulders, or the patient can perform a partial push-up to elevate the chest while maintaining the pelvis on the support surface.

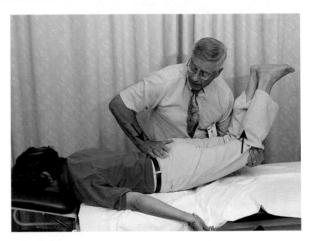

Fig. 6-44   Lumbar extension.

Lumbar Rotation

Position the patient supine with the hips and knees flexed and the feet on the support surface in a hook-lying position. Move the thighs to the left and to the right with one hand by applying a rotational force to the pelvis on the side opposite to the movement of the thighs, using your other hand to stabilize the chest. The right side of the pelvis should become elevated when the thighs are moved to the left and vice versa. Pictured is an alternative method for lumbar rotation. Caution: This activity should be performed carefully for a patient with a known hip abnormality or lumbar spine dysfunction; it is contraindicated for a patient with a recent total hip replacement or other similar surgery.

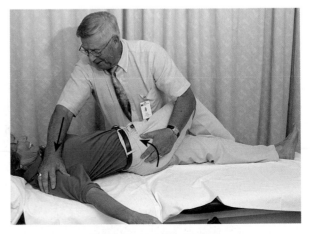

Fig. 6-45   Lumbar rotation.

Continued

Thoracic Spine

Stand at the side of the patient at the level of the upper thorax. The patient's upper extremities should be folded over the chest or abdomen, and the body should be close to the near edge of the support surface.

Thoracic Rotation

With the patient supine and with the hips and knees extended, grasp under the right scapula with one hand; use your other hand to stabilize over the right anterior superior iliac spine. Lift and rotate the upper trunk to the left, and then perform the motion in the opposite direction with your hands positioned under the left scapula and over the left anterior superior iliac spine. Ask the patient to lift and control his or her head while this motion is performed.

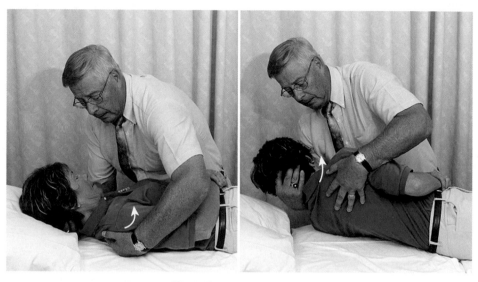

Fig. 6-46   Thoracic rotation.

Table 6-2 Diagonal Patterns: Component Positions

Extremity	Body part	Diagonal 1 Flexion	Diagonal 1 Extension	Diagonal 2 Flexion	Diagonal 2 Extension
Upper	Scapula	Elevation, abduction, upward rotation	Depression, adduction, downward rotation	Elevation, adduction, upward rotation	Depression, abduction, downward rotation
	Shoulder	Flexion, adduction, external rotation	Extension, abduction, internal rotation	Flexion, abduction, external rotation	Extension, adduction, internal rotation
	Elbow	Flexion, extension	Flexion, extension	Flexion, extension	Flexion, extension
	Forearm	Supination	Pronation	Supination	Pronation
	Wrist	Flexion, radial deviation	Extension, ulnar deviation	Extension, radial deviation	Flexion, ulnar deviation
	Fingers	Flexion, adduction	Extension, abduction	Extension, abduction	Flexion, adduction
Lower	Hip	Flexion, adduction, external rotation	Extension, abduction, internal rotation	Flexion, abduction, internal rotation	Extension, adduction, external rotation
	Knee	Flexion, extension	Flexion, extension	Flexion, extension	Flexion, extension
	Ankle	Dorsiflexion, inversion	Plantar flexion, eversion	Dorsiflexion, eversion	Plantar flexion, inversion
	Toes	Extension	Flexion	Extension	Flexion

Text continued from page 107

placements will be similar to those described previously, and the motions will be the same as those described for the UE patterns with the elbow extended.

Lower Extremity

Flexion and Extension with the Knee Extended. These four patterns can be performed with the knee flexed. Hand placements will be similar to those described previously, and the motions will be the same as those described for the LE patterns with the knee extended.

PRINCIPLES OF ACTIVE RANGE OF MOTION EXERCISE

Some of the advantages, uses, and goals associated with AROM have been described previously. For patients who are capable, it is important that the exercise program progress from passive to active because normal function requires muscle strength and endurance. Because numerous resources that provide detailed explanations of the effects of active exercise are available, such explanations are not provided in this book.

Many combinations or types of muscle contractions and assistance or resistance can be used in an AROM exercise program. The ingenuity and experience of the caregiver, the ability of the patient, and the goal of the exercise or program affect the selection and application of techniques. This book does not describe or present information related to resistive exercise using mechanical equipment; sources of such information can be found in the Bibliography.

Types of Muscle Contraction and Exercise

The three basic types or forms of muscle contraction are (1) isotonic, (2) isometric, and (3) isokinetic. Isotonic contractions can be subdivided into eccentric contractions and concentric contractions. Visible joint motion occurs when the muscle contracts isotonically. The load, or resistance, against which the muscle contracts can remain constant or can vary. When the muscle contracts concentrically, its fibers produce a relative shortening of the muscle. When the muscle contracts eccentrically, its fibers allow a relative lengthening of the muscle. An example of a concentric contraction is contraction of the biceps to produce elbow flexion when a person is sitting or standing. An example of an eccentric contraction is contraction of the biceps to control elbow extension when the forearm descends from 90 degrees of elbow flexion to a completely extended position when the person is sitting or standing.

The position of the patient, especially in relationship to gravity, affects the type of contraction produced and the muscles that produce the contraction. For example, when a person is supine and performs active shoulder flexion through the shoulder's full normal range, the shoulder flexors function concentrically from 0 to 90 degrees of flexion and the shoulder extensors function eccentrically from 90 to 180 degrees of flexion. When the extremity is returned to the patient's side, the shoulder extensors function concentrically from 180 to 90 degrees of extension and the shoulder flexors function eccentrically from 90 to 0 degrees of extension. The concepts of concentric and eccentric muscle contractions can be applied to different muscles or muscle groups as the position of the patient is varied.

Isotonic exercise can be used to maintain or increase strength, power, and endurance; promote local circulation; enhance cardiovascular efficiency; create hypertrophy of muscle fibers; maintain the physiological elasticity of a muscle; maintain joint motion; and maintain or enhance coordination. An eccentric muscle contraction develops more tension in the muscle than a concentric contraction and thus may develop strength more rapidly. External resistance or assistance can be applied manually or mechanically to either the eccentric or the concentric contraction.

An isometric muscle contraction produces little or no observable joint motion and no significant change in the length of the muscle. An isometric contraction can be performed with or without external resistance. When no resistance is applied, the contraction is frequently termed "muscle setting" (such as "quad" set or "glute" set).

Isometric exercise can be used to maintain muscle tone or, when resistance is applied, to increase strength, to focus the muscle contraction at one or several specific portions of the total joint range, and to avoid the pain associated with joint motion. Isometric exercise also may economize the time spent to perform the exercise. This type of exercise does little to contribute to cardiovascular fitness or joint or muscle flexibility or to maintain coordinated movement, but it can improve the stability of the trunk or extremity joints. Resistance can be applied manually or mechanically; when resistance is applied, increased tension occurs in the muscle fibers, resulting in increased strength. Proper rehabilitation would incorporate multiple angle isometrics in which resistance is applied every 10 to 20 degrees throughout the ROM of the joint for 6 to 10 seconds. The patient should be permitted to rest for at least 6 seconds between contractions.

A third form of exercise, termed isokinetic exercise, is possible when specific equipment is used. Isokinetic exercise equipment controls the speed of the patient's contractions and produces a variable resistance to the muscle as it contracts through its arc or ROM. Some equipment provides resistance to only the concentric contractions, whereas other equipment resists both concentric and eccentric contractions. Published studies indicate that isokinetic exercise strengthens muscle more efficiently than other forms of resistive isotonic exercise.

Refer to the information presented previously in this chapter to review the possible benefits and uses of passive and active exercise. Several criteria or factors must be considered when you are performing passive or active exercise to obtain the greatest benefit from the exercise and to protect the patient from injury.

Maintain the exercise activities within the physiological capabilities of the patient, remember the goals of therapy, and encourage the patient to perform at maximally tolerated levels. The Valsalva maneuver should be avoided during exercise to prevent the possibility of serious complications that could lead to a cerebrovascular accident or even death. Therefore instruct and remind the patient to avoid holding his or her breath and to breathe normally during the exercise program, particularly when performing resisted isometric exercise. Use caution to avoid causing unnecessary or excessive trauma to a skeletal or soft tissue structure when resistance is applied, and protect unstable or vulnerable structures (e.g., the site of a recent fracture, a hypermobile joint, a recent muscle strain, or a recent surgical site) during exercise. Finally, carefully evaluate the safety and monitor the effects of exercise for a patient who has experienced a recent myocardial infarction or has a history of cardiac dysfunction.

During exercise with a patient who has an unprotected healing fracture, avoid applying resistance to the distal segment of the fracture. Exercise that produces pain during or after exercise for a period of 24 to 36 hours may be contraindicated, and this reaction should be considered a precaution for its future application. Exercise that produces abnormal results, such as an undesired or adverse change in the patient's symptoms or intensification of his or her condition, should be terminated and the program reevaluated before it is continued. Finally, certain exercise movements may be contraindicated after selected surgical procedures; an example is excessive hip movement, especially hip adduction, flexion beyond 90 degrees, and excessive external or internal rotation after total hip replacement surgery (Box 6-4). Caution: Active exercise is contraindicated by a

---

Box 6-4 Precautions Related to Active Exercise

Revision or cessation of an exercise program should be considered in the following circumstances:
- Pain occurs during or persists after exercise
- Undesired cardiopulmonary stress occurs
- The breathing pattern of the patient becomes abnormal (e.g., rapid or shallow)
- The patient exhibits an undesired, adverse response to exercise
- An unstable area or segment undergoes stress
- Undesired movements or movement patterns occur
- Undesired tone of muscle develops or increases
- The patient's condition or functional ability regresses

UPPER EXTREMITIES: DIAGONAL PATTERNS

Diagonal 1, Flexion with the Elbow Extended

Movement: Shoulder flexion, adduction, and external rotation. Start with the shoulder of the UE slightly abducted, internally rotated, and extended. The elbow is extended and the forearm is pronated with the wrist and fingers extended.

Hand placement and motion: For the right UE, use your left hand to support the patient's hand and wrist; use your right hand to support the distal aspect of the upper arm. Lift the extremity diagonally across the chest and over the face; simultaneously, externally rotate the shoulder, supinate the forearm, and flex the wrist and fingers. Perform diagonal flexion within the width of the shoulder. Reverse your hand placement and grip for the left extremity.

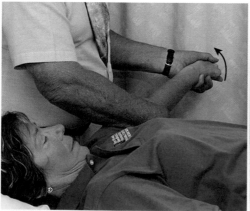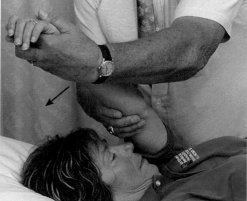

Fig. 6-47 Diagonal 1, flexion with the elbow extended.

Diagonal 1, Extension with the Elbow Extended

Movement: Shoulder extension, abduction, and internal rotation. Start with the shoulder of the UE adducted, flexed, and externally rotated. The elbow is extended, the forearm is supinated, and the wrist and fingers are flexed (see Fig. 6-47).

Hand placement and motion: For the right UE, use your left hand to grasp the patient's hand and wrist; use your right hand to grasp the posterior distal aspect of the upper arm. Move the extremity diagonally away from the face; simultaneously, internally rotate the shoulder, pronate the forearm, and extend the wrist and fingers. Perform the diagonal extension within the width of the shoulder. Reverse your hand placement and grip for the left extremity.

Diagonal 2, Flexion with the Elbow Extended

Movement: Shoulder flexion, abduction, and external rotation. Start with the shoulder of the UE positioned diagonally across the patient's body and internally rotated. The elbow is extended, the forearm is pronated, and the wrist and fingers are flexed.

Hand placement and motion: For the right UE, use your left hand to grasp the dorsum of the patient's hand; use your right hand to grasp the dorsal surface of the forearm or the lateral surface of the upper arm. Lift the extremity diagonally up from the body into flexion, abduction, and external rotation. Perform diagonal flexion within the width of the shoulder. Reverse your hand placement and grip for the left extremity.

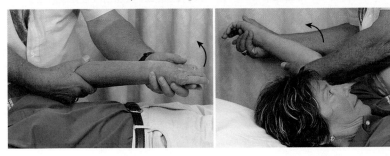

Fig. 6-48   Diagonal 2, flexion with the elbow extended.

Diagonal 2, Extension with the Elbow Extended

Movement: Shoulder extension, adduction, and internal rotation. Start with the shoulder of the UE flexed, abducted, and externally rotated. The elbow is extended, the forearm is supinated, and the wrist and fingers are extended (see Fig. 6-48).

Hand placement and motion: Retain your grasp as described for the diagonal 2 flexion pattern, and move the UE diagonally toward the body into extension, adduction, and internal rotation. Perform diagonal extension within the width of the shoulder.

LOWER EXTREMITIES: DIAGONAL PATTERNS

Diagonal 1, Flexion with the Knee Flexed

Movement: Hip flexion, adduction, and external rotation. Start with the hip of the LE slightly abducted, extended, and internally rotated and the knee extended.

Hand placement and motion: Use one hand to grasp and support the patient's heel; use your other hand to grasp and support the posterior distal aspect of the thigh by reaching over the thigh. Lift the extremity diagonally toward the abdomen and the opposite shoulder; simultaneously, externally rotate the hip and dorsiflex the foot. Perform diagonal flexion within the width of the hip. When this motion is performed with the knee extended, the full range of hip flexion will not be available.

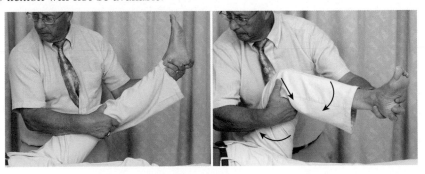

Fig. 6-49   Diagonal 1, flexion with the knee flexed.

Continued

Diagonal 1, Extension with the Knee Extended

Movement: Hip extension, abduction, and internal rotation. Start with the hip of the LE flexed, adducted, and externally rotated and the knee extended (see Fig. 6-49).

Hand placement and motion: Maintain your hand placement as used for the diagonal 1 flexion pattern, and return the extremity diagonally so the hip is extended, abducted, and internally rotated. Perform diagonal extension within the width of the hip.

Diagonal 2, Flexion with the Knee Extended

Movement: Hip flexion, abduction, and internal rotation. Start with the hip of the LE slightly adducted, externally rotated, and extended and the knee extended.

Hand placement and motion: Use one hand to grasp the lateral dorsal surface of the foot; use your other hand to grasp the posterior distal aspect of the thigh. Lift the extremity diagonally up and away from the body; simultaneously, internally rotate the hip. Perform diagonal flexion within the width of the hip.

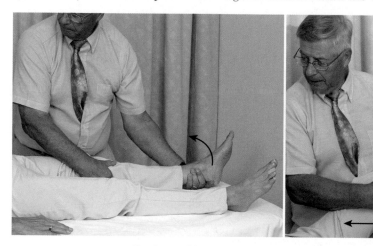

Fig. 6-50   Diagonal 2, flexion with the knee extended.

Diagonal 2, Extension with the Knee Extended

Movement: Hip extension, adduction, and external rotation. Start with the hip of the LE flexed, abducted, and internally rotated and the knee extended.

Hand placement and motion: Maintain the hand placement used for the diagonal 2 flexion pattern, and return the extremity diagonally toward the opposite LE; simultaneously, externally rotate the hip. Perform diagonal extension within the width of the hip (see Fig. 6-50).

patient who has unstable angina or has had a myocardial infarction within the past 30 days. According to the American Heart Association, a patient whose resting heart rate is higher than 120 beats/min, whose systolic blood pressure is higher than 180 mm Hg, or whose diastolic blood pressure is higher than 110 mm Hg must be monitored very closely during any physical activity and should seek medical attention.

Types of Active Exercise

The three common forms of active exercise are active assistive, active or active free, and active resistive. Before performing any form of exercise, introduce yourself to the patient, explain the activity, inform the patient of the desired outcome or purpose of the activity, obtain consent to participate in the program, and provide specific instructions. Once the exercise has been initiated, the caregiver should observe the patient and correct improper performance or posture (Procedure 6-4). Proper exercise performance includes but is not limited to performing the motion through the full available range slowly and correctly without extraneous motions.

Isotonic Exercise Application

Active Assistive Exercise Active assistive exercise requires the patient to actively contract the muscles

PROCEDURE 6-4

Application of Active Exercise

- Position the patient for support, stability, and the type of active exercise to be performed, provide access to the area or segment to be exercised, and drape the patient as necessary.
- Explain the purpose and goals of the exercise, obtain consent for treatment, and select equipment if necessary.
- Position the patient to promote the use of proper body mechanics by the patient and caregiver.
- Grasp the part to be treated to provide support, stability, control, or resistance as necessary; orally instruct and guide the patient to perform the exercise. Refer to the photographs and instructions in this chapter for specific information about this step.
- The patient performs the exercises smoothly and slowly through the complete, unrestricted range of motion with a pause at the start and end positions of the exercise.
- The caregiver observes for proper performance of the exercise and provides verbal cues/corrections when needed.
- The patient performs the predetermined number of repetitions and frequency of exercises based on predetermined abilities, needs, and goals.
- At the conclusion of the treatment, position the patient for proper alignment, support, and safety; drape or replace clothing for modesty and body temperature control.
- Evaluate the patient's response to treatment and document important findings such as tolerance of the exercises and any change in pain level.

involved in the exercise maximally while receiving assistance from another source to perform the exercise. The assistance may be provided manually or by a mechanical or gravitational force. It is important that the patient contract the muscles maximally during the exercise, and the caregiver should alter the assistance provided according to the patient's performance. The greatest amount of assistance should be given when the patient has the greatest difficulty performing the activity. Conversely, assistance should be reduced when the patient has the least difficulty performing the activity. An eventual goal for most patients is to progress from active assistive to active exercise.

Assistance or resistance to motion can be affected by the patient's position and the relationship of the effects of gravity. The effect of gravity as a resistance force can be eliminated with the use of external assistance or patient positioning. For example, although the patient may not be able to perform full hip flexion when supine, he or she may be able to perform the activity when assistance is provided manually or mechanically or when lying on his or her side with the LE supported on an elevated smooth surface such as a powder board. The resistance of gravity to the movement of hip flexion or extension or knee flexion or extension will be eliminated when the side-lying position is used. However, friction between the LE and the surface it rests upon will be created when the LE is moved actively over the surface. This friction can be reduced by placing a towel under the extremity so it can slide along the surface.

Before initiating an exercise, position the patient to provide stability and comfort. When you initiate the exercise, be certain to support, protect, stabilize, and control the segment being exercised, using the same hand placements described for passive exercise. Instruct the patient to actively contract the appropriate muscles through the available ROM, and establish an appropriate exercise speed or rate. Your instructions may include touching, tapping, or stroking the muscle to be contracted; having the person initially perform the contraction with the opposite uninvolved muscle; demonstrating the contraction yourself; and using terms such as "bend," "lift," or "straighten." Provide assistance only to the extent necessary to allow the patient to smoothly complete the movement through the available ROM and to avoid undesired motions. The external assistance you provide can be decreased gradually as the patient demonstrates an increase in strength. The patient should progress to active free exercise when he or she is able to complete the desired movement smoothly through the available ROM without undesired motions and assistance. The exercises may be performed in traditional anatomic planes or in the diagonal patterns described previously.

Active Free Exercise Active free exercise is performed by the patient without any assistance or resistance other than gravity and the weight of the extremity or segment involved in the exercise. The patient must have sufficient strength to perform the activity against the resistance provided by gravity. The position of the patient will affect the resistance provided by gravity. You can demonstrate to yourself how the effect of gravity is altered by attempting the same exercise while supine, sitting, standing, or prone. The more exercises you attempt and the more positions you use, the better you will be able to determine how to position a patient to obtain maximal effort while avoiding undesired motions.

Before initiating an exercise, position the patient depending on how you want gravity to affect the exercise and the movement to be performed. For example, do you want gravity to resist, assist, or be neutral during the exercise? Instruct the patient to perform the desired movement through the available ROM smoothly and without any undesired motions (e.g., elevating the shoulders when performing shoulder flexion). If necessary, encourage or guide the patient as the activity is performed.

Establish an appropriate exercise speed to produce a smooth, controlled movement, and require that the patient maintain that speed. The patient should be encouraged to briefly pause (hold) at the end and start positions during each repetition. A brief rest between each series of repetitions usually will be necessary to reduce the effects of fatigue (e.g., two sets of 10 repetitions with a rest between the two sets).

The exercises may be performed in traditional anatomic planes or in the diagonal patterns described previously.

Active Resistive Exercise Active resistive exercise requires the addition of a resistive force other than gravity, which can be done manually or mechanically. The resistance should require the patient to use a maximal contraction to perform the activity, but the movement should be able to be completed slowly, smoothly, and through the entire available ROM. Because gravity will have a resistive effect, as described previously, the position of the patient should be considered. Furthermore, the length of the lever arm and the amount of torque the patient can develop will affect the location of the resistance. For example, greater resistance to the shoulder flexors will be required or need to be applied if the resistance is positioned above the elbow, whereas less resistance will be required if the resistance is located in the patient's hand. The shorter the lever arm, the greater the torque the patient can develop and the more the resistance the muscles will be able to overcome. The longer the lever arm, the less force will be needed to provide resistance. To illustrate this concept, apply resistance at various locations on a seated person's UE as the person performs shoulder flexion with the elbow extended. Apply the resistance at the wrist, then at the elbow, and then at the proximal humerus, and sense the difference in the force you must develop to provide resistance as the person performs shoulder flexion. This concept can be applied to other body segments. A goal for many patients is to progress from active free exercise to active resistive exercise, especially when a gain in muscle strength is desired.

When the patient performs an isotonic contraction, the maximal resistance able to be used is the resistance that can be overcome through the part of the range where the muscle has the weakest contractile capacity. Most muscles have the weakest contractile capacity at the beginning and the end of the ROM, and most muscles tend to develop their greatest tension during the mid portion of the range. (These last two statements are general statements and may not be accurate for all body positions or exercise activities. However, they do explain the general concept of the length-tension curve of a muscle.) Although the load (resistance) remains constant, the effect of the resistance on the muscle will vary at different points within the range as the muscle lengthens and shortens as a result of a change in the lever arm relationships of the body segments involved.

Before initiating an exercise, position the patient depending on how you want gravity to affect the exercise, the movement required, and the amount or type of support or stabilization the patient requires. Instruct the patient to perform the desired movement through the available ROM smoothly and without any undesired motion as resistance is applied perpendicular to the extremity or segment. You will need to determine the most appropriate site or location for the resistance to be applied based on the patient's condition, ability, and exercise goals and your awareness of the concept of lever arm length.

The body segment to which the proximal component or origin of the muscle being exercised is attached should be stabilized. The patient's body weight or position may accomplish this stabilization, or an external strap or firm surface may be required. It may be necessary to vary or adjust the resistance during the exercise to allow the patient to complete the available ROM smoothly and without undesired motions.

If manual resistance is used, the site of the application of the resistance and the amount of resistance applied can be revised during the exercise to provide maximal resistance while allowing the patient to complete the movement through the available ROM smoothly and without motions; that is, the resistance lever arm can be lengthened or shortened, a new location can be used to avoid discomfort or to avoid an unstable area, or the applied resistance can be increased or decreased depending on the point in the range where the muscle is contracting.

The exercises may be performed in traditional anatomic planes or in the diagonal patterns described previously.

Isometric Exercise Application

Isometric Exercise Isometric exercise may be used when a muscle is immobilized, when a joint or soft tissue is painful when moved through its range, or when inflammation is present in the area. No observable joint motion should occur when an isometric muscle contraction is performed. Gravity has less effect on the muscle contraction when this type of exercise is used, and the patient's position is not as important as it usually is for isotonic exercise. The segment may be positioned at any point within the ROM depending on the patient's condition and the goal of the exercise. Manual or mechanical resistance can be applied, or a patient can isometrically contract the muscles using a stationary object, such as a wall, because resistance and the length of the lever arm can be varied. The benefits of resisted isometric exercise and the reasons to select them were presented previously.

Muscle setting is a form of isometric exercise that can be beneficial to maintain some muscle tone, to maintain contractile awareness, and to allow exercise to an immobilized, innervated muscle. Before initiating the exercise, position the patient to provide a stable, comfortable position and to have access to the muscle that will contract. Instruct the patient to contract or tighten (set) a specific muscle or muscle group without producing joint motion or changing the length of the muscle.

You may help the patient use mental imaging to initiate the contraction by describing the motion. The use of tactile or verbal cueing to initiate the contraction by touching the muscle or telling the patient what movement the muscle will perform is another teaching method. For example, you can instruct a supine or prone patient to squeeze or pinch the buttocks together to set (contract) the gluteus maximus. If the patient squeezes the arms close to the side of the chest as if trying to hold a newspaper or small purse, the pectoral muscles will contract. When a patient has a full-length cast on one LE, you can instruct him or her to try to pull the kneecap of that extremity toward the hip by tightening the muscle on top of the thigh to isometrically contract the quadriceps. To facilitate this motion, have the patient perform it with the opposite, nonimmobilized quadriceps while you tactilely stroke upward on the quadriceps or gently push up on the patella. These examples describe a few techniques that can be used to initiate an isometric contraction; you may need to consider other methods to teach a patient to contract the muscles isometrically.

Instruct the patient to maintain and hold the contraction for approximately 5 to 8 seconds and then relax. The patient should be instructed to breathe normally to avoid the Valsalva phenomenon.

Isometric Resistive Exercise Isometric resistive exercise can be used to increase muscle strength through the addition of manual or mechanical resistance. The segment can be positioned at any point in the range depending on the patient's condition and the goal of the exercise. The amount of resistance and the length of the lever arm can be varied. It is particularly important to instruct the patient to breathe normally and avoid the Valsalva phenomenon when performing isometric resistive exercise.

Before initiating the exercise, position the patient to provide stability, comfort, and access to the muscle that will contract. Determine where you want to apply the resistance on the segment, and position the segment within the available joint ROM. Be certain that the resistance is applied perpendicular to the segment, and instruct the patient to maintain and hold the position selected for approximately 5 to 8 seconds, then relax for 5 to 8 seconds before repeating the contraction. Joint motion should not occur or be permitted. Additional information about the concept, use, and application of all forms of active exercise is contained in many of the references listed in the Bibliography.

SUMMARY

Exercise is used to manage a variety of conditions. Several types of exercise exist, including passive, active assistive, active, and active resistive. The caregiver requires knowledge and competence to select the type of exercise that will provide the most benefit to the patient.

The three primary types of muscle contraction are (1) isotonic (which can be subdivided into concentric and eccentric), (2) isometric, and (3) isokinetic. Exercise can affect a person's strength, endurance, joint flexibility, coordination, and cardiopulmonary system.

Exercises can be performed with the patient positioned supine, sitting, prone, lying on his or her side, or standing. The position selected should be based on the purpose of the exercise, the condition of the patient, the patient's ability to assume and maintain a specific position, and the equipment to be used.

The patient's response to exercise during and after each treatment session should be monitored and should include the observation of changes in the appearance of the segment exercised; evaluation of vital signs; goniometric assessment of any changes in ROM or movement (e.g., coordination, strength, quality, or control); and complaints or indication of pain by the patient. You should provide specific support and stabilization to any segments that are unstable or produce pain, such as a recent fracture site, areas of hypermobility or paralysis, or a wound or incision site. The extremity or segment should be moved through the entire unrestricted, pain-free, normal range of the associated joint or joints. Forceful movement into a restricted component of the range constitutes stretching and should be avoided when you are performing PROM exercise. A description of stretching techniques is beyond the scope of this textbook and is not presented here.

All exercises should be performed smoothly and slowly through the unrestricted range. A brief rest at the end and start position of the exercise also should be incorporated into the exercise.

The number of repetitions required to accomplish the goals of treatment will vary, just as the frequency of the exercises will vary. Some patients may benefit from or require the exercises to be performed two or more times per day for 10 or more repetitions. Other patients may benefit from or require one exercise session per day and fewer than 10 repetitions per joint or area. The patient's response to treatment, any change in the patient's condition, and the judgment of the caregiver are the factors used to determine the parameters of the exercise program.

You may apply the exercises using traditional anatomic planes, diagonal planes, or a combination of planes by using functional movement patterns or by combining two or more of these techniques. At the termination of the treatment, the patient should be repositioned with proper support, security, and alignment. Any equipment or assistive devices that were used should be cleaned and stored, and the treatment area should be prepared for other patients. Information about the patient's response to treatment or any change in condition should be documented.

self-study ACTIVITIES

- Describe some factors you would consider when determining the type of active exercise to select for a patient.
- How would you determine whether a patient had performed active exercise maximally?
- Describe how you would determine whether a patient performs active exercise properly.
- Describe the actions you would use to enhance proper active exercise motions.
- Explain what happens when you lengthen or shorten the lever arm used to apply manual resistance.
- List at least one body position you would use to place each of the following muscles in a maximal gravity-resisted position, in a maximal gravity-assisted position, and in a gravity-neutral position: middle deltoid, biceps, triceps, pectoralis major, upper trapezius, quadriceps, hamstrings, gluteus maximus, erector spinae, and abdominals.
- Explain how you would decide that a patient is ready to progress from passive to active exercise.
- Describe some reasons or patient conditions for which you would perform passive exercise.
- Demonstrate the positions and motions you would use to perform concentric and eccentric contractions of the quadriceps, hamstrings, anterior deltoid, triceps, and abdominal muscles.

problem SOLVING

1. A 28-year-old patient with a C5 quadriplegia is being seen for exercises as an inpatient. What passive range of motion exercises for this patient should be avoided, and for what reason?

2. A 53-year-old woman with general muscle weakness due to prolonged immobility from 3 weeks of bed rest arrives in the department on a wheeled stretcher (gurney). What are two short-term and two long-term goals for her? What type of exercises would you use to initiate the program and have it progress?

3. A 20-year-old man with paralysis of all his extremity and trunk muscles below the level of his waist is referred for "exercise." What are two short-term and two long-term goals for this patient? What exercises would you use, and what is your rationale for their use?

CHAPTER 7

Features and Activities of Wheelchairs

objectives *After studying this chapter, the reader will be able to:*

- List the standard measurements for an adult wheelchair.
- Measure a patient for a wheelchair and confirm the fit of the chair.
- Teach a person to propel a wheelchair using both upper extremities or one upper extremity and one lower extremity.
- Name the components of a standard wheelchair and describe the purpose of each component.
- Teach various functional activities to a wheelchair user.
- Perform various wheelchair functional activities with a person in the chair by providing assistance.

key terms

Ascend   To go or move upward.

Condyle   A rounded projection on a bone.

Crash bar   The metal bar on a door that disengages the door latch when it is pushed.

Descend   To go down; to proceed from a higher level to a lower level.

Femoral   Pertaining to the femur (thigh bone).

Independent   Able to function or perform without assistance from another person.

Locomotion   The ability to move from one place to another.

Pedal   Pertaining to the foot or feet.

Pneumatic   Of or containing air or gases.

Popliteal   Pertaining to the area behind the knee.

Propulsion   The act of propelling; movement of a wheelchair by the person in the chair or by another person.

Restraint   The forcible confinement or restriction of movement of a person through the use of belts, straps, or other similar items.

Self-closing device   A device attached to a door that closes the door through the use of compressed fluid or air.

Semipneumatic   Partially containing air or gases.

INTRODUCTION

Persons who use a wheelchair as their primary mode of mobility should have a chair that fits properly to provide maximum function, comfort, stability, safety, and protection of body structures. The initial measurement and subsequent confirmation of fit must be done carefully. Information about special seating needs, chairs designed for special activities (e.g., chairs for recreation or sports participation), or chairs designed to fulfill special patient needs is not presented in this book. However, it may be important to consider whether the person using the wheelchair will require a cushion, a reclining back, an elevating or swing-away front rigging (leg rests), adjustable armrests, or other similar adaptations. Figure 7-1 are illustrates the major components of a standard wheelchair and the nomenclature of the components.

The type of wheelchair selected and its components will depend on the patient's decrease in body function; activity limitations; participation limitations; size and weight; the expected use of the chair; and the prognosis for change in

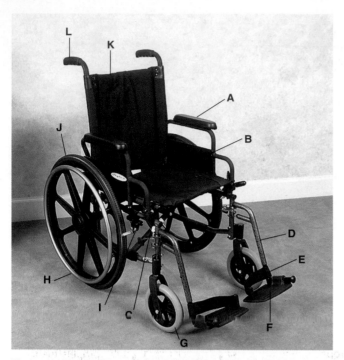

Fig. 7-1   Wheelchair components. *A,* Armrest. *B,* Clothing guard. *C,* Front rigging release. *D,* Front rigging. *E,* Heel loop. *F,* Footplate (footrest). *G,* Caster wheel. *H,* Hand rim. *I,* Wheel lock. *J,* Drive wheel. *K,* Back upholstery. *L,* Push handle.

<table>
<tr><td>Box 7-1</td><td>Factors Associated with the Selection of a Wheelchair Type and Components</td></tr>
</table>

- Patient's impairment, activity limitations, and participation restrictions
- Patient's age, size, stature, and weight
- User's functional skills or preference
- Portability/accessibility
- Reliability/durability
- Expected use or patient needs of the wheelchair (e.g., indoors, outdoors, recreation, transfer needs, ability to transport the chair)
- Temporary versus permanent use of the wheelchair
- Potential or prognosis for change in the patient's condition, especially as it affects mobility
- Mental and physical condition or capacity of the patient
- Cosmetic features
- Options available
- Service
- Cost

the patient's condition. Proper fit of the chair becomes more important if the patient has decreased sensory awareness, limited ability to alter a position, decreased subcutaneous soft tissue (especially over bony prominences), impaired peripheral circulation in the lower extremities, or abnormal skin integrity or condition, or if the chair needs to be used for extended periods. Any of these factors individually or in combination could cause a serious secondary problem or complication for the patient (Box 7-1).

Several wheelchair types and designs are available (Table 7-1). The more common or frequently prescribed types are described briefly. Product and accessory catalogs can be obtained from the manufacturers of wheelchairs. These catalogs contain information about the styles and types of wheelchairs that each company manufactures.

WHEELCHAIR SEATING AND POSITIONING

The type and features of a wheelchair prescribed for a person will depend on the person's needs, abilities, and goals. Generally, wheelchairs are considered to be a means of transportation or mobility, but they also provide support, safety, and stability to enable the user to perform functional activities. Proper seating and positioning should promote function, prevent deformity, improve body alignment, prevent tissue damage, and prevent additional complications. Items such as a headrest, lateral trunk support panels, seat pan or cushion, back panel, armrest trough with adjustments, and

lower extremity supports can be added to a chair to accomplish specific positioning goals.

A careful evaluation of the wheelchair user should be performed by knowledgeable, skilled individuals. The person's sitting balance, stability, reaching ability, method of propulsion, transfer method, ability to change positions, and sitting posture should be evaluated. The position of the pelvis, knees, feet, trunk, and head should be observed to determine which items may need to be added to the chair to maximize the person's function. A desirable posture minimizes energy expenditure, promotes function, reduces discomfort, and maintains trunk stability.

It is important to be aware that posture may be affected by the type of chair seat. For example, a sling or hammock seat tends to cause internal rotation of the femurs, posterior pelvic tilt, a forward head position, and a tendency for the pelvis to slide forward. These undesirable factors may adversely affect the person's function. In addition, lateral sitting transfers may be more difficult to perform from this type of seat.

The use of a cushion may reduce or eliminate some of these negative outcomes. However, the use of a cushion may elevate the person in the chair, making it difficult to position the chair under a table, use the armrests for support, or receive adequate support from the back upholstery, and it may require the footrests to be adjusted upward. Additional problems associated with the use of a cushion may arise as a result of individual patient needs. The majority of cushions are composed of foam, air (i.e., inflatable cushions), or a gel. Gel cushions are heavy and bulky to handle; foam and air cushions are lighter but also may be bulky and difficult to manage for some persons. All cushions require careful handling to prevent them from being damaged. The wheelchair user should try different cushions to find one that

Table **7-1**　Types of Wheelchairs

Type	Description
Standard adult	Designed for persons who weigh less than 200 lb and for limited use on rough surfaces; not designed for vigorous functional activities
Heavy-duty adult	Constructed for persons who weigh more than 200 lb or for those who perform vigorous functional activities
Ultralight wheelchair	Designed to be lightweight, may have a rigid or folding frame, and can be made with titanium in a rigid or folding frame; weighs from 12 to 30 lb; benefit is efficiency in propulsion and reduction in cumulative trauma in the upper extremities; weight capacity to 300 lb
Intermediate or junior	Designed for persons with a body build smaller than that of an adult but larger than that of a child
Growing	Designed to permit adjustments in the frame to accommodate the growth of the user
Child or youth	Designed for persons up to the approximate age of 6 y
Indoor	Constructed for use indoors, with the larger drive wheels placed at the front of the chair and the caster wheels at the rear; it functions better in confined areas but is more difficult to propel and makes it more difficult for the user to perform many functional activities
"Hemiplegic"	The seat is lowered approximately 2 inches to allow better use of the user's lower extremities to propel the chair; however, the lower seat may make it more difficult for the user to perform a standing transfer
"Amputee"	The rear wheel axles are positioned approximately 2 inches posterior to their normal position to widen the base of support of the chair and compensate for the loss of the weight of the user's lower extremities
One-hand drive	Two hand rims are fabricated on one drive wheel, and the two drive wheels are connected by a linkage bar; the smaller hand rim propels the near drive wheel, the large hand rim propels the far drive wheel, and when both rims are moved simultaneously, both wheels are propelled
Externally powered	The chair is propelled by a deep-cycle battery system, and various types of controls are used to operate the chair (e.g., a joystick, a chin piece, or a mouth stick)
Sports	A low-profile, fixed frame, lightweight (15-24 lb) chair with features such as a low back, canted rear wheels, fixed or adjustable axles, and fixed or adjustable seat and backrest; it can be bought or customized for various sports activities
Reclining	Used for persons who need to partially or fully recline at some time when they are in the chair; the chair may be a semireclining or fully reclining chair; semireclining chairs recline to approximately 30 degrees from vertical, and fully reclining chairs can recline to a horizontal position; elevating leg rests and headrest extensions are necessary components for these chairs

provides the best support and stability, enables him or her to maintain balance, and is manageable for various activities.

It is important to note that using a cushion does not provide adequate pressure relief, and thus frequent position changes should be performed by the wheelchair user while he or she is seated to relieve pressure on various body sites. Positioning and seating features must be evaluated so the user will have the best possible support and posture for the performance of functional tasks while seated in the chair.

STANDARD WHEELCHAIR MEASUREMENTS

The initial measurements should be made with the patient seated on a firm, flat surface such as a wood chair or a piece of plywood placed on a mat. The patient should wear clothing that is similar to the clothing he or she usually wears. The patient should sit with the trunk erect in a comfortable position and posture. If a seat cushion or backrest (e.g., a cushion or posture panel) is to be used, it should be in place when the measurements are made. A tape measure that can be read easily is recommended for measurements (Table 7-2).

The patient's age, weight, diagnosis, and activity limitations; the expected use of the chair; participation limitations; and specific features such as adjustable armrests, desk arms, reclining back, swing-away front rigging, elevating leg rests, and caster wheel locks should be specified when the chair is ordered.

Confirmation of Fit

The fit of a wheelchair should be determined with the patient seated in the wheelchair and wearing his or her usual clothing, including shoes. Any cushions or other components that would affect the fit should be in place. The importance of proper fit of the chair must be ensured to enable the patient to attain maximal comfort, stability, function, and safety. You should be able to confirm the fit of the wheelchair in a brief period (Procedure 7-1). When

Table **7-2** Standard Wheelchair Measurements for Proper Fit

Measurement	Instructions	Average Adult Size
Seat height/leg length	Measure from the user's heel to the popliteal fold, and add 2 inches to allow clearance of the footrest	19.5 to 20.5 inches
Seat depth	Measure from the user's posterior buttock, along the lateral thigh, to the popliteal fold; then subtract approximately 2 inches to avoid pressure from the front edge of the seat against the popliteal space	16 inches
Seat width	Measure the widest aspect of the user's buttocks, hips, or thighs, and add approximately 1.5 inches; this will provide space for bulky clothing, orthoses, or clearance of the trochanters from the armrest side panel	18 inches
Back height	Measure from the seat of the chair to the floor of the axilla with the user's shoulder flexed to 90 degrees, and then subtract approximately 4 inches; this will allow the final back height to be below the inferior angles of the scapulae (Note: This measurement will be affected if a seat cushion is to be used; the person should be measured while seated on the cushion, or the thickness of the cushion must be considered by adding that value to the actual measurement)	16 to 16.5 inches
Armrest height	Measure from the seat of the chair to the olecranon process with the user's elbow flexed to 90 degrees, and then add approximately 1 inch (Note: This measurement will be affected if a seat cushion is to be used; the person should be measured while seated on the cushion, or the thickness of the cushion must be considered by adding that value to the actual measurement)	9 inches above the chair seat

PROCEDURE 7-1

Wheelchair Fit Confirmation

The chair should be on a level, smooth surface, and the patient must sit erect with the pelvis in contact with the back upholstery.

Seat height and leg length
- A proper fit will allow you to place two or three fingers easily under the thigh, with your hand held parallel to the floor, from the front edge of the seat to a depth of approximately 2 inches (**A**).
- The bottom of the footrest must be at least 2 inches from the floor with the chair on a level surface when this evaluation is performed (**B**).
- Two inches provide adequate distance from the bottom of the footplate to the floor so the chair can be maneuvered easily and safely on most surfaces.
- Note: The footplate can be adjusted to the proper position by means of the adjusting bolt or nut located on the shaft of the front rigging (see Fig. 7-3).

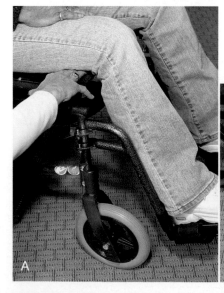 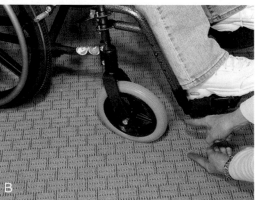

Fig. 7-2   Fitting a wheelchair. **A,** Proper fit allows two or three fingers to be placed under the thigh from the front seat edge. **B,** The footrest must be at least 2 inches from the floor.

PROCEDURE 7-1

Wheelchair Fit Confirmation—cont'd

Seat depth
- Proper fit will allow two or three fingers to be placed between the front edge of the seat and the user's popliteal fold with your palm horizontal to the seat (**C**) with your hand held parallel to the floor.
- It is important that the person be seated well back in the chair with the posterior area of the pelvis in contact with the seat back when this component is evaluated. If the person is not positioned back in the chair, the seat will appear to be too short and the thighs may not have sufficient support.

Seat width
- Proper fit will allow the placement of your hand, held vertically, between the user's greater trochanter, hip, or thigh and the armrest panels with your hand positioned vertically to the seat.
- Your hand should be in slight contact with the user and the armrest panel or wheelchair hand rims when the user is seated in the center of the seat.
- Both hands should be used in evaluation, one hand on the side of each hip, to ensure there is sufficient space between each hip and each armrest panel when the user is in the center of the seat (**D**).

Back height
- A proper fit for a standard seat back will allow you to place four fingers, with your hand held vertically, between the top of the back upholstery and the floor of the user's axilla.
- The inferior angles of the scapulae should be positioned approximately one fingerbreadth above the back upholstery when the user sits with an erect posture (**E**).

Armrest height
- Observe the angle made by the posterior aspect of the upper arm and the back post when the elbows rest on the armrest approximately 4 inches in front of the back post.
- Observe the position of the shoulders; they should be level.
- Observe the position of the trunk; it should be erect.
- The user should be able to sit with the trunk erect, the back against the upholstery, and the shoulders level when bearing weight on the forearms as they rest on the armrest (**F**).
- While the user is in this position, a triangle should be formed by the posterior aspect of the user's humerus, the top of the armrest, and the frame of the chair back.

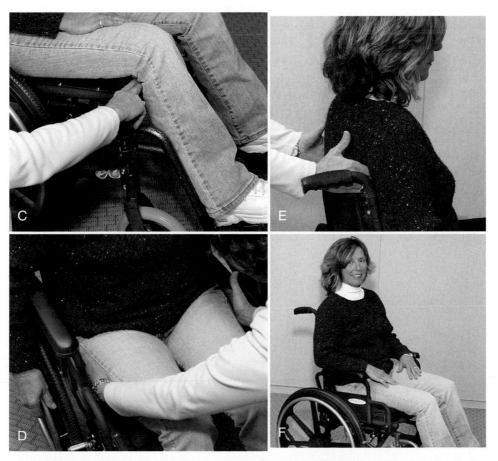

Fig. 7-2, cont'd   **C,** Proper fit of seat depth. **D,** Proper fit of seat width. **E,** Proper fit of back height. **F,** Proper fit of armrest height.

confirming wheelchair fit, the following parameters should be measured:
- Seat height
- Leg length
- Seat depth
- Seat width
- Back height
- Armrest height

Potential Adverse Effects of an Improper Fit

Some deviations in the proper fit may not cause a problem for the patient, but other deviations may cause or create serious problems. Thus each component of the fit must be evaluated to ensure that comfort, security, stability, and safety are maintained. By observing the patient when he or she maneuvers the wheelchair or performs functional activities, you may be able to detect problems associated with the fit of the chair.

Seat Height If the seat is too high, the wheelchair user may experience (1) insufficient trunk support because the back upholstery will be too low; (2) difficulty positioning the knees beneath a table or desk; (3) difficulty propelling the wheelchair because of the difficulty in reaching the hand rims on the drive wheels; or (4) poor posture when the forearms rest on the armrests.

If the seat is too low, the wheelchair user may experience difficulty performing a standing or lateral swing transfer because his or her center of gravity (COG) will be lower, making it difficult to elevate the body. A low seat also may cause improper weight distribution while the person is seated. If the footplates are lowered to compensate for the low seat, they may contact objects on the floor or ground, leading to decreased mobility and unsafe use of the chair.

Leg Length If the footplates are too low, the wheelchair user may experience increased pressure on the distal posterior aspect of the thigh, decreased function of the upper extremities when propelling the chair, and unsafe mobility because of a lack of sufficient clearance of the footplate from the floor or ground surface (Fig. 7-3).

If the footplates are too high, the user may experience increased pressure to the ischial tuberosities, difficulty positioning the chair beneath a table or desk, or decreased trunk stability caused by a lack of support by the posterior area of the thighs.

Seat Depth If the seat is too short from the front to the back, the wheelchair user may experience (1) decreased trunk stability because less support will be provided under the thighs; (2) increased weight bearing on the ischial tuberosities because the body weight will be shifted posteriorly as a result of the lack of support to the thighs; or (3) poor balance because the base of support (BOS) has been reduced.

If the seat is too long from the front to the back, the user may experience increased pressure in the popliteal area, leading to skin discomfort or compromise of circulation because the seat upholstery is longer than the thighs.

Seat Width If the seat is too wide, the wheelchair user may experience (1) difficulty propelling the chair when using the upper extremities because the distance to the hand rims is increased; (2) difficulty performing a standing or lateral swing type of transfer because the distance between the armrests is increased and the user will need to move the body over a greater distance; (3) difficulty moving through narrow hallways or doorways or using public restroom facilities because the overall width of the chair is increased; or (4) postural deviations because it may be necessary to lean to one side of the chair for support.

If the seat is too narrow, the user may experience (1) difficulty changing position because insufficient space is present to adjust position; (2) excessive pressure to the greater trochanters because they are likely to contact the armrest panel; and (3) difficulty wearing bulky outer garments, orthoses, or braces because insufficient space is present for the object to fit between the user's hip or thigh and the armrest panel.

Back Height If the back is too high, the wheelchair user may experience difficulty propelling the chair because it will be more difficult to use the arms comfortably. In addition, excessive irritation to the skin over the inferior angles of the scapulae may occur as they rub against the upholstery, and the user may experience difficulty with balance because the trunk may be inclined forward by the high back.

If the back is too low, the user may experience decreased trunk stability or postural deviations because less support will be available from the chair back. (Note: The current trend in many wheelchair styles is to have a low back to maximize function, as in Fig. 7-4. However, many patients may require and desire the traditional higher back for safety, stability, and support.)

Armrest Height If the armrest is too high, the user may experience (1) problems propelling the chair because it will be difficult to reach over the high armrest to grasp the hand rims; (2) difficulty performing a standing transfer because the armrest height will require the arms to be positioned in a poor functional position to push to stand; (3) postural deviation as a result of elevated shoulders when resting the forearms on the armrest; or (4) limited use of the armrests caused by discomfort when trying to use them, leading to decreased trunk stability and fatigue.

If the armrest is too low, the user may experience (1) poor posture or back discomfort caused by excessive forward trunk inclination when leaning forward to place the forearms on the armrest; (2) increased abdominal discomfort when leaning forward; (3) inadequate balance; or (4) difficulty

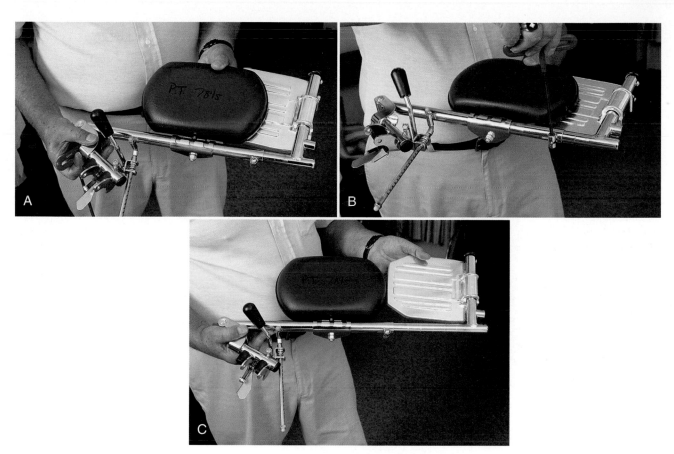

Fig. 7-3   The footrest can be adjusted for a proper fit.

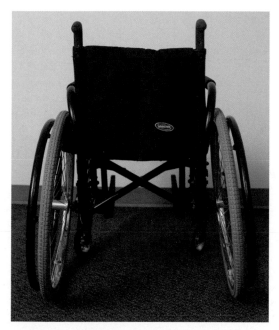

Fig. 7-4   A wheelchair with a low back height.

rising to a standing position from the chair because the armrests are too low to offer support when pushing to stand.

PATIENT AND FAMILY EDUCATION

The wheelchair user and his or her family should be instructed to inspect the user's skin after periods of prolonged sitting. It is important to routinely inspect the skin that overlies bony prominences such as the vertebral spinous processes, inferior angles of the scapulae, ischial tuberosities, greater trochanters, lateral femoral condyles, sacrum, and medial humeral epicondyles, especially for persons who have diminished sensation in those areas. Instructions should be given to the patient, family, or personal care attendant so each person will know how and when to relieve weight bearing. The importance of pressure relief must be emphasized, and compliance with a relief schedule or program should be encouraged. Some users will need to perform several sitting push-ups each hour, and some will need to elevate one buttock at a time by leaning to one side and then to the other side several times each hour they are in the wheelchair to relieve pressure from the ischial tuberosities.

Some persons who perform repetitive sitting push-ups may cause stress to the wrist structures, which may lead to a condition similar to carpal tunnel syndrome. As a preventive measure, an alternative pressure relief method may need to be used. Other patients will need to adjust their position by shifting the trunk forward, backward, or to each side several times each hour they are in the chair. Some users may need to be removed from the chair after sitting for 1 to 4 hours or lifted briefly from the seat by another person several times per hour. The user and his or her family members should be informed that sitting on a cushion or pillow does not eliminate the need to frequently relieve pressure on the buttocks by any of the methods described.

The patient and his or her family should be instructed to watch for the following signs or symptoms of decreased circulation in the lower extremities:

- Ankle edema
- Color changes in the toes, feet, or legs
- Decreased sensory response to surface stimuli
- Loss of hair follicles

Other similar conditions that cannot be explained or that are not associated with the person's illness or condition should be reported to a physician. If any of these signs or symptoms occur, it may be necessary to reduce the amount of time the person sits in the wheelchair. Prevention of a severe secondary problem is extremely important and should supersede the user's desire to sit in the wheelchair. Evaluation of the femoral, popliteal, and pedal pulses and observation of the legs should be performed frequently. Evidence of venous stasis or ischemic skin (e.g., dark skin over the malleolus) and soft-tissue ulcers should be reported to a physician. It is particularly important to perform such evaluation and observation for persons whose illnesses or conditions may lead to circulatory changes, such as patients with a spinal cord injury, diabetes mellitus, or a kidney disorder, or persons who use nicotine or alcohol excessively.

WHEELCHAIR COMPONENTS AND FEATURES

Many styles and types of wheelchairs have similar features, but the operation of these features may vary. The more common features and their operation are described, and some are illustrated in this section. The components or features that are appropriate and necessary for one patient may be unnecessary or inappropriate for another patient (see Appendix A). Decisions about the components and features selected for a patient's chair will depend on the criteria described previously.

Armrests

Fixed Armrests Fixed armrests, which are permanently attached to the chair frame, are recommended for users who will be performing standing transfers and have no need to remove the armrest.

Removable or Reversible Armrests Removable or reversible armrests are recommended for users who will perform a lateral swinging or sliding transfer in a sitting posture. The armrest can be reversed to temporarily narrow the distance between the armrest panels and is usually secured to the frame by a pin and lock (Fig. 7-5, A).

Desk or Cutout Armrests Desk armrests are recommended for persons who wish to position the wheelchair close to a permanent surface such as a desk, table, or countertop. The armrests usually can be reversed to improve anterior support when the wheelchair user performs a standing transfer (Fig. 7-5, B).

Adjustable Armrests Adjustable armrests are used by persons who need to adjust the armrest height for different activities or when cushions with different thickness or bulky outer garments are used. Typical adjustments include a friction adjustment, which is accomplished by loosening and tightening a knob, or a pin-in-hole adjustment. Hand function is necessary to adjust the armrest height (Fig. 7-5, C).

Wheels and Tires

Caster Wheels Caster wheels are usually located at the front of the chair to permit changes of direction and turns. They are usually 5 or 8 inches in diameter and may have solid rubber, pneumatic (air-filled), or semipneumatic (partially air-filled) tires (Fig. 7-6, A). Compared with solid rubber tires, pneumatic or semipneumatic tires provide a smoother, more comfortable ride and function better on rough and soft surfaces such as sand, gravel, and grass, but they may require greater energy expenditure by the user to propel the chair because they are wider than solid tires and create more friction, especially on carpeting.

Drive or Rear Wheels Drive wheels, which are used to propel the chair, may have solid rubber, semipneumatic, or pneumatic tires. Some pneumatic tires are manufactured to specifically reduce or prevent the occurrence of a flat tire. The hand rim may be molded to the wheel rim or separated from the rim. In addition, the hand rim may have vertical, horizontal, or angled projections, or it may be coated with plastic to enable the user to propel the chair more easily when the user has decreased hand function. Note: A power-assist device may be added to the axle to allow the chair to be propelled with minimal effort (Fig. 7-6, B).

One-Arm-Drive Chair A one-arm-drive chair may be used for independent propulsion when the user has only one functional upper extremity and no functional lower extremities. Two hand rims are attached to the same wheel. The outer, larger rim propels the far-drive wheel and the inner, smaller rim propels the near-drive wheel. When the user grasps and moves both hand rims simultaneously, the chair is propelled in a straight line forward or backward. Use of one hand rim independently causes the chair to turn. A linkage bar connects the two drive wheels. This chair is heavier and more difficult to fold than a standard chair.

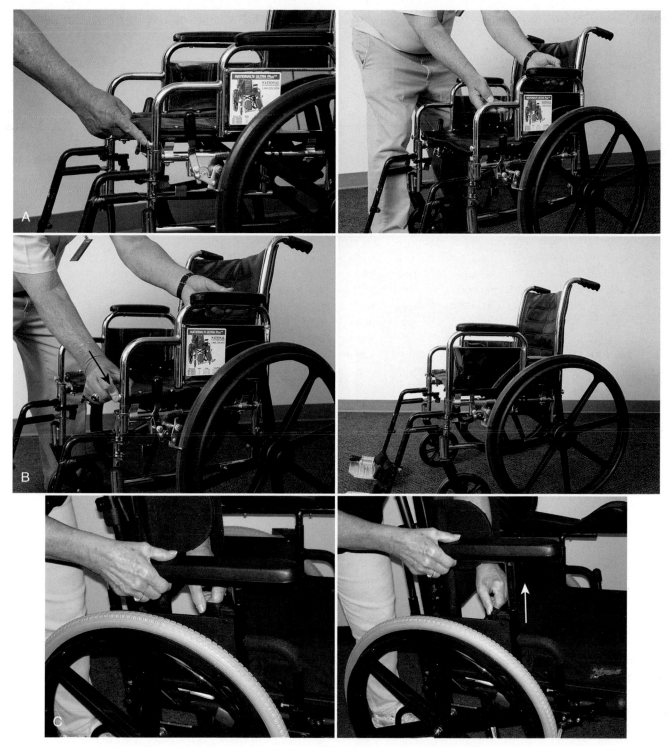

Fig. 7-5   Armrests, all with pin and lock releases. **A,** Removable arm. **B,** Desk (or cutout) arm. **C,** Adjustable arm.

Wheel Locks

Toggle Lock A toggle lock can be engaged either by pushing it forward or backward (Fig. 7-7, A). Although the lock should be engaged before any patient transfer is undertaken to stabilize the chair and to add to safety, persons who become proficient and can safely perform a transfer may prefer not to engage the locks before the transfer. The toggle lock should not be used as a brake to stop the chair or to retard the motion of the chair, as when ascending or descending an incline. A special device can be added to the

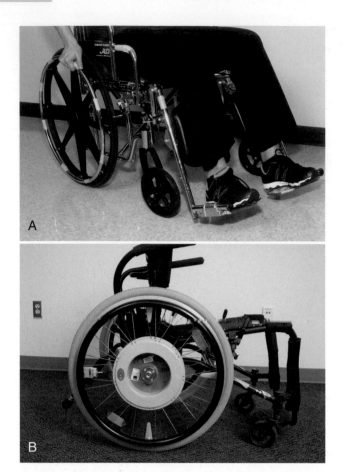

Fig. 7-6 Wheelchair tires. **A,** Caster and drive wheels. **B,** Power-assisted axle.

Caster Locks Caster locks are used to lock the caster wheels to prevent them from turning. Usually these locks have a pin or small flat metal bar that engages a hole or notch located in a metal ring attached to the caster wheel. Caster locks are an optional item for most wheelchairs.

Front Rigging, Leg Rest, and Footrest Components

Fixed Footrests Fixed footrests are attached permanently to the chair frame. The footrest or footplate can be elevated or raised from a horizontal to a vertical position when the user rises, sits, or desires to place his or her feet on the floor. This type of footrest prevents the chair from being positioned close to and directly in front of most objects.

Swing-Away or Removable Leg Rests With swing-away or removable leg rests, release of a locking mechanism allows the front rigging to be pivoted outward, and lifting the leg rest removes the front rigging from the chair frame (Fig. 7-8, *A*). Several different locking mechanisms are available, including a pin lock and a pressure release lever. This feature is used to allow the user to position the chair closer to objects and to provide greater unimpaired space at the front of the chair for the feet during transfers.

Elevating Leg Rest With an elevating leg rest, the entire front rigging can be elevated and maintained at different heights. This feature is useful for patients who are unable to fully flex their knees or when knee flexion must be avoided (e.g., in cases of a fused knee or a long leg cast). A calf panel is attached to the leg rest to support the lower leg (Fig. 7-8, *B*). The leg rest remains elevated by a serrated cam or small gear, which engages a serrated piece of metal on the leg rest. Lowering of the leg rest is usually accomplished by operating a lever that releases the adjustment lock (see Fig. 7-8, *B*). The speed of the leg rest as it lowers must be controlled by supporting the leg rest as it descends. It is important to protect the patient's lower extremity when the leg rest is lowered because the weight of the leg will cause it to descend rapidly if the patient cannot control its descent. This precaution is especially important when a lower extremity has a cast applied.

The front rigging usually can be pivoted outward or removed from the chair to aid transfer activities, and the length of the leg rest can be adjusted to accommodate the patient's lower extremity when it is elevated. When one or both lower extremities are elevated, the chair will have a greater tendency to tip backward because the COG of the chair is altered; therefore the user must be careful when propelling the chair up an incline. Too strong or too rapid movement of the rear wheels is likely to cause the caster wheels to be lifted from the surface. A weight added to the front of the chair frame may help reduce this problem.

wheelchair to prevent the chair's backward motion when the user ascends an incline or ramp (Fig. 7-7, *B*).

A vertical extension can be attached to the lock to help persons with poor trunk control or limited function of an upper extremity to operate the lock without leaning or reaching excessively (Fig. 7-7, *C*).

Z or Scissors Lock The Z lock is located beneath the chair seat (Fig. 7-7, *D*) toward the front of the seat rail. The wheelchair user must be able to reach under the seat to operate the lock. Because of the location, propulsion of the chair can be performed without interference from a lock positioned on the side of the seat rail and in front of the drive wheel.

Auxiliary Lock for a Reclining Back Chair An auxiliary lock is necessary to release the back and to increase the wheelbase when the back is reclined. An attendant is needed to engage and disengage the lock, unless a custom electric wheelchair with a reclining back system is used (Fig. 7-7, *E*).

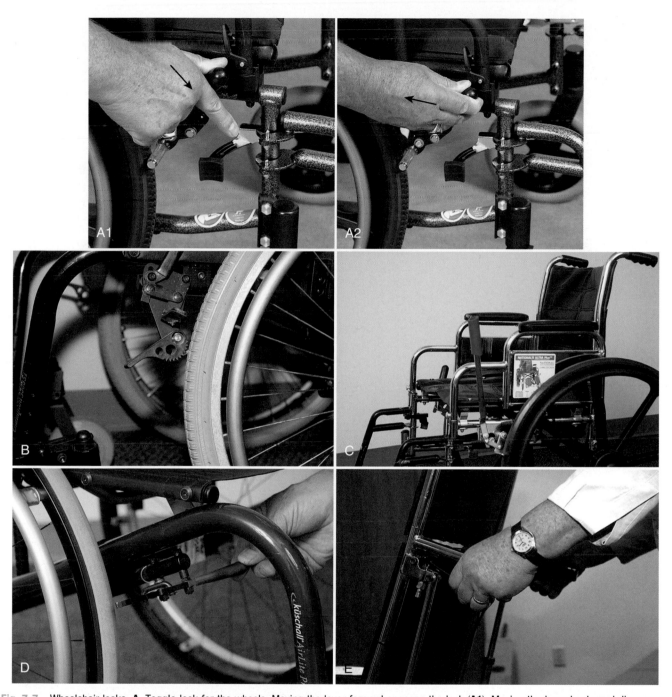

Fig. 7-7 Wheelchair locks. **A,** Toggle lock for the wheels. Moving the lever forward engages the lock (**A1**). Moving the lever backward disengages the lock (**A2**). **B,** Accessory to prevent the chair from rolling backward when it is propelled up a ramp or incline. **C,** Toggle lock extension. **D,** Z, or scissors, lock. **E,** Auxiliary lock for the back of a reclining wheelchair.

Footrest The footrest, also called a footplate, is available in various shapes and sizes depending on the patient's needs. It may have a toe or heel loop to help maintain the foot on the footrest (Fig. 7-8, C). The heel loop prevents the foot from sliding backward, and the toe loop prevents the foot from moving forward. The heel loop should be moved forward before the footrest is raised to prevent damage to the heel loop fabric and to allow the footrest to be fully

raised before a standing transfer or folding of the chair is attempted (Fig. 7-8, C). It is important to note that the footrests should always be elevated before a standing transfer and before movement of a patient into or out of the chair.

A strap rather than heel loops may be used between the two leg rests to prevent posterior movement of the patient's legs. These straps may have various shapes or

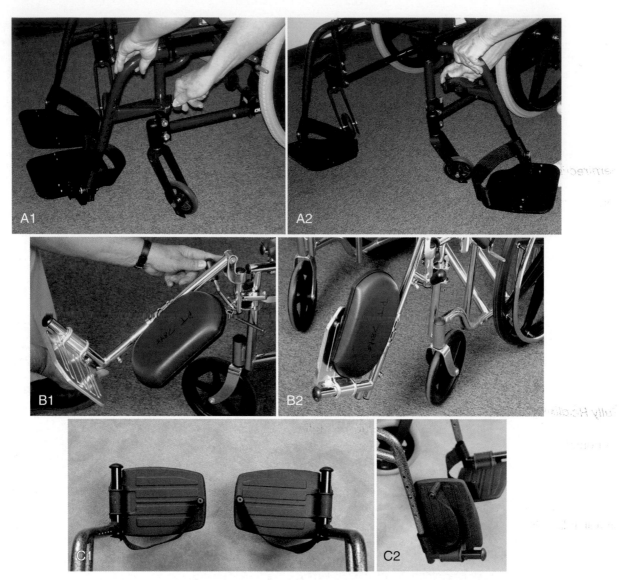

Fig. 7-8 Leg rests. **A1** and **A2,** Swing-away with release and lock control. **B1** and **B2,** Elevating leg rest. **C1** and **C2,** Footrests (footplates) with heel loops.

configurations (e.g., a single strap, a double strap, or an H strap).

Body Restraints

Lap (Waist) Belt A lap belt (i.e., restraint), which is attached to the frame of the chair, is designed to prevent the patient from falling out of the chair or sliding forward in the chair. As the name implies, this strap crosses the wheelchair user's lower abdomen or pelvis, similar to an airplane or automobile lap belt (Fig. 7-9). The buckle may be located in back of the chair to prevent the patient from having access to it.

Chest Belt A chest belt is attached to the frame of the chair at the mid-chest level to increase trunk stability, prevent the wheelchair user from falling out of the chair,

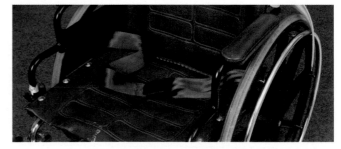

Fig. 7-9 A wheelchair lap belt.

and maintain the body upright. It may be combined with a lap belt for greater security. The buckle may be located in the back of the chair to prevent the patient from having access to it, or it may be built into the sides of the chair. A chest harness provides even greater security in maintaining trunk stability. (Note: These belts are provided to protect patients who have inadequate balance or trunk stability while seated. They are not appropriate for use as a method to restrain a patient in the chair for a prolonged period. Federal, state, and accrediting agency regulations and guidelines regarding the use of belts or straps as restraints must be followed.)

Reclining Wheelchairs

Semireclining Semireclining wheelchairs allow the back of the chair to be adjusted to various positions from fully upright to 30 degrees of extension (Fig. 7-10, A). Usually, two adjustment knobs or levers located on either side of the back frame are used to release and adjust the position of the back. The chair back usually is higher than that on a standard chair, and a removable head component is necessary to support the wheelchair user's head when he or she is in a reclined position. Elevating leg rests are necessary components of this chair for user comfort and to maintain the chair's stability. If the leg rests do not elevate, the chair will tend to tip backward when it is reclined because of a shift in the relative position of the user's COG and the BOS of the chair. A bar across the back adds support to the back frame.

Fully Reclining Fully reclining wheelchairs allow the back to be adjusted to various positions from vertical to fully horizontal (Fig. 7-10, B). Adjustment knobs or levers located on either side of the back frame are used to adjust the position of the back. A headrest and elevating leg rests are necessary components, as described previously. In addition, the rear wheels will be located more posteriorly than on a standard chair, or they may move back as the chair is reclined to increase the BOS and stability of the chair. (Note: The reclining wheelchair is used for persons who must recline periodically while seated in the chair. Persons with lower extremity circulatory problems who cannot tolerate an upright position because of decreased circulation or who need to relieve skin pressure but cannot perform pressure relief independently may find a reclining or tilt-in-space chair beneficial.)

The tilt-in-space wheelchair can be adjusted to position the user at various angles and can be wheeled with the user positioned at any angle (Fig. 7-10, C). Proper seating and positioning should promote function, prevent deformity, improve body alignment, prevent tissue damage, and prevent additional complications. Items such as a headrest, lateral trunk support panels, a seat pan or cushion, a back panel, an armrest trough and adjustments, and lower extremity supports can be added to a chair to accomplish specific positioning goals.

Externally Powered Wheelchair

An externally powered wheelchair is powered by one or more deep-cycle batteries that provide stored electrical energy to one or more belts that drive or propel the chair. The motorized chair is available for persons with insufficient strength or motor control of the extremities to propel a standard chair. Various controls are available to operate the chair, including those operated by the patient's hand, chin, head, tongue, or mouth. Sophisticated microprocessor control systems also are available (Fig. 7-11). The chair may have a proportional drive system in which the speed is directly related to the pressure applied to the control device (i.e., as more pressure is applied, greater speed is generated), or it may have a microswitch system, in which the speed is preset so the chair will move only at a fixed speed regardless of the amount of pressure applied to the control.

Three main battery types are available for electric wheelchairs. Wet batteries, which typically are the cheapest battery, use a chemical reaction between lead and sulfur to create a charge. Gel batteries contain a mixture of phosphoric acid, sulphuric acid, fumed silica, and pure water and tend to be heavier and more expensive than wet batteries. AGM batteries, which are costly, feature an absorbent glass mat between plates soaked with an acid electrolyte. Charging the wheelchair battery depends on the type of battery that is on the chair. The manual for the wheelchair and attached battery must be checked to determine charging instructions. The battery charger is specific to the wheelchair battery and should be purchased when the wheelchair is purchased. The wheelchair battery should be removed according to the instructions in the user's manual, and the battery charger should be plugged into the battery according to the charger's instructions. The charger should be plugged into an electrical wall outlet and the battery should be allowed to charge until it is at full capacity. Most batteries fully charge in less than 8 hours.

Sport or Recreational Wheelchair

Sport or recreational wheelchairs have specific features such as low backrests, solid, lightweight frames, canted (angled) rear wheels, low and narrow seats, and an overall low profile to make the chair more functional for the user. The engineering and design of sports mobility chairs enable them to be tough, highly maneuverable, responsive, and stable. In addition, they are built to withstand the impact and jarring that occurs with different types of competitive and recreational sports. Many of these chairs are custom fabricated, depending on the sport or recreational activity in which the user participates. The chair pictured in Figure 7-12, A, is an example of a basketball sport wheelchair. One feature of a sport wheelchair may be an adjustable back and/or seat height.

Lightweight or Ultralight Wheelchair

The most popular lightweight wheelchair model is the rigid wheelchair (Fig. 7-12, B). Rigid mobility chairs are lighter

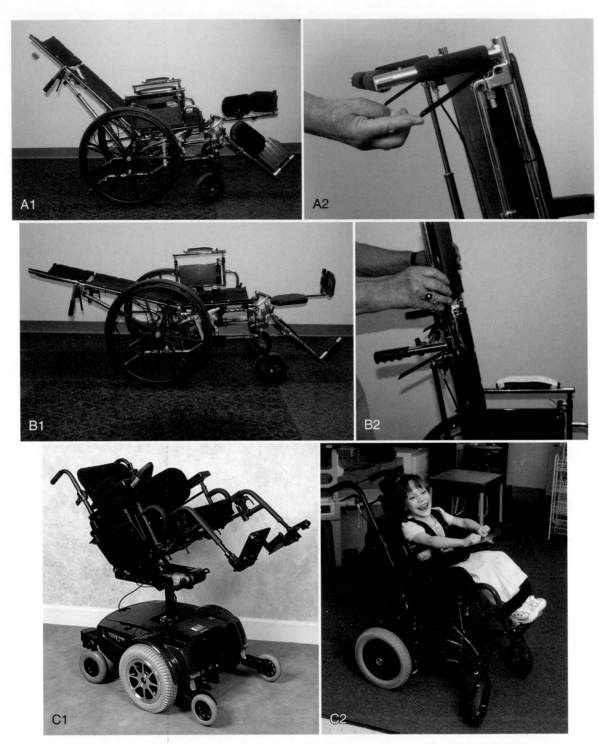

Fig. 7-10   Reclining wheelchairs. **A1** and **A2,** Semireclining. **B1** and **B2,** Fully reclining. **C1** and **C2,** Tilt-in-space.

than folding wheelchairs because they don't feature the additional hardware and mechanisms that folding wheelchairs require. The backrest of a rigid wheelchair can fold for transport. Unlike folding wheelchairs, the middle of a rigid wheelchair seat does not fold. Lightweight or ultralight wheelchairs also can have removable legs, arms that swing up or swivel (Fig. 7-12, C) and adjustable backs, as seen in Figure 7-12, D.

Standard lightweight wheel chairs are normally made of aluminum, but titanium is the material of choice for lightweight mobility aids. Titanium is not only a lighter metal, but it is more durable and features built-in shock

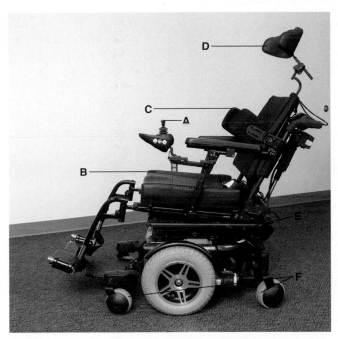

Fig. 7-11 An adult externally powered wheelchair. **A,** "Joystick" control. **B,** Molded seat cushion. **C,** Side panels. **D,** Head support. **E,** Swing-away leg rests. **F,** Pneumatic tires.

absorption. Titanium wheelchairs are available in both rigid and folding models and are more expensive than aluminum wheelchairs. Most long-term users select an ultra-light wheelchair to reduce the amount of energy required for propulsion and to reduce the trauma to the upper extremities. This type of chair is very durable, has higher quality wheel bearings, and has several adjustment features. It weighs from 12 to 30 lb.

Folding Wheelchairs

Many wheelchairs can be folded for storage or transport (Procedure 7-2). A folded chair can be wheeled (transported) most easily by elevating the caster wheels and wheeling the chair on the rear wheels, while using the push handles for control. When the folded chair is to be lifted, the fixed or solid portion of the frame should be used.

Caution must be exercised so the chair is not lifted by any of the removable components, such as the armrests or front rigging, because they may disengage from the chair.

FUNCTIONAL ACTIVITIES

A person who uses a wheelchair for mobility should be instructed in the proper use and care of the chair. The caregiver should instruct the wheelchair user's family regarding the proper use of good body mechanics while pushing or transferring the patient and should teach them how to use the wheelchair properly. The projected use of the chair should be based on the patient's goals, needs, and anticipated lifestyle. Many functional activities should be practiced by the new wheelchair user with the use of proper safety and protective guarding techniques. Visiting the environment where the user resides may be necessary to identify the usual, unusual, and special activities of the patient and related instruction that will be required.

Operation of Wheelchair Components

Each wheelchair user should be taught to perform the following maneuvers: (1) operate the wheel locks and tighten them when necessary; (2) remove and replace the armrests; (3) swing away, remove, and replace the front rigging; and (4) elevate and lower the footplates before performing other activities. The instructions may be oral, demonstrated, written, or illustrated, or a videotape can be used. The user should not be expected to inherently understand how to perform these activities. Instructions should be given to each user, along with an opportunity to practice and demonstrate the ability to perform these maneuvers.

Persons with functional use of the upper and lower extremities, normal trunk control, and normal balance should not experience difficulty learning and performing these tasks. However, persons with functional loss of use of one or more extremities, decreased trunk control, and decreased balance may require several practice sessions to learn to perform these tasks safely and proficiently.

Independent Propulsion

Bilateral Upper Extremities To move the wheelchair independently, the user grasps the hand rims at the top of the wheels (at the 12-o'clock position) and pushes forward or pulls backward with equal force on each wheel (Fig. 7-14, A). To perform a turn, instruct the user to hold one hand rim and pull or push on the opposite hand rim; to turn more quickly, he or she should simultaneously push forward on one hand rim and pull back on the opposite hand rim.

One Upper Extremity and One Lower Extremity To move the wheelchair independently with one upper extremity and one lower extremity, the user grasps the hand rim at the top of the wheel and pushes forward or pulls back, using the functional foot to pull or push simultaneously (Fig. 7-14, B). The foot also serves as a rudder to assist with turning while the user holds the hand rim (Fig. 7-14, C). The use of one upper extremity and one lower extremity, usually on the same side, is an excellent method for a person with hemiplegia.

Bilateral Lower Extremities To move the wheelchair independently with bilateral lower extremities, the patient uses the heels and soles of the feet or shoes to propel the chair forward and backward and as a rudder to turn to the left or right. This method is rarely used, but it would be of value for any person with reduced function of both upper extremities or with poor trunk control or for a user who is unable to ambulate.

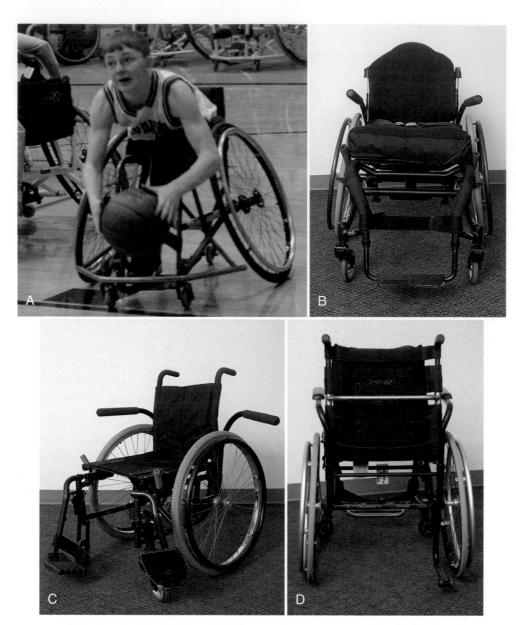

Fig. 7-12 **A,** Sport-style wheelchair with canted drive wheels, solid frame, low backrest, and fixed footplate. **B,** An ultralight wheelchair with a fixed frame and custom back. **C,** An ultralight chair with swing-away front rigging (left), swivel armrest (left), and wheel locks applied. **D,** Adjustable back upholstery on a fixed-frame chair.

Any person who uses a wheelchair should be instructed orally and by demonstration how to propel the chair forward and backward, turn to the left and to the right, and turn the chair in a half or complete circle. Practice of these techniques is required for the person to become independent and operate the wheelchair safely. These activities should be practiced initially on a smooth, flat surface rather than on a carpet and in a space free of objects. Eventually, the user should practice on carpeting or a rough surface and should attempt to maneuver around objects, in a congested area, and on a sidewalk or other outdoor surfaces.

Assisted Functional Activities

Assisted Propulsion on a Level Surface When assisting a person in a wheelchair, make sure you use proper body mechanics in all of the following maneuvers. When propelling a patient in a wheelchair, use the push handles to move and control the chair. To turn the chair, hold one push handle and push or pull on the other push handle. For example, to turn to the left, hold the left push handle and push on the right push handle, or hold the right push handle and pull on the left push handle. Do not push the chair and then release the push handles; always maintain control of the chair when it is moving and you are propelling it,

PROCEDURE 7-2

Folding a Wheelchair

- To fold the chair, the footrests must be raised after the heel loops have been moved forward.
  - Pull up on the seat rails or on hand loops attached to the seat rails (**A1** and **A2**).
  - An alternative method is to grasp the midline of the front and back of the seat upholstery and lift upward, though this method may cause damage to the upholstery if it is used excessively.
  - After the chair has been folded, the seat upholstery can be positioned downward between the seat rails.
- The back support bar of a reclining chair must be released or removed before this chair is folded. You will need to examine the bar to determine how to release it.

The bar must be replaced and secured in place before a patient is placed into the chair.
- To unfold the chair, lift the rear wheels from the floor by lifting on the push handles and gently begin to move the push handles away from each other. When the chair is partially unfolded, replace the rear wheels on the floor and complete the unfolding by pushing down evenly on each seat rail (**B1** and **B2**).
- If the chair is to be unfolded on a carpet, it may be necessary to unfold it with the rear wheels elevated throughout the entire process because the rear wheels will be difficult to separate when on carpet.

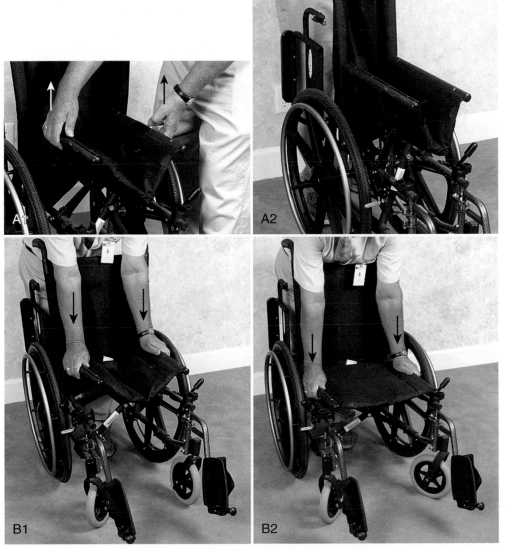

Fig. 7-13   Folding and unfolding a wheelchair.

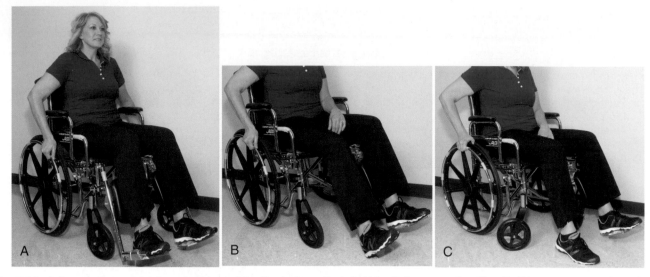

Fig. 7-14 Independent propulsion in an environment familiar to the patient. **A,** Using both upper extremities. **B,** Using one upper and one lower extremity. **C,** Turning to the left.

particularly when moving on an incline or ramp. Start and stop chair movement smoothly, and avoid a sudden or abrupt start or stop. In most settings and environments, use the right side of the corridor or sidewalk when propelling the chair. Use caution when you reach the corner of a wall, especially when no mirror is available to view oncoming traffic or hazards that might be around the corner. Also use caution when you move the chair through any doorway because the patient's feet and chair footrests project in front of the chair, making them susceptible to being struck and injured.

When it is necessary or desirable to tip the patient and propel the chair on its rear wheels, be certain to inform the patient of your intentions before you tip the chair.

Finally, be certain that the chair is secure and stable, with the footrests elevated, before the patient enters or exits the chair using a standing transfer. The chair wheels should be locked, or you should hold the push handles if the patient can enter or exit the chair independently and safely.

Elevation of the Caster Wheels The person in the chair should be warned before being tipped, and the entire procedure should be described before it is performed (Procedure 7-3). Reverse the procedure to lower the caster wheels to the floor and retard the effect of gravity as the caster wheels descend. You must be certain you have the physical strength to perform this procedure and control the chair when it is tipped; your use of proper body mechanics is very important.

Anti-tipping extensions can be added to prevent the chair from tipping completely backward (Fig. 7-16).

Ascending and Descending a Curb Practice the forward and backward methods for ascending and descending curbs to determine which is the most efficient and safest for you to perform. Perform each method with persons of different sizes and weights in the chair. By trying each method, you will be able to offer alternatives to a family member or other person who eventually may assist the user.

Methods for ascending a curb are found in Procedure 7-4, and methods for descending a curb are found in Procedure 7-5. Usually, ascending while facing forward and descending in a backward position are the movements that are the easiest to control and the safest to use.

Ascending a Curb While Facing Forward. The easiest way to ascend a curb is to face forward; this method provides the greatest control of the chair and requires the least effort by the caregiver (see Procedure 7-4).

If the patient is able to do so, he or she can provide assistance by leaning forward slightly and pushing on the hand rims until the rear wheels are on the sidewalk surface. The patient must have control of the trunk musculature, adequate balance, and functional use of the upper extremities to assist with this activity.

Ascending a Curb in the Backward Position. It is more difficult to ascend a curb in the backward position than in the forward position because of the effort needed to pull the chair up the curb and to control the chair (see Procedure 7-4).

If the person in the chair is able to do so, he or she can provide assistance by pulling back on the hand rims as the chair is pulled up and over the curb. The chair should be maintained in a tipped position until all four wheels are positioned over the surface above the curb.

Descending a Curb in the Backward Position. The easiest way to descend a curb is in the backward position because it provides the greatest control of the chair

PROCEDURE **7-3**

Elevation of the Caster Wheels

- Stand behind the chair.
- Push down and forward with one foot on one tipping lever (**A**) while pushing down and back with both hands on the push handles.

- Once the caster wheels are elevated, you will need to control the chair with the push handles.
- The chair can be propelled while the caster wheels are elevated (**B**).

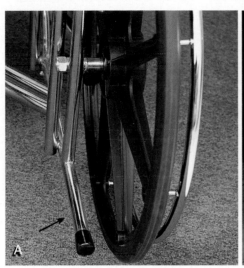 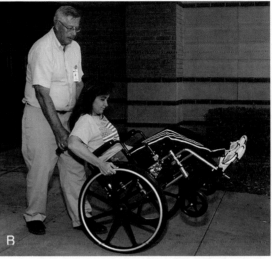

Fig. 7-15   Elevation of the caster wheels. **A,** Tipping lever for elevation of the caster wheels. **B,** Propelling a wheelchair while it is reclined on the drive wheels.

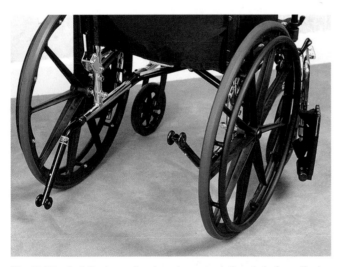

Fig. 7-16   Anti-tipping extensions to prevent the chair from tipping backward. The extensions can be rotated upward or removed.

and requires the least effort by the caregiver (see Procedure 7-5).

If the person in the chair is able to do so, he or she can provide assistance by providing friction with the hands against the hand rims and by leaning the trunk forward as the chair rolls over and down the curb.

Descending a Curb While Facing Forward. Descending a curb while facing forward is a difficult procedure; before attempting it, you must be certain you have the strength and ability to control the chair (see Procedure 7-5). Use of proper body mechanics is very important when performing this procedure.

The person in the chair can assist by providing friction with his or her hands against the hand rims as the chair rolls over and down the curb.

Ascending and Descending Stairs Just as with curbs, you should practice the forward and backward methods for ascending and descending stairs to determine which is the most efficient and safest method for you to perform. You should perform each method with persons of different sizes and weights in the chair. By trying each method, you will be able to offer alternatives to a family member or another person who eventually may assist the user.

Methods for ascension and descension of stairs are found in Procedure 7-6.

Ascending Stairs in the Backward Position. At least two persons other than the patient are needed to safely ascend stairs in the backward position; three persons may be required for a heavy or severely incapacitated patient.

PROCEDURE 7-4

Assisted Ascending of a Curb

For these activities, explain the activity to the patient, instruct how and when he or she should assist, and alert the patient as you begin the activity.

Ascending while facing forward

- Position the chair facing the curb.
- Stand on the street surface.
- Tip the chair back using the push handles and tipping lever (**A**).
- Wheel the chair forward until the rear wheels contact the curb; lower the caster wheels to the sidewalk surface (**B**).
- Lift up using the push handles and wheel the chair forward over the curb (**C**).

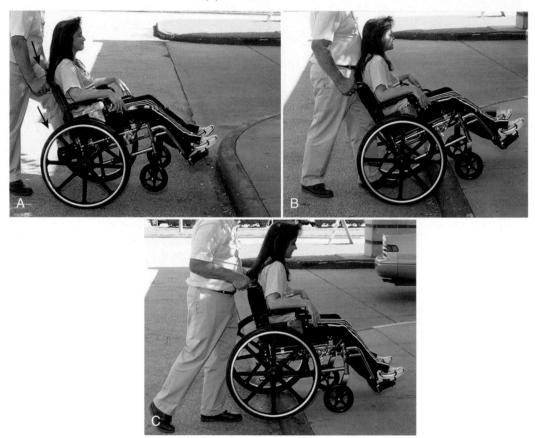

Fig. 7-17   Ascending a curb while facing forward.

It is important to caution assistants not to grasp any of the removable items of the chair such as the armrests or front rigging, because these items could become disengaged from the chair.

Descending Stairs While Facing Forward. Descending stairs while facing forward is performed most safely if at least two persons assist (three persons will be required for a heavy or severely incapacitated patient).

Assistants should be cautioned not to grasp any of the removable items of the chair such as the armrests or front rigging, because these items could become disengaged from the chair.

Ascending or Descending a Slope The techniques for ascending or descending a slope can be found in Procedure 7-7. Caution should be used when traversing any elevation, but for steep elevations it may be necessary to zigzag up or down the incline by angling the chair to the left and then to the right. The person in the chair can help propel the chair as described previously.

PROCEDURE 7-4

Assisted Ascending of a Curb—cont'd

Ascending in the backward position

- Position the chair so the rear wheels contact the curb.
- Stand on the sidewalk surface.
- Tip the chair back using the push handles; maintain this position (**A**).
- Pull the chair over the curb on its rear wheels (**B**).
- Back up or turn the chair to one side until the caster wheels are above the sidewalk surface.
- Lower the caster wheels using the push handles and tipping lever.

Note: You will need to stoop or bend down while using this method.

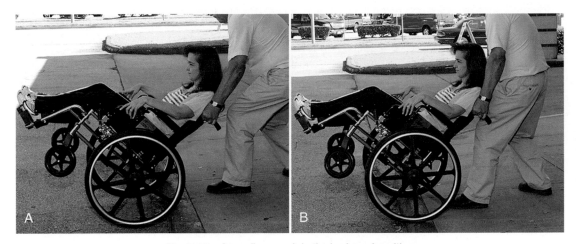

Fig. 7-18   Ascending a curb in the backward position.

Allowing the chair to ascend or descend a slope with the chair facing downhill with all four wheels in contact with the surface is not recommended because the patient may fall forward.

Moving Across Rough or Soft Surfaces The most effective way to control and propel a wheelchair over an uneven or soft surface is to elevate the caster wheels so that only the rear wheels contact the surface. The chair must be maintained in this tipped position as it is propelled over the surface.

Entering and Exiting Elevators Elevators may be entered with the chair facing forward or in the backward position. Many persons prefer to enter backward so they can access the selector panel, avoid facing the back wall of the car, and avoid turning the chair around to exit the car. However, entering the elevator backward and leaving the elevator forward places the lower extremities at risk if the door panels close prematurely or if access to the corridor into which the person exits is limited. Furthermore, when leaving the elevator facing forward, the caster wheels may lodge in the space

between the elevator floor and the corridor surface, and the traffic in the corridor cannot be observed until the patient has completely left the elevator. When the patient exits the elevator backward, the lower extremities are still at risk of being struck by the door panels, and turning in the corridor may be difficult because of limited space or traffic. However, the patient will be able to view the traffic in the corridor easily, and it will be easier to move the rear wheels over the space between the surface of the floor and the elevator car surface. Be certain the chair is completely out of the elevator car before attempting to turn it; this step is particularly important when one or both of the patient's lower extremities are elevated. You may need to position your body against the edge of the door or ask someone in the car to use the control button to keep the door open as the patient enters or leaves the elevator car.

Many elevator locations have exterior wall mirrors that enable you to view the corridor before you exit the elevator. You should be familiar with the safety devices in the elevator car, such as the panel control to maintain the door in the open position, along with the emergency door control items, such as a photoelectric beam or pressure sensors in the edge

PROCEDURE 7-5

Assisted Descending of a Curb

For these activities, explain the activity to the patient, instruct how and when he or she should assist, and alert the patient as you begin the activity.

Descending in the
backward position

- Position the chair with the rear wheels at the edge of the curb; the caster wheels should remain in contact with the sidewalk surface.
- Stand on the street surface.
- Allow the rear wheels to roll over the edge of the curb until they contact the street; control the movement of the chair with one hip against the back of the chair (**A**).
- Elevate the caster wheels until they have cleared the curb; back up or turn the chair to one side (**B**). Caution: Maintain the chair in a reclined position until the caster wheels and front rigging clear the curb.
- Lower the caster wheels onto the street surface using the push handles and tipping lever.

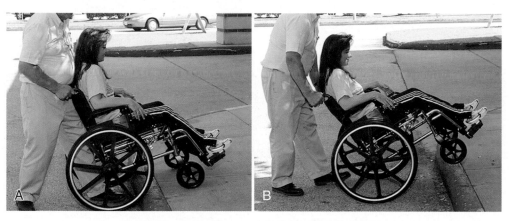

Fig. 7-19   Descending a curb in the backward position.

Descending while facing
forward

- Position the chair with the caster wheels at the edge of the curb; the patient should be seated back in the chair.
- Stand on the sidewalk surface.
- Tip the chair onto its rear wheels using the push handles and tipping lever (**A**).
- Wheel the chair forward, and allow it to roll over the edge of the curb as you pull back on the push handles (**B**). If the patient is able to do so, he or she can help control the movement of the chair by providing friction to the hand rims with the hands.
- After the rear wheels are on the street, gently lower the caster wheels using the push handles and tipping lever.

Note: You will need to stoop or bend down while using this method.

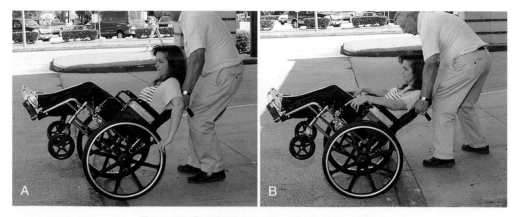

Fig. 7-20   Descending a curb while facing forward.

PROCEDURE 7-6

Ascending and Descending Stairs

For these activities, explain the activity to the patient, instruct how and when he or she should assist, and alert the patient as you begin the activity.

Ascending in the backward position
- Position the rear wheels so they contact the bottom step and elevate the caster wheels (**A**). The chair must be maintained in this tipped position as it is moved up the stairs.
- Pull the chair up onto each step as described for ascending a curb backward.
- The persons who assist should stand on one or both sides of the chair and grasp the frame of the chair (**B**).
- On the command of the leader, all persons should help roll the chair up the stairs, one step at a time. The leader should indicate when the next step is to be ascended so all persons work together.
- At the top of the steps, turn the chair 90 degrees or roll it backward until it can be lowered onto its caster wheels.
- The person who controls the chair by grasping the push handles must use proper body mechanics by partially stooping, widening the base of support, and pulling (rather than lifting) on the push handles.
- When this activity is being performed without additional assistance, the person in the chair can assist by pulling back on the hand rims on command (**C**).

Descending while facing forward
- Position the caster wheels at the edge of the top step, and tip the chair onto its rear wheels.
- Slowly and carefully roll the chair until its rear wheels are at the edge of the step.
- The persons who assist should stand on one or both sides of the chair and grasp the frame of the chair. They should not grasp any of the removable items of the chair (**D**).
- On the command of the leader, all persons retard the motion of the rear wheels down to the next step. The chair must be maintained in this reclined position as it moves down the stairs.
- Stop the chair on each step to avoid developing momentum.
- Lower the chair onto its caster wheels at the bottom of the steps.
- The person who controls the chair by grasping the push handles must use proper body mechanics as described previously.

Note: The person in the chair can assist by providing friction against the hand rims as the chair descends each step.

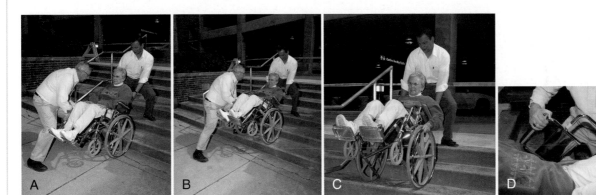

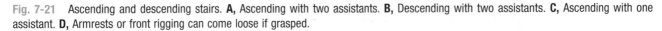

Fig. 7-21   Ascending and descending stairs. **A,** Ascending with two assistants. **B,** Descending with two assistants. **C,** Ascending with one assistant. **D,** Armrests or front rigging can come loose if grasped.

PROCEDURE 7-7

Ascending or Descending a Slope

Two approaches can be used to ascend and descend slopes: a two-wheeled approach and a four-wheeled approach.

Ascending a slope   On two wheels:
- Elevate the caster wheels and push the chair forward (**A**) or backward (**B**) with only the drive wheels in contact with the ground.
- Propel the chair forward or backward on the rear wheels.

On four wheels:
- Push the chair forward with all four wheels in contact with the ground.

Descending a slope   On two wheels:
- Elevate the caster wheels and retard the motion of the chair by holding the push handles as the chair descends forward.

On four wheels:
- Allow the chair to descend backward with all four wheels in contact with the ground.
- As the chair descends, retard the motion of the chair with the side of your body against the back of the chair and your feet in a widened base of support (**C**).
- The person in the chair can assist in retarding the motion of the chair by providing friction with the hands against the hand rims.

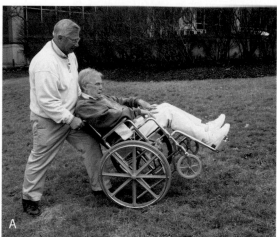
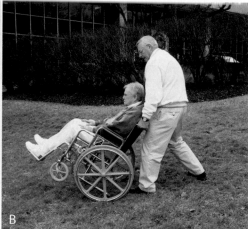
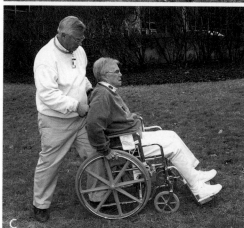

Fig. 7-22   Ascending or descending a slope. **A,** Forward on two wheels. **B,** Backward on two wheels. **C,** Forward or backward on all four wheels.

of the door. Observing whether the floor of the elevator car and the corridor surface are level is important. If the two surfaces are not level, you may need to elevate the caster wheels to safely enter or leave the elevator.

Ascending and Descending Escalators Persons in a wheelchair should avoid using an escalator *except in an extreme emergency*. When the escalator must be used because it is the only means to ascend or descend from one level to another, extreme caution is required to maintain the safety of the wheelchair user.

The person in the chair, assisted by a caregiver, can ascend the escalator while facing forward so the caster wheels are on the step above the rear wheels. Instruct the person in the chair to lean forward and grasp the moving handrails if the width of the escalator permits this maneuver. The caregiver remains behind the chair to prevent it from tipping backward. When the level surface at the top of the escalator is reached, the caster wheels will contact it so the chair can be propelled forward.

The person in the chair, assisted by a caregiver, can descend in the backward position by positioning the rear wheels on the first step and positioning the caster wheels on the step above the rear wheels. The wheelchair user grasps the escalator handrails and leans forward; the caregiver remains behind the wheelchair, for protection. At the bottom of the escalator, the person in the chair wheels backward until the front rigging clears the side of the escalator and turns the chair to proceed.

Ascending and descending an escalator should not be considered an ordinary activity for a person in a wheelchair, and extreme care must be used to prevent possible injury. The caregiver should remain behind the wheelchair as the person ascends or descends to provide control and protection. Use of an escalator by a wheelchair user may be prohibited by many facilities.

Entering and Exiting Doors and Doorways A wheelchair user may be moved through a doorway while facing forward or while in the backward position (Procedure 7-8). Remember that problems or situations similar to those described for entering and leaving an elevator may occur when moving through a doorway. (Note: If a raised threshold is present, it may be easier to move the chair through the doorway backward because the larger rear wheels will roll over the threshold more easily than the caster wheels. If you are pushing the chair while leading with the caster wheels, it may be necessary to elevate the caster wheels to clear the threshold.)

Independent Functional Activities

Elevation of the Caster Wheels Elevation of the caster wheels (otherwise known as a "wheelie" or "pop-up") is necessary so the wheels can clear objects on the floor, side-

---

PROCEDURE 7-8

Entering Doorways

For all procedures, observe the area for traffic or other hazards before you move the patient into the room or corridor.

Entering while facing forward
- If the door opens toward you:
  - Position the chair at a slight angle so the patient faces the edge of the door with the handle. Leave room for the door to open outward.
  - Open the door wide enough so the chair will pass between the door frame and the door edge. If the door has a self-closing device, use one foot or one hand to hold the door open as the chair moves through the doorway.
  - Push the chair through the doorway.
- If the door opens away from you:
  - Position the patient at a slight angle so the patient faces the edge of the door with the handle.
  - Open the door wide enough for the chair to pass through; hold the door open if it has a self-closing device.
  - Push the chair through the doorway.

Entering in a backward position
- If the door opens toward you:
  - Position the chair so the back is toward the opening edge of the door with the chair at a slight angle away from the door edge.
  - Open the door wide enough for the chair to pass through.
  - Pull the chair through the doorway.
  - After the chair has passed completely through the doorway, turn the chair so it faces forward.
- If the door opens away from you:
  - Position the chair so the back is toward the opening edge of the door with the chair at a slight angle toward the door frame.
  - Open the door wide enough for the chair to pass through.
  - Pull the chair through the doorway.

walk, or ground and to ascend or descend curbs and curb cutouts. The wheelchair user must have sufficient bilateral upper extremity strength and coordination and the ability to maintain sitting balance when performing the activity. Practice is required, and the user should be protected from falling backward during practice sessions. A demonstration of the technique by another person or by you is usually helpful and should be performed for all patients (Procedure 7-9).

During practice sessions, stand behind the patient initially, tip the chair to find the balance point, and protect the person from falling backward (Fig. 7-24). You must be alert when the patient attempts to perform the "wheelie" independently so you are prepared to prevent the chair from tipping back too far. A rope properly measured to prevent the chair from tipping backward too far, attached to the push handles and running through a ceiling pulley or eye bolt, can be used to protect the patient as this activity is practiced. A patient with only one functional upper extremity probably will not be able to perform this activity because it will not be possible to generate sufficient force to generate rearward momentum of the chair frame and still safely control the chair.

The caster wheels will lift off the floor because of the abrupt stopping of the rearward motion of the chair. This action will occur because of the principles associated with Newton's first law of motion (i.e., a body will remain at rest or in motion in a straight line until acted on by a force). Once the chair and the person in it start in motion backward, they will continue to move backward even when a force (e.g., the hands grasping the hand rims) stops the motion. The patient's first attempts may only briefly lift the caster wheels a few inches. Over time and with continued practice, while being guarded and protected, many patients will be able to balance on the rear wheels and may be able to propel the chair in this position.

A proficient wheelchair user will be able to perform a wheelie while the chair is moving and maintain the wheelie to descend a curb, cutout, or ramp or to clear an obstacle on the ground or floor (e.g., a threshold, an uneven sidewalk, or a hose). To elevate the caster wheels when the chair is moving, the user must grasp the hand rim or tire at a point well behind the hips and pull forward with the upper extremities as described previously.

The wheelchair user may lean the trunk and head backward slightly to help elevate the caster wheels. This activity requires a great deal of practice, and the user must be guarded from behind the chair continuously. If the patient is unable to master this procedure, teach him or her to perform the wheelie from a stationary position and then propel the chair with the caster wheels elevated.

Ascending and Descending Ramps or Inclines It may be necessary to instruct the person in the chair to zigzag

PROCEDURE 7-9

Elevation of the Caster Wheels

- Instruct the patient to pull back quickly and equally on both hand rims and then abruptly stop the rearward motion of the rear wheels by firmly grasping the hand rims.
- The patient should not attempt to propel the chair backward but should develop a rearward movement momentum of the chair.
- Once the chair and the person in it start in motion backward, they will continue to move backward, with the axles of the rear wheels acting as a fulcrum, and the chair frame with the person seated in it will rotate backward, causing the caster wheels to become elevated.
- When the caster wheels are elevated, small forward movements of the hand rims will cause a rearward movement of the chair frame and seat, and small backward movements of the hand rims will cause a forward movement of the chair frame and seat. The patient should be taught and should practice these motions by sliding the hands forward or backward on the hand rims and using slight head movements to maintain a balanced position.
- Experienced users will be able to perform a wheelie without the initial rearward motion of the chair.
  - The user positions the hands on top of the hand rims or tires slightly posterior to the hips (i.e., a 2-o'clock position) with the trunk inclined forward slightly.
  - The user simultaneously leans the trunk back and pulls forward on the hand rims or tires by bending the elbows without propelling the chair forward.
  - The head can be moved backward slightly to assist in elevating the caster wheels.3

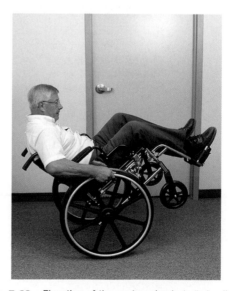

Fig. 7-23 Elevation of the caster wheels (a "wheelie").

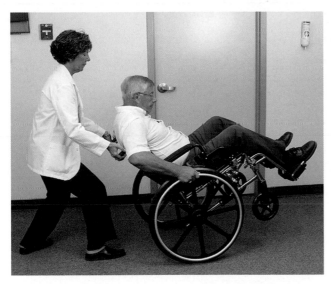

Fig. 7-24 Practicing elevation of the caster wheels with close guarding.

or angle up or down an incline, especially if the incline is particularly steep. This maneuver is done by propelling up or down the incline at an angle to the right for several feet and then propelling at an angle to the left for several feet. This pattern is continued until the top or bottom of the incline is reached.

Ascending an Incline While Facing Forward. When the wheelchair user is using a lower extremity and an upper extremity to move forward on an incline (Procedure 7-10), the chair is likely to move to the left or right depending on the position of the caster wheels and the extremities used to propel the chair. If the user propels the chair with the right extremities, the chair may deviate to the left; the chair may deviate to the right if the user's left extremities propel the chair.

It is important for the user to lean forward to move the COG forward and to decrease the possibility of tipping backward.

Descending an Incline While Facing Forward. Some persons may be able to descend an incline while using a wheelie position. This technique requires advanced skills, and the patient must be guarded during all practice sessions.

As is the case with ascent of an incline while using one lower and one upper extremity, the wheelchair user will need to use his or her functional foot to guide the chair. Friction on only one hand rim will cause the chair to drift or roll toward the side to which the friction is applied (e.g., when friction is applied to the right hand rim, the chair will tend to deviate to the right; when the friction is applied to the left hand rim, it will deviate to the left). This activity may be difficult for a patient to perform and master safely.

Ascending an Incline in the Backward Position. Ascending an incline in the backward position is recommended for a person who uses one upper and one lower extremity for propulsion. Instruct the patient to pull back on the hand rim and push with the functional foot and lower extremity (Fig. 7-26). He or she should maintain the trunk erect and positioned back in the chair seat. One complication with this procedure is that the patient is unable to see the rearward progress of the chair directly. He or she can be instructed to look behind the chair periodically or to locate a fixed object in front and use it as a guide to maintain the chair's direction.

Ascending and Descending Curbs Before the skills involved in ascending and descending curbs can be attempted, the wheelchair user must be able to perform a wheelie and be comfortable performing it. These techniques require a great deal of practice, and the user should be protected by someone standing behind the chair throughout the activity (Procedure 7-11).

Ascending a Curb While Facing Forward. If the caster wheels are not elevated high enough or if they are not placed on the upper level of the curb, the footrests are likely to strike the front of the curb. When they strike the curb, the patient's body will move forward, and he or she may fall out of the chair. When the caster wheels are placed on the upper level, the patient must maintain his or her body weight forward to avoid tipping backward.

Descending a Curb While Facing Forward. Descending a curb while facing forward creates a risk that the wheelchair user may tip backward or the chair may drop forward if the wheelie position is not maintained; thus it should be attempted only by persons who are able to control the balance and position of the chair. The person in the chair should be guarded very closely when descending or ascending the curb while facing forward.

Descending a Curb in the Backward Position. When a curb is descended in the backward position, the footplates will probably strike and rest on the curb as the chair is moved away from the curb, which can misalign or damage the footplates.

Independent ascent and descent of a curb requires excellent strength, balance, and coordination and a great amount of practice before the wheelchair user is able to perform the activity safely and independently. Guard the user during the practice sessions by remaining behind the chair and being ready to react to excessive forward or backward movement of the chair or the person to prevent a fall or injury. Persons who use one upper extremity and one lower extremity to propel the chair probably will not be able to ascend or descend a curb independently.

It is important to be aware that the person in the chair may tip backward as the wheelie is performed or when the footrests are on the upper level of the curb. He or she must lean the body forward to reduce this danger.

PROCEDURE 7-10

Ascending and Descending Inclines While Facing Forward

Ascending while facing forward

- Using both upper extremities:
  - Instruct the patient to move the hips forward in the chair, lean the trunk forward, and push equally on the hand rims, using a smooth forward motion (**A**).
  - The hands will need to be repositioned on the hand rims to progress up the ramp.
- Using one upper extremity and one lower extremity:
  - Instruct the patient to move the hips forward in the chair, then lean the trunk forward.
  - The upper and lower extremities should be used the same way they are used on a level surface, though it will be necessary to use the lower extremity for more power than is required on a level surface (**B**).
  - This activity can be performed more easily by patients if they ascend backward or if a handrail is available to grasp and pull on.

Descending while facing forward

- Using both upper extremities:
  - Instruct the patient to position the hips to the rear of the seat and maintain the trunk erect to avoid falling forward (**C**).
  - The patient should retard the forward motion of the chair by applying equal friction with the palms of the hands on the hand rims (and avoid catching the fingers in the spokes of the wheel). He or she can accomplish this by a maneuver using only the palms against the side of the hand rims and keeping the fingers extended. If uneven pressure is applied by the person's hands on the hand rims, the chair will turn toward the wheel to which the greatest pressure is applied.
- Using one upper extremity and one lower extremity:
  - Instruct the patient to position the hips to the rear of the seat and maintain the trunk erect.
  - The patient should retard forward motion of the chair by applying friction with the palm of the hand against the hand rim. Additional friction can be performed when the sole of the shoe is applied to the surface.

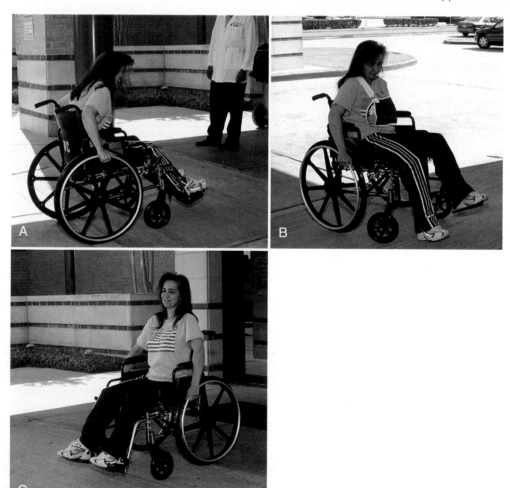

Fig. 7-25   Ascent or descent of a ramp unassisted. **A,** Ascent using both upper extremities. **B,** Ascent using one upper and one lower extremity. **C,** Descent using both upper extremities.

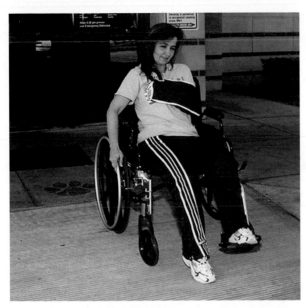

Fig. 7-26   Backward ascent of an incline using one upper and one lower extremity.

Ascending and Descending Curb Cutouts   Many curb cutouts have a relatively narrow area where the cutout meets the street. If the person in the chair does not align the caster wheels of the chair properly with this area, it may be difficult to ascend the cutout while facing forward because the footrests may contact the surface, the chair may tip back when the caster wheels contact the surface, or the chair may stop abruptly when the footplate or caster wheels contact this area. The person in the chair should be instructed to observe the cutout before attempting to use it to prepare for the difficulties that could occur because of the construction of the cutout.

Ascending a Curb Cutout While Facing Forward.   To ascend a curb cutout while facing forward, instruct the person in the chair to use the same positions and techniques described for ascending an incline or ramp (Fig. 7-27, A). Some persons may be able to perform a wheelie and ascend the cutout on the rear wheels. This method requires advanced skills, and you will need to guard the person during practice sessions by being behind the chair. If the cutout is steep or uneven with the street surface, it may be necessary for the user to perform a partial wheelie to elevate the footplates over the edge of the cutout so the caster wheels will rest on the cutout surface. A person who uses one upper and one lower extremity to propel the chair may find it easier to ascend in the backward position. It is important to be aware that if the user ascends forward and the footplates strike the cutout surface before the caster wheels rest on it, a fall or loss of balance forward may occur.

Descending a Curb Cutout While Facing Forward.   To descend a curb cutout while facing forward, instruct the

---

PROCEDURE 7-11

Ascending and Descending a Curb

Ascending a curb while facing forward	• Position the chair close to and facing the curb. • Perform a partial wheelie to elevate the caster wheels onto the upper surface of the curb. • Lean forward and propel the chair onto the curb by pushing strongly and equally on the hand rims. • Occasionally, only one drive wheel ascends the curb. When this occurs, the person must shift the body weight to the side opposite to the trailing drive wheel and push forward on both hand rims to propel the trailing drive wheel onto the curb.
Descending a curb while facing forward	• Approach the edge of the curb. • When the caster wheels reach the edge, perform a wheelie. • Roll the drive wheels over the edge of the curb until they rest on the surface below the curb. • Lower the caster wheels onto the support surface.
Descending a curb in the backward position	• Turn the chair so the curb edge is behind the chair. • Push the chair to the edge of the curb, lean the trunk forward, and allow the rear wheels to slowly and gradually roll over the edge of the curb. • Retard the movement of the chair with hand friction on the hand rims. • When the rear wheels are on the lower surface, perform a wheelie and roll back from the curb to clear the footrests from the curb. • Lower the caster wheels to the surface. • If the patient is unable to perform a wheelie, he or she can wheel the chair backward until the caster wheels are on the same level as the rear wheels.

---

patient to use the same positions and techniques described for an incline or ramp (Fig. 7-27, B). Some persons may be able to perform a wheelie and descend on the rear wheels of the chair. This technique requires advanced skills, and you will need to guard the user from behind the chair during practice sessions. If the cutout is steep or uneven with the street surface, the footplates may strike the street surface before the caster wheels rest on it, which may cause the user to fall or lose balance forward.

Descending a Curb Cutout in the Backward Position.   To descend a curb cutout in the backward position, instruct the person to use the same positions and techniques described for descending a curb or incline in the backward

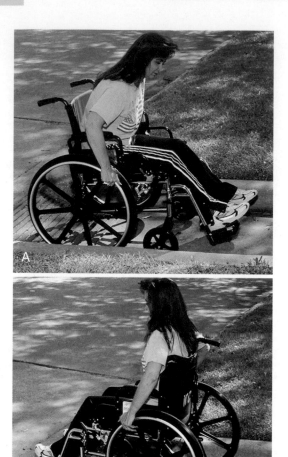

Fig. 7-27 Use of both upper extremities to ascend (**A**) and descend (**B**) a curb cutout.

position, that is, by keeping all four wheels in contact with the cutout. (Note: Patients who use one upper extremity and one lower extremity to propel the chair should use the same techniques described for an incline or ramp.) If the cutout is steep, the person in the chair should lean forward during the descent.

Ascending and Descending Stairs **Descending Stairs While Facing Forward.** Some persons may be able to descend multiple steps using a wheelie. This technique requires very advanced skills, and the wheelchair user must be guarded closely during all practice sessions. The same techniques that were used to descend a curb while facing forward are used; balance and control of the chair must be maintained.

Entering and Exiting Doors and Doorways The user of a wheelchair should be taught to open a door, proceed through a doorway, and close a door with and without a

self-closing device (Procedure 7-12). Propelling the chair through the doorway should be practiced until the activity can be accomplished safely and efficiently.

A door with a self-closing device poses problems for the wheelchair user because it offers resistance when it is opened and will be closing as the chair proceeds through the doorway. Therefore the user will need to learn specific techniques to open the door, keep it open while moving through the doorway, and avoid personal injury from the force of the self-closing device. If the resistance of the self-closing device or the size or weight of the door is excessive, or if the space available to open the door and maneuver the chair is limited, it may be necessary for the user to request assistance. Because of the resistance offered by the self-closing device, the wheelchair may need to be stabilized so it does not roll backward before pushing on the door. This stabilization can be accomplished by holding one hand rim, locking one wheel, or holding onto the door frame.

If the user intends to pass through an automatic, self-opening door (i.e., an electronically operated door) that swings on its hinges and opens toward the user, he or she must be cautioned to remain far enough away from the door so the front rigging of the chair or the feet will not be struck by the door as it opens. The patient should practice propelling the chair over a raised threshold, which often is associated with exterior doors. It may be necessary to have the patient enter and leave backward to lead with the rear wheels of the chair and make it easier to cross the threshold. When entering while facing forward, it may be necessary to perform a partial wheelie to elevate the caster wheels over the threshold.

A Self-Closing Door Opening Outward. When pushing a self-closing door open, it may open wider than necessary with the initial push, but it also may need to be opened with a series of short pushes to enable the chair to pass through the doorway. (Note: Some self-closing devices provide greater resistance when a forceful push is used to open the door.)

A Self-Closing Door Opening Inward. A self-closing door may need to be opened with a series of short pulls until it is opened wide enough for the chair to pass through the doorway (see Procedure 7-12). The same techniques and precautions described previously to keep the door open, stabilize the chair, and propel the chair through the doorway can be applied to this activity. (Note: This task will be extremely difficult for a patient who does not have functional use of both upper extremities and good trunk control.)

A Regular Door with No Self-Closing Device. If the patient can move through the doorway at an angle, the door will not need to be opened as wide as it would if moving straight through the doorway. However, if a wall or other obstruction is present in the area where the person enters, it may be necessary to open the door fully to provide adequate space for the wheelchair.

PROCEDURE 7-12

Propelling a Wheelchair Through a Door

Self-closing
door opening
outward (away
from the
patient)

- Position the wheelchair to face the door at an angle, toward the side of the door frame without hinges. If space does not permit angling of the chair, approach the door forward and as near as possible to the door edge that will open.
- Reach for the doorknob, latch, or crash bar to open the door with a quick, firm push (**A**).
- You may be able to quickly propel the chair through the doorway before the door closes, but it is more likely the door will need to be kept open to move through it (**B**). The door can be held open by using the distal portion of the front rigging, by holding the crash bar, or by using a series of pushes on the door or crash bar to keep the door open to pass through the doorway (**C**).
- Protect the foot and hand nearest to the door when proceeding through the doorway (**D**).

Self-closing
door opening
inward
(toward the
patient)

- Position the wheelchair to face the door at an angle toward the side of the door frame with hinges. If space does not permit angling of the chair, approach the door forward as near as possible to the door edge that will open.

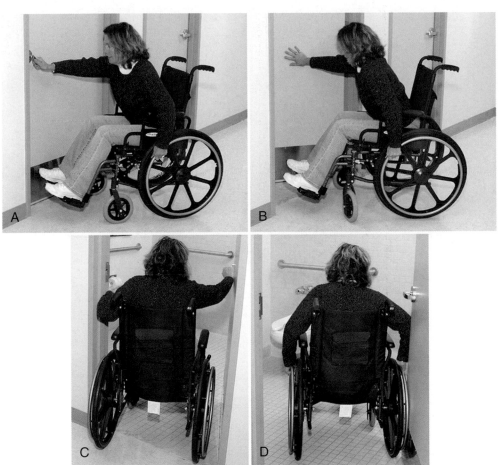

Fig. 7-28   Patient in a wheelchair negotiating a self-closing door that opens away from her.

Continued

PROCEDURE 7-12

Propelling a Wheelchair Through a Door—cont'd

- Reach for the doorknob or latch to open the door with a quick, firm pull (**A**).
- You may be able to quickly propel the chair through the doorway before the door closes, but it is more likely the door will need to be kept open to move through it (**B** and **C**).
- The patient can use one hand or both hands on the door frame to pull the chair quickly through the doorway, and the rear wheels can be used to prevent the door from closing until the chair is completely through the doorway (**D**).

Regular door, no self-closing device
- Position the wheelchair as described for the door that opens outward or inward.
- Reach for the doorknob or latch to open the door.
- Because there is no self-closing device, strong force may not be needed to open the door, and the door should be opened only wide enough for the chair to pass through the doorway.
- It will be necessary to turn the chair, or turn the body, to close the door once the chair has passed through the doorway.

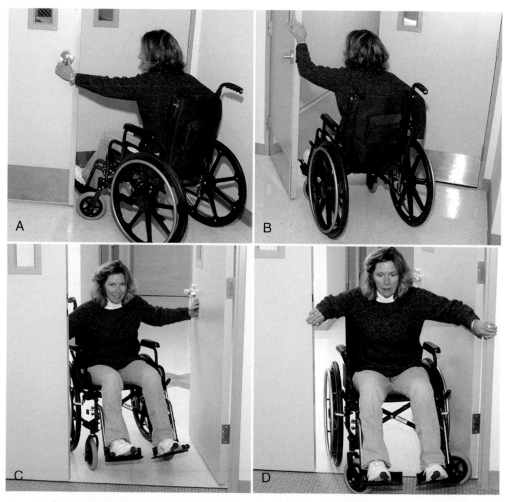

Fig. 7-29 Patient in a wheelchair negotiating a self-closing door that opens toward her.

Entering and Exiting Elevators The wheelchair user should be taught how to enter and leave an elevator car and should practice this maneuver. He or she may enter and exit while facing forward or in the backward position, depending on the space available in the car and in the area outside the car, such as the corridor or entryway. You should caution the user to observe and be aware of some specific problems associated with an elevator. For instance, the floor of the elevator and the surface of the corridor or entryway may be uneven; that is, the elevator car may stop slightly above or below the outside surface. This uneven surface may make it difficult for the person to enter or exit the car because the caster wheels may not roll over the elevated surface, or the chair could stop abruptly or tip forward. To avoid this scenario, the user should enter and leave by leading with the rear wheels.

A second problem can occur when a large space is present between the front edge of the car floor and the outside surface. The caster wheels may drop into this space if they are turned to the side, and extracting them may be difficult for the patient. Because this problem may occur, the user should enter and leave the car with the caster wheels directed straight forward. Most of the information provided previously in the section on assisted propulsion of a wheelchair with regard to the use of an elevator also applies to the independent use of an elevator; the user will need to decide whether to enter and exit while facing forward or in the backward position. Instruct the user to approach the external panel where the control pads or buttons are located with the wheelchair positioned at an angle or parallel to the wall that contains the panel so he or she can reach the control pads or buttons more easily. If the user approaches the wall directly forward, the front rigging will prevent the chair from being close to the control panel and he or she will need to lean forward to reach the panel. Furthermore, it may not be possible to reach the pads or buttons that are located at the top of the panel, and assistance from another person may be required.

Once the wheelchair user is inside the car, it may be necessary to ask another passenger to press the desired floor pad and to activate the door-open control so he or she can have more time to exit safely.

The user should be taught to recognize automatic door-opening devices such as a photoelectric beam or pressure sensors in the edge of the elevator doors. Remind him or her that the feet and lower extremities project in front of the chair and are relatively unprotected from various objects in the environment, including the doors of an elevator. Therefore the user must be aware of the potential hazards or objects that could cause an injury to the feet and lower extremities. Also remind the user that the hand rims and rear wheels can provide protection when the hands and arms are placed within the area between the two wheels (as in the lap or on the armrests). The rear of the chair is protected by the push handles and by the posterior position of the rear wheels. The front of the chair is somewhat protected by the distal portion of the front rigging; however, the feet may project beyond the foot plate.

Reaching an Object on the Floor in Front of the Chair Reaching an object on the floor in front of the chair should be considered a relatively unsafe maneuver and should be used primarily in an emergency. If the object weighs more than 5 to 10 lb, the chair is likely to tip forward onto the footplates when the object is lifted from the floor, especially if the caster wheels are positioned backward (Fig. 7-30, A), or the wheelchair user may have difficulty lifting the object and returning to an erect posture. It is imperative to have the caster wheels positioned forward (Fig. 7-30, B) before the user attempts this task. A safer procedure is to teach the user to reach for and lift the object with the chair positioned to the side and parallel to the object.

It is important to instruct the patient how to position the caster wheels and how to maintain trunk control while reaching forward. The caster wheels can be positioned by maneuvering the chair until they face forward to increase the distance between the back of the caster wheel and the front of the rear wheel. The wheelchair user may need to control the trunk by holding onto a push handle, the back frame, the seat frame, the armrest, or the upper position of the front rigging. The specific site chosen will depend on the user's condition and abilities (Procedure 7-13).

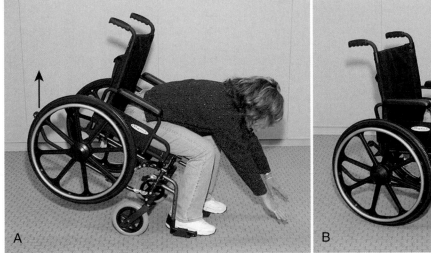
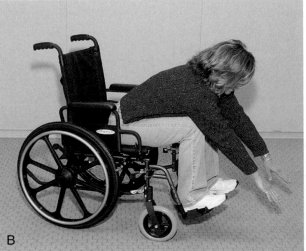

Fig. 7-30 Person reaching forward with caster wheels in (**A**) improper position and (**B**) proper position.

PROCEDURE 7-13

Reaching for an Object on the Floor in Front of the Chair

- The patient should position the caster wheels in a forward position to increase the base of support of the chair.
- The rear wheels should be locked and the patient's hips should be shifted forward in the chair.
- Some persons may prefer to place their feet on the floor, but it is possible for the feet to remain on the footplates while the activity is performed and the person reaches forward for the object.

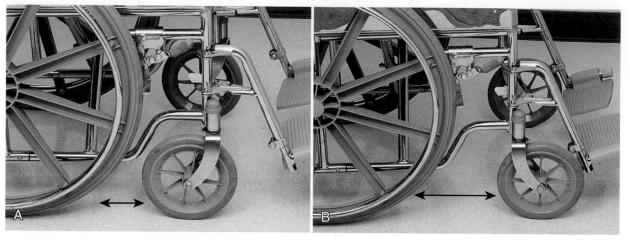

Fig. 7-31   **A,** Improper position of wheels while reaching forward. **B,** Proper position of wheels while reaching forward.

Falls in the Wheelchair Persons using a wheelchair as a mobility aid can sometimes experience falls and be thrown either backward or forward from the chair. Fall and recovery strategies for persons using a wheelchair can help reduce injury (Procedure 7-14).

Backward Fall. When the chair tips backward, instruct the patient to prevent the knees and thighs from hitting the face by placing one forearm across them with the hand holding the opposite armrest. The patient should not attempt to reach backward for protection because this maneuver will increase the speed of the fall and the possibility of injury to the upper extremities and head. The push handles of the chair will strike the ground before the back of the chair, but it is important for the patient to keep the head and trunk forward. Grasping an armrest with one hand will help keep the body in the chair. The feet are likely to fall off the footrests, and the lower legs may dangle below the seat when the chair tips back.

Forward Fall. If the caster wheel strikes an object while the chair is moving, the patient may fall forward. If this scenario occurs, instruct him or her to hold an armrest with one hand and reach toward the floor with the other hand. This technique may cause the chair to fall on top of the person if the armrest is held too long; therefore some patients prefer to reach forward with both hands simultaneously for protection. Instruct the patient to absorb the force of the fall by flexing the elbows when the

hands strike the floor. The knees may strike the floor with excessive force, and injury may result unless the patient is taught to turn the body to land on the lateral area of a hip.

Returning to an Upright Sitting Position. Returning to an upright sitting position after a fall is an advanced activity that will require much practice. A lap belt may be necessary during the practice sessions, and an assistant may be needed to help the patient attain an upright position. Many patients may not be able to perform this activity independently. Some persons may fall out of the chair when it tips; therefore it may be necessary to instruct them to place the chair upright and enter the chair forward or backward as described in Chapter 8.

Moving from the Wheelchair to the Floor and Returning to the Wheelchair Techniques that enable a person to move from the wheelchair to the floor and then return to the wheelchair are presented in Chapter 8. These techniques allow the patient to plan and somewhat control the movement from the wheelchair to the floor and return to the wheelchair. These techniques should not be confused with the information related to falling forward or backward while seated in a wheelchair. However, a review of that material may provide some ideas you could offer the patient to assist him or her develop methods of self-protection should a fall from the chair occur.

PROCEDURE 7-14

Protected Fall from a Wheelchair

These procedures should be described and demonstrated by the caregiver before the patient attempts them; you should guard closely when the patient practices the activity, and protective mats should be placed on the floor.

Backward fall
- The patient quickly grasps an opposite armrest with one hand, allowing the forearm to rest on or above the thighs.
- The chin is lowered toward the chest, and the free upper extremity reaches forward (**A**).
- A semi-flexed trunk position is maintained; the free hand should grasp the hand rims as the push handles and chair back contact the floor.
- To return to an upright position, the person remains in the chair, locks the rear wheels, places one hand on the floor behind the chair, grasps an opposite armrest with the free upper extremity, and "walks" the hand on the floor forward while keeping the head and trunk flexed (**B**).
- The fingers and upper extremity are used to push strongly, and the opposite upper extremity reaches forward simultaneously to move the chair to an upright position.
- An alternative method is to remove the body from the chair, position the chair on all four wheels, and reenter the chair using one of the techniques presented in Chapter 8, providing no serious injury has occurred.

Returning to an upright sitting position
- The patient should remain in or return to the chair and lock the rear wheels.
- One hand should be placed on the floor behind the chair before reaching with the other arm across the body to the opposite seat rail or armrest.
- The patient then uses the hand on the floor to "walk" forward, keeping the head and trunk flexed to move the chair to an upright position (**B**).
- When the chair has been elevated to its highest point, a rapid, strong push with the hand on the floor while reaching forward with the other arm and flexing the head and neck will help tip the front of the chair down.

Forward fall
- The patient reaches forward with both upper extremities.
- When the hands contact the floor, the elbows are flexed to absorb some of the force of the fall.
- The person attempts to turn or pivot the pelvis to land on one hip or, if the knees contact the floor first, attempts to side sit on one hip.
- To return to the chair, the chair is positioned on all four wheels and the person reenters the chair using one of the techniques presented in Chapter 8, providing no serious injury has occurred.

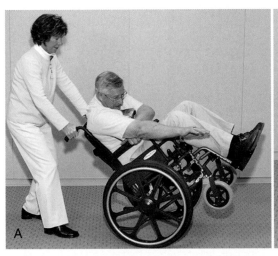 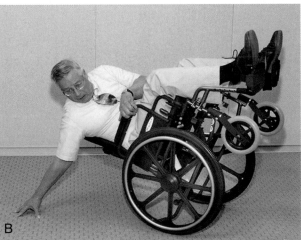

Fig. 7-32   Instructing a patient in a wheelchair how to fall backward (**A**) and return to an upright position (**B**).

GENERAL CARE AND MAINTENANCE OF A WHEELCHAIR

A wheelchair functions best when it is maintained properly. The user should be encouraged to read and follow the instructions contained in the maintenance manual supplied by the manufacturer or distributor. Periodic cleaning of exposed metal with a nonabrasive metal polish or automobile wax and cleaning of the upholstery with use of an appropriate fabric cleaner or damp cloth is recommended. The chair should not be immersed in water or sprayed with a hose, and it should be wiped dry after exposure to rain, snow, or other types of moisture. The cross-brace center pin should be lubricated with molybdenum-based grease every 6 months. Light oil should not be used because it will collect dirt particles and will not provide long-lasting lubrication. The armrest insert posts and the front and rear post slides (i.e., the open tubing into which the armrest posts insert) should be lubricated periodically with a silicone spray, such as WD-40, or a small amount of paraffin. The wheel bearings can be lubricated only if they are removed from the wheels. High-quality bearing grease should be used as the lubricant. The bearings should not be oiled, because oil will decrease the effectiveness of the grease that is in the bearings and the overall lubrication will be decreased. It may be best to have these items inspected and lubricated by a reputable dealer or repair service.

Frequent visual inspection of the frame, upholstery, wheels, joints, tires, brakes, and other parts of the wheelchair will enable early detection of signs of wear or disrepair. Pneumatic tires should be checked for proper inflation at least monthly. Wheel spokes should be tested for tightness, and loose spokes should be tightened to maintain proper rim shape and support. It is important to note that improper tightening of the spokes may distort the shape of the rim, and thus it may be best to have this adjustment performed by a reputable dealer or repair service. The user and family members should be encouraged to read the owner's manual periodically for information about proper maintenance. The facility where the chair was purchased and the manufacturer are additional sources of information about proper chair maintenance. In many large cities, wheelchair repair or service facilities are available and can be found in a telephone directory or online; additional information may be available from a health care facility. The patient and the family should be encouraged to perform proper maintenance and repair the chair promptly to enhance its function and longevity.

SUMMARY

When a wheelchair is a person's primary means of locomotion, it must fit and function properly to enhance independence and safety. The caregiver should evaluate and confirm the fit of the wheelchair and determine its mechanical and functional condition. The potential adverse effects of an improperly fitting wheelchair should be recognized by the caregiver and explained to the user. These problems should be corrected or modified as soon as possible to avoid injury, discomfort, or reduced independent function.

The caregiver should become competent in the management and handling of the chair to be able to demonstrate and instruct others in proper techniques or procedures. The person using the chair should be instructed to use the chair independently, including how to perform as many functional activities as possible within his or her established abilities. Instruction in the proper maintenance and care of the chair should be provided.

self-study ACTIVITIES

- Discuss the potential adverse effects on the user of an improperly fitted wheelchair in relation to seat width, seat depth, leg length, armrest height, seat height, and back height.
- Describe how you would teach a patient to propel a standard wheelchair on a level surface using both upper extremities, then one upper extremity and one lower extremity.
- Demonstrate how the patient will turn and move backward.
- List the primary components of a standard wheelchair.
- Demonstrate how you would confirm the fit of the wheelchair with the patient seated in the chair.
- Describe how you would teach a patient to elevate the caster wheels (i.e., perform a wheelie or pop-up).
- Outline what type of wheelchair and components are required, and explain your rationale for your selection, for persons with (1) hemiplegia of the left upper and lower extremities; (2) paralysis below the level of T10; (3) bilateral transfemoral amputations (no prostheses); and (4) paralysis below the level of C3.

problem SOLVING

1. You are preparing a wheelchair user for reentry to her job, and she informs you that she will need to use an elevator and must be able to turn the wheelchair using a small radius. Describe the instructions or directions you would provide to enable her to perform these activities safely and effectively.

2. A 25-year-old woman with weakness in her right upper and lower extremity because of a severe head injury is beginning to use a wheelchair; she is unable to use her right extremities for propulsion. How would you teach her to (1) propel the chair; (2) open and close a door without a self-closing device; and (3) ascend and descend a curb cutout and ramp?

3. A 15-year-old male adolescent uses a wheelchair for mobility, and he has functional strength of his trunk and upper extremity muscles. To attend school, he must be able to ascend and descend a ramp and enter and leave through several doors that are self-closing; some open toward him, and some open away from him. What techniques would you use to teach him how to perform these activities independently?

Transfer Activities

objectives *After studying this chapter, the reader will be able to:*

- Teach a patient how to perform independent bed mobility and functional activities in preparation for a transfer.
- Adjust the position of a person who is recumbent with or without the assistance of another person in preparation for a transfer.
- Instruct another person in how to perform various transfer techniques and assist in performing these techniques.
- Instruct one or more assistants in how to perform a safe lift transfer.
- Properly guard and protect a patient while a transfer is being performed.

key terms

Anteroposterior   From the front to the rear of an object or a living being.

Bariatric   Field of medicine that is concerned with weight loss or that deals with causes, prevention, and treatment of obesity.

Contralateral   On the other—or opposite—side.

Dependent   Requiring some level or type of assistance, which may be human or mechanical. The patient is unable to assist with transfers.

Exacerbation   An increase in the severity of disease or any of its symptoms.

Graft   Any tissue or organ for transplantation or implantation.

Hemiplegia   Paralysis of one side of the body.

Ipsilateral   Homolateral; on the same side.

Lateral   Indicates a position away from the median plane or midline of a body or structure.

Medial   Related or located toward the midline of a body or structure.

Mobility   The ability to move in an environment with ease and without restriction.

Osteoporosis   A decreased mass per unit volume of normally mineralized bone when compared with that in age-matched and sex-matched control subjects; loss of bone mass.

Paralysis   Loss of power of voluntary movement in a muscle through injury or disease of its nerve supply.

Paresis   Partial or incomplete paralysis.

Plinth   A padded table for a patient to sit or lie on while performing exercises, receiving a massage, or undergoing other physical therapy treatment.

Safety belt   An adjustable belt or strap that is secured around a person's waist and is used to protect and control the person; also referred to as a guard, transfer, ambulation, or gait belt.

Syncope   A temporary suspension of consciousness as a result of cerebral anemia; fainting.

Transfer   The moving of a patient from one surface to another surface.

Vertigo   A sensation of rotation or movement of one's self or of one's surroundings.

INTRODUCTION

A transfer is the safe movement of a person from one surface or location to another or from one position to another. Depending on the mental and physical ability of the patient, a transfer may be performed either independently, with assistance (minimal, moderate, maximal, or standby supervision), or dependently. A variety of terms are used for transfer assistance. The list in Table 8-1 is not meant to be all-inclusive, but it provides a good introduction. Additional terminology and a discussion of the International Classification of Functioning, Disability, and Heath Performance Qualifiers can be found in *DeLisa's Physical Medicine and Rehabilitation: Principles and Practice* (see the Bibliography).

Adjusting the patient's position and bed mobility activities are included in the broad definition of a transfer. The ability to move upward, downward, or from side to side and the ability to roll, turn over, and move to a sitting position from a recumbent position are important activities for a patient to be able to accomplish for independence. Often these movements are preliminary to the actual transfer from a bed* or mat table to a wheelchair or to a standing position. These movements also are necessary to permit patients to alter their position for comfort and to avoid the development of contractures or skin breakdown. The caregiver should not overlook teaching the patient how to perform these movements and should emphasize their importance to the patient and family. Preparatory activities may be required, such as muscle strengthening, development of joint and muscle flexibility (i.e., range of motion), and development of endurance.

The caregiver also will need to know how to properly document a patient transfer in the medical record as follows:

*Where "bed" is referred to in all subsequent procedures, you may infer that a bed, mat, or plinth can be used.

- The type of transfer performed
- Information on the amount or type of assistance the patient requires to perform the transfer
- The amount of time required to complete the transfer
- The level of safety demonstrated
- The quality of movement demonstrated
- Precautions for transfer (e.g., spinal, total knee replacement, or total hip replacement)
- The level of consistency of the performance
- The equipment or devices used

ORGANIZATION OF PATIENT TRANSFERS

Planning and organization are required before a patient attempts to perform any transfer. The patient should be informed about the transfer and taught how to assist with or perform the maneuver before attempting it. A demonstration of the activity by another patient or by the caregiver may help the patient learn how to perform the transfer. Careful attention to the safety precautions associated with each transfer will enhance the patient's confidence and lead to a more effective transfer.

You must be certain to obtain and use sufficient assistance or equipment to ensure a safe procedure. When the patient is able to assist more fully with the procedure, external assistance can be reduced or eliminated, leading to increased patient independence. Although patient independence is a frequent goal associated with transfer activities, your primary responsibility during the practice of a transfer is to guard and protect the patient to avoid injury.

Before the Transfer

You will need to prepare the patient, the environment, yourself, and possibly other persons before performing a transfer activity. Initially you should review the medical record and interview the patient for information to help you

Table **8-1** Terminology for Transfer or Ambulation Assistance	
Independent	The patient can perform a transfer without any type of verbal or manual assistance (Note: In some situations, specific equipment or devices may be used)
Assisted	The patient requires assistance from another person to perform the activity safely in an acceptable time frame; physical assistance, oral or tactile cues, directions, or instructions may be used
Standby (supervision) assistance	The patient requires verbal or tactile cues, directions, or instructions from another person positioned close to, but not touching, the person to perform the activity safely and in an acceptable time frame; the assistant may provide protection in case the patient's safety is threatened
Contact guarding	The caregiver is positioned close to the patient with his or her hands on the patient or a safety belt; it is very likely the patient will require protection during the performance of the activity
Modified independent	The patient uses adaptive or assistive equipment to perform a task independently (e.g., a transfer board, bed rail, grab bars, or furniture); the patient may have safety or timeliness issues
Minimal assistance	The patient performs 75% or more of the activity; assistance is required to complete the activity
Moderate assistance	The patient performs 50% to 74% of the activity; assistance is required to complete the activity
Maximal assistance	The patient performs 25% to 49% of the activity; assistance is required to complete the activity
Dependent	The patient requires total physical assistance from one or more persons to accomplish the activity safely; special equipment or devices may be used

Table 8-2   Patient Considerations While Planning a Transfer

The patient's experience	What has the patient accomplished previously?
	How does the patient transfer now?
	What are the patient's activity limitations and abilities?
	How much assistance is required to move the individual in bed or to perform a transfer?
	Does the patient need to use orthotics or splints during the transfer to ensure safety?
	Must specific precautions be used to protect the patient or to avoid further injury?
The patient's physical ability	You should have an understanding of the following characteristics of the patient:
	Muscle strength
	Joint and soft-tissue flexibility
	Sitting and standing balance
	Endurance
	Tolerance of sitting and standing positions
	Motor control

plan the activity (Table 8-2). Your assessment or evaluation of the patient will help determine the person's abilities and activity limitations.

A decision regarding the appropriate transfer or activity to be performed will need to be made on the basis of four general parameters:

- Your evaluation
- The available written information
- Information from the patient and/or family members
- The goals of treatment

As you mentally plan and organize the activity, you can consider whether mechanical or human assistance will be needed. Equipment such as a transfer board, a hydraulic or pneumatic lift, an electric hoist, a rope, a bed rail, or an over-the-bed frame or bar (trapeze) may be required to assist with a transfer. Because these devices can perpetuate dependence in a patient, they are recommended only for patients who are unable to perform a safe transfer without them or when the caregiver is unable to safely assist the patient without using equipment. If equipment is needed, the caregiver must obtain, position, and stabilize it and be certain it functions properly before beginning the transfer. (Note: A trapeze should not be used in transfers if at all possible; its primary use is for repositioning the patient in the bed.)

During the Transfer

After these planning activities have been completed, you will need to apply certain concepts and principles to ensure a safe and successful outcome. You must analyze each component part of the transfer, such as the position of the equipment, the operation of the equipment by the patient or caregiver, the position of the patient's body, and the movements the patient will need to perform.

The transfer procedure should be explained to the patient before the transfer is begun. Even if you believe the patient has consented to the proposed treatment, obtain consent after you have explained the activity and the possible risks, if any, that are associated with it. It may be necessary for

the patient to practice and accomplish the component activities before the total transfer is attempted. After you have instructed the patient, ask him or her to repeat your instructions. Avoid asking the patient, "Do you understand the instructions?" Most patients will answer "yes" when asked such a question, even if they have not understood the instructions. Instead, ask the patient to explain the procedure to you to verify what he or she understands. Verbalizing the steps of the procedure allows the patient to mentally practice the skill that he or she is about to perform, which is helpful for motor learning. Persons who are to assist also must be informed of and understand their roles and must be instructed how to assist with the transfer.

Your instructions to the patient and to any persons who assist you should be brief, concise, and action oriented. Try to avoid lengthy instructions (e.g., "Now, the first thing I want you to do is. ...") Many patients will still be processing these nondirective words when you are beginning to state the actual instructions. You might instruct the patient in this manner: "First, lock your chair; now lift the footrests, move your hips forward, place your right foot closer to the chair and your left foot farther from the chair," and so on.

Encourage the patient to participate in the transfer mentally and physically to the fullest extent possible and within the limits of safety. The more the patient assists in the maneuver, the easier it will be to become independent. The caregiver must prepare for the transfer and always use proper body mechanics when performing any patient transfer to reduce the possibility of injury (Procedure 8-1).

Safety Concerns in Transfers

Several precautions should be considered when assisting a patient with a transfer, especially a standing transfer, regardless of the patient's condition. The patient should wear proper shoes to perform a standing transfer. Slippers, sandals, shoes with smooth leather soles, or socks without shoes will decrease safety and should be avoided. A safety belt or transfer sling provides a secure object to grasp and decreases

PROCEDURE 8-1

Overview of the Transfer Procedure

PREPARATION FOR TRANSFER

- Check the patient's chart for precautions such as weight-bearing status, postsurgical procedure orders, joint disease, or osteoporosis.
- Plan the transfer across the shortest distance.
- Plan to move the patient toward his or her strongest side and assist the weak side.
- Obtain necessary equipment or assistance if needed.
- Ensure the patient is properly dressed for the transfer. Excessively loose clothing, long trousers, slacks, or pajamas should be avoided. Shoes with nonskid soles should be worn.
- Wash your hands and don gloves if appropriate.
- Introduce yourself to the patient
- Explain the transfer procedure to the patient and demonstrate it if necessary. Explain the patient's role in the procedure; provide simple, concise commands and help carry them out.
- Obtain the patient's consent after you have explained the activity and the possible risks, if any, associated with it.

PERFORMING THE TRANSFER

- Lock all the wheels on the wheelchair, bed, or gurney.
- Be alert to paraphernalia such as intravenous lines, cardiac leads, and catheters if you are in a hospital setting and ensure that this equipment is of an adequate length so it is not pulled out in the process of the transfer.
- A safety belt or a transfer sling, sheet, or towel under the buttocks should be used if the patient will move from one surface to another, especially during the early treatment sessions.
- Use a safety belt or sling and the patient's knees, pelvis, or upper thorax for stabilization or control.
  - Do not use the patient's upper extremity or clothing for guidance or stability because this technique will not enable you to control the patient adequately and you may injure the extremity.
- Remain close to the patient and guard him or her properly.
- The caregiver and any assistants should use proper body mechanics:
  - Lift with your legs and avoid twisting
  - Avoid trunk flexion and rotation
  - Position your center of gravity (COG) as close to the patient's COG as possible
  - Increase your base of support (BOS) (lower your COG and maintain your vertical gravity line within your BOS)
- Continue to instruct the patient and those assisting with the transfer by using short statements; it may be possible to incorporate some patient teaching while the activity is performed.

the need to use the patient's clothing or extremities. You should anticipate and be alert for unusual patient actions or equipment that may create unexpected risks. Any bandages or equipment attached to or used by the patient should be protected, including casts, drainage tubes, intravenous tubes, and dressing sites. When using a wheelchair, be certain the drive wheels are locked during the transfer.

Anticipate the need for an assistant and, if necessary, have someone available before attempting the initial transfer. You must determine the best position to use to protect the patient. To prevent injury to the patient as the result of a fall, it is usually best to be in front of and slightly to one side of the patient when he or she stands. Your body mechanics may be compromised when you are in this protective position, but it will enable you to provide maximal protection for the patient. At the conclusion of the transfer, you may protect the patient by applying a lap belt when he or she is seated, engaging the bed rails, positioning the person in the center of the bed, or using other similar methods. Do not leave the patient unattended unless adequate support, stabilization, and protection is in place to prevent injury.

When a patient performs a transfer, it is important that the environment be free of unneeded equipment such as bedside trays, telephones, intravenous line poles, and other hazards. The area needed for the transfer should be accessible to all caregivers and assistants. When transfers are performed in an area protected by curtains or drapes, you should know what is on the other side of the curtain when it is closed.

Conditions Requiring Special Precautions

When assisting patients with certain conditions while they are in bed, on a mat, or performing a transfer, special care and precautions must be used to avoid additional trauma or exacerbation of their condition. Examples of some of these patient conditions are listed in Table 8-3.

TYPES OF TRANSFERS

Transfers are designated by a variety of terms. Some transfers may be described according to the number of persons required to assist the patient (such as "plus 1" or "plus 2"); however, most descriptions indicate whether the patient requires assistance or can function independently. The designation of the transfer is important because it is part of the documentation to which other caregivers will refer. All caregivers in the same facility should use the same terminology when describing the transfer, and a consensus should be reached regarding the terminology that will be used (see Table 8-1). Once the transfer method or type has been selected, it is important that all caregivers perform each transfer the same way with a particular patient to enhance learning and competence. If modifications are made to the transfer, each caregiver should be made aware of these modifications either verbally or through patient documentation.

Table **8-3**   Conditions Requiring Special Precautions During Transfers

Total hip replacement, especially within the initial 2 weeks after surgery*	The surgically replaced hip should not be adducted or rotated, flexed more than 90 degrees, or extended beyond neutral flexion-extension
	Do not cross the ankle of the surgically affected extremity over the opposite extremity, pull on the surgically affected extremity, or allow the patient to lie on the surgically replaced hip
	Maintain the surgical extremity in abduction when moving into a side-lying position and during side lying, require the patient to sit in a semireclining position, and require the patient to maintain the surgically affected extremity in abduction when moving from side to side; if an abduction pillow is available, apply it after the patient returns to bed
Low back trauma or discomfort	Excessive lumbar rotation, trunk side bending, and trunk flexion should be avoided
	When turning, patients may experience less discomfort if they "logroll" (i.e., roll the entire body simultaneously) rather than roll segmentally (i.e., rolling the shoulders and upper trunk first, then the pelvis, and then the lower extremities); they also may be more comfortable with the hips and knees partially flexed with a pillow under or between the knees when they are in a supine or side-lying position
Spinal cord injury	For a patient with a recent spinal cord injury, the injury site may be protected by an external appliance (e.g., a brace, plaster or plastic body jacket, or halo device), internal fixation (e.g., bone graft, metal rods, or wires), or a combination of the two methods
	Because distracting and rotational forces should be avoided, do not move the person downward by pulling on the lower extremities; logroll the person when turning
	Protective positioning or restraints will be required when this patient is in a side-lying position or sits without a back support
	Caution: For a person with an injury that occurred several months or years earlier, be aware that osteoporosis, especially in the long bones of the lower extremities and the vertebral bodies, may be present; even mild to moderate stress or strain to these bones may lead to a fracture; some patients could experience a fracture when turning over or transferring from a wheelchair to the floor or to other objects
	Also be aware that this patient may experience syncope when transferred from a supine to a sitting position because the blood pressure may not adapt quickly to the positional change
Burns	The primary precaution is to avoid creating a shear force across the surface of the burn wound, graft site, or area from which the graft was taken; sliding creates a shear force, causing friction and disruption of the healing process
	The patient should be instructed to elevate the body or extremities when moving an area with a burn to avoid the effect of shear forces
Hemiplegia	Pulling on the involved or weakened extremities should be avoided to control or move the patient; this precaution is particularly important for the affected shoulder because the muscles will not provide adequate support to the joint as a result of the effects of paralysis
	Many patients will experience pain or discomfort when they lie on or roll over the involved shoulder

*These precautions also can be used for patients with a recent hip fracture or dislocation to decrease the possibility of dislocation or additional trauma to the site.

The patient's family should observe the transfer and practice providing assistance while being guided by the appropriate caregiver before the patient's discharge. Box 8-1 lists general transfer principles.

Standing, Dependent Pivot

The standing, dependent pivot transfer requires at least one person to transfer the patient. The patient is elevated to a standing position, usually from a bed, plinth, toilet seat, or wheelchair, and is pivoted so his or her back is toward the object to which the person is lowered. You may be required to lift the patient to a standing position, stabilize the knees and hips for the pivot, and help the patient to sit.

Standing, Assisted Pivot

With a standing, assisted pivot, the caregiver provides assistance for the patient to stand, pivot, and transfer to another object such as a bed, wheelchair, plinth, or toilet seat. The patient must be able to provide minimal (up to 25%) to maximal (75% or more) physical effort during the transfer. Safety often is an issue with this transfer, and thus the caregiver must be alert at all times.

Standing, Standby Pivot

The standing, standby pivot requires the standby presence of a person. Patients using this transfer may be able to stand, pivot, and sit as they move from one object to another. The assistance required may vary from verbal cueing to close or

Box **8-1** General Transfer Principles

- Predetermine the patient's mental and physical capabilities to perform the transfer, including weight-bearing status.
- The patient's clothing and footwear should be suitable for the transfer.
- Mentally preplan the activities and sequence associated with the transfer; teach and practice components of the transfer before attempting the transfer.
- Assess the patient's pain status prior to and at the completion of the transfer.
- Instruct the patient slowly, clearly, and concisely; allow time for the patient to process and apply the information.
- Select, position, and secure any needed equipment; apply a safety belt or use a sling.
- Be alert for unusual events that may occur, such as patient dizziness or distractions.
- Do not guard the patient by using clothing or grasping the arm; use a safety belt or a sling and the trunk.
- Position yourself to guard, guide, direct, and protect the patient throughout the transfer.
- Ask the patient to initiate and perform the transfer in simple directive terms; assist as necessary.
- At the conclusion of the transfer, position the patient for comfort, stability, and safety and document changes in the patient's performance.

casual guarding. Safety is still a concern with this type of transfer, and you must be alert to provide protection when it is needed.

Standing, Independent Pivot

With a standing, independent pivot, the patient is able to perform the entire transfer safely and consistently without any physical or verbal assistance from another person.

Sitting or Lateral Assisted Transfer

In a sitting or lateral assisted transfer, the patient is able to move from one surface to a second surface while in a sitting position with the assistance of at least one person. This transfer may require the use of a transfer (sliding) board, an overhead bar or frame, overhead straps, or other equipment. These items are used to bridge the space between the two objects or to permit the patient to use the upper extremities for assistance. The patient may be able to physically assist with the transfer but may require physical assistance and must be guarded and protected throughout the transfer.

Sitting, Independent Transfer

In a sitting, independent transfer, the patient is able to move safely and efficiently from one surface to a second surface while in a sitting position without assistance from another person. It still may be necessary for the patient to

use a transfer or sliding board, an overhead bar or frame, overhead straps, or other equipment.

Sitting, Dependent Lift

In a sitting, dependent lift, one, two, or three persons may be required to lift and move the patient from one surface to a second surface. A mechanical lift may be used instead of multiple persons. If a mechanical lift is used, only one caregiver is usually needed to perform the transfer. This transfer is used when the patient is totally unable to physically assist with the transfer and other persons or equipment are required.

Recumbent, Dependent Lift

The recumbent, dependent transfer is used with patients who are physically unable to assist with the transfer and are unable to be placed in a sitting position. One, two, or three persons or special equipment are required to lift and move the patient from one surface to a second surface. The equipment may be a mechanical lift, a mechanical transfer stretcher, a mattress pad, a bed liner (e.g., a draw sheet or plastic liner), or a plastic transfer board.

MOBILITY ACTIVITIES

Mobility activities are used to adjust the recumbent patient's body position. The activities may be performed independently by the patient, with assistance from another person or persons, or with the use of various types of equipment. The most common movements are turning from a supine to a side-lying position and returning to the original position; turning from a supine to a prone position and returning to the original position; moving upward, downward, or from side to side and returning to the center; and moving from a lying to a sitting position and returning to the original position. Equipment used in these mobility activities may include bed rails; an overhead bar or frame; loops attached to the bed, mat, or mattress; and linen items such as a draw sheet.

These activities should be taught to patients to improve independence and assist in preventing the development of skin problems or contractures as a result of lying in one position too long. The patient must become independent in all phases of bed or mat mobility to become independent in sitting and standing transfers. Remember to raise the bed, if possible, lock the wheels on the bed, and use proper body mechanics as you assist and guard the patient.

The patient should mentally and physically participate in these activities even when being assisted. Initiate patient involvement by asking the patient to control his or her head, position the upper or lower extremities, or use the upper and lower extremities to help with the activity. The patient should perform these assistive movements to promote independent movement as his or her condition improves. You and the patient may need to problem solve together to determine the most effective way to use the person's abilities so that independent movement is encouraged and decreased assistance is required.

To perform mobility activities with greater ease, you should attempt to reduce friction between the patient's body and the surface of the bed or mat, centralize the weight of the patient, reduce the effects of gravity, or use gravity as an assistive force. In all of the following activities, to the extent possible, raise the level of the bed or mat to a position that is comfortable and causes less stress to your back and ensure that the bed wheels are locked and/or that the mat is secure. Each of these techniques will reduce the energy expenditure of both you and the patient, increase safety, and enhance the patient's ability to move. You can discover and apply many "tricks of the trade" by using your problem-solving skills and ability; some of these techniques are presented later in this chapter.

Knowledge of many of the basic principles of physics and body mechanics will help you develop innovative and safe ways to adjust a patient's position or perform a transfer. Role playing with a friend, classmate, or coworker and simulating specific patient conditions or activity limitations are excellent ways to start the problem-solving process. The better you mimic a patient's condition, the better you will be able to devise techniques to alter your position on the bed or mat.

Dependent or Assisted Mobility Activities

To move a supine or prone patient, you should move individual body segments to reduce the effort required and to provide greater control. Begin by positioning yourself close to the side of the patient or the bed or mat table. This step will allow you to use your upper extremities with short lever arms to reduce strain and increase the mechanical advantage of your muscles. Kneeling on the mat or flexing your hips and knees as you treat the patient will minimize strain to your back. If it is possible to adjust the height of the bed or mat, position it at the most comfortable and most beneficial level for you to function. Ensure that the bed wheels are locked before you perform any of these transfers. Apply the principles of body mechanics to reduce stress and strain to your muscles, joints, and ligaments.

Be certain to explain the activity to the patient and encourage him or her to assist with each of the movements. You should continue to guide and encourage the patient throughout the activity to promote motivation and increased independence.

Side-to-Side Movement, Patient Supine To perform a side-to-side movement with the patient supine, position one forearm under the patient's neck or upper back and one forearm under the middle of the back. Gently slide the upper body and head toward you without lifting the upper body. It may be necessary to support the patient's head with your upper arm as you move him or her. Next, position your forearms under the patient's lower trunk and just distal to the pelvis; gently slide that body segment toward you. Finally, position your forearms under the thighs and legs and gently slide them toward you (Fig. 8-1). When you slide

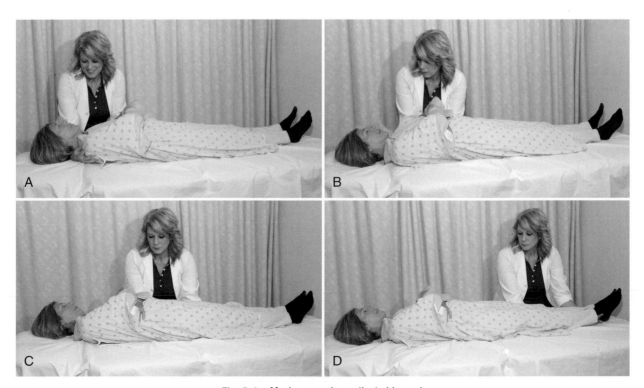

Fig. 8-1   Moving a supine patient sideward.

rather than lift the patient toward you, the amount of energy required and the stress to your upper extremities and back muscles are reduced. The force you use to pull and slide the patient should be applied parallel to the surface of the bed or mat to further reduce the energy required.

Remember to lower your trunk by flexing your hips and knees before moving the patient if the height of the bed or mat cannot be adjusted. This movement will position your center of gravity (COG) as close to the patient's COG as possible. Position your feet to widen your base of support (BOS) by placing one foot in front of the other. These actions allow you to control the patient better, reduce stress and strain to your arms and back, and reduce the energy required to move the patient. When it is necessary to move the patient sideward over a long distance, it will be easier if each body segment is moved several times. Moving the patient closer to one side of the bed or mat is necessary before you perform an exercise or a transfer. Having the patient close to you allows you to take advantage of the use of proper body mechanics. (Note: If the patient is too large to move comfortably, use an assistant to help and/or use a transfer sheet.)

Upward Movement, Patient Supine Before attempting to move a patient upward, bring him or her closer to the near edge of the bed or mat, especially if the patient is lying in the center of the bed or mat. If the patient is on an adjustable bed, be certain the portion that raises the head and trunk is flat, and remove any pillows from under the head and shoulders. This position will allow you to use the muscles of your upper extremities more effectively by using short lever arms. Short lever arms can develop greater force than long lever arms, require less energy expenditure, and provide better patient control.

To initiate the move, ask the patient to perform a bridging exercise by flexing the patient's hips and knees so the feet rest flat on the bed or mat. This step will reduce friction between the extremities and the bed or mat surface and will position the patient so he or she can assist by lifting the pelvis or pushing with the legs. It may be necessary to support the thighs with one or more pillows if the patient is unable to maintain the position. You should face toward the patient's head and stand approximately opposite the patient's midchest level with the foot that is farthest from the bed in front of your other foot (i.e., in stride in an anteroposterior position). Support the patient's head and upper trunk with your arms, and lift until the inferior angles of the scapulae clear the bed or mat; your chest should be close to the patient's chest so you use short lever arms with your arms. This position will reduce the friction of the patient's trunk on the bed or mat but should not place excessive strain or stress on the structures of your back. If you are unable to lift the patient's trunk or if the lift creates excessive strain or stress to your back, ask another person for assistance and use a draw sheet (Fig. 8-2). (Note: Several

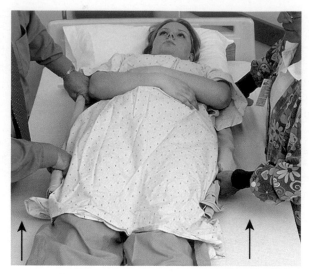

Fig. 8-2 Moving a supine patient upward using a draw sheet.

types of movement transfer products are available that are safer to use and require less effort than a draw sheet; they can be found in equipment product catalogs.)

Slide the lower trunk and pelvis upward approximately 6 to 10 inches. Do not attempt to move the patient over a long distance unless the patient is able to provide assistance. To move the patient farther, reposition yourself and the patient's lower extremities and repeat the process. Some patients may be able to grasp your trunk to help elevate their trunk. However, doing so may increase stress or strain to your back, and you must determine whether it is a safe technique. If an over-the-bed frame, bar, or trapeze is available, the patient can grasp it and elevate his or her upper body. After you have moved the patient upward to the final position, reposition him or her in the center to reduce the possibility of rolling off the bed or mat.

Downward Movement, Patient Supine To move a supine patient downward, initially move him or her closer to the near edge of the bed or mat and partially flex the hips and knees. If necessary, use a pillow to support the thighs. Position yourself approximately opposite to the patient's waist or hips or at the patient's feet (Fig. 8-3). Cradle and lift the pelvis slightly before you slide the patient's upper body and head downward. Move the patient approximately 6 to 10 inches and then reposition yourself and the patient's lower extremities if further movement is required. Reposition the patient in the center of the bed or mat.

Movement of a recumbent patient upward, downward, or sideward can be accomplished more easily if a small sheet or linen pad is placed beneath the patient. This item is frequently called a draw sheet; it usually extends from the upper back to the buttocks or midthigh area. Two persons, one on each side of the bed or mat, grasp the sheet or pad and, on command by the leader, they simultaneously move the patient by sliding. Some lifting may be required, but the

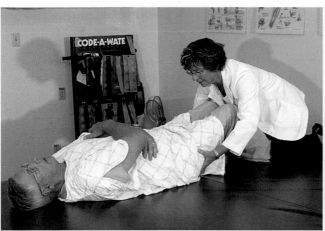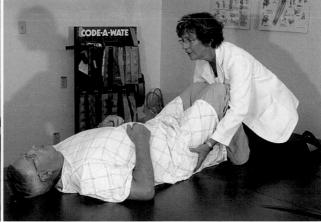

Fig. 8-3 Moving a supine patient downward.

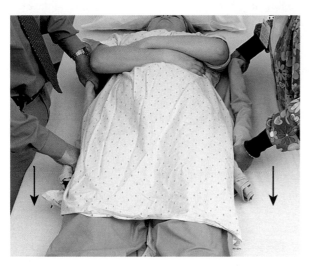

Fig. 8-4 Moving a patient downward using a draw sheet.

primary force used is sliding (Fig. 8-4). The patient should be encouraged to assist by using his or her upper or lower extremities to partially elevate the trunk or pelvis. When the patient is moved upward or sideward, the upper portion of the bed should be lowered; when he or she is moved downward, the upper portion of the bed can be raised. Use of a draw sheet may create friction with the patient's heels, sacrum, spinous processes, and back of the head, so it should be used only for short movements. (Note: A commercially available fabric tube sheet or a plastic transfer sheet, which creates a low coefficient of friction between it and the surface on which the patient lies, can be used instead of a draw sheet to reduce the effort necessary to reposition the patient. These sheets also can be used for lateral transfers.)

Move to a Side-Lying Position, Patient Supine When moving a supine patient to a side-lying position, to ensure that sufficient space is available on the bed or mat, it may be necessary initially to position the patient close to the far

edge of the bed or mat. Because this position is potentially dangerous, you, another person, a bed rail, or a wall must protect the patient from rolling off the bed or mat. Be certain the bed wheels are locked or blocked to prevent the bed from moving.

Stand facing the patient so you can roll (or turn) him or her toward you to a side-lying position. When it is absolutely necessary to roll the patient away from you, be certain he or she is protected from rolling off the bed or mat table (i.e., elevate the bed rail, block the edge with pillows, or position another person at the opposite side of the bed). If you plan to roll the patient toward the right, place the left lower extremity over the right lower extremity, place the left upper extremity on the chest, and place the right upper extremity in straight abduction. Roll the patient toward you by pulling gently on the left posterior scapula (shoulder) and the left posterior pelvis. Do not pull on the upper or lower extremity to initiate the roll, because you will not be able to properly control or initiate movement of the trunk and the extremity may be injured.

When the patient is in a side-lying position, flex the hips and knees and place a pillow under the head, between the knees and ankles, and along the front and back of the trunk. The lowermost upper and lower extremities should be positioned for comfort. Refer to the description of the side-lying position in Chapter 5 for more complete information about this position. If the patient is to remain in this position unattended, it may be necessary to apply trunk restraints or engage the bed rails.

It is important to be careful when readjusting the patient's position when he or she is side lying. Lying on the side is an unstable position, and the patient can easily roll forward or backward. Inform the patient when you move from one side of the bed or mat to the other side. It is recommended that you maintain manual contact with the patient as you move. You should roll the patient toward you and guard the edge of the bed or mat to prevent him or her from rolling too far. This maneuver will require you to stand close to the side of the bed or mat toward which you roll the patient, with at least one thigh against the edge of the bed or mat. These precautions must be followed when you are moving the patient from a supine to a prone position or from a prone to a supine position to protect the patient and maintain control of the maneuver.

Move to a Prone Position, Patient Supine When moving a supine patient to a prone position, with the bed wheels locked, move the patient closer to one side of the bed or mat and prepare to roll him or her to a side-lying position as described previously, with one modification. The arm over which the patient will roll should be positioned in one of two ways: (1) close along the side with the shoulder externally rotated, the elbow straight, the palm up, and the hand tucked under the pelvis, or (2) with the shoulder flexed so the arm rests next to the ear with the elbow straight. The other contralateral upper extremity remains by the side (Fig. 8-5).

Stand facing the patient and roll the patient to a side-lying position. Determine whether sufficient space exists to allow the roll to a prone position to be completed. If the space is insufficient, move the patient backward while lying on his or her side until sufficient space is available to complete the roll to the prone position. Because the patient is very insecure while in a side-lying position, you must guard him or her closely.

Roll the patient toward you and protect the near edge of the bed or mat by placing one of your thighs against it. This maneuver will prevent the patient from rolling off the bed or mat.

Move to a Supine Position, Patient Prone To move a prone patient to the supine position, first move the patient close to one edge of the bed or mat. If the patient is going to roll toward the right side, cross the left leg over the right leg. Position the right upper extremity close to the side with the elbow straight, the palm up, and the hand tucked under the pelvis; alternately, the right shoulder can be flexed and the arm can be positioned close to the patient's ear, with the other upper extremity placed next to the patient's side. Stand on the far side of the table and roll the patient

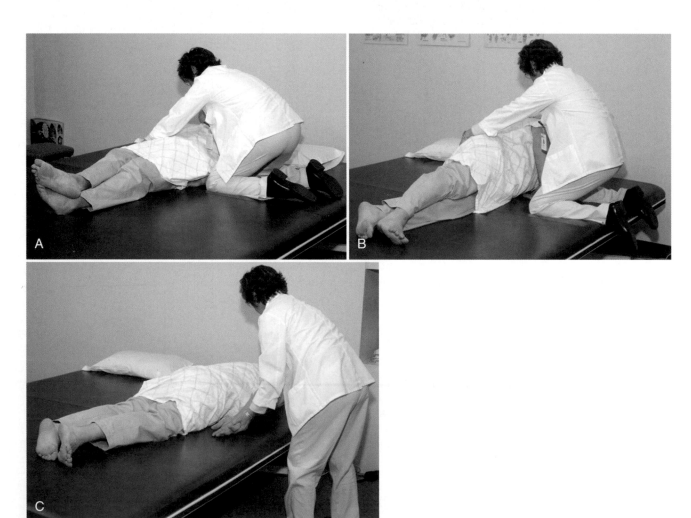

Fig. 8-5   Moving a supine patient to a prone position.

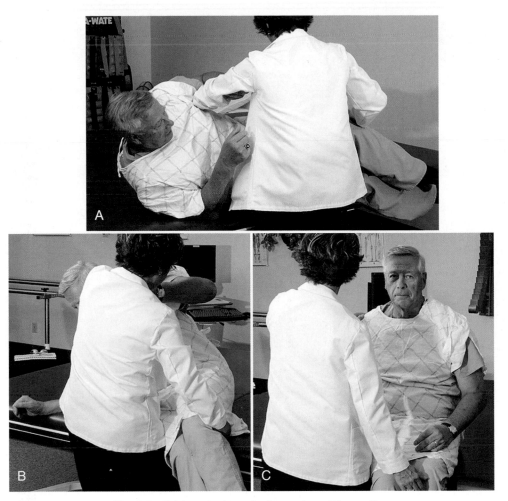

Fig. 8-6   Helping a supine patient move to a sitting position.

toward you to a side-lying position. Determine whether sufficient space is available to allow the patient to be rolled to the supine position. If the space is insufficient, move the patient forward while lying on his or her side until sufficient space exists to complete the roll to a supine position.

Guide the patient from a side-lying to a supine position by resisting against the posterior left shoulder and pelvis to retard the movement to a supine position. Protect the near edge of the bed or mat by placing your thighs against it. After the patient is supine, reposition him or her in the center of the bed or mat.

Move to a Sitting Position, Patient Supine   To move a supine patient to a sitting position, move the patient close to one edge of the bed or mat (using the length of the patient's thigh as a guide to where the patient's buttocks should be) and roll the patient to a side-lying position with the lower extremities partially flexed. Elevate the trunk by lifting under the shoulders or by instructing the patient to push up using either or both upper extremities. To assist in this maneuver, ask the patient to look in the direction of

movement and to engage neck and trunk muscles during the activity (Fig. 8-6).

Pivot the lower extremities over the side of the bed or mat as the trunk is raised. If the patient is not able to control the lower extremities to put them on the floor, you may need to assist or guide the lower extremities to prevent pain or injury. Do not allow the patient to sit unattended or unsupported.

This method is recommended for patients who have a lower back condition that might be aggravated by trunk flexion or for patients who have functional use of only one upper and lower extremity. The patient's body weight will be concentrated closer to the COG, which will make it easier for you to lift the trunk. Position your feet in an anteroposterior position to widen your BOS and to avoid twisting your back as you lift the patient.

Alternative Method.   For an alternative method of moving a supine patient to a sitting position, move the patient close to one edge of the bed or mat and flex the hips and knees with the feet flat on the bed or mat (Fig. 8-7). The trunk can be elevated by using an over-the-bed frame,

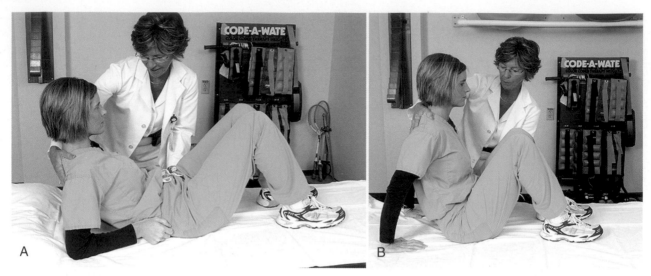

Fig. 8-7   Alternative method of helping a supine patient move to a sitting position.

bar, or trapeze. If this equipment is unavailable, place one or both of your arms under the patient's upper back and head and have the patient push with the upper extremities to elevate the trunk until a long sitting position is attained.

Pivot the patient by supporting him or her under the thighs and behind the back to a short sitting or dangling position. (Caution: Do not allow the patient to sit unattended or without support, even briefly. Some patients may experience vertigo or syncope [i.e., become dizzy or faint] when they are moved quickly from a supine to a sitting position. Other patients may lack sufficient strength or balance to remain sitting without some form of support.)

Move to Supine Position, Patient Sitting   To move a sitting patient to the supine position, reverse the sequence of activities described in the preceding section to move from a supine to a sitting position. Reposition the patient in the center of the bed or mat when he or she is supine.

Independent Mobility Activities

Each patient should be taught and encouraged to independently perform or assist with all bed or mat mobility activities to the extent of his or her abilities. Initially these activities can be used while dependent or assisted bed or mat mobility activities are practiced. Instruct and guide the patient in the activities to be performed. Assistive equipment such as bed rails or overhead bars should not be used unless the patient is unable to safely perform the activity without equipment. Remember that these activities are necessary to enable the patient to perform transfers and avoid soft-tissue pressure and the development of contractures as a result of prolonged immobilization.

Side-to-Side Movement, Patient Supine   To have a supine patient perform a side-to-side movement, instruct

the patient to do the following: (1) flex his or her hips and knees and place the feet flat on the bed or mat; (2) position one upper extremity next to the trunk; and (3) abduct the other upper extremity approximately 4 inches from the trunk.

Instruct the patient to (1) push down with the lower extremities (i.e., perform a bridging maneuver) to lift the pelvis and move it toward the abducted upper extremity and (2) elevate the upper trunk by pushing into the bed with the elbows and the back of the head to move toward the abducted elbow. The patient should then reposition the lower and upper extremities to move again or for comfort.

An alternate method is to elevate the pelvis and upper trunk by simultaneously pushing down with the legs and the back of the head and shifting the body toward the abducted upper extremity. The patient should be taught to move to the left and to the right.

Upward Movement, Patient Supine   To have a supine patient perform an upward movement, instruct the patient to fully flex the hips and knees, position the feet flat on the bed or mat with the heels close to the buttocks, and position the upper extremities with the elbows flexed and next to the trunk with the shoulders (scapulae) pulled up toward the ears (Fig. 8-8).

The patient elevates the pelvis using the lower extremities and elevates the upper trunk by simultaneously pushing into the bed or mat with the elbows and the back of the head, and then he or she moves upward by pushing with the lower extremities and depressing the shoulders (scapulae). The patient then repositions the lower and upper extremities for successive movements. Many patients may find this maneuver difficult. If the bed is adjustable, the upper portion should be flat and the wheels should be locked.

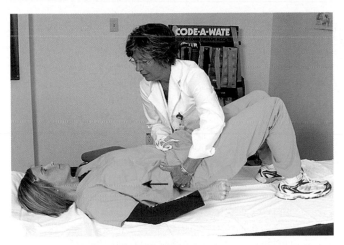

Fig. 8-8   Helping a supine patient move upward.

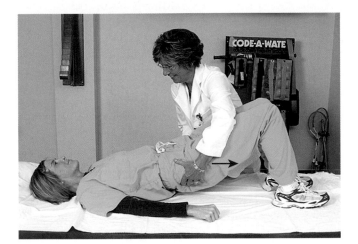

Fig. 8-9   Helping a supine patient move downward.

Downward Movement, Patient Supine To have a supine patient perform a downward movement, instruct the patient to partially flex his or her hips and knees to position the feet flat on the bed or mat; the heels should be 8 to 12 inches distal to the buttocks. The upper extremities should be positioned next to the trunk with the elbows flexed and the shoulders (scapulae) depressed (Fig. 8-9). If the bed is adjustable, the upper portion should be elevated slightly and the wheels should be locked.

The patient elevates the pelvis using the lower extremities and elevates the upper trunk by simultaneously pushing into the bed or mat with the elbows and the back of the head, and then he or she moves downward by pulling with the lower extremities, simultaneously pushing up with the shoulders (scapulae) and pulling downward with the elbows or forearms. The lower and upper extremities are repositioned for successive movements.

Move to a Side-Lying Position, Patient Supine To have a supine patient move to a side-lying position, first instruct the patient to move to the far side of the bed or

mat. To roll toward the right, the patient simultaneously reaches across the chest with the left upper extremity and lifts the left lower extremity diagonally over the right lower extremity; he or she then uses head flexion and the abdominal muscles to roll onto the side or uses the left hand to grasp the edge of the mattress, draw sheet, or bed rail to pull to a side-lying position.

Instruct the patient to maintain the side-lying position by using the left hand on the bed or mat and by flexing the lower extremities. A pillow will be needed for the head.

To roll to the left, the patient performs the same process with the opposite extremities.

Alternative Method. An alternative method can be used to have a supine patient move to a side-lying position. First, instruct the patient to move to the far side of the bed or mat. To roll to the right, the patient pushes with the left upper extremity and the left lower extremity before reaching across the body. Some patients may prefer to reach with an upper extremity and push with a lower extremity to initiate the roll. To roll to the left, the patient performs the same process with the contralateral extremities.

It is important to inform the patient about the relative insecurity of the side-lying position. Instruct the patient to flex his or her hips and knees and place the uppermost hand in front of the chest on the bed or mat to increase stability. In addition, you may need to teach the patient to reposition his or her body in the center of the bed or mat to provide as much bed area in front of the body as behind the body.

Move to a Prone Position, Patient Supine To have a supine patient move to a prone position, first instruct the patient to move to one side of the bed or mat. To roll to the right, the patient positions the right upper extremity under the right side of the body or flexes the shoulder so it is positioned next to the right ear and then moves to a side-lying position. If the space is insufficient to roll to a prone position, the patient should reposition his or her body away from the near edge of the bed or mat. As the patient rolls to the prone position, the left upper extremity is used to protect and lower the body. The person then adjusts the position as desired for comfort.

Move to a Supine Position, Patient Prone To have a prone patient move to a supine position, first instruct the patient to move to one side of the bed or mat. To roll to the right, the patient positions the right upper extremity under the right side or flexes the right shoulder so the upper arm is positioned next to the right ear. The left hand is placed flat on the bed or mat near the anterior left shoulder; the left hip and knee can be partially flexed or extended.

The patient pushes with the left upper extremity, lifts the left lower extremity over the right lower extremity, and moves to a side-lying position. If space on the bed or mat is insufficient to roll to a supine position, the patient should reposition his or her body away from the near edge of the bed or mat and then roll to a supine position, adjusting the body as desired for comfort.

You must instruct the patient to determine the body's position on the bed or mat before any rolling activities are attempted. Depending on the width of the bed or mat, it may be necessary for the patient to adjust his or her position by moving forward or backward while in a side-lying position.

Move to a Sitting Position, Patient Supine To have a supine patient move to a sitting position, first instruct the patient to move toward one edge of the bed or mat, but leave sufficient space to roll to a side-lying position. The position of the patient on the bed should be about a thigh's length away from the edge, so that when he or she comes to a sitting position, the thighs will be supported on the bed. The patient rolls to a side-lying position and flexes the hips and knees to maintain this position briefly, then positions the hand of the uppermost upper extremity on the bed or mat at the midchest level (Fig. 8-10, A).

The patient pushes with the upper extremity to raise the trunk and maintains this position by resting on the elbow and forearm of the lowermost upper extremity, then elevates the trunk fully by pushing with both upper extremities to a side-sitting position (Fig. 8-10, B). The lower extremities can be pivoted simultaneously over the edge of the bed or mat (Fig. 8-10, C). This technique is beneficial for the patient with low back dysfunction or pain because less stress is directed to the lumbar spine by avoiding rotation and flexion. The patient can return to a supine position by performing the movements in reverse sequence. Occasionally a patient with low back dysfunction may want to move

to the floor and return to standing. Procedure 8-2 presents techniques designed to accomplish the movements safely and with reduced stress and discomfort.

Alternative Method. An alternative method can be used to have a supine patient move to a sitting position. First, instruct the patient to move to the near edge of the bed or mat. If the bed is adjustable, raise the upper portion to approximately 45 degrees. Start with the hips and knees flexed and the feet flat on the bed or mat; the upper extremities are slightly abducted, with the shoulders internally rotated and the forearms resting on the bed or mat (Fig. 8-11, A).

The patient lifts the head and pushes with the upper extremities to elevate the trunk using a tripod support, with the hands placed on the bed or mat behind the hips with the elbows extended. By alternately moving the hands forward, the patient attains a sitting position (Fig. 8-11, B). The patient can then pivot the lower extremities over the edge of the bed or mat (Fig. 8-11, C).

It may be necessary to alter or modify these activities for patients who have reduced strength or reduced function of one or more of the extremities. For example, the paralysis or paresis of the ipsilateral upper and lower extremity that results from a cerebrovascular accident (i.e., a stroke) will require the patient to use the remaining (contralateral) functional extremities to adjust position and to be mobile in bed or on a mat. Patients who have limited function as a result of joint disease or trauma will need to rely on the noninvolved or least involved joints to adjust position. Finally, patients with paralysis of the lower extremities and lower trunk (i.e., paraplegia) or with paralysis of all four extremities and trunk (i.e., quadriplegia) will require a

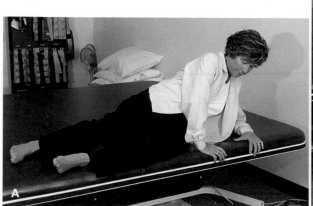
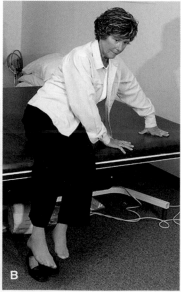
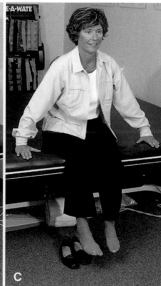

Fig. 8-10 Independent movements to rise from the supine position.

PROCEDURE 8-2

Protective Transfer to and from the Floor for a Person with Low Back Dysfunction

The patient should be encouraged to use a firm, stable object for support to reduce stress to the back as these activities are performed.

MOVEMENT FROM STANDING TO THE FLOOR

- The patient places one hand on a firm object and moves to a single knee (half-kneeling) position, keeping the trunk erect.
- The patient briefly kneels on both knees (high kneeling), then moves to all fours (hands and knees).
- The patient moves the hands forward until he or she is prone or gently side sits, if this is not painful, and then lowers onto one elbow to a side-lying position.
- The patient adjusts his or her body position as desired.

MOVEMENT FROM THE FLOOR TO STANDING

- The patient starts in the prone position and pushes to his or her hands and knees or logrolls to a side-lying position.
- If the patient is on all fours, he or she moves to a half-kneeling position, then to standing; a firm object may be used for assistance.
- If the patient is lying on his or her side, he or she pushes to a side-sitting position, moves to a hands-and-knees position, and then performs the movements listed in the previous step.

longer period of training and practice to learn how to safely and efficiently adjust position. Quadriplegic patients may require aids such as loops attached to the mattress or to an overhead bed frame, bed rails, an overhead trapeze, or loops of cloth sewn to clothing to assist in altering position. The techniques or procedures that must be learned and practiced by patients with multiple injuries or severe paralysis are beyond the scope of this book. Refer to the Bibliography for sources of information about these types of patient conditions.

TRANSFER ACTIVITIES

Transfers, Wheelchair and Bed

Independent Standing Transfer Before an independent standing transfer is performed, the wheelchair should be positioned (angled at approximately 45 degrees), locked, and prepared as previously described. In many situations, the wheelchair will need to be repositioned so a return transfer can be performed safely. When a significant difference exists in the strength of the extremities, it usually will be easier for the patient to transfer while leading with the stronger extremities. These transfers should only be performed by a patient who has the mental and physical abilities to accomplish them consistently and safely. It is the responsibility of the caregiver to determine whether the patient meets these criteria. In preparation for these transfers, the patient must be able to manipulate and maneuver a wheelchair, rise from a supine to a sitting position and return from a sitting to a supine position, move from sitting to standing and from standing to sitting, and ambulate a short distance. Independent transfer from a wheelchair to a

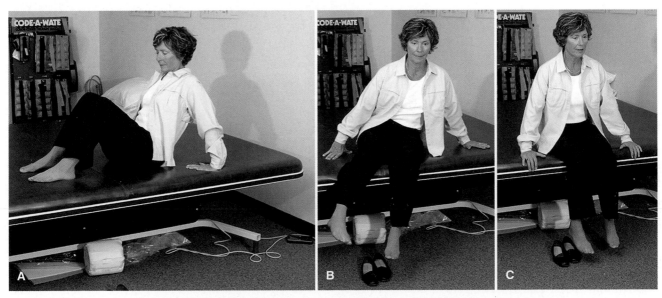

Fig. 8-11   Alternative method of rising independently from the supine position to a sitting position.

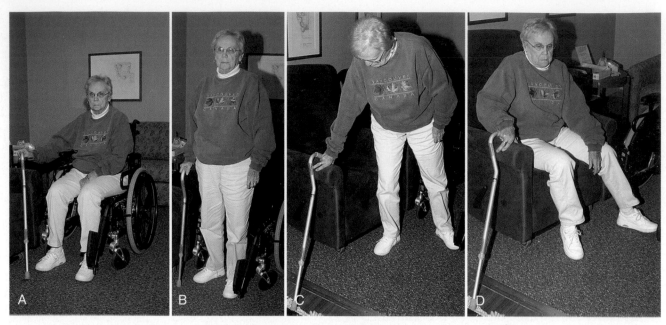

Fig. 8-12   Modified independent standing transfer from a wheelchair to a chair.

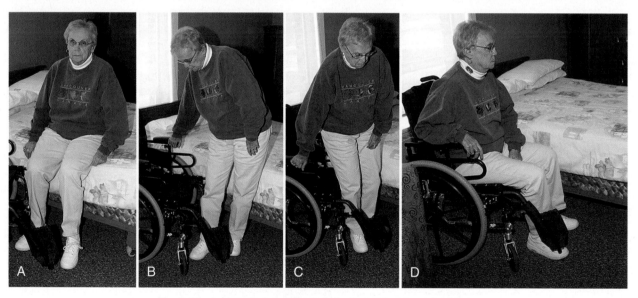

Fig. 8-13   Independent standing transfer from a bed to a wheelchair.

chair is shown in Fig. 8-12; independent transfer from a bed to a wheelchair is shown in Fig. 8-13; and independent use of a cane to get to a toilet is shown in Fig. 8-14. (Note: The caregiver should be at the patient's side for protection or assistance when the patient initially attempts any type of independent standing transfer.)

For patients with a recent total hip replacement, care must be taken to avoid adduction of the surgically replaced hip beyond a midline position, excessive internal or external hip rotation, and excessive hip flexion, which is usually restricted to 60 to 90 degrees. The patient must not pivot on that extremity when standing, flex the surgical hip or the trunk past 90 degrees, or adduct the hip past neutral at any time during the transfer.

Standing, Dependent Pivot   A standing pivot should not be attempted with a dependent patient unless the patient is small and the caregiver has sufficient strength for the maneuver. Instead, a lateral or sitting transfer can be performed if a standing pivot transfer requires maximal assistance. A safety belt or transfer sling placed under the buttocks should be applied before any sitting or standing transfer is attempted, particularly during the early treatment sessions. The patient should be instructed in the procedures

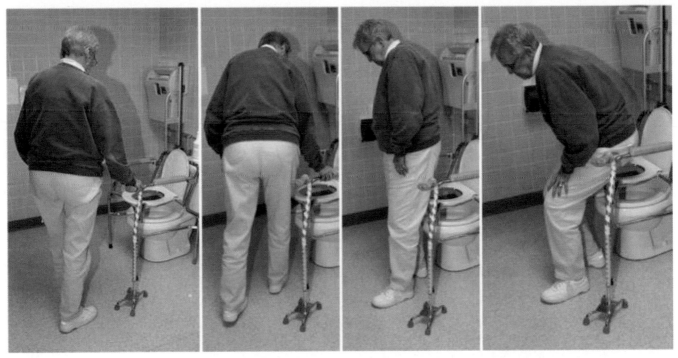

Fig. 8-14   Modified independent standing transfer to a toilet with a four-footed cane.

required to maneuver, position, and operate the wheelchair and its components. These procedures are described in Chapter 7.

Position the wheelchair parallel or at a 45- to 60-degree angle to the bed midway between the head and foot of the bed (Fig. 8-15, A). Apply a safety belt or use a large towel or sheet as a sling under the buttocks and lock the wheelchair with the caster wheels positioned forward to increase the BOS of the wheelchair. (Note: The caster wheels may pivot or turn to one side when the patient performs the transfer. That movement does not cause a safety problem, and the patient can continue to perform the transfer. However, the caster wheels should not be permitted to be directed backward because that position reduces the stability of the chair, particularly when the patient moves to the front portion of the seat.) Remove the patient's feet from the footrests and elevate the footrests; remove or swing away the front rigging, and place the patient's feet flat on the floor. Remove the armrest nearest to the bed if the top surface of the bed is lower than the armrest. Move the patient forward in the chair by grasping the posterior area of the pelvis and guiding it so that the buttocks slide forward, position the feet parallel to each other, and position the trunk over the pelvis. Some patients can be taught to move the hips forward by using the upper trunk to push back against the upper portion of the seat back and sliding the pelvis forward. The trunk will need to be repositioned over the pelvis before you begin the transfer. Partially stoop and position your knees and feet outside and touching the patient's knees and feet. The patient should be discouraged

from holding onto the caregiver during transfers, but if the patient insists or is in the habit of doing so, he or she can hold your middle or upper back with the upper extremities. (Caution: Do not allow the patient to hold you around your neck. You must use proper body mechanics to prevent undue strain on your back.)

Grasp the safety belt at the sides of the patient's waist or the sling and inform the patient when and how to move to standing. If necessary, you may rock the patient to develop momentum before standing (Fig. 8-15, B).

Instruct the patient using terms such as "ready, stand" or "one, two, three, stand." Instruct the patient to move his or her head forward and shift his or her weight forward, if possible, so as to unload the weight from the backside to begin the transfer. As you lift on the safety belt or sling, simultaneously straighten your lower extremities and stabilize the patient's knees by pushing in and forward with your knees. Elevate the body high enough to clear the wheelchair wheel and stand the patient to the height necessary to elevate the pelvis above the level of the surface of the bed. Pivot by sliding your feet and the patient toward the bed and lower the patient onto the surface when the buttocks (pelvis) are turned and directed toward the bed. (Note: A commercially available rigid or flexible fabric disk that allows the patient to be pivoted without moving the feet can be placed under the patient's feet before standing, thus reducing the effort required by the caregiver to perform the transfer.) Set the patient on the edge of the bed (Fig. 8-15, C to F; Procedure 8-3). Then help the patient perform sitting activities or help him or her into a supine position. To prevent a fall, you

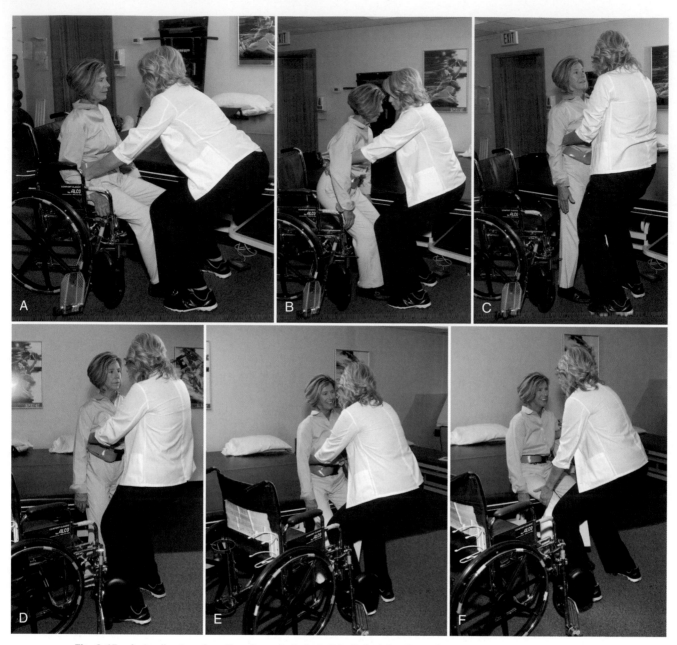

Fig. 8-15   A standing transfer with a dependent pivot. **A** to **F,** Assisting the patient to stand, pivot, and sit on the bed.

should not leave the patient sitting unattended or without sufficient support.

The return to the wheelchair is performed using the same procedures in reverse, but the wheelchair position may need to be reversed if the patient needs to lead with a stronger or less involved side. The patient should be transferred toward the left and right side for practice and should be asked to assist as much as possible with the transfer. As the patient gains strength, the assisted standing transfer should be attempted.

If a safety belt or sling is not used, the assistant may lift the patient by grasping under the buttocks. However, this procedure may be difficult to perform on large patients, and some patients may prefer that you not use this method. Your hands may slip or slide over the patient's clothing, and it may not be as easy to control the patient as it would be with a safety belt. (Caution: You should not use the patient's clothing, including the belt, to lift or protect the patient. You could soil and tear the clothing, or the belt may unbuckle or cause patient discomfort if you use it as a means of control.)

Standing, Assisted Pivot When performing a transfer with a patient who has greater strength in one upper and

PROCEDURE 8-3

Procedures Associated with a Standing Transfer

- Examine and evaluate the patient's mental and physical capacities to perform or assist with the transfer.
- Position, secure, and stabilize the wheelchair and other items involved with the transfer, swing away the front rigging or elevate the foot plates, and apply a safety belt or transfer sling to the patient.
- Instruct the patient in the steps of the transfer, indicate the activities he or she is expected to perform, and demonstrate the transfer. Instruct the patient to move forward in the chair and angle his or her backside so that the thighs are parallel to the surface to which he or she is transferring. Provide assistance if needed; position the patient's feet flat on the floor parallel or anteroposterior to each other.
- The patient initiates the transfer with trunk momentum or by inclining the trunk forward ("nose over toes"); the caregiver is positioned in front and slightly to one side of the patient to protect and guard him or her.
- The patient uses the upper and lower extremity or extremities to rise to a standing position; assistance is provided by the caregiver as needed using the knees and the safety belt.
- The patient stands briefly to establish balance and to acclimate to the upright position, then turns or pivots toward the object to which he or she is transferring.
- The patient contacts the object using the upper and lower extremity or extremities before lowering onto the object; assistance is provided by the caregiver as needed.
- The patient's position is adjusted for proper support, stability, and safety; any reaction and physiological response to the activity are evaluated by the caregiver.
- Remove the safety belt and document the patient's performance and amount of assistance needed.

lower extremity than in the contralateral extremities, you should decide in which direction the patient will transfer. Initially it will be easier and safer for most patients to transfer by leading with the stronger extremities. However, the patient also should learn to lead with the weaker extremities. When the patient leads with the weaker extremity and uses the weaker upper extremity to assist with the transfer, proprioception and kinesthesia in those extremities may be improved, and the patient is more likely to sense or feel them in a functional way. In addition, if the patient learns to transfer using both the left and the right extremities, he or she will be better prepared to move in either direction at home or in the community regardless of the location of a bed, toilet, or bathtub. The patient should learn to transfer by leading with both the weaker and the stronger extremities to increase independence and encourage use of the weaker extremities.

When you determine that the patient is able to support weight on the stronger lower extremity safely and independently, you may choose to stabilize the weaker extremity. This method will allow the patient to increase use of the lower extremities and improve independence. When the patient transfers by leading with the left (stronger) extremities, grasp the safety belt with both hands and stabilize the weaker (right) knee by placing your left foot next to the lateral area of the right foot and by placing your left knee on the medial side of the right knee (Fig. 8-16). An alternative method to control the patient's trunk is to grasp the safety belt with your left hand and place your right hand on the left shoulder or on the posterolateral area of the thorax by reaching under the left upper extremity. The patient positions the wheelchair parallel or at a 45- to 60-degree angle to the bed, with the stronger extremities nearest the bed. The chair should be at the midpoint between the head and foot of the bed or mat (see Fig. 8-16).

The patient locks the wheelchair with the caster wheels directed forward, removes the feet from the footrests, and removes or swings away the front rigging. Armrests of the desk chair type should be reversed so the highest part is forward. The patient moves forward to the center or forward part of the seat by shifting weight off one buttock, elevating the pelvis on that side, and moving it forward to the desired position in the chair or by leaning against the chair back and pushing the pelvis forward to the desired position in the chair (the thighs are parallel to the surface to which they are transferring) and then moving the trunk to an erect or forward-inclined position to move the COG over the feet.

The patient positions the feet with the stronger foot posterior to the weaker or most affected foot. This position allows a stronger lower extremity to raise the body most effectively. However, that extremity will need to be advanced so it is anterior to the opposite lower extremity before the patient pivots. (Note: An elderly patient may perform better with the feet positioned parallel rather than anteroposterior.) The patient places the hands forward on the armrests and simultaneously pushes down with the upper and lower extremities while inclining the trunk forward slightly ("nose over toes") to stand. Some trunk motion can be initiated by rocking the trunk forward and back to develop momentum before attempting to stand. You may need to stabilize one or both of the knees as described previously when the patient begins the stand while you maintain control using the safety belt and the shoulder or the posterior neck. (Caution: Do not use the patient's upper extremity or clothing for control, as stated previously.)

Allow the patient to stand briefly to establish balance and to determine whether lightheadedness or a dizzy sensation occurs. The patient pivots by taking small steps with the lower extremities toward the bed so the back is nearest to the bed (the lower extremities are touching the bed), and he or she then reaches with the nearest upper extremity to

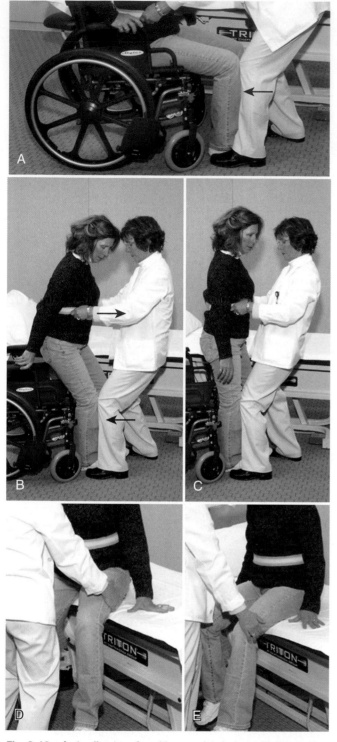

Fig. 8-16 A standing transfer with an assisted pivot with the weaker (right) knee stabilized.

the surface of the bed and lowers to sitting on the bed. The caregiver may need to assist with weight shifting to allow the patient to step in the process of pivoting. The patient places the lower extremities onto the bed and then lies down; if necessary, you may need to lift the lower extremities onto the bed and help the patient recline.

Alternative Method. Occasionally it may be necessary for a patient to use a footstool to elevate the hips to the height of a nonadjustable bed. The important principle to remember is that the patient should step onto the stool with the stronger lower extremity and that it may be necessary to guard the opposite extremity. The footstool should have four legs, and the feet of the legs should be located beyond the edges of the top. For maximal stability, the feet should have rubber tips and the top should have a nonskid surface. The footstool should be between 8 and 12 inches high.

As with other transfers, the chair must be angled properly and the patient should initiate the transfer with the stronger extremities nearest to the bed. The preliminary steps are the same as those listed for a standing transfer with an assisted pivot. The caregiver guards the weaker knee as the patient steps onto the footstool with the stronger lower extremity. That extremity is used to lift the body high enough to position the buttocks slightly above the surface of the bed. The caregiver helps the patient pivot so the buttocks are turned toward the bed or plinth. The person sits on the edge of the bed and establishes balance (Fig. 8-17, A to D). Another method is to have the patient pivot after standing and sidestep up onto the footstool with the stronger lower extremity. The caregiver can help the patient lie down by controlling the trunk and the lower extremities.

You can also instruct the patient to place the stronger foot on the footstool and to stand with assistance (Fig. 8-17, E to G). When this method is used, the weak lower extremity is not stabilized. (Caution: The patient must be instructed to push down onto the footstool and not to push forward to avoid sliding or tipping the footstool.)

Usually it is not necessary to use a footstool to transfer from the bed or plinth to a wheelchair, particularly if the bed or treatment table can be lowered. The caregiver helps the patient sit with the legs over the edge of the bed or plinth and the stronger lower extremity slightly forward of the opposite extremity. The wheelchair is positioned at a 45-degree angle and nearest to the stronger lower extremity. Guard the patient and help him or her move forward, leading with the stronger lower extremity so that it contacts the floor before the opposite lower extremity. When the leading foot is secure on the floor, the weaker foot is placed onto the floor. The patient grasps the far armrest of the wheelchair, partially pivots on the stronger lower extremity so the back is toward the chair seat, completes the pivot, and is helped to sit. If necessary, the knee of the weaker lower extremity can be stabilized by the caregiver.

Remember to apply and use a safety belt or sling for these transfers and have another caretaker in the room if assistance is required. If it becomes apparent you will not be able to control or protect the patient throughout the transfer, return the person to the object from which the transfer was initiated. Transferring a patient from a wheelchair to a motor vehicle also will require a safety belt (Fig. 8-18).

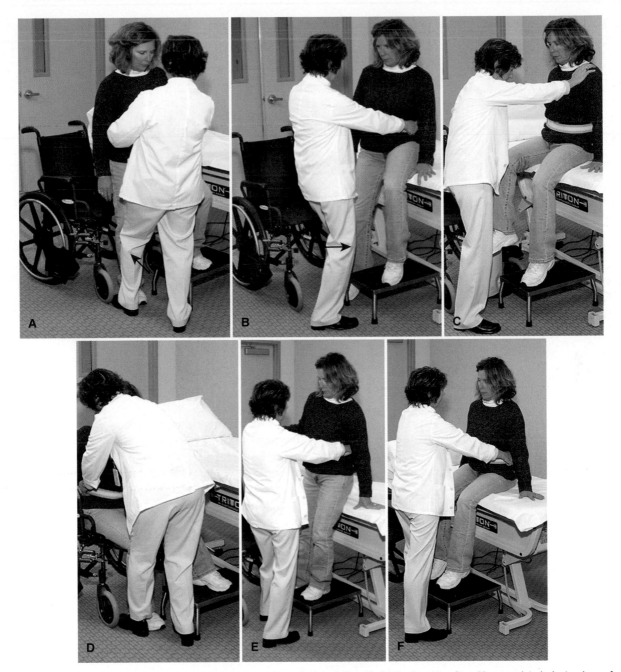

Fig. 8-17 **A** to **C,** A standing transfer with an assisted pivot using a footstool. **D** to **F,** A standing transfer with an assisted pivot using a footstool (alternative method).

Sitting, Assisted For an assisted transfer from a wheelchair to the sitting position on a bed, instruct the patient to position the wheelchair at an angle to the bed and midway between the head and foot of the bed or mat. With the caster wheels forward and the bed wheels locked, apply a safety belt to the patient. Instruct the patient to lock the wheelchair, remove the feet from the footrests, swing away or remove the front rigging, and place his or her feet on the floor. Instruct or help the patient to move forward in the chair and to remove the armrest nearest to the bed or mat.

The transfer board is positioned under the patient's thigh, in front of the drive wheel, so it extends from the wheelchair seat to the bed (Fig. 8-19). (Note: Do not place the transfer board just under the buttocks, which can result in the patient sliding forward off the transfer board in the process of the transfer. The board needs to be under the thighs.)

If the patient is going to move to the left, the left hand is placed on the board 4 to 6 inches from the left thigh and the right hand is placed next to the right thigh. The patient

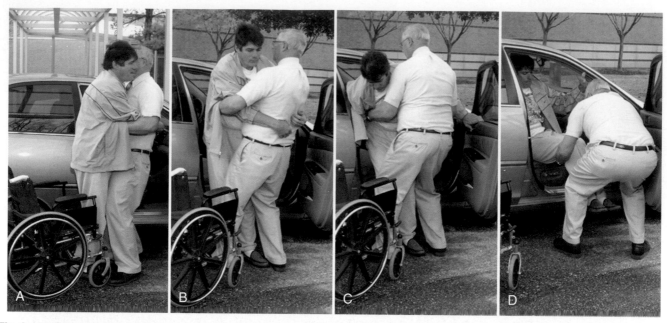

Fig. 8-18 An assisted transfer into a motor vehicle. **A,** The caregiver protects the person's knees and helps him stand; the chair is prepositioned and locked. **B,** The knees are protected as the person pivots. **C,** The caregiver uses the safety belt to help the person to sit. **D,** The lower extremities are placed inside the car.

performs a push-up with the upper extremities to elevate the body and begins to move toward the bed by quickly moving the head to the left and pushing toward the right with the left arm simultaneously. This procedure is repeated until the hips are on the bed. To move to the right, the position of the patient's hands is reversed. (Note: Some patients will be able to totally elevate the pelvis and move across the board without assistance. However, other patients will not be able to totally elevate the pelvis and must slide their buttocks, using a series of small movements, to progress across the board.) You should guard the patient's knees and use the safety belt to assist in elevating the body or moving the buttocks across the board. You can protect the patient's loss of balance by placing your hand on the upper trunk. The patient will need to shift weight off of one hip so the transfer board can be removed when he or she is seated securely on the bed. The caregiver may need to assist with the removal of the board, but the patient will need to learn how to remove the board in order to be independent with this transfer. The patient then lies down independently or is assisted to a lying position. (Caution: Do not leave the patient sitting unattended.)

The return to the wheelchair is performed using the same techniques in reverse order. The patient should learn to transfer to the left and right to maximize independence.

This transfer is most commonly used for patients who are unable to stand (e.g., because of the effects of severe orthopedic or neurologic conditions) but have functional upper extremities. A similar transfer can be performed by a patient with weakness in one upper and lower extremity and normal strength in the other extremities but who is unable to stand safely. Some patients will require the use of a transfer board at all times, whereas other patients will develop the balance, strength, and skill to permit them to perform the transfer without the board (Procedure 8-4).

Sitting, Independent For an independent transfer from a wheelchair to sitting on a bed, instruct the patient to position the wheelchair at an angle to the bed and midway between the head and the foot of the bed or mat and lock the wheelchair. The caster wheels should be positioned forward to expand the BOS of the chair. Instruct the patient to remove his or her feet from the footrests, remove or swing away the front rigging, and place the feet on the floor.

Instruct the patient to move forward in the chair to clear the buttocks past the drive wheel and remove the armrest nearest to the bed. The patient then moves the buttocks to partially pivot the body so the back is toward the bed. If the patient is going to move to the right, the right hand is placed on the edge of the bed and the left hand is placed on the armrest on the seat of the chair or on the back of the chair, depending on the patient's strength, size, and skill. The patient pushes with the upper extremities to elevate the body and swings the buttocks onto the edge of the bed by moving the head quickly to the left and pushing toward the right with the left arm simultaneously, then repositions the hands and moves farther onto the bed. The patient then stabilizes the body on the edge of the bed, places the lower extremities onto the bed, and lies on the

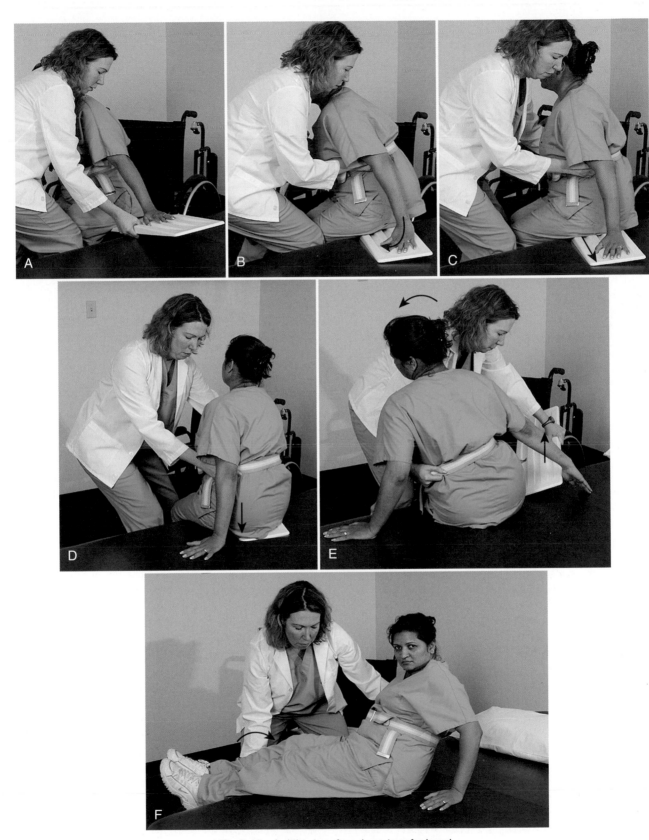

Fig. 8-19   A sitting transfer using a transfer board.

PROCEDURE 8-4

Transfer with a Transfer Board

If the bed height can be adjusted, it should be positioned as near to the height of the wheelchair seat as possible before the transfer is attempted, and the bed wheels should be locked.

BED TO WHEELCHAIR

- Position the wheelchair at an angle next to the bed, facing the foot of the bed with the caster wheels forward and opposite the patient's hips. Lock the chair, remove the armrest nearest the bed, and swing away the front rigging.
- Help the patient into a long-sitting position, apply a safety belt, and help the patient move to the edge of the mattress. The lower extremities may be positioned over the edge of the mattress/mat or remain parallel.
- Position one end of the transfer board under the patient's upper thighs and buttocks; the other end rests on the chair seat. Position yourself slightly in front and to the near side of the patient to guard and protect him or her throughout the transfer.
- Help the patient move across the board onto the chair seat. Guard and protect the trunk if the lower extremities need to be lowered from the bed; help the patient shift his or her weight away from the board, and remove the board.
- Place the feet on the footrests, position the body for safety and comfort, and remove the safety belt.

WHEELCHAIR TO BED

- Position the chair at an angle next to the bed, facing the foot of the bed and midway between the head and foot of the bed. Lock the chair and remove the armrest nearest the bed. Swing away the front rigging with the caster wheels forward.
- Help the patient move forward in the chair. Place one end of the board under the thighs and buttocks; the other end should rest on the bed surface. Position yourself slightly in front of and to one side of the patient to guard and protect him or her.
- Help the patient move across the board onto the bed; the legs may dangle over the edge before they are lifted onto the bed. Guard and protect the patient as the lower extremities are placed onto the surface.
- Help the patient shift his or her weight away from the board and remove the board; help the patient move toward the center of the bed and lie down.
- Position the patient's body for safety and comfort and remove the safety belt.

bed. It may be necessary to help some patients place their lower extremities onto the bed and lie down (Fig. 8-20).

The return to the wheelchair is performed by using the same techniques in reverse order. The patient should learn to transfer to the left and right to maximize independence.

Sitting, Dependent

One-Person Dependent. The one-person lift transfer (sometimes referred to as the "quad pivot") can be used when a patient is unable to stand or is unable to perform any type of assisted transfer and when the assistant is sufficiently strong and skilled to perform the lift. The caregiver must use proper body mechanics and perform the lift over the shortest possible distance (Fig. 8-21). (Caution: This transfer needs to be learned and practiced with able-bodied persons before attempting it with a patient. Repeated practice is helpful and necessary to develop competence and confidence in moving a patient who is not able to assist. If necessary, have another individual present in the room for further assistance.)

Position the wheelchair at an angle to and touching the other surface, and use a commercial transfer sling, large towel, or sheet under the patient's buttocks to perform the transfer. Position the caster wheels forward, lock the chair, and remove the patient's feet from the footrests. Elevate the footrests, remove or swing away the front rigging, and place the feet on the floor. If the wheelchair has a removable arm, remove the armrest nearest to the object to which the patient is to be transferred and move the patient forward to the front of the chair.

Stand in front of the patient, flex your hips and knees, and position your knees and feet on the outside, but next to, the patient's knees and feet. Lift the patient's thighs and hold them between your knees or the lower area of your thighs so the patient's feet are off the floor. Flex the patient's trunk with his or her head positioned on the side of your body that faces away from the direction of the transfer (see Fig. 8-21, A), because this position will make it easier for you to swing the patient's buttocks in the direction of the transfer. Ideally, the patient's arms should be folded in the lap or across the chest.

Grasp the transfer sling, towel, sheet or buttocks on each side of the patient (you can cross your arms if you use a sheet, towel or transfer sling to ensure a better grasp and further cradle the patient) and lift from the chair (see Fig. 8-21, B). Pivot your body by moving your feet and turn the patient's buttocks toward the transfer object. Lower the patient onto the transfer object (see Fig. 8-21, C), place the patient's feet on the floor, and straighten the trunk to an upright, sitting position. Be certain to protect the patient while sitting, and then reposition as necessary.

The return to the wheelchair is performed by using the same techniques in reverse order. (Caution: Do not leave the patient sitting unattended on the edge of the bed, mat, chair, or plinth. If you have returned the patient into the wheelchair, be certain that his or her hips are positioned back on the seat so the trunk will be supported by the chair back.)

An alternative method is to lift the patient's thighs, flex the hips, and hold the thighs between your knees or place the flexed lower extremities against your chest so the feet

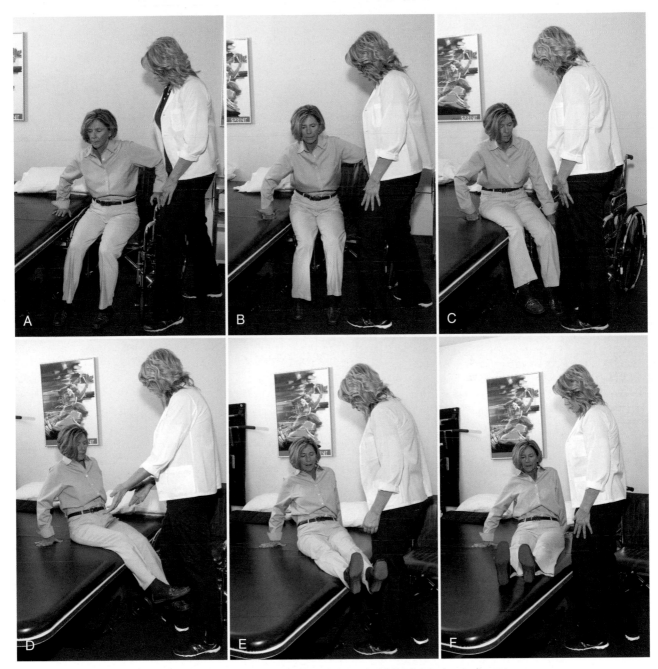

Fig. 8-20 A sitting transfer with an independent lateral swinging movement.

are off the floor. Follow the aforementioned procedure to complete the transfer.

Two-Person Dependent: Chair to Bed. The two-person lift transfer can be used when the patient is unable to stand, when the transfer is performed from two surfaces of unequal height, or when the patient is unable to assist with the transfer. The use of proper body mechanics for the persons performing the lift is extremely important. Each person should mentally review and plan how the lift will be performed, and one person must assume the role of the leader. The leader will instruct the patient and the assistant so all

three can work together. The transfer procedure should be explained to the patient and to the person assisting so everyone will understand what is planned. This information should be provided before you perform any of the lifting transfers to reduce possible fears or apprehensions the patient may have. (Caution: This transfer can cause back strain for the persons lifting and should be used only in an emergency or when mechanical equipment is not available.)

Proper technique for this procedure is described in Procedure 8-5. Note that a safety belt can be used instead of

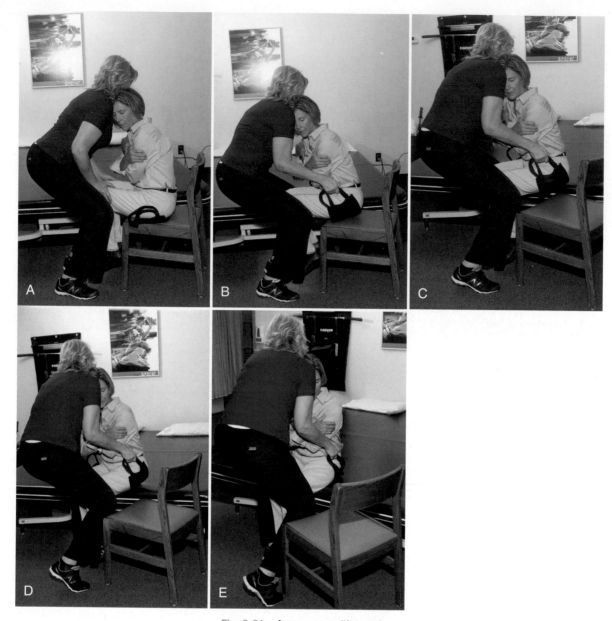

Fig. 8-21   A one-person lift transfer.

the patient's forearms, but it must be secured tightly and firmly below the flair of the rib cage so it will not slip upward when the lift occurs.

Alternative Method. Several other two-person lifts can be used depending on the size of the patient and the strength of the persons who will perform the lift. This alternate method distributes the patient's weight more equally but requires the patient to be lifted and carried over a longer distance than that of the previous lift. It also may require the assistants to step and turn while carrying the patient. The wheelchair is positioned and locked either parallel to and approximately 2 feet from the head of the bed or facing the center of the bed approximately 3 feet from the side of the bed, with both armrests and the front rigging removed.

The persons performing the lift approach the patient from each side. Each lifter uses one forearm to cradle the patient's thighs while the other upper extremity crosses the patient's posterior upper trunk and grasps the other lifter's forearm. The patient's upper extremities are placed over each lifter's upper back or shoulders, but not around their necks. One person gives the command to lift and the lifters walk forward, away from the chair, carrying the patient (Fig. 8-23). They turn so the patient's back is toward the bed and move backward toward the bed. The patient is seated on the edge of the bed, assisted to a supine position, and centered in the bed. (Caution: Do not allow the patient to sit unattended or unsupported. To transfer the patient from a bed/mat to a chair, reverse the procedure.)

PROCEDURE **8-5**

Two-Person Lift Transfer

WHEELCHAIR TO BED

- Position the wheelchair parallel to the side and midway between the head and foot of the bed; lock the bed wheels.
- Lock the chair and raise the foot plates or swing away front rigging; the armrest nearest to the bed should be removed only if it is higher than the surface of the bed.
- The taller and stronger person stands behind the chair. The patient crosses his or her arms over the abdomen, and the person behind the chair reaches through the axillae and grasps either the patient's forearms near the wrists or a safety belt placed firmly below the rib cage (**A**).
- A second person stoops or squats at the side of the patient's lower extremities, facing the bed, and positions one forearm under the thighs and one forearm under the lower legs to cradle the lower extremities. (Caution: One

forearm must be under the patient's thighs to assist in lifting the pelvis/buttocks and to avoid strain to the posterior aspect of the knees.)

- The person standing behind the patient instructs the patient to push down and hold the position with the shoulder muscles.
- On command from the person standing behind the patient (e.g., "One, two, three, lift"; "Ready, lift"; "Prepare to lift"; or "Lift"), the two persons simultaneously lift and place the patient on the near side of the mattress; the patient's knees should be straight during the lift (**B** to **D**).
- The patient is maintained in an upright position (long-sitting position) by the person at the patient's back while the other person moves the wheelchair.
- The two persons partially lift and move the patient to a safe position on the bed; the person holding the forearms or safety belt helps the patient lie down and adjust the body position for safety and comfort.

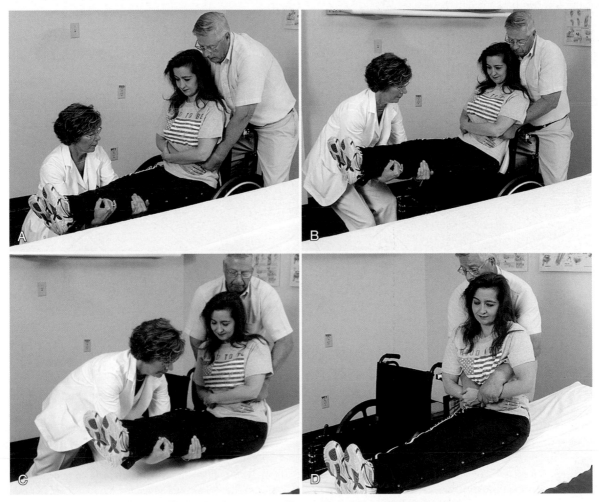

Fig. 8-22   A two-person lift transfer from a wheelchair to a bed.

Continued

PROCEDURE 8-5

Two-Person Lift Transfer—cont'd

BED TO WHEELCHAIR

- Move the patient to the near edge of the bed.
- Position the wheelchair parallel to the bed and opposite the patient's hips, lock the chair, raise the foot plates or swing away the front rigging, and remove the armrest nearest the bed.
- Elevate the patient's trunk to a long-sitting position; guard and protect the patient as necessary.
- One person stands behind the patient, and the patient crosses his or her arms over the abdomen; the caregiver reaches through the axillae and grasps either the patient's forearms near the wrists or a safety belt firmly applied below the rib cage.
- A second person stands at the side of the patient's lower extremities, facing the bed, and positions one forearm under the thighs and one forearm under the lower legs to cradle the lower extremities.
- On command from the person standing behind the patient, the two persons simultaneously lift and lower

the patient into the wheelchair; the patient's knees should be straight during the transfer. The person holding the lower extremities must stoop or squat to lower the patient.

- The patient's body is moved to the rear of the chair seat, and the front rigging is replaced or the front plates are lowered; the patient's feet are placed on the footrests. If necessary, a lap or chest belt is applied to protect or stabilize the patient.
- The patient's position is adjusted for safety and comfort.

Note: If the bed height can be adjusted, it should be lowered to as near the height of the wheelchair seat as possible before either transfer is attempted. The person at the head of the bed should use caution not to run into the push handles of the wheelchair in the process of the transfer. If the bed is not adjustable and the person lifting the trunk is too short, a secure stool to stand on can be used.

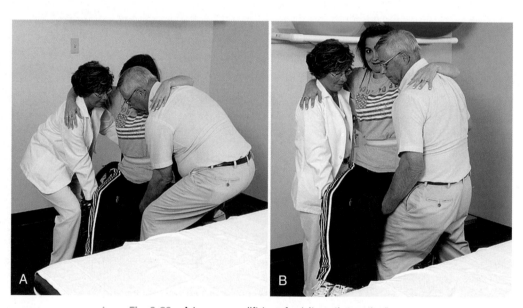

Fig. 8-23 A two-person lift transfer (alternative method).

Two-Person Dependent: Bed to Chair To perform a two-person dependent transfer from a bed to a chair, the patient is moved toward the near edge of the bed or mat, and the wheelchair is positioned and locked as described in Procedure 8-5. This transfer is the reverse of the two-person chair to bed dependent lift. (Caution: Both persons performing the transfer must use proper body mechanics to lower the patient into the chair by flexing at the hips and knees, keeping a neutral spine, and avoiding excessive trunk flexion. Some trunk rotation may be required by the person who stands behind the patient during the lift, and this

person must be prepared to pivot using the hips and feet to avoid lower back strain.)

Alternative Method. In an alternative method, the wheelchair is locked and positioned as described previously, and the patient is positioned sitting on the edge of the bed with the lifters positioned on each side of the patient. This transfer is the reverse of the alternative chair to bed two-person dependent lift.

The patient is supported by the lifters as described previously. One lifter gives the command to lift, and the patient is lifted and carried to the wheelchair. The patient is lowered into the chair and properly positioned. The lifters must use proper body mechanics to lower the patient into the chair. The armrests and front rigging are replaced, the feet are positioned on the footrests, and a lap or chest strap is applied, if necessary, to protect or stabilize the patient.

Bariatric Patient. A dependent transfer can be performed when a bariatric patient is transferred and no mechanical equipment is available. A technique that requires two persons and a sheet can be used. The sheet is applied to cradle, control, and move the patient from one surface to another as shown in Fig. 8-24, A. With the patient supine, roll the patient to a side-lying position and place a folded sheet next to the body from midchest to midthighs (Fig 8-24, B). Roll the patient to the opposite side, extending the sheet under the body (Fig. 8-24, C). Help the patient to a sitting position by moving the legs over the edge of the mat and using the sheet to get the patient to an upright position (Fig. 8-24, D and E). Both caregivers brace the patient's knees with their knees and use the sheet in a cradlelike fashion to help the patient stand (Fig. 8-24, F). The caregivers then pivot the patient and help him or her to sit, using the sheet to lower the patient into the chair (Fig 8-24, G). Position the feet on the footrests and apply a lap or chest strap, if necessary, to protect or stabilize the patient. The persons assisting with the transfer must use proper body mechanics throughout the activity, and they should discontinue the transfer at any time if they are unable to safely control the patient. Transfer from a wheelchair to a bed or mat is accomplished by reversal of the sequence described for transferring the patient from a bed to a wheelchair.

Two-Person Dependent: Chair to Floor To perform a two-person dependent transfer from a chair to the floor, position the wheelchair parallel to the area on the floor to which the patient is to be transferred. One person stands behind the patient, and another person stands at the side of the lower extremities. The patient is lifted from the chair as described previously, and the lifters move sideward away from the chair. On command, both lifters stoop to lower the patient to the floor (Fig. 8-25). (Caution: The lifters must flex their hips and knees and avoid trunk flexion as the patient is lowered to the floor.) The patient is assisted to a lying position or maintains a sitting position, using the upper extremities to form a tripod with the hips.

To return the patient to the chair, the person is positioned in a long sitting position. The two lifters stoop and grasp the patient as described previously. On command, the lifters stand simultaneously to lift the patient and then step toward the chair. The patient is lowered into the chair and properly positioned. Caution must be used around the wheelchair push handles.

Three-Person Dependent: Bed to Stretcher The three-person lift transfer can be used to transfer a patient from one flat surface to another (as from a wheeled stretcher to a bed, or vice versa) with the patient supine. It is used when no other type of transfer can be used, in an emergency, when mechanical equipment is not available, and when the patient cannot sit or stand. To decrease injuries to employees and increase patient safety, health care facilities are evolving to a "No Lift Environment." Ergonomic equipment such as mechanical lifts, lateral transfer and repositioning mats, slip and roller sheets, and standing pivot transfer discs are being used to replace manual lifting. (These policies can be reviewed at www.osha.gov.)

When it is necessary to perform a three-person lift transfer, before lifting the patient, it is important to properly position the stretcher in relation to the bed or item to which the patient is to be transferred. The two stronger and taller of the three persons should be positioned at the patient's head, shoulders, and pelvis. The third person is positioned to control the lower extremities. One person becomes the leader (usually the person at the patient's head) to instruct and give commands to the lifters. This process is outlined in Procedure 8-6. To transfer the patient from the stretcher to the bed, the process described previously is performed in reverse sequence.

Proper body mechanics must be used to prevent possible injury to the lifters. They should flex their hips and knees before lifting and when lowering the patient, and they should be close to the patient and cradle the patient's body in their arms by flexing their elbows to use short lever arms throughout the transfer. (Note: Rather than lift a patient, a plastic spine board placed under the patient may be used to slide the patient to or from a stretcher or bed when the patient is positioned parallel [side by side]) (Fig. 8-27).

Transfers, Wheelchair and Floor

When performing transfers from the wheelchair and floor, initially the patient will need to be protected or guarded using the general guarding principles and techniques described previously. The activity should be practiced in an area free of hazards, and mats may be placed on the floor to protect the patient. Some patients may benefit from the use of incremental steps or small platforms when they initially perform and practice some of these transfers. Instruction will be necessary for the patient to learn how to properly and safely perform these transfers. Eventually the patient should be taught how to move down to the floor and return to the chair without any additional equipment to maximize independence. Not all patients will be able to accomplish this transfer, and for those who are able to perform it, it is generally taught near the end of the patient's length of stay.

Strong Right Extremities and Weak Left Extremities (Hemiplegia)

Wheelchair to Floor. To move from a wheelchair to the floor, the patient first must position the caster wheels forward, lock the chair, remove the feet from the footrests,

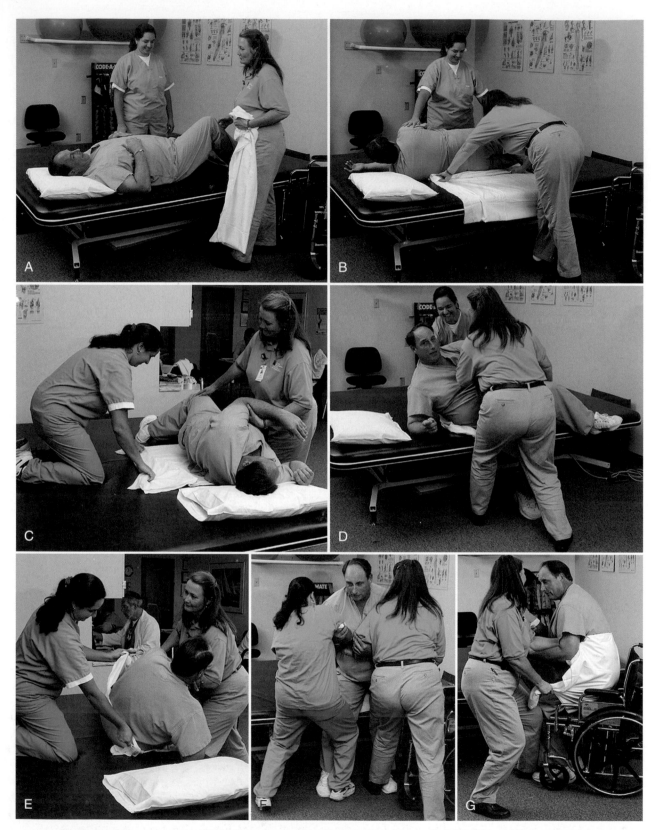

Fig. 8-24 A two-person dependent lift transfer of a bariatric patient by using a sheet from the mat to the wheelchair.

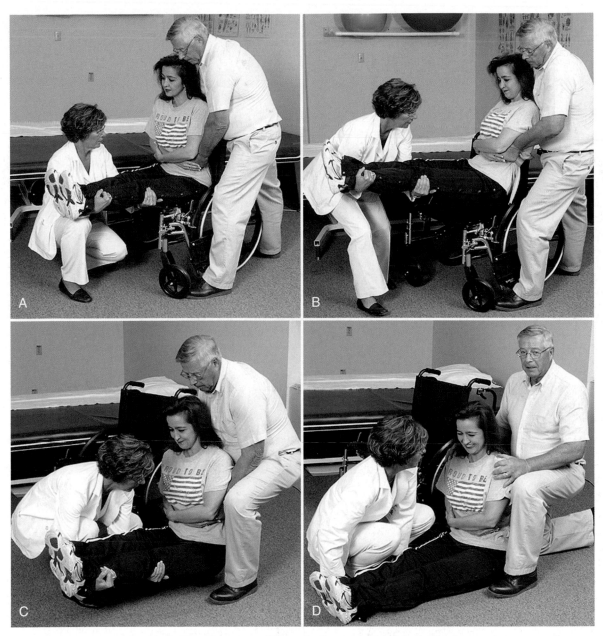

Fig. 8-25   A two-person lift transfer from a wheelchair to the floor.

and remove or swing away the front rigging or elevate the footrests. The patient moves forward in the chair with his or her body pivoted or turned slightly so the right extremities are forwardmost (Fig. 8-28, A).

The patient shifts the weight onto the right lower extremity and reaches toward the floor with the right upper extremity (Fig. 8-28, B). When the right hand is on the floor, the patient uses the right upper and lower extremity to lower the body to the floor and sit on the right buttock or both buttocks (Fig. 8-28, C). The body position can be adjusted as desired.

Floor to Wheelchair. To move from the floor to a wheelchair, the patient sits on the right hip facing the locked wheelchair with its caster wheels positioned forward. The lower extremities should be flexed at the hips and knees (Fig. 8-29, A).

The patient reaches to the back of the seat or the armrest and pulls up to a kneeling position. The patient moves to a half-kneeling position with the right foot forward and flat on the floor, and he or she kneels on the left knee (Fig. 8-29, B and C). The patient places the right upper extremity on the near armrest or on the seat of the chair and uses the right extremities to push to a partial or full standing position (Fig. 8-29, D). (Note: The caster wheels may pivot or turn to one side when the patient uses the chair for support. That movement does not create a safety problem, and the patient can continue to perform the transfer. However, the caster wheels should not be directed backward during these

PROCEDURE 8-6

Three-Person Lift Transfer

FROM A BED TO A NEW SUPPORT SURFACE (e.g., stretcher, bed, or tilt table)

- Select one person to lead the lift process.
- Position the head of the new support surface perpendicularly (i.e., at a right angle) to the foot of the bed and lock it in place.
- The lifters place their respective upper extremities in the following positions:
  - Under the patient's head and upper trunk
  - Just above and below the pelvis
  - Under the upper thigh and lower leg to maintain the knees straight (**A**)
- Move the patient close to the near edge of the bed to position the patient's center of gravity closer to the centers of gravity of the lifters.
- On command from the lead lifter, roll the patient to a side-lying position facing the lifters and cradle the patient with your flexed elbows (**B**).
- On command from the lead lifter, lift the patient, keeping the person on one side (**C**).

- On command from the lead lifter, step back from the bed and pivot so the patient's back is toward the surface onto which the patient will be placed.
- The lifters should use short steps and sidestep rather than use a crossover step to avoid stepping on another person's foot.
- Once the patient is positioned over the stretcher, and on command from the lead lifter, lower the patient to the new support surface by bending your knees and hips; keep the body cradled until your elbows rest on the support surface (**D**).
- On command, lower your forearms to the support surface to place the patient flat (**E**).
- Move the patient toward the center of the support surface, position the body for comfort and safety, and apply security straps, pillows, and towel rolls as necessary.

RETURN TO BED

- Reverse the sequence of the transfer from the bed to a new support surface to return the patient to the bed.

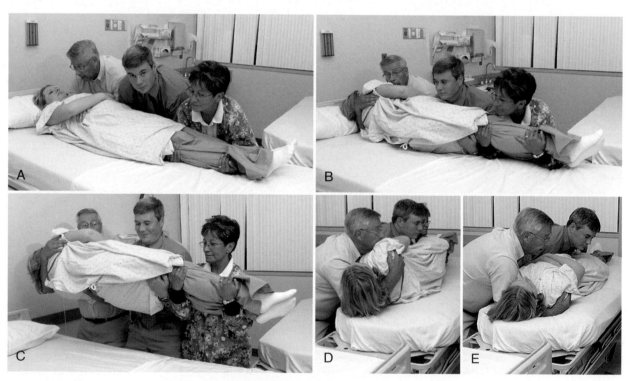

Fig. 8-26　A three-person lift transfer from a bed to a stretcher.

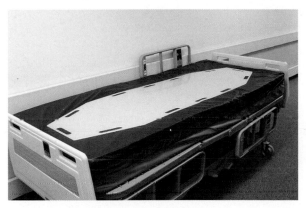

Fig. 8-27 The flexible plastic item on the stretcher is used to transfer a supine patient to or from a bed or stretcher.

transfers because that position reduces the stability of the chair. The patient should be taught not to allow the caster wheels to be directed backward, or a chair with caster wheel locks may be recommended.)

The patient reaches for the far armrest with the right upper extremity and pivots on the right lower extremity so the back is toward the chair, then lowers into the chair using the right extremities.

Strong Upper Extremities and Weak or Paralyzed Lower Extremities (Paraplegia)

Wheelchair to Floor Forward or Sideward. To move from the wheelchair to the floor forward or sideward, the patient positions and prepares the chair as previously described. The patient moves to the front of the chair and positions the lower extremities to one side with the knees extended or under the chair with the knees flexed.

The patient maintains one hand on the armrest or chair seat rail and reaches toward the floor with the other upper extremity while flexing the head and trunk (Fig. 8-30, A). After the hand has contacted the floor, the patient releases the grasp on the wheelchair and lowers onto the floor (Fig. 8-30, B). An option is to have the patient reach with both arms simultaneously toward the floor with the knees flexed and legs under the chair (similar to falling forward) to establish a hands-and-knees position. However, if the knees contact the floor forcefully, trauma could occur to the hips, femur, or patella, so this method must be used with caution. The patient repositions the body as desired. During practice sessions it may be helpful to place pillows on the floor to reduce the trauma to the knees during practice until the patient gains control of the descent.

Alternative Method. In an alternative method for moving from a wheelchair to the floor forward or sideward, the patient positions and prepares the wheelchair as described previously, except one or both front riggings remain in place with the footrests elevated (Fig. 8-31, A). The patient moves forward in the chair and positions the lower extremities away from the chair with the knees extended. Instruct the patient to place one hand on the top of the front rigging and one hand on the chair seat and then perform a push-up with the upper extremities to elevate the buttocks from the chair seat while extending the head and upper trunk (Fig. 8-31, B). The patient lowers the body to the floor with the buttocks between the footrests of the front rigging (Fig. 8-31, C). Patients with wide hips will need to swing away, but not remove, one front rigging to have sufficient space for the hips when they descend to the floor. (Note: This method can be used to move from the floor to the chair backward, but the patient's head and trunk will need to be flexed as the pelvis is elevated by the upper extremities that are positioned with one hand on the seat and one hand on the upper portion of the front rigging. The patient must have excellent flexibility in the shoulders and maximal strength in the upper extremities to perform this technique.)

It is important to note that many inactive or paralyzed patients may have osteoporosis in the lower extremities and vertebral bodies. Some of these transfer methods may be unsafe for these patients because of the floor-reaction force the patient may experience when dropping onto the knees or hip. This force may be sufficient to cause a fracture in weakened bone. Therefore the patient may need to be assisted down to the floor to avoid injury.

The wheelchair-to-floor-and-return transfer methods described may be interchanged to meet the needs, strength, preference, flexibility, agility, balance, size, and skill of a given patient. For example, a patient may prefer or find it easier to transfer to the floor while facing forward and return to the chair in the backward position, or to transfer to the floor in the backward position and return to the chair while facing forward. The patient should be given the opportunity to attempt any of the methods to determine the most suitable, safe, and efficient method for him or her. Guard and assist the patient during practice sessions until the patient is able to perform the transfer independently in a safe manner. A safety belt should be used, and you should not use the patient's clothing or upper extremities to control or guard the patient when these transfers are performed for the reasons explained elsewhere in this book.

Floor to Wheelchair Forward Push-up. To perform a floor to wheelchair forward push-up, the patient sits on one hip close to and facing the wheelchair with the hips and knees flexed (Fig. 8-32, A). The chair must be locked and the front rigging should be swung away, with the caster wheels positioned forward or turned to one side. Some patients may prefer to initiate this transfer from an all-fours position (i.e., on the hands and knees). The patient moves to the front of the chair and places one hand on the armrest or on the seat (Fig. 8-32, B). The patient grasps the armrest or the seat of the chair and pushes down on the chair to a high kneeling position and maintains balance (Fig. 8-32, C). The patient grasps both armrests or places one hand on

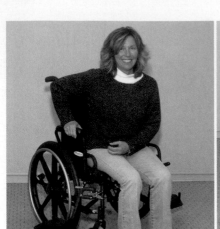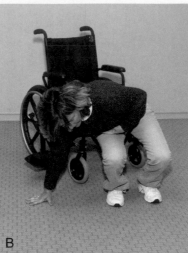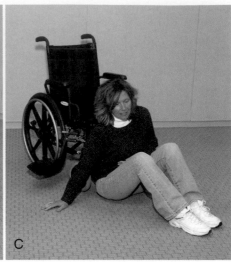

Fig. 8-28   A transfer from a wheelchair to the floor for a patient with strong right upper and lower extremities.

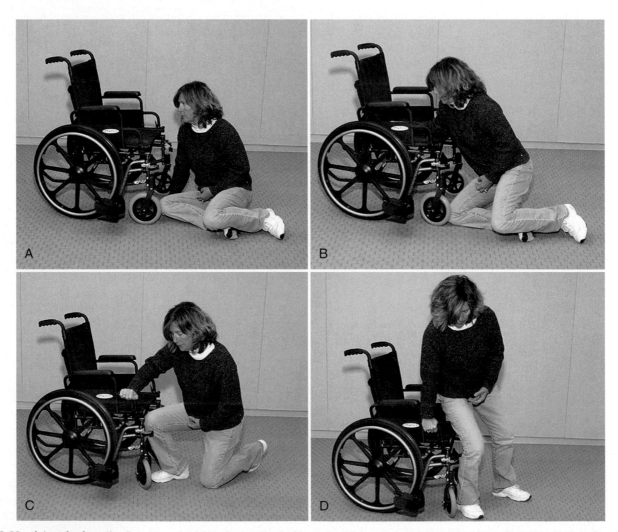

Fig. 8-29   A transfer from the floor to a wheelchair for a patient with strong right upper and lower extremities. (Note that for transfers from a wheelchair to the floor with a return to the chair, the caster wheels will probably pivot or turn to one side when the patient uses the chair for support unless the wheels can be locked in the forward position. If the caster wheels pivot, there is no safety problem and the patient can continue to perform the transfer. However, the patient should not allow the caster wheels to be directed backward because that position reduces the stability of the chair.)

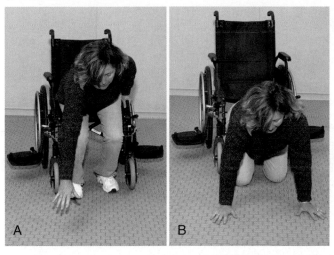

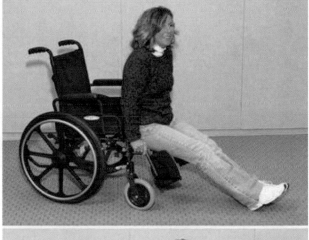

Fig. 8-30 A transfer from a wheelchair to the floor, facing forward, for a patient with strong upper extremities.

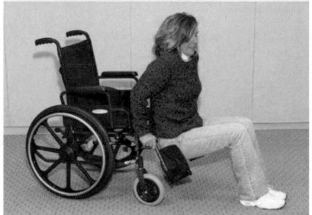

the seat of the chair and one hand on the armrest and then performs a push-up to elevate the hips above the seat level (Fig. 8-32, *D*). At the peak of the lift, the patient pivots so one hip is over the seat and moves the hand to allow one hip onto the chair (Fig. 8-32, *E*). The patient repositions the hands on the armrests (Fig. 8-32, *F*) and performs a push-up to position the body in the chair.

Some patients may be able to elevate their pelvis (buttocks) onto the front edge of the chair using an initial push-up with one hand on the chair seat or armrest and the other hand on the upper portion of the front rigging. This method requires exceptional upper extremity strength and trunk control, and the patient must have the ability to maintain balance while in a high kneeling and push-up position. The patient can reverse this method to move from the wheelchair to the floor. This maneuver is a safe and secure activity, and many patients will be able to perform it efficiently.

Wheelchair to Floor in a Backward Position. To move from the wheelchair to the floor in a backward position, the patient positions and prepares the wheelchair as described previously. The patient moves to the front of the chair, pivots onto the right or left side of the hip, and grasps the armrests. If the patient is sitting on the right side of the hip, the right hand grasps the left armrest and the left hand grasps the right armrest to rotate the upper body so the patient now partially faces the back of the chair.

The patient performs a partial push-up to clear the pelvis from the seat and then uses the upper extremities to lower onto the knees to a high kneeling position facing the front of the chair. Then the patient lowers to a side-sitting position or onto all fours and then onto one hip.

This method is the reverse of moving from the floor to a chair in the forward position. It requires exceptional upper extremity strength, trunk control, and balance, and the

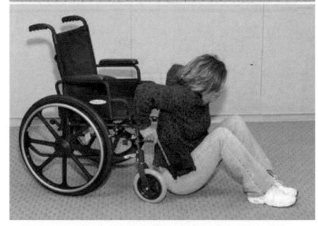

Fig. 8-31 A transfer from a wheelchair to the floor (alternative method). The movements are reversed to move from the floor to a wheelchair.

patient must be flexible and agile to perform this maneuver.

Standing Dependent Pivot from a Lift Chair to a Wheelchair. A Lift Chair is a commercially manufactured electric chair with a switch to raise and lower it. To perform a standing dependent pivot from a Lift Chair to a wheelchair, the caregiver puts a gait belt on the patient or uses a sling under the buttocks in preparation for the transfer. An assistant raises the lift chair and then stabilizes the

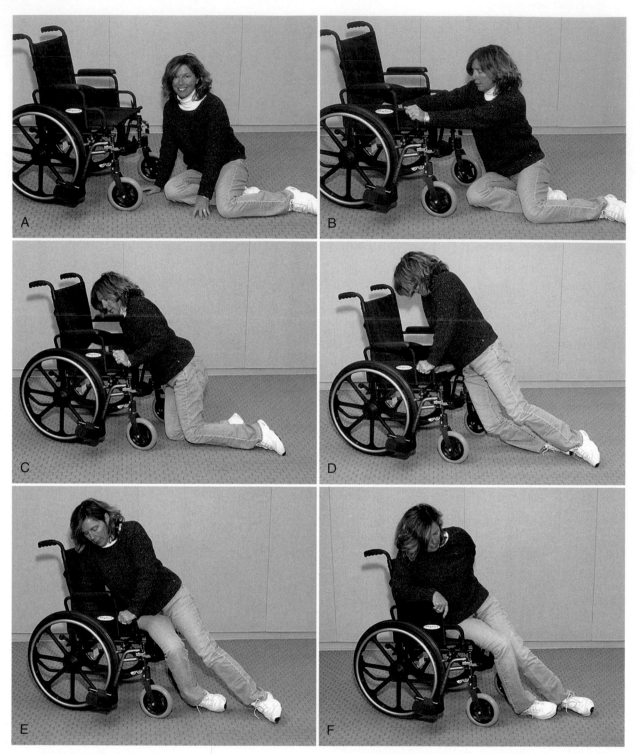

Fig. 8-32 A transfer from the floor to a wheelchair with a forward push-up for a patient with strong upper extremities. The procedure is reversed to move from a wheelchair to the floor. (Note that the caster wheels may pivot during this transfer if they cannot be locked in a forward position. The transfer can be performed safely as long as the caster wheels do not pivot completely rearward.)

wheelchair during the transfer. The caregiver stands in front of the patient, grasps the gait belt or sling, and with proper body mechanics raises the patient the rest of the way to standing (Fig. 8-33, A). The patient is then pivoted toward the wheelchair and lowered onto the chair (Fig. 8-33, B).

Fig. 8-34, A, shows a patient in the home setting with a bar installed in the wall just below a window so the patient may stand and look outside. In this photo, the caregiver is using a gait belt to help the patient to stand; the caregiver is unable to use a transfer sling because of the inability to

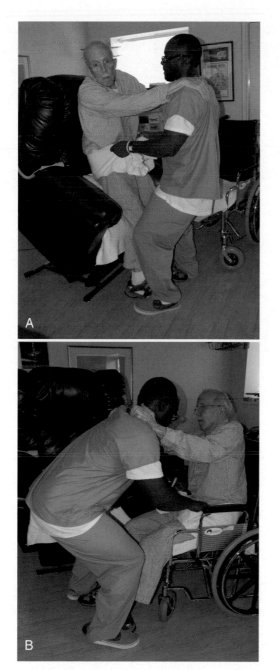

Fig. 8-33   A dependent pivot transfer from a lift chair to a wheelchair.

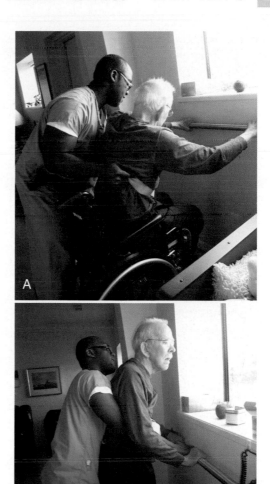

Fig. 8-34   **A,** Helping a patient stand with a gait belt. **B,** A patient being supported at a window.

stand in front of the patient. Fig. 8-34, *B*, shows the patient being braced by the caregiver at the window.

MECHANICAL EQUIPMENT

When a heavy or dependent patient needs to be lifted or transported, the safest and most effective device to use is a manual (hydraulic) or an electrical (battery powered) mechanical lift. Either of these devices can lift a patient who weighs up to 450 lb, depending on the specifications for the lift. Neither of the lifts should be used for any patient whose body weight exceeds the maximum load approved for the lift; a medical error (i.e., a sentinel event) may occur if

the weight of the patient is greater than the load capacity of the lift. Failure of the equipment leading to patient injury is a possible outcome if the person's weight exceeds the load capacity of the lift.

These devices have a U-shaped base supported on four caster wheels. The legs of the base usually can be widened for increased stability and to position the lift around a large piece of furniture, a toilet, or a wheelchair, and they can be narrowed for transport. A vertical metal support column (mast) extends from the base and has a movable arm with a spreader bar attached to it; this is the uppermost component of the lift. A body sling or similar item is used to support the patient during the lift once it is attached to the spreader bar.

Manually Operated Lift

A manual mechanical lift uses a hydraulic fluid system to raise and lower the patient. A valve on the cylinder that contains the fluid controls the containment or release of pressure developed in the cylinder. When the valve is opened, pressure is released; when it is closed, the pressure can be increased. A manually operated lever is used to control the fluid in the cylinder. When the valve is closed and the lever is "pumped," the fluid compresses and the arm with the spreader bar is raised. When the valve is opened, pressure in the cylinder is released and the arm and spreader bar are lowered. The patient's weight and the amount the valve is opened determine the rate of descent of the patient. The valve must be closed to raise the patient, and it must remain closed while the patient is elevated. After the patient has been lowered to a final position, the valve must be closed so the arm and spreader bar do not continue to descend and strike the patient's head. It is important to adhere to the manufacturer's instructions for the proper use of the lift. Guidelines for using this type of lift are outlined in Procedure 8-7.

Wheelchair to Bed

Transfer from a wheelchair to a bed or mat is accomplished by reversal of the sequence described for transferring the

---

PROCEDURE 8-7

Mechanical Lift Transfer, Manually Operated Lift

BED TO WHEELCHAIR
- Explain the activity to the patient the first time it is performed.
- Place the individual slings or body sling under the upper trunk and buttocks and upper thighs by rolling the patient onto one side and then onto the other side.
- The sling attachments should be exposed with the outside seams of the sling directed away from the patient.
- Position the lift perpendicularly to the patient and close to the bed with the legs of the base spread wide and the spreader bar over the chest; attach the chains or web straps to the spreader bar.
- Partially open the control valve to slowly lower the spreader bar until the chains or web straps can be attached to the sling or slings. Close the valve so the spreader bar does not continue to lower.
- Attach the rings of the web strap or the S hook of the chain to the sling: attach the shortest segment of the chain or web strap to the upper part of the sling, and attach the longest segment to the lower part of the sling. These positions will ensure that the patient will be lifted into a sitting position.
- When S hooks are used, they should be directed away from the body to prevent injury to the skin.
- Before you attempt to lift the patient, check all the attachments; adjust the slings and attachments as necessary.
- Caution the patient not to reach for or grasp the spreader bar when he or she is being raised.
- Fold the patient's arms over the abdomen and elevate the body using the pump handle.
- Elevate the patient until the buttocks clear the surface of the bed; reevaluate the position, the location of the slings, and the security of the attachments before moving away from the bed.
- Assist in the lift by moving the patient's lower extremities from the bed so the patient sits properly in the slings. The knees can be allowed to flex or can be kept extended as you carefully move the lift away from the side of the bed and then turn the patient to face the support column.

- Transport the patient to the wheelchair using the cross-handles on the center post.
- Maneuver the patient so his or her buttocks are over the front or the middle of the seat of the locked wheelchair.
- Partially open the control valve to slowly lower the patient into the chair; move the body toward the back of the seat by pushing on the knees before the buttocks contact the seat. Close the valve when the person is seated.
- Remove the sling attachments and move the lift away from the chair; the slings remain under the patient to permit a transfer back to bed. If the slings are removed, they will be difficult to reposition under the patient.
- Position the feet on the footrests, and apply a lap or chest strap, if necessary, to protect or stabilize the patient.

WHEELCHAIR TO BED
- Reverse the sequence of the activities of the transfer from the bed to chair. Position the patient on the mattress and remove the sling.
- Be certain to check the position of the sling or slings and the security of the chains or web straps before lifting the patient from the chair.
- Remember to close the valve after the spreader bar has been positioned to attach or remove the chains or web straps.

BED TO WHEELCHAIR
When using a manually-operated lift, all of the following steps must be performed:
- Ensure that the valve that controls the adjustable arm is closed as you position the lift.
- Ensure that the floor is free of objects and sufficient space is available to maneuver the lift. Objects that could interfere with or block the caster wheels from moving smoothly, such as a throw rug, door threshold, or line cord, should be avoided.
- The valve must be closed as soon as the patient is properly positioned in the chair so the adjustable bar does not continue to lower and strike the patient's head.

patient from a bed to a wheelchair. After the patient has returned to the bed, the slings are removed by rolling the patient to one side, rolling the sling into a tube that is placed as close to the patient's body as possible, and then rolling the patient to the opposite side and removing the sling.

Having multiple slings available will be helpful if this equipment is to be used for several patients. In addition, the slings must be laundered periodically or when they become soiled; therefore more than one sling should be available for use when one is being laundered.

Patients are likely to be apprehensive the first few times a mechanical lift is used. To help overcome any fear or apprehension, explain the procedure to the patient and provide information about the safety of the unit before using it. Before a transfer is performed, it may be helpful to allow the patient to observe the unit being used with another person.

Electrical Lift

The electrical mechanical lift uses power from rechargeable batteries that are connected to a control unit that accompanies the lift. The patient can be raised and lowered by pressing a button on the control unit. The remainder of the features of the lift are similar to those of the manual lift. Guidelines for using this lift are outlined in Procedure 8-8; Fig. 8-35 shows the use of this lift.

OTHER TYPES OF TRANSFERS

Totally Dependent Patient: Stretcher to Bed or Bed to Stretcher

When transferring a totally dependent patient from a stretcher to a bed or vice versa, when the two surfaces are at approximately the same height, position the stretcher (gurney) parallel to and touching one edge of the bed. Be certain the stretcher and the bed wheels are locked or secured so the two objects will not separate during the transfer.

If the stretcher has a loose pad, slide it and the patient onto the bed and then remove the pad; if a draw sheet is available, use it to slide the patient from the stretcher onto the bed.

The patient can be rolled from the stretcher toward you onto the bed, or you can slide the patient, by segments, from the stretcher to the bed as you kneel on the bed, using your forearms for support under the patient to avoid skin irritation.

Extreme care must be used when any of these techniques are attempted, because the stretcher and bed could separate and the patient could fall. Another person may be needed to hold the two objects together or to assist with the transfer. In addition, you are advised not to use bed linen to lift and carry a patient from one object to another, because the linen could tear and the patient could fall. This technique should be used only in an emergency when no other option

---

PROCEDURE 8-8

Mechanical Lift Transfer, Electrical Lift

BED TO WHEELCHAIR

- Explain the activity to the patient the first time it is performed; obtain consent for the maneuver.
- Position and lock the wheelchair; ensure that sufficient space is available for the equipment.
- Apply the body sling under the patient by rolling the patient onto one side, then onto the other side.
- Position the lift perpendicular to the bed, open the base legs, and position the spreader bar over the shoulders or midchest.
- Lower the lift arm until the sling loops or clips can be attached to the spreader bar, with the shorter straps going at the shoulders and the longer straps by the hips. Securely attach the loops or clips to the spreader bars, fold the patient's arms over his or her chest, and check the sling position.
- Gradually elevate the patient until the body clears the surface of the bed; check the security of the sling attachments.
- Transport the patient to the wheelchair, turn the body so the back is toward the chair seat, and position the body over the midportion of the chair seat.
- Gradually lower the patient; push on the knees to direct the hips to the most posterior portion of the seat, guide the body into the chair, and adjust the body position as necessary.
- Lower the lift arm until the sling loops or clips can be removed from the spreader bar.
- Ensure that the patient is clear of the lift and move the lift away; check the body position for safety and security. The sling may be removed or remain in place for the return transfer.

WHEELCHAIR TO BED

- Reverse the sequence of the previous transfer; check the security of the sling attachments before lifting the patient.
- Position the patient on the bed or mat for safety and security.

---

is possible or when the situation requires a rapid transfer. Using a sheet to transfer a patient by sliding is relatively safe because even if the sheet tears, the patient remains supported by a firm surface. However, this technique should not be used if contraindications exist to sliding the patient or when the shear forces associated with sliding are likely to cause skin irritation (e.g., to a burn, pressure ulcers, or sutures).

Patient with a Total Hip Replacement

Assisted Standing Transfer Special precautions or considerations should be used with a patient who has undergone surgery for a total hip replacement. Each surgeon will

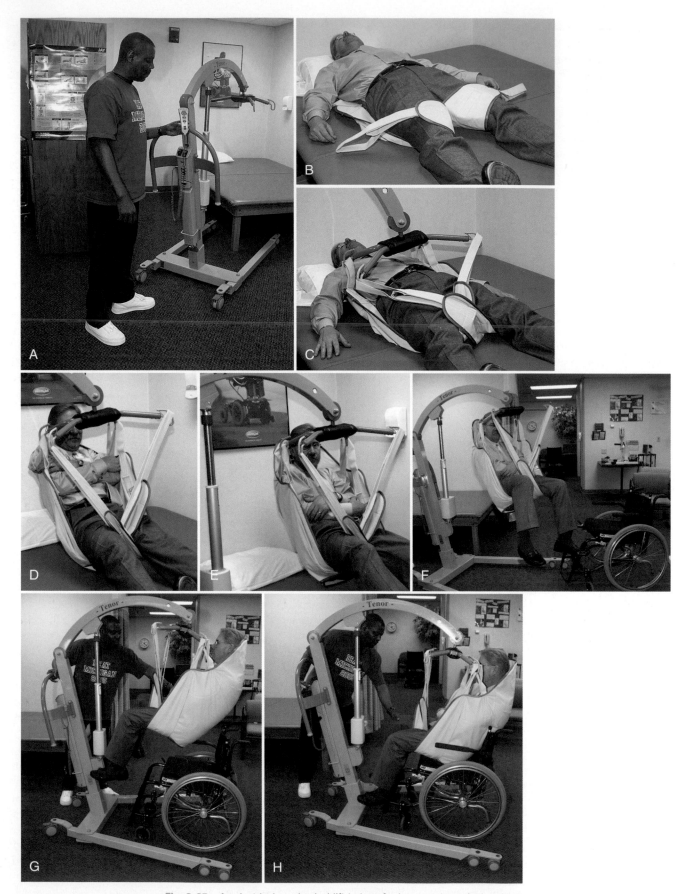

Fig. 8-35 An electrical mechanical lift to transfer large or dependent patients.

have instructions or preferences for the amount of weight bearing allowed, the movement or activities to be permitted, and the alignment of the trunk in relation to the surgically replaced hip. The patient and the person who assists the patient must be aware of these specific precautions, instructions, and preferences. Most of the precautions or contraindications are designed to reduce the possibility of hip dislocation during the first 10 to 14 days of postoperative care. Some of the generally and widely accepted precautions or contraindications for this patient condition are listed in Box 8-2.

Movement from the Bed to a Walker Most patients who have had a hip replacement use a walker initially to improve stability and support, although bilateral axillary crutches also may be used. Before allowing the patient to stand, measure and adjust the walker for the patient (refer to Chapter 9), apply a safety belt, apply footwear, lock the bed, adjust the height of the bed slightly higher than its lowest position, and partially elevate the head of the bed to help the patient come to a sitting position before standing. Instruct the patient to move to the edge of the bed using the upper extremities and the normal lower extremity to elevate the body. The patient should move toward the normal lower extremity to maintain

---

| Box **8-2** | Precautions for Patients with a Total Hip Replacement |

- When the patient is supine, maintain the surgical hip abducted from the midline of the body (some facilities use abduction pillows) and in neutral rotation (i.e., the patella and toes are positioned toward the ceiling). The hip should not be adducted beyond the midline of the body when the patient lies, sits, or stands.
- Maintain the surgical hip in neutral extension. The hip should not be extended beyond the midposition of flexion and extension.
- Maintain hip abduction and neutral rotation while the patient is in a side-lying position on the unaffected hip by supporting the surgical lower extremity with pillows or a bolster. The surgical extremity must be in the uppermost position.
- Avoid external hip rotation when an anterior or anterolateral surgical approach was used.
- Avoid internal hip rotation when a posterior or posterolateral surgical approach was used.
- Avoid rotating or twisting the upper body with the lower extremity fixed or immobile (as when reaching for an object on a bedside stand while lying in bed); such activity indirectly causes hip rotation.
- Avoid hip flexion beyond a range of 60 degrees. This guideline means that the patient should not sit erect in a wheelchair or in bed, because bringing the trunk closer to the thigh produces hip flexion.
- Avoid excessive trunk flexion while the patient is sitting; use an elevated toilet seat and an elevated chair when available.

---

the surgically replaced hip in abduction. The trunk should be maintained so the surgical hip is in no more than 60 degrees of flexion by semireclining on the arms positioned behind the body. You should help control the surgical hip and its lower extremity in slight abduction as the patient pivots and positions the lower extremities over the edge of bed. Instruct the patient to place the normal foot on the floor as you assist in lowering the surgical lower extremity to the floor. The patient maintains the trunk in a semireclining position by resting on the extended upper extremities, which are placed posterior to the hips. (Caution: The patient may need to sit on the edge of the bed for a short time to avoid dizziness or syncope and to accommodate being upright before standing. Do not allow the patient to sit unattended or unprotected.)

The patient pushes up from the bed, stands, and grasps the hand grips on the walker while you maintain control of the safety belt and shoulder. You may guard or stabilize the patient's normal foot so it does not slide as the person rises. The patient maintains balance and takes time to accommodate to standing before ambulating. You should monitor the patient's pulse rate and ask him or her about any adverse reaction to standing, look for signs of orthostatic hypotension, and take the patient's blood pressure if warranted.

The patient ambulates using a three-one pattern (refer to Chapter 9). Instruct him or her to turn by pivoting on the normal lower extremity and stepping around the normal lower extremity with the surgically affected lower extremity. (For example, a patient with a right hip replacement will be taught to turn toward the left.) These procedures are explained in Chapter 9. (Caution: The patient must not pivot or twist the hip while standing on the lower extremity of the surgical hip.)

Return to Bed When a patient with a hip replacement returns to bed, be certain that the bed is locked and will not roll, and adjust the bed so it is slightly below the patient's buttocks. The patient backs toward the bed until the posterior area of the thigh of the normal lower extremity touches the edge of the mattress; the surgical lower extremity should remain slightly forward of the opposite lower extremity.

The patient reaches back to the mattress and shifts the body weight onto the normal lower extremity while allowing the surgical lower extremity to slide forward. The patient sits on the edge of the bed in a semireclining position as you control the surgical hip and lower extremity.

The patient then pivots toward the center of the bed, leading with the normal lower extremity and keeping the surgical hip abducted. You should assist in controlling the surgical hip and lower extremity to maintain abduction and to limit flexion of the hip.

The patient uses the normal lower extremity and the upper extremities to shift the body toward the center of the bed while you guide the surgical lower extremity, until a proper position is attained. A pillow or hip abduction accessory should be placed between the legs. Note that some patients may return to the center of the bed leading with the surgical lower extremity so that it moves in abduction. The position of the bed and the ability to have access to either side of the bed may dictate how the return-to-bed transfer is accomplished.

Patient with One Non–Weight-Bearing Lower Extremity, Standing Transfer

The standing transfer for a patient with one non–weight-bearing lower extremity is described in Procedure 8-9.

SUMMARY

Transfer activities are necessary to alter a patient's position, move a patient from one surface to another, and promote independent functional activities. Some patients may require various amounts of assistance or may depend on other persons or mechanical equipment to perform or complete a transfer. Whenever possible, mechanical or ergonomically designed equipment should be used to move, lift, or transfer a patient, especially a large, heavy, or dependent individual. Other patients will be able to accomplish transfers without assistance or with only standby assistance. Transfers can be performed with the patient lying, standing, or sitting. Regardless of the technique used, the caregiver must guard and protect the patient during all transfers. A safety belt, a commercial sling, or a sheet/towel should be used with all patients when they transfer initially until the transfer can be performed safely and independently.

The procedures or techniques used to assist or teach the patient will vary depending on his or her condition, abilities, and needs. The philosophy and preferences of the caregiver also may affect the way the transfer is taught or performed. The caregiver and patient may need to problem solve together to develop the most efficient and safest transfer technique. Observing other patients as they perform a specific transfer may help the patient learn a transfer technique. Practicing the transfer and using the same technique consistently should improve the patient's skill and efficiency.

self-study ACTIVITIES

- Describe five different types of transfers.
- Explain the rationale for teaching a patient bed-mobility activities.
- Describe at least five specific precautions that should be followed when you are transferring a patient who has recently undergone a total hip replacement.
- Explain the wheelchair positions you might use for a standing transfer and for a transfer-board transfer to and from a bed or mat, and indicate why these positions are necessary and important for the transfer.
- Demonstrate two different methods for moving from a wheelchair to the floor and returning to the wheelchair for a person with lower extremity paralysis.

PROCEDURE 8-9

Patient with One Non–Weight-Bearing Lower Extremity, Standing Transfer

BED TO WHEELCHAIR

- Position the wheelchair at an angle on the side next to the hip of the full weight-bearing (FWB) lower extremity, facing the foot of the bed; lock the chair and swing away the front rigging or elevate the footplates.
- Help the patient move to the edge of the mattress and sit up; apply a safety belt or sling.
- Position yourself in front of the patient to guard and protect him or her; assist in moving the non–weight-bearing (NWB) extremity to the edge of the mattress. (Caution: Avoid excessive hip flexion and adduction if the patient has had a total hip replacement.)
- Help the patient stand on the FWB lower extremity; assist in controlling or supporting the NWB lower extremity.
- Instruct the patient to reach for and grasp the far armrest of the wheelchair and pivot on the FWB foot to position the hips in preparation to sit.
- Instruct the patient to use the upper extremities and FWB lower extremity to slowly lower the body into the chair; maintain control and support of the NWB lower extremity.
- Position the NWB lower extremity on an elevated leg rest as necessary; place the other foot on the foot plate.
- Position the patient for safety and comfort and remove the safety belt.

WHEELCHAIR TO BED

- Position the wheelchair at an angle next to the bed, facing the foot of the bed and midway between the head and foot of the bed; either lower extremity can be nearest the bed. Lock the chair, swing away the front rigging, and apply a safety belt.
- Help the patient move forward in the chair; maintain control of and support the NWB lower extremity. Position yourself in front of the patient to guard and protect him or her throughout the transfer.
- Instruct the patient to stand by pushing with the upper extremities and FWB lower extremity.
- Instruct the patient to pivot so that the buttocks are toward the bed. Control and support the NWB lower extremity as the patient sits on the edge of the mattress.
- Assist in lifting the NWB lower extremity onto the mattress as the patient lifts the FWB lower extremity. (Caution: Avoid excessive hip flexion and adduction if the patient has had a total hip replacement.)
- Instruct the patient to move toward the center of the mattress and lie down.
- Position the patient for safety and comfort; remove the safety belt.

- Describe how you would reduce friction between a patient's body and the surface of the bed or mat, center the patient's weight, reduce the effects of gravity, and use gravity as an assistive force during bed mobility activities.
- What patient diagnoses do you think would be used for a transfer using a mechanical lift?

problem SOLVING

1. You need to help a 72-year-old man with weakness in his left upper and lower extremities perform a standing transfer from the bed to a wheelchair. Describe the procedures/techniques you will use, the preparatory actions you will take, the instructions you will give to the person, and how you will assist with the transfer.

2. A 35-year-old woman with a 3-day-old postoperative surgical abdominal incision needs to transfer from a wheelchair to a bed. What instructions will you give her? What precautions will you take before and during the transfer? What will be your role during the transfer?

3. A 22-year-old man with paralysis of his lower trunk and lower extremities resulting from a spinal cord injury is referred for "transfer training" while using a wheelchair. Outline the sequence of the training from the first day until he can independently transfer from the wheelchair to a bed or mat and return to the chair. In addition, indicate the techniques and equipment you will use and the precautions you will consider during the training.

4. A 52-year-old man who weighs 220 lb has had a left cerebrovascular accident. You are seeing him for the first time 3 days after this incident. He has not yet transferred from his bed to a chair at this time. Describe the methods you will use to examine the patient before making the transfer, your instructions to the patient and safety precautions you will take, and the method of transfer you will use.

Assistive Devices, Patterns, and Activities

objectives *After studying this chapter, the reader will be able to:*

- Identify various types of assistive devices.
- Describe the advantages and disadvantages of various types of assistive devices.
- Describe and perform the two-point, four-point, three-point, three-one–point, and modified gait patterns.
- Describe the advantages and disadvantages of the previously cited gait patterns.
- Teach a patient to perform any of the gait patterns cited using appropriate equipment for his or her condition.
- Describe and perform various functional activities when using assistive devices.
- Teach a patient to perform the functional activities appropriate for his or her condition using proper assistive devices.

key terms

Affected   Attacked by disease; afflicted.

Ambulation   Act of walking or being able to walk.

Assistive device   A piece of equipment (e.g., a crutch, cane, or walker) used to provide support or stability for a person when he or she is walking.

Axillary crutches   Wooden or metal crutches, adjustable or nonadjustable, that fit under a person's upper arms and into the axilla and have a handpiece to grasp.

Bilateral   Pertaining to two sides.

Quad cane   A cane with three or four feet that forms a wider base of support than the single crutch tip; also referred to as a crab, three- or four-footed, or hemi cane.

Forearm crutches   Wooden or metal crutches with a full or half cuff that fits over a person's forearms and that have a handpiece to grasp; also known as Lofstrand or Canadian crutches.

Four-point gait   The repetitive, alternate, reciprocal forward movement of an assistive device (e.g., a crutch or cane) and a person's opposite lower extremity.

Functional activities   Activities identified by an individual as essential to support the person's physical and psychological well-being and to create a personal sense of well-being.

Immobilizer   An object or apparatus that immobilizes or prevents motion, such as a cast or brace.

Monitor   To check on a given condition or phenomenon, such as blood pressure or heart or respiration rate.

Parallel bars   Adjustable or nonadjustable wooden or metal bars that are horizontal and parallel to each other and attached to vertical uprights to provide a stable, nonmobile support for a person who requires an assistive device.

Platform attachment   Wooden or metal crutches with an adjustable or nonadjustable platform for a person's forearm to rest on and aid in weight bearing.

Reciprocal   Corresponding but reversed on both sides.

Riser   A vertical piece of wood joining two steps; the back of the step.

Three-one–point gait (partial weight bearing [PWB])   One lower extremity is full weight bearing, and the opposite lower extremity is PWB; the patient uses bilateral canes, crutches, or a walker to partially support body weight as he or she bears weight on the PWB lower extremity; the full weight-bearing lower extremity advances independently, and the assistive devices and PWB lower extremity advance simultaneously.

Three-point gait (non–weight bearing [NWB]) One lower extremity is full weight bearing, and the opposite lower extremity is non–weight bearing; the patient uses bilateral crutches or a walker to support his or her weight when the weight-bearing lower extremity advances.

Tripod position The use of three points as supports, such as a cane or crutch tips and a person's feet, with the tips in front of and to the side of the person's feet to form a base of support when the person stands.

Two-point gait The repetitive, simultaneous, reciprocal forward movement of an assistive device (e.g., a crutch or cane) and a person's opposite lower extremity.

Unilateral Pertaining to one side.

Walker An assistive device that usually has four contacts that are placed on the floor and a frame to support the patient's weight and provide stability during ambulation.

INTRODUCTION

A person may require assistive devices for the following reasons: (1) to compensate for impaired balance, decreased strength, alteration in coordinated movements, pain during weight bearing on one or both of the lower extremities, absence of a lower extremity (with or without prosthetic replacement), or altered stability; (2) to improve functional mobility; (3) to enhance body functions; and (4) to assist with fracture healing. Selection of the proper ambulation devices or aids and gait pattern is important to provide optimal security and safety and to function with the least expenditure of energy.

Normal ambulation can be described as consisting of gait patterns. A normal gait pattern has a swing and a stance phase because during the gait cycle a given foot is either in contact with the ground (stance) or is in the air (swing). The stance phase comprises approximately 60% of the cycle, and the swing phase comprises approximately 40% of the cycle. Included in these values is a brief period when both feet are in contact with the ground simultaneously (i.e., a period of double support). A person's walking speed affects the amount of time the body remains in double support. The faster the person walks, the less time will be spent in double support. The gait cycle is defined as the time from the initial contact (heel strike) of a given foot to the next initial contact (heel strike) of the same foot.

Each major gait phase has subphases. In 1974, Perry suggested the use of new terminology to describe the subphases. Using her system (with other terms that are used in parentheses), the stance subphases are initial contact (heel strike), loading response, midstance (foot flat), terminal stance (heel off), and preswing (toe off). The swing subphases are initial swing (acceleration), midswing, and terminal swing (deceleration).

Another factor related to ambulation is the expenditure of energy. In the early 1950s, Saunders et al. contributed information to explain the way the body functioned to reduce energy expenditure during ambulation. They described six determinants of gait that affect the overall vertical and horizontal displacement of the center of gravity (COG) of the body that occur during gait. The determinants they identified were transverse pelvic rotation, pelvic tilt, knee flexion during midstance, foot and ankle motion, knee motion, and lateral pelvic rotation. It was their assertion that the interaction of these determinants functioned to limit the lateral and upward or downward displacement of the COG of the body, thus reducing the expenditure of energy. This information has been examined several times since it was introduced, and some disagreement exists about the premise that these determinants are the only factors involved with the conservation of energy during ambulation. Further study in this area appears to be warranted.

The major muscles or muscle groups of the lower extremity have an important role in gait and act at specific times during the gait cycle. Examples of the major phase of function and purpose are shown in Table 9-1.

MUSCLE ACTIVITY

The primary phases of gait are the stance and swing phase. When a lower extremity is in contact with the floor or other surface (i.e., weight bearing), it is in the stance phase; when it is not in contact with the floor, it is in the swing phase. The upper extremities are used for support, stability, and movement when ambulation-assistive devices are used. The scapular stabilizers; the shoulder depressors, flexors, and extensors; the elbow flexors and extensors; and the finger flexors are the primary upper extremity muscles involved in supporting the body's weight and assisting in propelling the body. In the weight-bearing phase, the hip extensors and abductors, the knee flexors (which function as hip extensors in the stance phase), the knee extensors, and the plantar flexors are the primary lower extremity muscles involved in supporting the body's weight. The hip flexors, knee flexors, and ankle dorsiflexors are used to elevate the extremity and, with momentum, move the extremity during the non–weight-bearing (NWB) (swing) phase. Other muscles of the upper and lower extremities also are used during gait and should not be overlooked during the assessment of the patient's strength. Trunk musculature (especially the trunk

Table **9-1** Major Phase of Function and Purpose of Lower Extremity Muscle Groups

Muscle/Group	Phase	Purpose
Gluteus maximus	Initial contact to foot flat	Stabilize limb
Gluteus medius/minimus	Terminal stance to preswing	Stabilize the pelvis in the frontal plane
Hip flexors/adductor	Preswing to midswing	Accelerate limb
Quadriceps	Loading response	Absorb shock, eccentric contraction stabilizes the knee
Hamstrings	Midswing to initial contact	Decelerate limb
Tibialis anterior/ peroneals	Initial contact to midstance and preswing to initial contact	Absorb shock, elevate foot
Gastrocnemius/soleus	Midstance, terminal stance to preswing	Knee stability at terminal stance, push off
Erector spinae	Initial contact to initial contact	Stabilize trunk

Box **9-1** Major Muscle Groups Used for Non–Weight-Bearing Ambulation

- Upper trunk: scapular depressors, scapular stabilizers
- Lower trunk: trunk extensors, trunk flexors
- Upper extremity: shoulder depressors, shoulder extensors and flexors, elbow extensors, finger flexors
- Weight-bearing lower extremity: hip abductors, hip extensors, knee flexors (which function as hip extensors), knee extensors, ankle dorsiflexors, and plantar flexors

Note that strength, flexibility, endurance, and motor control of these groups should be evaluated before ambulation training is begun, and deficiencies should be corrected so ambulation can be performed safely.

Box **9-2** Preparation for Ambulation Activities

- Review the patient's medical record for information to assist in planning the ambulation activities. What information will be particularly important to you?
- Assess, examine, and evaluate the patient to determine limitations and capabilities to plan the preambulation activities and gait pattern.
- Determine the appropriate equipment and gait pattern based on the medical record, your assessment, and the goals of intervention.
- Prepare the patient for ambulation (e.g., obtain consent) and explain the gait pattern.
- Remove items in the area that may interfere with ambulation to maintain a safe environment.
- Confirm the initial measurement of the equipment to ensure a proper fit and determine that the equipment is safe (e.g., tighten loose nuts and bolts, be certain spring adjustment buttons are secure, and examine rubber tips for dirt or cracks in the rubber).
- Apply a gait belt to the patient.
- Be certain the patient is mentally and physically capable of performing the selected gait pattern.
- Explain and demonstrate the gait pattern for the patient; require that the patient describe the pattern, how it is to be performed, and what is expected of him or her.
- Use the gait belt and the patient's shoulder or trunk as points of control when guarding the patient.
- Maintain proper body mechanics for yourself and the patient.

extensors) is necessary to maintain an erect position and proper posture (Box 9-1).

This introductory material is meant to provide a brief description of basic information about ambulation and gait patterns. An in-depth presentation about this subject is beyond the scope of this textbook. Please refer to the Bibliography for references related to this material.

ORGANIZATION OF AMBULATION ACTIVITIES

Planning and organization must be conducted before ambulation activities are initiated. The caregiver must be aware of the patient's health condition, activity limitations, participation restrictions, and environmental and personal factors as well as the goals and expectations of ambulation; the selection, measurement, and fit of the equipment; and the selection, practice, and progression of specific gait patterns and functional activities required by each patient (Box 9-2). The caregiver must provide safety and protection for each patient through the use of proper guarding techniques, precautions, and instructions (Box 9-3). The caregiver may need to prepare the patient physically or mentally to perform the activities that the patient and caregiver decide are important.

Usually it is beneficial and necessary to provide a period of preparation and training for a patient who will ambulate

with assistive aids. Providing such preparation and training is especially true for persons who have been immobile; those whose condition has affected their balance, coordination, strength, flexibility, or ability to tolerate an erect position; who are elderly; or those whose physical capacity to learn or perform motor skills has been diminished.

The purposes of preambulation procedures and activities are to provide safe and stable practice sessions, improve the patient's ability to use assistive devices safely and effectively, determine the type of assistive aids and functional skills the patient will require, and allow the patient to develop

Box 9-3 Precautions for Ambulation Activities

- Ensure that the patient wears appropriate footwear; do not allow the patient to ambulate while wearing loose-fitting shoes or slippers or when barefoot. These conditions can lead to patient insecurity and injury.
- Monitor the patient's physiological responses to ambulation frequently and evaluate vital signs, general appearance, and mental alertness during the activity. Compare your findings with normal values to determine the patient's reaction to the activity.
- Avoid guarding or controlling the patient by grasping his or her clothing or an upper extremity.
- Anticipate the unexpected and be alert for unusual patient actions or equipment problems; anticipate that the patient may slip or lose stability or balance at any time.
- Guard the patient by standing behind him or her and slightly to one side, and maintain a grip on the gait belt until the patient is safe to ambulate independently.
- Do not leave the patient unattended while he or she is standing.
- Protect patient appliances (e.g., a cast, drainage tubes, intravenous tubes, and dressings) during ambulation.
- Be certain that the area used for ambulation is free of hazards, such as equipment or furniture, and that the floor or surface is dry. Maintain safe conditions to reduce the risk of injury to the patient.

confidence in the use of the assistive aids. Equipment such as a tilt table to help accommodate the patient to an erect position, parallel bars for safety and security when practicing a gait pattern or to improve balance, standing frames to acclimate patients who are wheelchair bound, and various other preambulatory assistive devices can be used to facilitate the performance of mobility and functional tasks.

Interventions to strengthen muscles of the upper and lower extremities, improve cardiopulmonary function and endurance, improve sitting and standing balance, and teach and practice ambulation patterns and functional skills may need to be performed. The selection of specific equipment, including assistive devices and the procedures or activities to be used, is based on the findings of the patient's examination and evaluation and the goals of treatment related to the desired functional outcomes. The caregiver must be aware of the home, workplace, and social environments to which the patient will return to be certain that all functional needs can be determined and practiced. Often it will be helpful for a family member or coworker to observe the patient performing the ambulation pattern and primary functional activities before discharge. If necessary, the family member should be instructed in and should practice guarding techniques. Specific oral or written instructions regarding safety, precautions, or contraindicated activities should be given to the patient and family member.

ASSISTIVE DEVICES

Assistive devices are designed to improve a person's stability by expanding the base of support (BOS), reduce weight bearing on one or both lower extremities, and permit mobility. Stated another way, they help the patient compensate for decreased balance, strength, coordination, or a decreased ability to bear weight on one or both lower extremities, and they help relieve pain during ambulation. Although a tilt table is not an assistive device, it can be used for patients who must physiologically acclimate to an erect position before they can initiate ambulation.

The basic categories of assistive devices, given in order from greatest to least in the amount of support or stability provided, are walkers, bilateral crutches, single crutches, bilateral canes, quad canes, hemi canes, and single canes (Fig. 9-1). A patient may need to initiate ambulation with an aid that provides maximal stability or support but restricts mobility. As the patient's ability or condition improves, he or she may be able to progress to an aid that provides less stability or support and allows greater mobility. Decisions regarding the type of aid to use, when to change to a different aid, and the type of gait pattern to use are made by the caregiver (Table 9-2). Many factors are involved in determining whether a patient is an appropriate candidate for an assistive device. These factors include the patient's cognitive judgment, function, vestibular function, vision, physical endurance, upper body strength, and living environment. Impairments in any of these functions, depending on their severity, may make it impossible for a patient to safely use a device.

Criteria to consider include information such as weight-bearing status and diagnosis, the expected or desired ambulation activities, and the prognosis for improvement or regression of the patient's condition and abilities.

PREAMBULATION DEVICES

Parallel Bars

Parallel bars can be used for balance training, to teach specific gait patterns, and to provide support while measuring an assistive device. The bars should be adjusted so their width permits the hips and trunk to pass through them with clearance on both sides and the height is at the level of the greater trochanters when the patient stands erect. Each bar should be adjusted to provide 20 to 25 degrees of elbow flexion when the patient stands erect and grasps the bars approximately 6 inches anterior to the hips. Each bar should be approximately 2 inches wider than the patient's greater trochanters when he or she is centered between the bars. Elbow flexion can be estimated by adjusting the bar so its top is even with the patient's greater trochanter or with the patient's wrist crease or ulnar styloid process when the patient stands erect and the upper extremity is straight along the side.

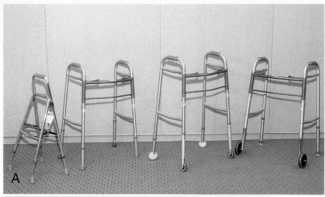

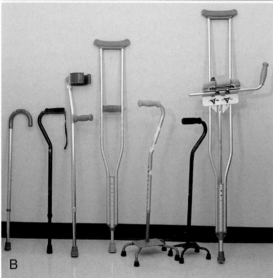

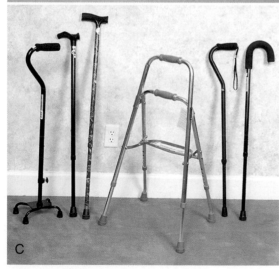

Fig. 9-1 Assistive devices. **A,** Types of walkers. **B,** An assortment of canes and crutches. **C,** An assortment of canes and a walker.

Parallel Bar Method for Measurement of Axillary Crutches To measure a patient for axillary crutches, have him or her stand inside the parallel bars with the head erect, the shoulders level and relaxed, the upper extremities grasping the parallel bars, the trunk erect, the hips straight, the pelvis level, the knees slightly flexed, and the

feet flat on the floor. Use this position to measure from a point at the anterior axillary fold to a point on the floor approximately 2 inches lateral and 4 to 6 inches anterior to the patient's toes for the overall crutch length. (It will be necessary to ask the patient or another person to hold one end of the tape at the axilla as you extend the tape to the floor.)

To determine the handpiece height, the crutch should be positioned in the patient's axilla with the tip forward and lateral to the patient's toes. The patient should have approximately 20 to 25 degrees of elbow flexion when grasping the handpiece while keeping the shoulders level and relaxed. The slight amount of elbow flexion will allow the patient to lift or support the body by extending the elbows during the NWB phase of the three-point gait pattern and to maintain a comfortable elbow position when other gait patterns are used. To obtain the most accurate measurement and fit, the axillary pad, handpiece pad, and crutch tip should be applied before all measurements are made and the fit is confirmed. The patient should wear shoes.

Alternative Method. For an alternative method of measuring a patient for axillary crutches, position the patient in the parallel bars as described previously. Using a crutch with push-button ("quick fit") length and handpiece adjustments, position the crutch in the axilla and along the patient's side. Adjust the handpiece at the level of the wrist crease, greater trochanter, or ulnar styloid process; then position the tip approximately 2 inches lateral and 4 to 6 inches anterior to the forefoot (toes) and adjust the length so that approximately two fingerbreadths are present between the axillary rest and the bottom of the axilla. Have the patient grasp the handpiece and evaluate the amount of elbow flexion and the length of the crutch with the crutch in the proper forward, tripod position. Readjust the crutch as necessary to obtain the proper length and handpiece position.

Tilt Table

A tilt table may benefit persons who need to physiologically acclimate to an upright position as a result of a variety of conditions, such as prolonged recumbence, disturbance in balance, decreased proprioception, kinesthesia, lower extremity circulation, or generalized weakness. A tilt table is particularly useful because it can be elevated gradually and maintained at any position between horizontal and completely vertical. Changes in elevation levels are accomplished manually or mechanically; an angular scale or protractor attached to the frame can be used to measure the elevation angle the person attains and tolerates. The ability to gradually elevate a person from a horizontal to an upright position and to allow him or her to adapt or adjust to any given elevation provides a safe method for the body to accomplish physiological accommodation for upright activities (Fig. 9-2). If the patient is NWB on one lower extremity, a low wooden box or platform may be placed under the

Table 9-2 Assistive Devices

	Use	Characteristics	Disadvantages
Walkers	Used when maximal patient stability and support are required	Various styles are available, and most have four support legs or feet; some may have two or four wheels, and most can be adjusted for proper fit Most walkers are lightweight, and some can be folded for storage Types include standard, child, bariatric (which are wider, support more weight, and are either adjustable or nonadjustable), reciprocal, stair-climbing, wheeled, folding, and one-handed ("hemiplegic") (see Fig. 9-1, *A*)	May be difficult to store or transport Difficult or impossible to use on stairs Reduces the speed of ambulation May be difficult to perform a normal gait pattern Can be difficult to use in narrow or crowded areas
Axillary crutches	Used for persons who need less stability or support than is provided by parallel bars or a walker; they allow greater selection of gait patterns and ambulation speed and provide stability and support	Most crutches are composed of wood or aluminum and can be easily adjusted for proper fit; they can be stored and transported and can be used in narrow or crowded areas or for stairs Types include standard (adjustable and nonadjustable), offset, and triceps (elbow extension) (see Fig. 9-1, *B*).	Are less stable than a walker Can cause injury to axillary vessels and nerves if used or measured improperly Require good standing balance Elderly patients may feel insecure with them Functional strength of the upper extremities and trunk muscles is required
Forearm crutches (also referred to as Lofstrand or Canadian crutches)	Used when the stability and support of an axillary crutch are not required, but when more stability and support than can be provided by a cane are needed; they eliminate the danger of injury to axillary vessels and nerves and are more functional on stairs and in narrow, confined areas	They are easy to store and transport, and the forearm cuff retains the crutch on the forearm when the patient reaches for an object Types include aluminum or wood, adjustable, and nonadjustable (see Fig. 9-1, *B*)	Provide less stability and support than axillary crutches, a walker, or parallel bars Require functional standing balance and functional upper body and upper extremity strength for many gait patterns Forearm cuff can make it difficult to remove the crutch Elderly patients may feel insecure with them
Platform attachment	Used for persons who are unable to bear weight through their wrists and hands, have severe deformities of the wrists or fingers that make it difficult to grasp the handpiece of a regular crutch, have a below-elbow amputation, or are unable to extend one or both elbows	Types include a platform that can be attached to an axillary or forearm crutch or to a walker; it is sometimes referred to as a "trough" or "shelf" (see Fig. 9-1, *B*)	Patient loses the use of the triceps to elevate and maintain the body during the swing phase Another person may need to apply or remove them Are less effective on stairs
Canes	Used to compensate for impaired balance or to improve stability and are more functional on stairs and in narrow, confined areas	A cane can be stored and transported more easily than crutches or a walker Types include "J," "T," pistol grip, offset shaft, three- or four-legged or four-footed (sometimes referred to as a quad, hemi, or crab cane), and Walkane (walk cane) (see Fig. 9-1, *C*)	Provides very limited support because of its small base of support

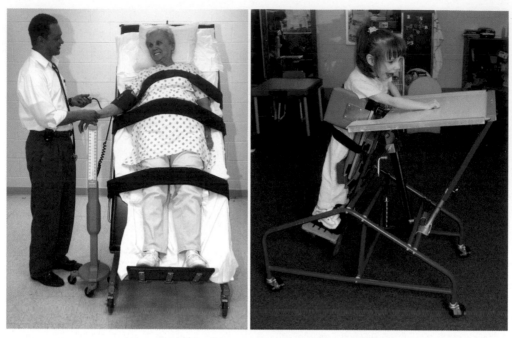

Fig. 9-2   Dependent standing devices (tilt table, standing table).

weight-bearing extremity so the NWB extremity is unable to contact the footboard of the tilt table.

The patient's vital signs should be measured before treatment to establish baseline values, especially for blood pressure and pulse rate, and they should be measured each time a progression to a higher elevation occurs; a log of the values should be maintained. Excessive increases or decreases in the blood pressure and pulse rate are usually indicators that the patient is experiencing difficulty in adapting to an upright position. Other indicators of the patient's intolerance include changes in consciousness, excessive perspiration, formation of edema in the lower legs, a decrease in or loss of pedal pulses, reports of nausea or numbness, a change in facial or limb color (i.e., flushed or pale), tingling in the lower extremities, and vertigo. A patient whose condition limits his or her capacity or ability to return venous blood from the lower extremities or abdomen to the heart may benefit from the application of elastic bandages or elastic hose to the lower extremities, or from an abdominal binder.

Although the circulatory system will be primarily conditioned, bowel and bladder function also may be affected because of the effect of gravity. In addition, it has been theorized that standing on a tilt table may assist in promoting or maintaining bone density in the lower extremities, especially for persons with a complete spinal cord injury. However, research studies have not provided conclusive evidence that this effect occurs.

Many persons who have used a tilt table have indicated that their mental outlook improved because they were able to assume a semi-upright or fully upright position, even if only for a brief period. Other activities can be performed by the person while standing, depending on the amount of function of the upper extremities, mental status or capacity, and the maximum elevation that is tolerated. An adjustable over-the-bed table or a lapboard attached to the frame of the tilt table can be used to support items such as reading or writing materials, food and utensils, communication devices, personal hygiene materials, games, cards, and similar items. Thus the person can be somewhat active while erect rather than merely standing. Strengthening and range of motion exercises can be performed, and lower extremity muscle groups can be positioned so a prolonged passive stretch force can be applied to them.

Usually it will not be necessary to elevate the table to 90 degrees to help the patient adapt to or become accommodated to an upright position. An elevation of approximately 70 to 80 degrees for 15 to 20 minutes, for several sessions, should be sufficient; however, each person must be considered individually. When the patient is elevated more than 80 degrees, the sensation of falling forward may occur because his or her COG will be shifted forward as a result of the pressure from the surface of the table against the back. The compensatory function of the anteroposterior curves of the body is negated by the table surface; thus the patient senses that a forward position change has occurred. If the patient is elevated beyond 70 degrees, a chest strap should be applied to prevent the upper body from falling forward. Using such a strap is particularly necessary if the patient does not have strong trunk extensors. The frequency and duration of treatment sessions with a tilt table vary depending on the person's condition or diagnosis, the response to the treatment, and the ability or capacity to adapt to, accommodate, or tolerate an upright position. A session

PROCEDURE 9-1

Tilt Table

- Explain the procedure to the patient and obtain consent; measure the patient's vital signs.
- Position the patient supine on the table and place a rolled towel beneath each knee. If the patient is bilaterally full weight bearing, position the feet flat on the footboard approximately shoulder width apart. The upper extremities may be positioned parallel to the sides of the body, may be placed beneath or remain free from the chest strap, may rest on an over-the-table support, or may be supported by slings attached to the table frame. A pillow under the head will add to the patient's comfort until he or she is elevated to approximately 75 degrees, at which time it may be more comfortable to remove it.
- Apply one restraint strap over the lower thighs (just proximal to the patellae) and one strap across the mid or upper thorax; a towel may be placed beneath each strap for protection and comfort, and the strap buckles should be positioned so they do not contact the patient. Note that when the lower strap is applied over the distal thigh rather than directly over the patellae, pressure to the patellae can be avoided. If desired, a third strap can be applied over the abdomen or pelvis. (Caution: An abdominal strap should not be used in place of a chest strap, especially for a person who lacks functional trunk and hip extensors. An abdominal strap without a chest strap will not prevent the upper body from falling forward at elevations where gravity has a forward force effect [i.e., approximately 65 degrees and higher]. If a chest strap is not in place, the patient must have sufficient strength and control of the trunk and hip extensors to maintain the body erect.)
- Elevate the table to a position tolerated by the patient, maintain that position for several minutes, measure and log the vital signs and tolerance time, and inquire about the patient's status (e.g., "Tell me how you feel." "Are you comfortable?").
- When the patient's condition is stable, raise the table to a new elevation, measure and log the vital signs and time, determine the tolerance to the new position, and maintain the position for several minutes.
- Repeat this process based on the patient's ability to tolerate and accommodate becoming more erect, continue to measure and log the vital signs and tolerance time, and decrease elevation of the table when it is apparent a given elevation is not tolerated. (Caution: Signs and symptoms of intolerance to being upright include syncope, tachycardia or hypotension, facial pallor or flushing, excessive perspiration, complaints of nausea or dizziness, or sensory or color changes in the lower extremities. Be observant for signs and symptoms of autonomic hyperreflexia and postural [orthostatic] hypotension.) (Refer to Chapter 12 for information about these conditions.) Note that several sessions may be required for the patient to adapt to an upright position.
- To conclude a treatment session, gradually return the patient to a horizontal position, observe the patient measure and log the vital signs, and observe and palpate the lower extremities for edema or circulatory responses (i.e., pedal pulses, color, and temperature).
- Document your activities and findings.

---

may be as brief as 5 or 10 minutes or as long as 1 hour, and sessions may occur once or twice per day or on alternate days (Procedure 9-1).

Supported Suspension Ambulatory Aid

A supported suspension device can be used for patients who need to be partially "unweighted" during gait training. This device uses adjustable suspension straps, a harness that fastens around the patient's trunk, optional thigh straps to avoid loads to the groin area, and a type of suspension with a Y-shaped yoke that supports the patient from directly over each shoulder to maintain posture and balance. Some indications for use of this device are cerebral palsy, some spinal cord injuries, Parkinson disease, and severe weakness that necessitates the use of bilateral leg braces. Benefits of using the supported suspension aid include controlled weight bearing and posture to correct asymmetric movement, facilitation of proper gait patterns, and the ability to work on balance, posture, and the sit-to-stand maneuver. In addition, this device can lift patients safely to the standing position from a chair or mat.

This book does not discuss patient training with the support suspension ambulatory aid, which "unweights" a person during ambulation. See the Bibliography for a video related to this equipment and its use.

MEASUREMENT AND FIT OF ASSISTIVE DEVICES

Several methods can be used to initially measure various assistive devices. If the initial measurement is performed with the patient in a position other than standing, the fit of the aid must be evaluated and confirmed when the patient stands. An aid that does not fit the patient properly will adversely affect his or her ability to perform a gait pattern and may result in an unsafe or unstable pattern. The position to use to confirm the fit of the aid is described on the following pages.

Walkers

The appropriate height of a walker can be determined with the patient standing or supine. The hand grip of the walker should be placed level with the patient's wrist crease, ulnar

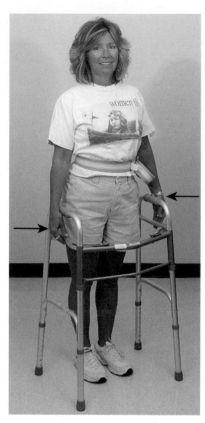

Fig. 9-3   Measurement for proper fit of a walker.

styloid process, or greater trochanter, with the walker positioned in front of and along the patient's sides and with the patient's arms straight along the sides (Fig. 9-3). The feet of the walker should be resting on the floor or even with the heels, the hips and knees should be straight, and shoes should be worn. A tape measure can be used to determine the distance from the patient's greater trochanter to the heel, with shoes on and with the hips and knees straight. This value is used to adjust the height of the walker by measuring from the floor to the top of the handpiece with the walker resting on its feet on the floor or on a higher surface, such as a treatment table, for convenience.

Axillary Crutches

Several methods can be used to measure axillary crutches. Any should provide an initial measurement, but you should not rely on these measurements to be exact or final. The fit must be evaluated and confirmed while the person is standing with the crutches properly positioned.

Length of Crutches If the height of the patient is known, multiply it by 77% (e.g., 70 inches × 77% = 53.90, or 54 inches) or subtract 16 inches from the height (e.g., 70 inches − 16 inches = 54 inches) and use the resulting value for the overall crutch length (i.e., axillary rest to tip).

With the patient supine, use a tape to measure the distance from the anterior axillary fold (i.e., the crease of the armpit) to a point approximately 6 to 8 inches lateral to the heel for the overall crutch length.

With the patient sitting and the upper extremities abducted at shoulder level, with one elbow extended and one elbow flexed to 90 degrees, measure from the olecranon process of the flexed elbow to the tip of the long finger of the hand of the opposite upper extremity; this measurement determines the overall crutch length.

These methods should provide similar results, but a difference in the measurements may be found. Select the method that provides the best result consistently. These measurements are only estimates of the length of the crutch; their fit must be confirmed with the patient standing.

Handpiece Height With the patient supine, measure from the greater trochanter, from the wrist crease, or from the ulnar styloid process with the arm by the side and the elbow extended to the heel of the shoe; hold the tape next to the side of the lower extremity. Use this value to position the handpiece by measuring up from the rubber tip of the crutch to the handpiece. An alternate method is to measure from the anterior axillary fold to the patient's trochanter or ulnar styloid with the arm along the side, with the elbow extended. Use this value to position the handpiece by measuring downward from the center of the axillary rest to the handpiece.

Forearm Crutches

The length of the crutch can be measured as for the cane (see the next section) to determine the height of the handpiece with the patient supine or standing (Fig. 9-4, A). The top of the forearm cuff should be located approximately 1 to 1.5 inches distal to the olecranon process when the patient grasps the handpiece with the cuff applied to the forearm and the wrist in neutral flexion-extension (Fig. 9-4, B).

Canes

The length of the cane can be determined with the patient standing or supine. The hand grip of the cane should be placed at the level of the patient's greater trochanter, the wrist crease, or the ulnar styloid process with the arm straight along the side. Place the cane parallel to the femur and tibia with the foot (tip) of the cane on the floor or at the bottom of the heel of the shoe (Fig. 9-5). A tape measure can be used to determine the distance from the patient's greater trochanter to the heel with the hip and knee straight, which determines the length of the cane when the patient is supine.

CONFIRMATION OF FIT

Improper fit is likely to cause decreased stability, increased energy expenditure, decreased function, and decreased safety for the patient.

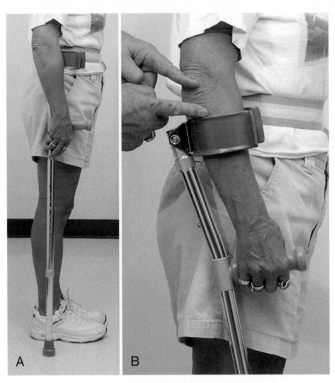

Fig. 9-4 Measurement for proper fit of a forearm crutch.

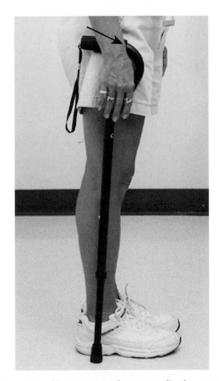

Fig. 9-5 Measurement for proper fit of a cane.

The initial fit of the aid may need to be revised after the patient has ambulated several times. As the patient becomes stronger, more skilled, and more proficient, the initial fit of the aid may no longer be comfortable or efficient. It will be necessary to observe the patient during ambulation to

determine whether the aid continues to fit properly. The aid should be readjusted if it does not provide proper function to avoid the development of bad gait habits or an unsafe gait pattern (Procedure 9-2).

When axillary crutches (as well as forearm crutches) fit properly, the patient's stance should form a triangle of the crutch tips and the patient's foot or feet, called the tripod position (Fig. 9-6). This position provides the best BOS and starting position for most crutch gait patterns, especially the three-point and three-one patterns. Common errors associated with the measurement or evaluation of fit of axillary crutches are listed in Box 9-4.

WEIGHT-BEARING STATUS

The patient may be required to perform the gait pattern with NWB, partial weight bearing (PWB), or full weight bearing (FWB) on one lower extremity. (Note that the term "weight bearing as tolerated" may be used to describe the weight bearing permitted.) If only PWB is permitted, the patient must learn to judge the optimal amount of weight to be placed on the restricted lower extremity. One method for learning how to judge this weight is to have the patient place the PWB extremity on a scale and bear weight up to the amount that has been predetermined. Afterward the patient will need to rely on proprioception to remember how much weight was applied and to repeat a similar amount of weight bearing during ambulation. It may be necessary to reevaluate the patient's ability to bear partial weight with the proper amount of weight. For some patients, a temporary device with a microswitch connected to an audible alarm can be attached to the shoe. The microswitch can be adjusted to cause the alarm to sound when the predetermined amount of weight bearing is reached or exceeded.

If a "touch-down" or "toe-touch" gait is desired, the patient should be encouraged to use a heel-strike gait or place the foot flat with PWB rather than using a toe-touch

PROCEDURE 9-2

Confirmation of the Fit of an Assistive Device

Each aid should be evaluated for fit with the patient standing with the head erect, shoulders relaxed and level, trunk erect, pelvis level, knees flexed slightly, and feet (foot) flat.

PARALLEL BARS

- Position the patient so he or she is standing erect between the bars.
- Adjust the height of the bar (rail) so it is level with the greater trochanter or even with the wrist crease with the upper extremity by the side.
- Observe the angle of elbow flexion when the patient grasps the bars; it should be approximately 20 to 25 degrees.
- Adjust the width of the bars, if possible, to provide approximately 2 to 4 inches of space between each of the patient's hips and the bar.

WALKERS

- Position the walker in front of the patient so the rear tips of the walker are placed opposite to the midportion of the feet (foot).
- Have the patient grasp the handpieces.
- Observe the angle of elbow flexion; it should be approximately 20 to 25 degrees when the patient grasps the handpiece and positions the device in preparation for ambulation.

AXILLARY CRUTCHES

- Position the axillary rest in the axilla; position the tips approximately 2 inches lateral and 4 to 6 inches anterior to the toe of the shoe(s).
- Have the patient grasp the handpieces with the wrists straight (avoid wrist flexion or extension).
- Evaluate for space between the top of the axillary rest and the floor of the axilla; it should be approximately 2 inches.
- Observe the angle of elbow flexion; it should be approximately 20 to 25 degrees when grasping the handpiece with the wrists in a neutral position.

FOREARM CRUTCHES

- Have the patient grasp the handpieces with the forearms inserted in the forearm cuffs.
- Position the crutch tips approximately 2 inches lateral and 4 to 6 inches anterior to the toe of the shoe(s).
- Observe the angle of elbow flexion; it should be approximately 20 to 25 degrees.
- Observe the position of the upper edge of the cuff; it should be approximately 1 to 1.5 inches below the olecranon process.

CANES

- Position the cane so the tip is approximately 2 inches lateral and 4 to 6 inches anterior to the toe of the shoe.
- Observe the angle of elbow flexion; it should be approximately 20 to 25 degrees.

gait. Although the toe-touch pattern can be used to decrease the amount of weight bearing a patient performs, it is an abnormal pattern because it positions the foot in plantar flexion rather than dorsiflexion at the beginning of the weight-bearing (stance) phase of the pattern. The normal gait pattern requires the heel to contact the floor first, so a heel-strike or foot-flat approach should be taught.

SAFETY CONSIDERATIONS AND PRECAUTIONS

Proper guarding techniques must be used to protect the patient during ambulation and associated functional activities. The caregiver must observe the patient and note any problems with balance, coordination, strength, or endurance and determine his or her ability to perform all activities safely. The judgment of the caregiver regarding the patient's ability to ambulate independently and safely is a critical determination.

When guarding a patient, many clinicians recommend that the caregiver initially stand to the side or at the back of the patient's affected or weakest side or lower extremity. However, a patient can be guarded safely and protected regardless of where you choose to stand. Therefore, as the patient's ability improves, you may want to change your position. Your personal preference, ability, or patient progress can be factors that determine the position you choose (Procedure 9-3).

Guarding from in front of the patient is not recommended because this position does not allow you to move smoothly with the patient, it blocks the patient's view, you cannot see objects or hazards behind you, and you must stay too far from the patient to have sufficient space for a step to be taken (Procedure 9-4).

A gait belt should be applied before and during all ambulation and functional gait activities for persons with decreased balance, strength, coordination, or a decreased ability to bear weight on one or both lower extremities; it also should be used when instructing a person for the first time. The belt should be applied securely around the waist. If the belt has a buckle, position the buckle so it will not injure the patient if tension is applied to it (i.e., position the buckle to the side or at the back) (Fig. 9-11). A gait belt is rarely used with small children because the caregiver usually can have full control of the child by placing the hands in guarding positions on the chest or waist. (Caution: Do not use the patient's clothing, upper extremity, or personal belt for control. These items are not sufficiently strong or secure to provide a safe grasping site.)

You should be alert for unexpected or unusual movements by the patient (e.g., misplacement of the assistive device, slippage of the aid, or a misstep) and be prepared to prevent or control a forward, backward, or sideward loss of balance. You must be prepared to control the shoulder and upper trunk quickly or move your forearm across the patient's chest to maintain optimal control of movement. It may not

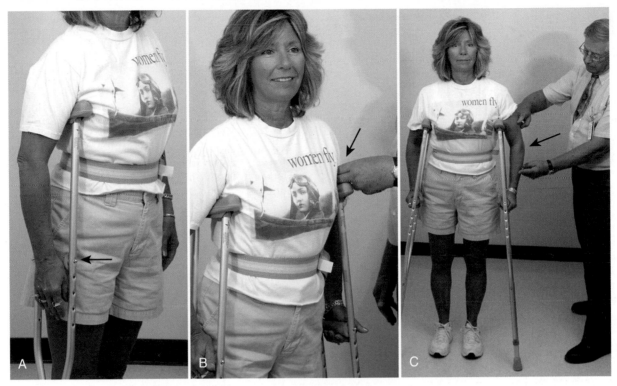

Fig. 9-6 Measurement and confirmation of the fit of axillary crutches.

be possible to totally prevent a fall, but you must be prepared to reduce the possibility of patient injury by helping the patient to a safe, secure position (e.g., onto the floor, ground, furniture, or a stair step). Additional specific instructions related to protection for loss of balance are presented in Procedure 9-4.

PREAMBULATION FUNCTIONAL ACTIVITIES

Parallel Bar Activities

For some patients, ambulation should be initiated with use of parallel bars to provide maximal security, stability, and safety. The gait pattern should be explained and demonstrated to the patient before it is attempted. Ambulation is a motor skill, so allowing the patient to practice the activity is necessary to reduce anxiety and fear and increase safety. The equipment selected must fit properly and be. When parallel bars are used, remain inside the bars to guard and assist the patient most effectively and reduce the risk of injury to yourself.

Moving from Sitting to Standing and Returning to a Sitting Position The necessary components of the activity of moving from a sitting to a standing position are forward movement of the body to the center or front portion of the seat, proper foot placement, forward inclination of the trunk with flexion of the hips, flexion of the neck and spine, forward movement of the pelvis to initiate an erect posture,

pushing with the upper extremities on the arms of the chair, extension of the neck and trunk, and extension of the hips and knees to attain the final standing posture. These activities help the patient shift his or her COG over and, within the BOS, align the trunk and move the COG from a lower to a higher position. To return to a sitting position, the patient needs to be positioned so the chair seat contacts one or both posterior thighs. He or she should (1) incline the trunk forward by flexing the spine and neck combined with hip and knee flexion, (2) move the pelvis rearward, (3) grasp the arms of the chair, and (4) flex the hips and knees to lower the body into the chair seat. These same principles should be applied when moving from a sitting to a standing position (Procedure 9-5).

Balance and Initial Gait Pattern Activities While standing in parallel bars, the patient should perform the following maneuvers:

- Slowly shift the body from side to side and forward and back while maintaining the shoulders and pelvis in line and the trunk erect, hold each position change for 3 to 5 seconds, and maintain the proper weight-bearing status on each lower extremity.
- Briefly and alternately lift the hands from the bars to promote a sense of the decreased support that will be experienced when the assistive device is moved; later, both hands may be lifted simultaneously.
- Perform a "push-up" using the bars to improve arm strength and to experience the sense of effort required

PROCEDURE 9-3

Position During Ambulation on Level Ground

- Stand behind and slightly toward the patient's weak or involved lower extremity; remain close.
- Use your hand nearest to the patient to grasp under the back of the gait belt with your forearm supinated. (Note: If the patient's balance and strength are good and the level of assistance is standby guard or better, you may choose not to use the gait belt.)
- Position your other hand above the patient's nearest shoulder, or allow your hand to rest lightly on the patient's shoulder (**A** to **C**). If you rest your hand on the shoulder, you must not restrict the patient's movement or cause an alteration in balance.
- Be certain that your arm does not contact the anterior neck or throat. If a great difference in height exists between you and the patient, it may be better to insert your arm between the patient's upper extremity and chest when you need to control the trunk (see Fig. 9-8).
- Place your feet in an anteroposterior stance with your most forward lower extremity behind the patient's lower extremity and the assistive device; position your opposite lower extremity posterior to the patient's nearest lower extremity (e.g., if you stand behind and on the patient's right side, your right foot will be positioned forward, between the assistive device and the right foot; your left foot trails behind). This technique will help you maintain a wide base of support.
- Move forward in step with the patient; your forward foot moves with the assistive device and your trailing foot moves forward as the patient moves.
- Avoid "cross steps" with your feet by allowing one foot to trail the other foot.

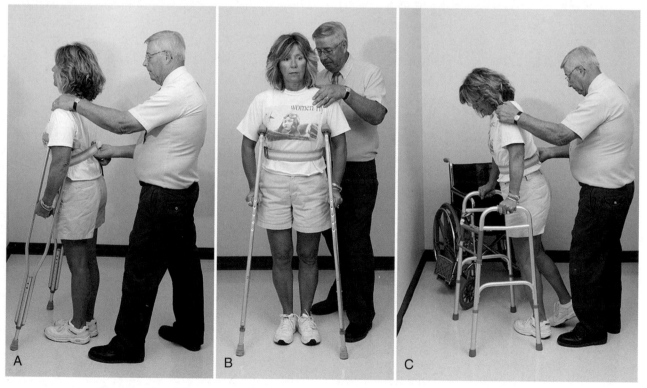

Fig. 9-7   One of the caregiver's hands grasps the gait belt; the other hand controls the shoulder.

to support the body when the lower extremities are not in contact with the floor or ground.

- Alternately or simultaneously lift the opposite upper and lower extremities to simulate a particular gait pattern or to increase balance when support and stability are decreased. Other exercises to improve the patient's strength, endurance, and coordination can be performed with the patient in the bars. The selection of specific exercises should be based on the patient's health condition and the particular gait pattern to be used. The exercises should be designed to improve the desired ambulation and coordination skills.

- Practice the selected gait pattern in the bars, including moving forward, backward, and sideward and turning to the right and left (Fig. 9-12).
- Practice the selected gait pattern using the proper assistive devices. The aids may be used with the patient

inside the bars, or the patient may use one bar and one assistive device.

Guard the patient using a gait belt and proper protective techniques. It is recommended that you remain inside the bars with the patient for optimal control and safety.

Basic Gait Patterns

Selection of the appropriate gait pattern will depend on the patient's balance, strength, coordination, functional needs, weight-bearing status, and energy level (Procedure 9-6) (Table 9-3). The advantages and disadvantages of several patterns are presented.

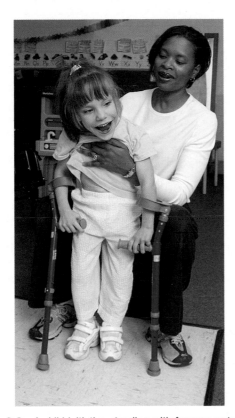

Fig. 9-8   A child initiating standing with forearm crutches.

Four-Point Pattern The four-point gait pattern requires the use of bilateral assistive devices. The pattern uses an alternate and reciprocal forward movement of the assistive device and the patient's opposite lower extremity (i.e., right crutch, then left foot; left crutch, then right foot) (Fig. 9-13). This pattern is very stable and can be performed slowly, and it is the safest pattern to use in crowded areas. It requires low energy expenditure and can be used when the patient requires maximal stability or balance. This pattern approximates a normal gait pattern, but the patient must ambulate slowly.

Two-Point Pattern The two-point gait pattern requires the use of bilateral assistive devices. The pattern uses a simultaneous, reciprocal forward placement of the assistive device and the patient's opposite lower extremity (i.e., right crutch and left foot; left crutch and right foot) (Fig. 9-14). This pattern is relatively stable and can be performed more rapidly than the four-point gait. It requires relatively low energy expenditure and is very similar to a normal gait pattern. However, it also requires coordination by the patient to move one upper extremity and its opposite lower extremity forward simultaneously. With the two-point pattern, the patient can ambulate more rapidly but with less stability than with the four-point pattern.

Modified Four-Point or Two-Point Pattern Modified four-point and two-point gait patterns are appropriate for the reduction of stress on an arthritic hip, for example, but they are not appropriate for a postsurgical patient who needs a true PWB gait. The patterns require only one assistive device and can be used for patients who have only one functional upper extremity or who have a lower extremity medical condition for which less stress is required. The aid is held in the upper extremity opposite to the lower extremity that requires protection, which widens the BOS and assists in shifting the patient's COG away from the protected lower extremity. This pattern is sometimes referred to as a "hemi" gait pattern. The patient performs the pattern in the sequences described for the four- and two-point

Table 9-3   Ambulation Pattern, Weight-Bearing Status, and Appropriate Walking Aids

Ambulation Pattern	Weight-Bearing Status	Walking Aid
Three-point	NWB	Walker, if indicated; progress to bilateral crutches
Four-point, two-point	WBAT to FWB	Reciprocal walker, bilateral crutches, bilateral canes
Three-one–point (modified three-point)	PWB as ordered by MD	Walker, bilateral crutches
Modified four-point, modified two-point	FWB	One crutch or one cane
Four-point, two-point, three-one–point	WBAT	Axillary crutches, if indicated, to bilateral canes
Modified four-point, modified two-point	WBAT	One crutch or one cane
Any of the aforementioned patterns may be chosen depending on the patient's abilities	FWB	Walker to axillary crutches to forearm crutches to bilateral canes to single cane to independent of walking aids

FWB, Full weight bearing; *MD*, physician; *NWB*, non–weight bearing; *PWB*, partial weight bearing; *WBAT*, weight bearing as tolerated.

PROCEDURE 9-4

Guarding Techniques: Standing and Ambulation on a Level Surface

GENERAL CONSIDERATIONS

- The size, stature, weight, and strength of the patient and caregiver may affect the techniques presented; modifications may be required.
- For some situations, two persons may be required to guard the patient; a gait belt must be applied before ambulation. If you are unable to maintain the patient in a stable upright position, help him or her to a safe position (e.g., onto the floor, ground, step, or piece of furniture).
- Teach the patient to use protective measures if his or her balance becomes unstable (see Procedure 9-11).

PATIENT STANDS WITH ASSISTIVE DEVICES

- Position yourself appropriately (see Procedure 9-3).
- Grasp the gait belt with one hand; your other hand guards at the shoulder or chest. Do not grasp the patient's arm or clothing.

When Balance Is Lost Forward

- Pull back on the gait belt, use your other hand to pull the trunk upward and back, and do not pull on the patient's clothing or upper extremity.
- It may be helpful to push forward against the pelvis as you pull back on the trunk.
- Help the patient regain a balanced position or help him or her to the floor or a chair.

When Balance Is Lost Backward

- Push forward on the pelvis and trunk to help the patient regain a balanced position.
- If the patient is unable to maintain an upright position, assist him or her to the floor or a chair.

When Balance Is Lost to One Side, Away from You

- Pull on the gait belt to move the patient toward you.
- Help the patient regain a balanced position or help him or her to the floor or a chair.

When Balance Is Lost to One Side, Toward You

- Move your body so you face the patient's side, widen your stance, and use your body to support the patient.
- Help the patient regain a balanced position or help him or her to the floor or chair.

AMBULATION ON A LEVEL SURFACE

- Position yourself somewhat behind and toward one side of the patient; position your outside foot behind the assistive device and the patient's foot; position your other foot so it trails as you walk.
- Grasp the gait belt with one hand. Be prepared to use your other hand to control the trunk; do not use it to grasp clothing or an arm.
- Initially, many caregivers prefer to be positioned to the side of the patient that is weakest or least functional.

When Balance Is Lost Forward

- Pull back on the gait belt, turn your body sideward, and widen your stance.
- Use your free hand to pull back on the upper trunk; position one hip against the patient's pelvis.
- Help the patient regain a balanced position or help him or her to the floor or to a stable object.
- If balance is lost beyond the point where standing can be maintained, take the following steps:
  - Instruct the patient to quickly release or remove the crutches and reach for the floor.
  - Slow the forward motion by pulling back gently, but firmly, on the gait belt and the patient's shoulders but do not stop the patient's movement.
  - Step forward with your outside foot as the patient is falling; gently slow the descent (**A** and **B**).

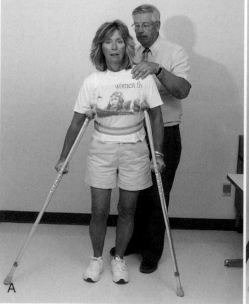
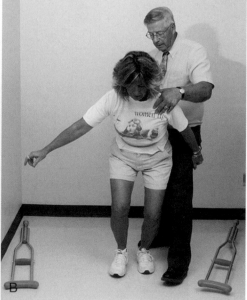

Fig. 9-9 The guarding position for a forward fall.

PROCEDURE 9-4

Guarding Techniques: Standing and Ambulation on a Level Surface—cont'd

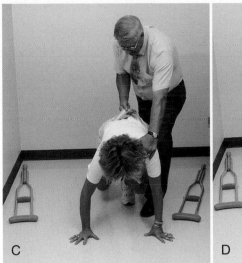
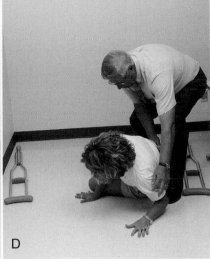

Fig. 9-9, cont'd

- If time permits and you are able to sufficiently retard the patient's fall, take the following steps:
  - Instruct the patient to cushion the fall by bending the elbows as the hands contact the floor and to lower the body to the floor (**C**).
  - Instruct the person to turn the head to one side to avoid injuring the face (**D**); check for any injuries.

When Balance Is Lost Backward

- Position your body so one side is toward the patient, widen your stance, and support the patient with your body.
- Use the gait belt and your other hand for control.
- Help the patient regain a balanced position or to the floor or a stable object; check for injuries.
- If balance is lost beyond the point of control:
  - Rotate your body so it is turned toward the patient's back and widen your anteroposterior stance.
  - Instruct the patient to release the crutches and allow him or her to briefly lean against your body.
  - It may be necessary to lower the patient onto the floor to a sitting position using the gait belt and proper body mechanics (see Procedure 9-4); check for injuries.

When Balance Is Lost to One Side, Away from You

- Pull on the gait belt to move the patient toward you.
- Push forward against the pelvis and pull back on a shoulder or the anterior chest.
- Allow the patient to lean against you for support.
- Help the patient regain a balanced position or to the floor or a stable object; check for any injuries.

When Balance Is Lost to One Side, Toward You

- Turn your body so that one side is turned toward the patient's back and your stance is widened; use the gait belt and your other hand for control.

- Help the patient regain a balanced position or to the floor or a stable object; check for any injuries.

Caution: When pulling on the gait belt, do not pull too quickly or use excessive force. Attempt to correct the movement of the patient by using a firm, smooth pull on the belt. Excessive force may cause further imbalance. Practice with an unimpaired individual who can simulate various loss-of-balance movements to help develop a sense of the control needed with a gait belt.

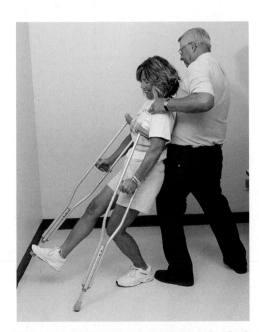

Fig. 9-10   Guarding a person when balance is lost backward.

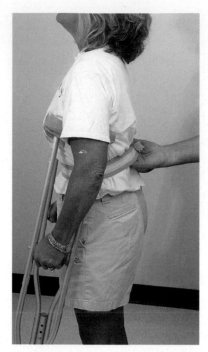

Fig. 9-11   A caregiver grasping a correctly applied gait belt.

patterns, but only one assistive device is used; thus the pattern is modified (Fig. 9-15).

Three-Point/Non–Weight-Bearing Pattern   The three-point NWB pattern requires bilateral assistive devices or a walker, but not with bilateral canes because the canes cannot support a significant amount of the body's weight. This "step to" or "step through" pattern is used when the patient is able to bear full weight on one lower extremity.

The walker or crutches and the NWB extremity are advanced, and then the patient steps up to the front rail of a walker or through the crutches (Fig. 9-16). It is a less stable pattern than the patterns described previously or than the three-one–point gait pattern, but it permits rapid ambulation. Use of this pattern requires good strength in the upper extremities, trunk, and one lower extremity, but energy expenditure is high because of the need to use the upper extremities to lift, support, and propel the body. The patient should be taught to step through rather than "swing through" the crutches and to control the movement of the trunk and lower extremities with normally functioning musculature, which will reduce energy expenditure and increase the patient's balance and stability.

Note: It is recommended that the terms "swing-to" and "swing-through" not be used in conjunction with the three-point pattern. These terms are better suited for patients who are unable to actively use the muscles of the lower trunk and lower extremities during ambulation and who must "swing" the trunk and lower extremities "to" or "through" the crutches to ambulate. These gait patterns are associated most frequently with patients who have a spinal cord injury

PROCEDURE 9-5

Standing in Parallel Bars and Returning to a Sitting Position

SITTING TO STANDING

- Position and lock the wheelchair in front of the bars.
- Remove the feet from the footrests, lift the footrests, swing away the front rigging, and position the caster wheels forward.
- Position desk-type arms with the armrest forward, if this is one of the features of the chair.
- Move the body forward to the middle or front edge of the seat by alternately lifting each hip and moving it forward or by leaning against the back of the chair and sliding the hips forward, then moving the trunk forward. Patients who can move each hip forward alternately will have more independence to stand.
- Position the foot of the stronger lower extremity slightly posterior to the foot of the weaker lower extremity. For some patients, it may be desirable to place the feet parallel to each other. Try each position with each patient to determine which position is most effective. Place both hands on the armrests of the chair with the trunk inclined forward (i.e., the "nose over toes" position).
- Simultaneously push down with the upper and lower extremity or extremities while leaning the trunk forward and continue to stand; alternately, place each hand onto the bars. Do not allow the patient to use the bars to pull to a standing position. The ability to stand independently is enhanced when the patient is taught to stand by pushing on the chair armrests while simultaneously using the lower extremity or extremities to elevate the body.

STANDING TO SITTING

- Turn so the back is toward the chair; position the stronger lower extremity approximately 4 to 6 inches from the front edge of the seat, or allow the thigh to contact the front of the seat.
- Release one hand from the bar and reach to an armrest; simultaneously, partially flex the hip and knee of the stronger lower extremity (or both lower extremities if they are both able to bear weight). (Note: It may be easier to release the hand on the side of the stronger lower extremity.)
- Release the other hand and grasp the other armrest.
- Flex both hips and knees and lean the trunk forward; lower into the chair.
- Move the pelvis and trunk back into the seat until they contact the back upholstery.
- Reposition the front rigging and footrests and replace the feet on the footrests when the treatment session concludes. (Note: For a short patient, it may be necessary to use the feet on the footrests to help move the body back to the back of the chair.)

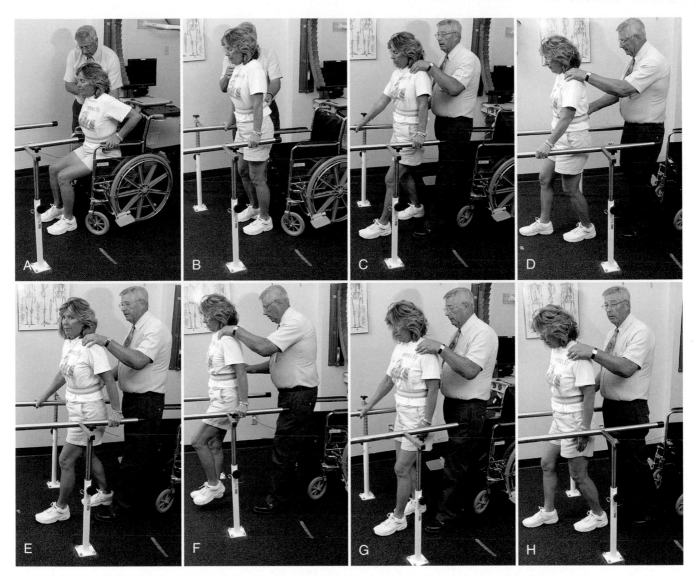

Fig. 9-12 Preparatory ambulation activities in the parallel bars. **A,** Preparing to stand. **B,** Gaining balance. **C** to **E,** Initiating a two-point pattern. **F,** Three point (non–weight-bearing) pattern. **G** to **H,** Modified two-point pattern.

or a developmental impairment that requires the patient to use the upper extremities to support and provide the force necessary to lift and move the body forward without assistance from the lower extremities.

Three-One–Point/Partial Weight-Bearing or Modi-fied Three-Point Pattern The three-one–point/PWB gait pattern requires the use of bilateral assistive devices that will support a significant amount of body weight (canes are not appropriate for this gait pattern) or a walker. The pattern is used when the patient is permitted to bear full weight on one lower extremity but only partial weight on the other lower extremity. The walker or crutches are advanced simultaneously with the PWB lower extremity (Fig. 9-17, *A*). Then the FWB lower extremity is advanced while the patient distributes the body weight onto the aid

and partially bears weight on the protected lower extremity (Fig. 9-17, *B* to *D*). This pattern provides more stability and requires less strength and less energy expenditure compared with the three-point pattern; however, movement with this pattern also is slower than with other patterns. It allows the affected lower extremity to function actively while maintaining some weight bearing on it. These features and benefits can be positive, depending on the patient's diagnosis or condition (see Procedure 9-6).

Preambulation Instruction

Instruction on how to perform the gait pattern to be used and how to perform various functional activities must be provided to each patient. Actual requirements may vary from patient to patient depending on each person's goals, needs, problems, and abilities. Patients will require

PROCEDURE 9-6

Ambulation Patterns with Assistive Devices

A. Four-point: The assistive aid and opposite lower extremity (foot) advance alternately; bilateral canes, crutches, or a reciprocal walker may be used.

B. Two-point: The assistive aid and opposite lower extremity (foot) advance simultaneously; bilateral canes, crutches, or a reciprocal walker may be used.

C. Three-point (non–weight bearing): The assistive aid advances simultaneously with the non–weight-bearing lower extremity; then the full–weight-bearing lower extremity (foot) steps through the aids. Bilateral crutches or a walker may be used.

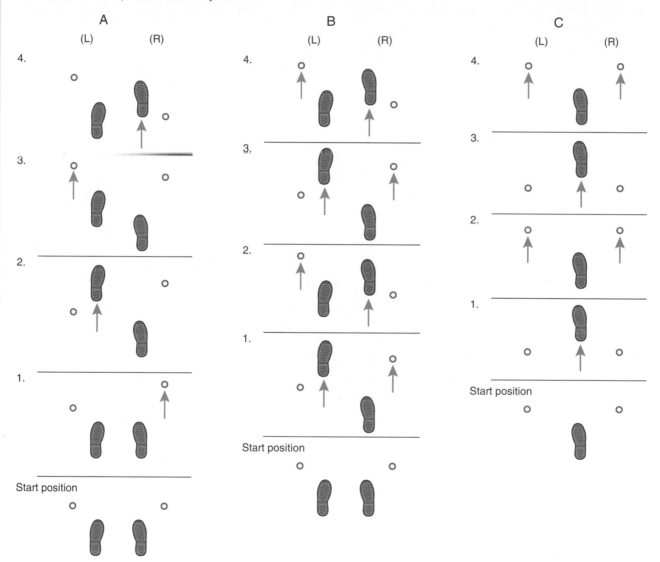

instruction and practice in various functional activities such as using stairs, curbs, inclines, ramps, and doors; sitting in and standing from different types of chairs or other seating items (e.g., armless chairs, low chairs and sofas, soft chairs and sofas, toilets, automobile seats, theater seats, and benches); ambulating on rough, soft, or uneven surfaces (e.g., grass, carpeting, gravel, or concrete); sitting on the ground or floor and returning to standing; and protecting oneself at the time of a fall. Using public transportation, crossing a street during the walk cycle of the traffic control system, and using an elevator and escalator also can be considered for inclusion in the gait training program. The specific activities selected will depend on the patient's needs, goals, anticipated activities, problems, assistive device used, and abilities.

The caregiver must explain and demonstrate the activities to the patient and protect or guard the patient during practice sessions to reduce the risk of injury. Videotapes,

PROCEDURE 9-6

Ambulation Patterns with Assistive Devices—cont'd

D. Three-one–point (partial weight bearing): The assistive aid and partial–weight-bearing lower extremity (foot) advance simultaneously; then the full–weight-bearing lower extremity steps through the aids. A bilateral cane, crutches, or a walker may be used.

E. Modified four-point: Only one assistive aid is used. The assistive aid and the opposite lower extremity (foot) advance alternately; the assistive aid is held in the hand opposite the affected lower extremity. One cane or crutch may be used.

F. Modified two-point: Only one assistive aid is used. The assistive aid and the opposite lower extremity (foot) advance simultaneously; the assistive aid is held in the hand opposite the affected lower extremity. One cane or crutch may be used.

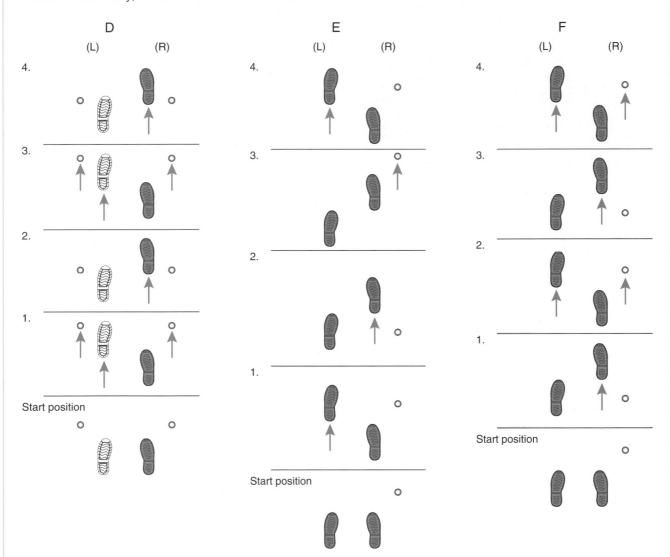

instructional booklets or manuals, and observation of other skilled and competent patients are other methods of instruction that can be used.

The goal for most patients will be the safe and independent performance of functional activities (Fig. 9-18). However, some patients may not become independent, in which case a family member, friend, or coworker should be instructed in the proper way to assist and protect the patient.

In addition, the patient should be made aware of any limitations and risk of injury that would accompany an attempt at independent performance of an activity for which assistance is required. The caregiver should document the activities the patient is able to perform safely and independently and any restrictions or limitations in ambulation activities. This information is especially important for family members of young or elderly patients or patients who have decreased

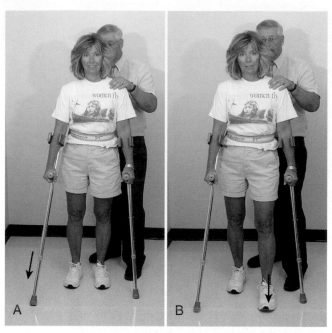

Fig. 9-13 The four-point gait pattern.

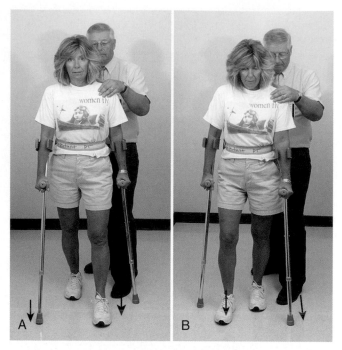

Fig. 9-14 The two-point gait pattern.

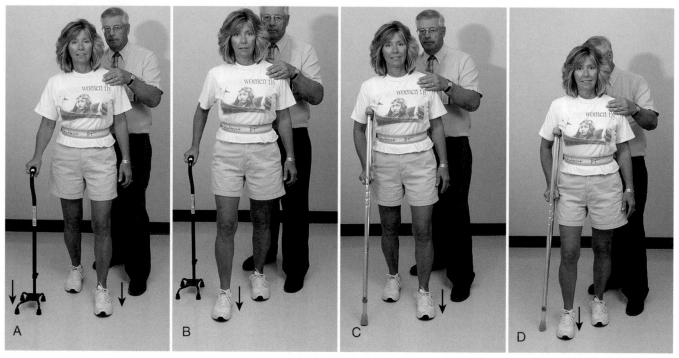

Fig. 9-15 Modified two-point gait patterns. **A** and **B,** Modified two-point gait with wide-based cane. **C** and **D,** Modified two-point gait with an axillary crutch.

mental competence that would interfere with the ability to make a competent decision or judgment.

The amount of time available to instruct the patient and practice ambulation activities may be extremely limited because of restrictions on the patient's length of stay in the hospital. Because many patients may be hospitalized for only a few days before they are discharged home, they may

not have access to multiple treatment or practice sessions, and their opportunities to become proficient in functional activities will be minimal. Patients who have not reached their maximal potential to ambulate independently, efficiently, and safely should continue with therapy either through home health (if they are unable to leave their home) or as an outpatient. You should provide written

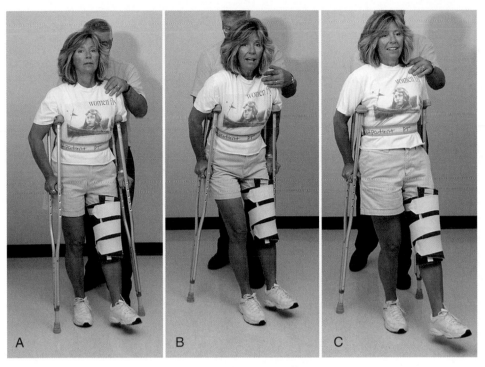

Fig. 9-16   The three-point gait pattern.

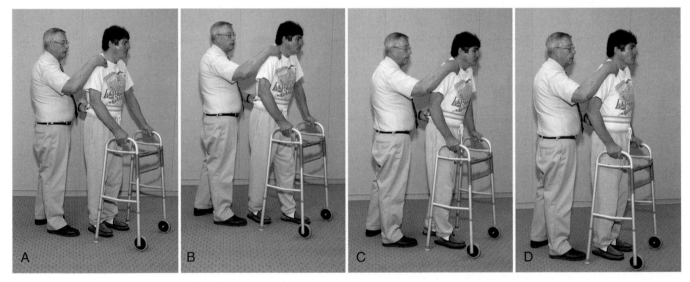

Fig. 9-17   The three-one–point/partial weight-bearing gait pattern.

instructions and precautions related to functional activities for the patient and family if the patient is deemed independent upon discharge.

These precautions may include suggestions for the proper maintenance of equipment (e.g., wheelchairs or walking aids), such as inspecting the support tips of the device for wear or damage or dirt in the grooves, checking wing nuts for tension, inspecting the item for cracks or broken parts, and checking all spring adjustment buttons to be certain they are securely positioncd in the holes provided. The patient should be cautioned that moisture on the support

tips or ambulation on a wet floor could cause the tips to slide. Loose objects, such as small area rugs, and waxed or polished floor surfaces also are threats to safety and should be avoided if possible. Extra care should be taken during ambulation on grass or on rough or uneven surfaces and in areas crowded with furniture or other people (e.g., a busy hallway, store, or sidewalk).

Sidewalks that are wet, icy, obstructed by snow, or in disrepair create special problems, and only the most proficient and cautious person should attempt to ambulate with assistive devices in these conditions. The patient should be

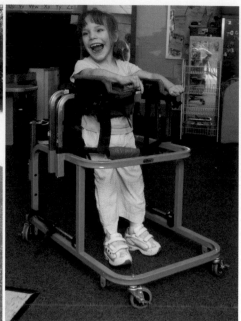

Fig. 9-18 Children ambulating with adjustable wheeled walkers.

made aware of the potential problems associated with doorway thresholds, the change from one type of surface to a different surface (such as from a linoleum surface to a carpeted surface), and the stair tread overhang (stair lip).

These precautions are most important for persons who use the assistive aid for maximal body support and stability, such as persons who are NWB on one lower extremity. However, all persons who use an assistive device should be instructed how to avoid or reduce the risks to their safety caused by the conditions or factors cited. It is the caregiver's responsibility to discuss these precautions with the patient during the ambulation training program. In addition, you should inform the patient or the family how you can be contacted for advice or assistance after the patient has been released from the facility. This information should be written and given to the patient's family upon discharge.

Standing and Sitting Activities

Each patient must be taught to stand and return to a sitting position while using the assistive device(s) safely, efficiently, and independently (Procedure 9-7). The techniques used may differ among patients, but many components should be taught to all patients. Weight-bearing and safety precautions must be reiterated to the patient.

Before a patient attempts to stand, he or she must move forward in the chair seat. This will position the COG nearer to the BOS (i.e., the feet and lower extremities) so the patient will be able to stand more easily and have better balance once standing. Most patients find it easier to stand if they place the foot of the stronger lower extremity slightly posterior to the foot of the opposite lower extremity. This anteroposterior position of the feet promotes a better "push-off" or lift from the stronger lower extremity as the patient begins to stand. The position also provides a wide BOS when the patient is standing and approximates the foot position most people use to stand from a chair. If both lower extremities have essentially equal strength and weight-bearing capacity, the foot of the dominant lower extremity is usually positioned most posterior (Fig. 9-25, A).

The patient uses the upper extremities to push simultaneously with the lower extremities to elevate the body. The hands should be placed on the chair armrests or on the appropriate part of the assistive device and initially should be positioned anterior to the hips. This hand placement allows the patient to push upward and forward to move the hips and trunk forward and toward the BOS (Fig. 9-25, B); it also enables the patient to use the most stable object for support as the movement to a standing position is initiated. A person who has normal or greater strength in the upper extremities, trunk, and at least one lower extremity and has normal balance and coordination may be able to stand using only the assistive devices (Fig. 9-25, C and D). (Note: A patient may initiate this activity independently. The patient should be cautioned that this method is less safe than the other methods presented. It is not recommended that this method be taught because it is too insecure.)

The patient inclines the trunk forward and pushes with the upper and lower extremities. This maneuver shifts the COG forward and eventually over the BOS, leading to a relatively stable standing position. (Note: When a patient stands from a wheelchair, the chair will be most stable when the caster wheels are positioned forward and the drive wheel locks are engaged, as described in Chapter 7.)

When the patient returns to the chair, the process is reversed. The patient approaches the chair and pivots so the back is toward the chair, with the foot of the stronger extremity nearest the chair seat. The patient lowers into the chair using the upper and lower extremities to control the movement. The trunk is inclined forward to maintain the COG over the BOS and to avoid striking the back of the chair with the upper back before the buttocks are on the chair seat. A person who attempts to sit without inclining the trunk forward will be unstable and have difficulty controlling the movement of the body into the chair.

Standing and Sitting with a Walker The proper procedures for standing and sitting with a walker that are outlined in Procedure 9-7 should be followed in most cases. The alternative methods described below should not be considered safe to use with wheeled walkers or for patients who are weak, mentally confused, or who have poor balance or decreased strength in the upper and lower extremities.

Alternative Methods. An alternative method for standing is to instruct the patient to preposition the body and feet as described previously and place one hand on one hand grip of the walker and the other hand on the chair armrest in front of the hips (see Fig. 9-19 B). However, this position can be unsafe if the patient attempts to pull to a standing position using only the walker because the walker is not secure on the floor. Furthermore, when the patient attempts to push down with both upper extremities on the hand grips, it may be difficult to stand because the upper extremities will be too high to exert a strong downward force and the walker may tip if the patient pulls on the handpieces.

An alternative method for sitting is to instruct the patient to reach one hand to the armrest while the other hand remains on the walker hand grip (Fig. 9-26). This method offers less stability than the previously described method because the walker is not as secure as the chair. However, some patients may perform better using this method. The patient lowers the hips onto the chair using the upper extremities and the stronger lower extremity and then positions the body in the chair by moving the hips back into the seat. If the chair does not have arms, the patient can be taught to use the hand grips of the walker to help raise or lower the body using the alternative methods previously described. It is important to teach the patient to push down on the walker hand grips and avoid pulling or pushing the walker when attempting to stand or return to sitting.

Standing and Sitting with Axillary Crutches Placing the crutches opposite to the foot of the stronger lower extremity widens the patient's BOS so when the patient stands, the body's vertical gravity line will be located between the crutches and the strong lower extremity (see Fig. 9-21, B).

Alternative Methods. An alternative method for standing is to hold the crutches with the hand on the same side of the body as the stronger lower extremity. This technique narrows the BOS but increases the force the patient is able to use to stand. The ipsilateral upper and lower extremities function simultaneously to lift the patient upward. The

Text continues on page 240

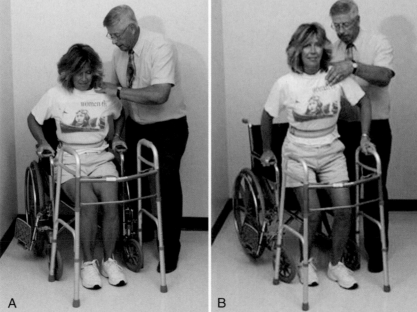

Fig. 9-19   A patient standing from a wheelchair using a walker.

PROCEDURE 9-7

Independent Standing and Sitting with Assistive Aids

WALKER

For descriptive purposes, assume the patient has generalized weakness in the lower extremities.

Rise to a Standing Position

- The walker is positioned directly in front of the chair with the open side toward the patient and close enough to be within the patient's reach.
- The patient moves the hips forward to the middle or front portion of the chair seat.
- The patient positions the foot of the unaffected lower extremity slightly posterior to the foot of the least functional extremity; the feet should be flat on the floor, and the hands should be placed on the front portion of the armrests.
- The patient grasps the chair armrests in front of the hips (**A**). This position provides the greatest stability and allows the patient to use his or her upper and lower extremities most effectively to stand.

- To rise, the patient leans the trunk forward, simultaneously pushes down with the upper extremities and the strongest lower extremity, and stands.
- When standing, the patient reaches one hand at a time to grasp the handpieces on the walker and establishes balance before ambulating.

Return to a Sitting Position

- The patient approaches the chair forward and pivots toward the chair on the stronger lower extremity until the back is toward the chair (**A** to **C**).
- The patient steps back until the front edge of the chair seat contacts the back of the stronger lower extremity.
- The patient reaches, one hand at a time, to grasp each armrest and lowers the body into the chair slowly using the upper and lower extremities, then moves back in the chair. This method provides the greatest stability for the patient (**D** to **E**).

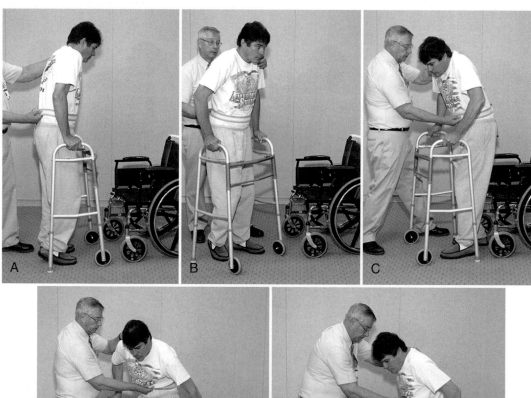

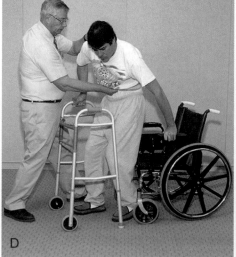
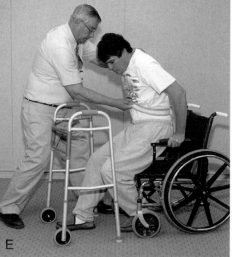

Fig. 9-20   A patient returning to a wheelchair from a walker.

PROCEDURE 9-7

Independent Standing and Sitting with Assistive Aids—cont'd

CRUTCHES

For descriptive purposes, assume the patient is non–weight bearing on the left lower extremity.

Rise to a Standing Position

- The patient moves toward the front of the chair seat and places the right foot approximately 6 to 8 inches forward. If the knee of the most affected lower extremity cannot be flexed, the patient should be taught to slide the heel forward before attempting to stand, or the caregiver can support the lower extremity as the patient stands (**A**).
- The handpieces of both crutches are grasped in the left hand and are positioned vertically slightly in front and to the side of the chair; the right hand holds the armrest (**B**).
- To rise, the patient leans the trunk forward and pushes with both hands and right lower extremity (**C**).

Standing with Axillary Crutches (See Fig. 9-21)

- The patient establishes balance and uses the right hand to place one crutch in the right axilla; the remaining crutch is placed in the left axilla using the left hand (**D**).
- The crutches are positioned to form a tripod before ambulating.

Standing with Forearm Crutches (see Fig. 9-22)

- The patient establishes balance and uses the right hand to grasp the handpiece of one crutch. The crutch is positioned lateral and anterior to the right foot. The crutch is positioned similarly on the opposite side.
- When each crutch is positioned, the forearm cuff is applied alternately to each forearm, unless the patient has reached through the cuff to grasp the handpiece.

Return to a Sitting Position

- The patient approaches the chair forward and pivots toward the right until his or her back is toward the chair.
- The patient steps back until the edge of the chair seat contacts the posterior thigh of the right lower extremity.
- The crutches are removed from the axillae; the patient holds the handpieces with the left hand to widen the base of support and increase stability. The crutches are positioned to the side and held vertically.
- The right hand reaches to the armrest, and the patient lowers the hips into the chair using the right upper and lower extremities. If the knee of the least affected lower extremity cannot be flexed, the patient should slide it forward to sit.
- The crutches can be placed on the floor, and the body moves back in the chair.

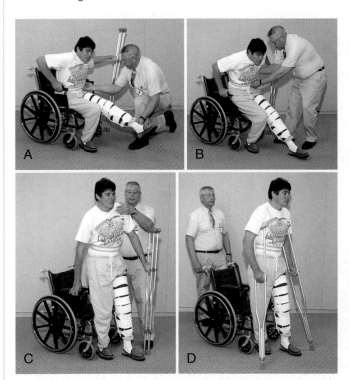

Fig. 9-21   A patient rising from a sitting position with axillary crutches.

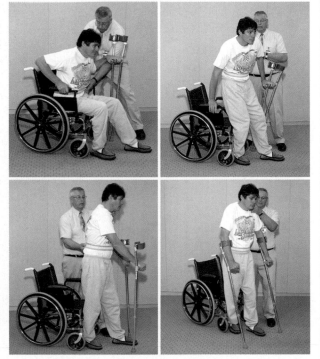

Fig. 9-22   A patient standing from a wheelchair using forearm crutches.

Continued

PROCEDURE 9-7

Independent Standing and Sitting with Assistive Aids—cont'd

CANE

For descriptive purposes, assume the left upper and lower extremities are affected or weaker.

Rise to a Standing Position

- Position the cane on the right side of the chair; a footed cane is placed slightly to the front and side of the right armrest, and a standard cane is hooked onto the front portion of the armrest.
- The patient moves toward the front of the chair seat and positions the right foot slightly posterior to the left. The patient places his or her hands on the armrests in front of the hips to be able to push with them to lift the body from the chair.
- To rise, the patient leans the trunk forward and pushes strongly with the right upper and lower extremities; if they

are capable of providing assistance, the left extremities can be used as well.
- The patient grasps the cane with the right hand (**A** to **C**) and establishes balance before ambulating.
- When using a self-standing (three- or four-footed, crab, or Walkane) cane for this procedure, the cane is placed next to the front of the armrest of the stronger upper and lower extremities, and the patient proceeds as described (**D** and **E**).
- Note: If the chair does not have arms, the patient can be taught to hold the cane in the hand opposite to the weaker or more affected lower extremity and use either one or both upper extremities to push down on the seat or back of the chair to assist in standing.

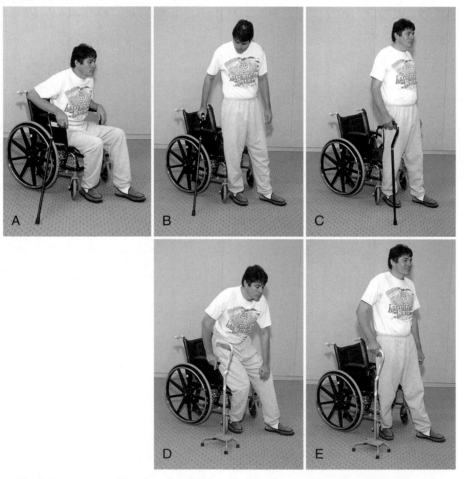

Fig. 9-23   A patient rising from a wheelchair to a standing position with two types of canes.

PROCEDURE 9-7

Independent Standing and Sitting with Assistive Aids—cont'd

Return to a Sitting Position

- The patient approaches the chair and pivots toward the chair, leading with the right upper extremities, until the right side is nearest the chair.
- The footed cane is placed in front and to the side of the right armrest; a standard cane is hooked onto the armrest.
- The patient reaches for the near armrest with the right hand and then, if he or she is able to do so, grasps the far armrest with the left hand and continues to turn until the back is toward the chair seat.

- The patient lowers into the chair slowly and then positions the body back in the chair.
- Note: If the chair does not have arms, the patient can be taught to release the cane, allowing it to fall sideward to the floor, and to reach to the chair seat or the back of the chair with the free upper extremity to help lower the body into the chair.

  For each of these activities, the patient should be instructed to lock the wheelchair, elevate the footplates or swing away the front rigging, and position the caster wheels forward before standing.

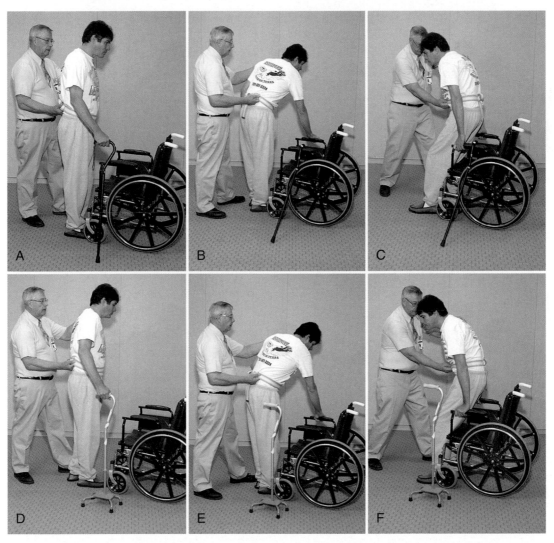

Fig. 9-24   A patient returning to a wheelchair from a standing position using two types of canes.

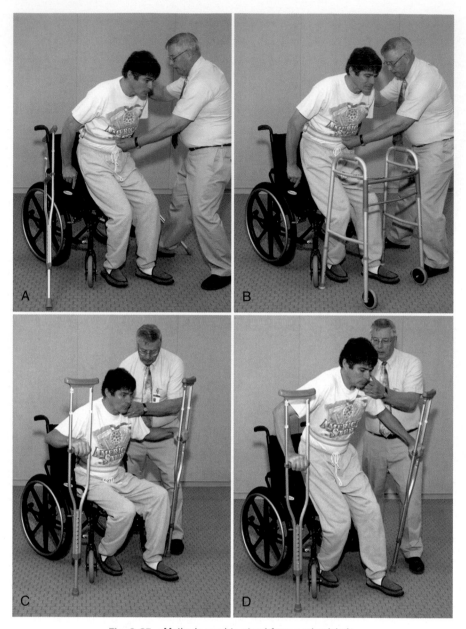

Fig. 9-25 Methods used to stand from a wheelchair.

patient pushes from the armrest, seat, or back of the chair with the opposite hand to assist with the stand (Fig. 9-27, A to E). If more leverage is needed to arise from a chair without arms, using the back of the chair to push off by sitting sideways in the chair is an alternative method (Fig. 9-27, F). (Note: The patient must push downward on the chair back so the chair does not tip or slide.)

Two alternative methods may be used for sitting:

1. Hold the crutches with the hand on the same side of the body as the stronger lower extremity, as described previously.

2. Place the crutch on the side of the least functional lower extremity over the push handle of the chair, and use the armrest while placing the other crutch over the push handle on the stronger side. Both hands are then free to use the armrests to pivot and assist to sitting (Fig. 9-28). To initiate standing, the patient may need to be taught to pivot toward the chair and to face the chair after standing to grasp the crutches, which have been hooked over the push handles or armrests to begin ambulation.

Patients should be instructed to avoid placing the crutches against a wall, table, or chair because they are likely to slide and fall to the floor, which could damage the crutches or injure someone nearby.

Standing and Sitting with Forearm Crutches The processes involved with standing and sitting while using forearm crutches are similar to those with axillary crutches (see Procedure 9-7).

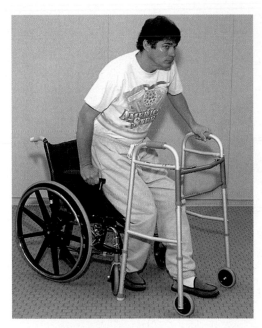

Fig. 9-26 A patient returning to a wheelchair from a walker (alternative method).

Alternative Methods. An alternative method for standing can be used for patients with good strength, coordination, and balance, but usually cannot be performed by elderly, weak, unstable, or debilitated patients. For this method, the patient moves the hips forward to the middle or front portion of the chair seat. The foot of the stronger lower extremity is positioned slightly posterior to the foot of the other lower extremity. The patient grasps the handpiece of each crutch in each hand and the crutch tips are positioned lateral and anterior to each foot. The person simultaneously pushes down with the upper extremities and the stronger lower extremity, leans the trunk forward, and stands (Fig. 9-29). (Note: It is not recommended that this method be taught because it is insecure.)

An alternative method for sitting is to instruct the patient to perform all activities described for sitting with axillary crutches before removing the crutches. Then the patient alternately removes the cuff from each forearm but continues to grasp each handpiece. The patient lowers into the chair using the upper and lower extremities, places the crutches on the floor, and moves back into the chair seat.

Standing and Sitting with a Cane By positioning the cane appropriately, the patient will be able to use the aid with the upper extremity opposite to the weaker or more affected lower extremity. This approach positions the cane in the proper hand, widens the patient's BOS, and allows some weight shift from the weaker lower extremity onto the cane when it is used during the weight-bearing (stance) phase of the gait pattern.

The methods described for standing from a chair and sitting into a chair should be safe and effective for the majority of patients who have average or normal strength, coordination, and balance. However, some patients may require the assistance of another person or the use of a firm, stable object (e.g., a chair with arms, a table, a handrail, grab bars, a vanity, a bed, or a counter) to help them to stand or sit. Observing the patient or attempting different methods may be necessary to determine which method will be the safest and most independent for the patient. You must protect the patient when any of these methods are taught by using proper guarding techniques, including the application and use of a gait belt (Fig. 9-30).

Guarding During Gait Training on Curbs, Stairs, and Ramps

The procedures involved in guarding a patient while ascending or descending an elevation are similar to those used for curbs, stairs, and ramps (Procedure 9-8). Understanding how to perform these procedures will allow you to tailor the steps to meet the particular needs of a patient and/or environment.

When ascending or descending stairs or a ramp, initially teach the patient to stop and gain balance on each step before progressing to the next step to avoid building momentum. Patients who gain too much momentum may be at risk for a fall.

Guarding from either the front or back can provide safety for the patient, but most patients have a greater sense of security when someone is in front of them as they descend from an elevation. If you are behind the patient and balance is lost forward, you can provide security by gently pulling back on the gait belt and the patient's shoulder (when descending stairs you may seat the person on the stair to prevent further injury). You must prevent the patient from pulling you forward if a serious loss of balance occurs.

If a handrail is not available when ascending an elevation, it is recommended that two persons guard the patient. One person is positioned in front of or slightly to one side of the patient, and another person is positioned behind or to the side of the patient.

When descending stairs, some caregivers prefer to widen their stride so the upper foot is on the step the patient is standing on and the lower foot is on the step below the step to which the patient will step (Fig. 9-31). This technique requires the caregiver to span two steps, which may not be possible for women who wear skirts or for a person with a short stride. (Caution: Do not stand with your feet parallel to each other and on the same step directly below and in front or to the side of the patient. This position will be unstable if the patient falls forward because it does not provide a wide anteroposterior BOS.)

Actions if the Patient Loses Balance or Falls You must be alert and be ready to act quickly in case the patient loses balance. Your protective reactions must be so well developed that you are able to react automatically to prevent

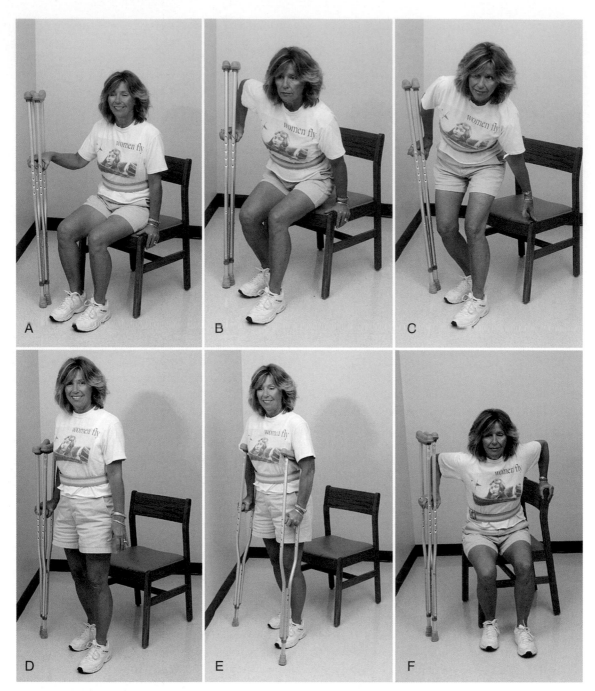

Fig. 9-27 A patient using axillary crutches to rise from a sitting position in a chair without arms.

or minimize injury. Proper guarding techniques must be practiced after you understand the rationale and basis for them. In many instances it will not be necessary or desirable to maintain the patient upright. Assisting the patient to the floor or onto a firm object is an accepted procedure, as long as proper techniques are used and injury to the patient is minimized. Your primary responsibility is to provide a safe environment and treatment and to protect the patient from injury to the best of your ability.

Procedure 9-8 covers guarding techniques and procedures in case of a fall during ascent or descent of an elevation. Steps for guarding and fall recovery techniques for patients ambulating on level ground can be found in Procedure 9-4.

AMBULATION FUNCTIONAL ACTIVITIES

Functional activities of ambulation with an aid are frequently overlooked during the ambulation training program. Before a patient can be fully independent, he or she must be taught how to move backward and sideward, to turn to

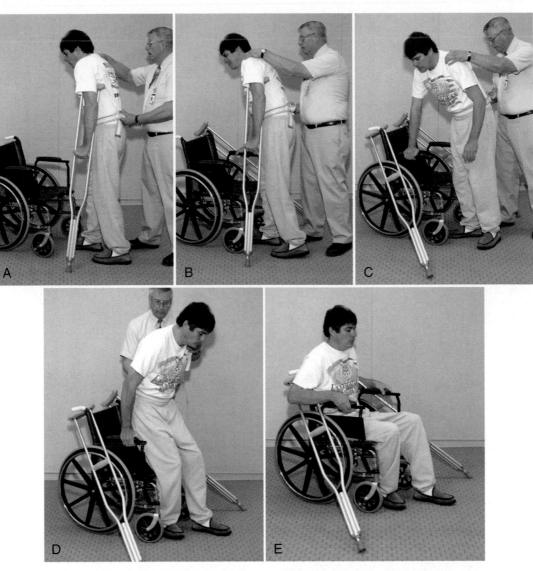

Fig. 9-28   A patient approaching a wheelchair using axillary crutches.

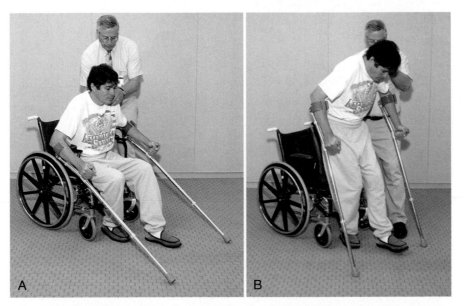

Fig. 9-29   A patient standing from a wheelchair using forearm crutches (alternative method).

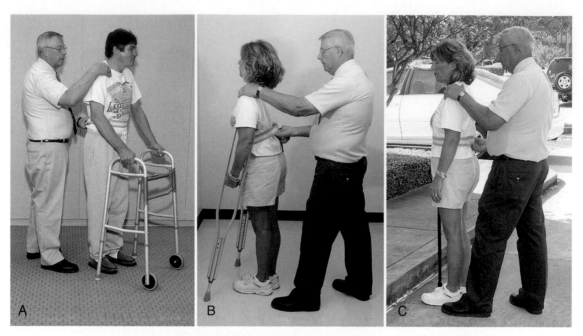

Fig. 9-30   Correct position of the caregiver behind a patient with an assistive device.

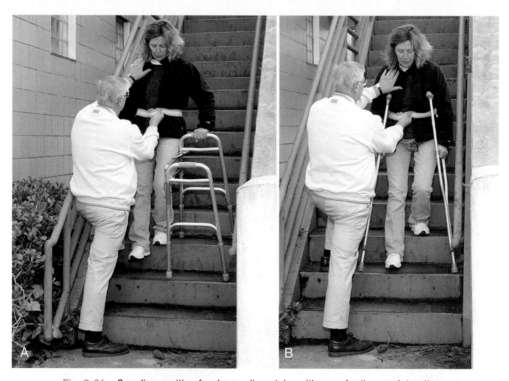

Fig. 9-31   Guarding position for descending stairs with use of a three-point pattern.

the left and to the right, and to perform a 180-degree arc. These movements are necessary because they are components of basic, functional ambulation activities. The patient will need to move backward to sit or to move away from a door that opens toward him or her. A sideward movement is required in narrow spaces (e.g., the area between two rows of seats in a theater or a narrow hallway or doorway).

Turning is required to change direction of movement or for positioning before sitting or performing other activities that require a change of direction. You should not assume that each patient is able to perform these activities without being taught how to do so. Failure to teach the patient these activities may result in decreased independence or an increased risk of injury for the patient.

PROCEDURE 9-8

Guarding Techniques for Stairs, Curbs, and Ramps

GENERAL CONSIDERATIONS

The size, stature, weight, and strength of the patient and the caregiver may affect how the techniques presented are applied; some modifications may be necessary, and in some situations, two persons may be required.

Regardless of the technique used to guard a patient on stairs, you must prevent the patient from falling down multiple steps or experiencing a fall. Therefore you must take the following steps:

- Maintain a wide stance with your feet; do not place both feet on the same step, and use one hand to grasp the gait belt.
- Properly position yourself to maximally protect yourself and the patient.
- Anticipate the actions you will perform in case balance is lost when ascending or descending the stairs.

The techniques presented for use on stairs also are appropriate for use with curbs and ramps.

ASCENDING A CURB, STAIR, OR RAMP: GUARDING THE PATIENT FROM THE BACK

- Position yourself behind and slightly to the side of the patient in the area where there is the least protection for the patient.
- If a handrail is used, position yourself to the side opposite it. If a handrail is not used, position yourself to the side at which the greatest danger or potential for injury exists in case the patient's balance is disturbed. (Note: Many caregivers prefer initially to be positioned to the patient's weakest side or the side of the least functional extremity.)

- Grasp the gait belt with one hand; be prepared to use your other hand to control the trunk or grasp the handrail when available. If a handrail is not available, guard with your opposite hand placed on the patient's shoulder.
- Use an anteroposterior stance with your outside foot on the step on which the patient is standing and your inside foot on the step below the step on which the patient is standing.
- Advance your feet up one step after the patient has advanced one step, but maintain your feet in an anteroposterior position as described. This process is repeated to ascend all the steps.

Balance Lost Forward

- Gently and firmly pull back on the gait belt and the trunk or shoulder; if a handrail is available, grasp the gait belt and use your other hand to grasp the handrail.
- Move closer to the patient, and maintain your anteroposterior stance as you help the person regain balance and stand erect.
- If you are unable to maintain the patient in a standing position, instruct the patient to release the crutches and reach for the handrail; then lower the patient to the stair using the gait belt, or maneuver the patient toward the wall of the stairway.

Balance Lost Backward

- Pivot your body sideward toward the patient and maintain a wide stance with your feet.
- Use one hand to press forward against the pelvis or trunk, and use your other hand to grasp the gait belt or handrail.

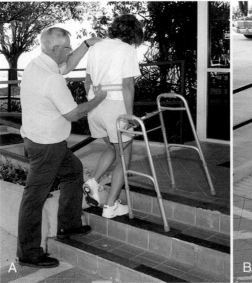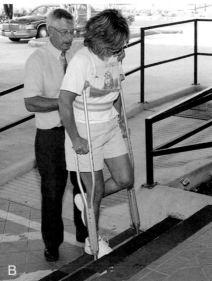

Fig. 9-32   Guarding position for ascending stairs with use of a three-point pattern.

Continued

PROCEDURE 9-8

Guarding Techniques for Stairs, Curbs, and Ramps—cont'd

- Help the patient regain a balanced position.
- If you are unable to maintain the patient in a standing position, instruct the patient to release the crutches and grasp the handrail or lean forward.
- Allow the patient to lean against your body or sit on your thigh, or maneuver the patient toward the wall of the stairway. Regardless of which technique you use, you must prevent the patient from falling backward and causing both of you to fall down the stairs.

Balance Lost to One Side, Toward You

- Use one hand or your shoulder to press against the patient's trunk; use your other hand to grasp the gait belt or handrail.
- Help the patient regain a balanced position or, if that is not possible, help lower the patient to the steps or move the body toward the handrail.

Balance Lost to One Side, Away from You

- Use the gait belt to pull the patient toward you; use your other hand to control the trunk or grasp the handrail.
- Help the patient regain a balanced position or, if that is not possible, lower the patient to the steps or move the body toward the handrail.

DESCENDING A CURB, STAIR, OR RAMP: GUARDING THE PATIENT FROM THE FRONT

- Follow the general considerations listed previously in this procedure.
- Stand in front and to the side of the patient in the area where there is the least protection.
- Place your outside foot on the step onto which the patient will step; place your other foot on the step below.
- Grasp the gait belt with one hand and the handrail, if available, with the opposite hand. If there is no handrail, grasp the gait belt with one hand and position your other hand to lightly touch the patient's shoulder. If your hand does touch the anterior shoulder, it must not restrain the patient's forward movement or cause the patient to alter his or her normal balance.
- Do not allow the patient to develop momentum when descending the stairs. A too-rapid descent is likely to lead to imbalance and increases the possibility of a fall.

Balance Lost Forward

- Move directly in front of the patient, but maintain a wide stance.
- Use one hand to gently but firmly push on the patient's shoulder or chest and on the gait belt; you may prefer to hold firmly to the handrail and the gait belt and move your body toward the patient's chest. Instruct the patient to look up and straighten the trunk or release the aid(s) and grasp the handrail.
- Help the patient regain a balanced position or sit on a step.

- If you are unable to maintain the patient in a standing position, instruct the patient to release the crutches and grasp the handrail, or push on the pelvis or chest while grasping the handrail to maneuver the person toward the wall of the stairway. Regardless of which technique you use, you must prevent the patient from falling forward and causing both of you to fall down the stairs.

Balance Lost Backward

- Pull forward on the gait belt and use your other hand to grasp the handrail. Move closer to the person while maintaining your anteroposterior stance.
- Help the patient regain a balanced position or sit on a step, or instruct the patient to release the aid(s) and grasp the handrail.
- If you are unable to maintain the patient in a standing position, instruct the patient to release the crutches and grasp the handrail, or instruct and help the patient to sit on a step.

Balance Lost to One Side, Toward You

- Use one hand or your shoulder to press against the side of the patient's chest to move the patient away from you; grasp the gait belt with one hand, and if necessary, use one hand to grasp the handrail.
- Help the patient regain a balanced position or, if that is not possible, help the patient to sit on a step or instruct the patient to release the aid(s) and grasp the handrail.

Balance Lost to One Side, Away from You

- Pull on the gait belt to move the patient toward you; use your other hand to grasp the handrail.
- Help the patient regain a balanced position or, if that is not possible, help the patient to sit on a step or instruct the patient to release the aid(s) and grasp the handrail.

DESCENDING A CURB, STAIR, OR RAMP: GUARDING THE PATIENT FROM THE BACK

- Follow the general considerations listed previously in this procedure.
- Stand behind and to the side of the patient in the area where there is the least protection.
- Place one foot on the step on which the patient stands; place the other foot on the step above.
- Grasp the gait belt with one hand and the handrail, if one is available, with your opposite hand. Descend one step with each foot after the patient has descended one step.
- Teach the patient to stop and gain normal balance on each step before progressing to the next step.

Balance Lost Forward

- Pull back on the gait belt, use your other hand to control the trunk or to grasp the handrail, and maintain a wide

PROCEDURE 9-8

Guarding Techniques for Stairs, Curbs, and Ramps—cont'd

stance with your feet. You also may pull back on the gait belt and on an anterior shoulder. The patient may briefly lean backward against you to regain balance and to stand erect.

- Help the patient regain a balanced position to sit on a step, or instruct the patient to release the aid(s) and grasp the handrail.
- If you are unable to maintain the patient in a standing position, instruct the patient to release the crutches and grasp the handrail, or pull back on the gait belt and instruct the patient to sit on a step. Regardless of which technique you use, you must prevent the patient from falling forward and causing both of you to fall down the stairs.

Balance Lost Backward

- Move so you are somewhat behind the patient, press forward at the pelvis or upper thorax, use your other hand to control the trunk or grasp the handrail, and maintain a wide stance with your feet.
- Help the patient regain a balanced position or, if that is not possible, help the patient to sit on a step or instruct the patient to release the aid(s) and grasp the handrail.
- If you are unable to maintain the patient in a standing position, instruct the patient to release the crutches and grasp the handrail or instruct and help the patient to sit on the step.

Balance Lost to One Side, Toward You

- Use your body to support the patient and to prevent him or her from falling to the side; use one hand to grasp the handrail.
- Help the patient regain a balanced position or, if that is not possible, help the patient to sit on a step or instruct the patient to release the aid(s) and grasp the handrail.

Balance Lost to One Side, Away from You

- Pull on the gait belt to move the patient toward you; use your other hand to control the trunk or to grasp the handrail.

- Help the patient regain a balanced position or, if that is not possible, help the patient to sit on a step or instruct the patient to release the aid(s) and grasp the handrail.

Caution: When you pull on the gait belt, do not pull too quickly or use excessive force. You should attempt to correct the movement of the patient by using a firm, smooth pull on the belt. If you pull with excessive force, you may cause further disturbance of the patient's balance. It is recommended that you practice with an unimpaired person who can simulate various loss-of-balance movements to help you develop a sense of the control needed when you use a gait belt.

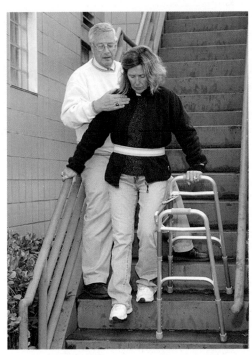

Fig. 9-33   Guarding position for descending stairs (alternative method).

Backward Movement

Four-Point Pattern To move backward in a four-point pattern, instruct the patient to move one assistive device backward and then to step back with the opposite lower extremity, and then move the other assistive device backward and step back with the opposite lower extremity. Continue to repeat the pattern as necessary.

Two-Point Pattern To move backward in a two-point pattern, instruct the patient to simultaneously move one assistive device and the opposite lower extremity backward and then move the opposite aid and lower extremity backward simultaneously. The pattern should be repeated as necessary.

Three-Point Pattern To move backward in a three-point pattern, instruct the patient to start with the crutch tips lateral to, but even with, the toes of the shoes, then step back approximately 6 inches and reposition the crutches. The pattern should be repeated as necessary.

An alternative advanced technique is to instruct the patient to place the crutches approximately 6 inches behind the heels to form a reverse tripod and then step back through the crutches to create a forward tripod. The crutches are repositioned, and the pattern is repeated as necessary.

The first technique is a more stable method because the crutches remain in front of the patient to preserve the forward tripod position. The second pattern should be used only with patients who have excellent balance and coordination.

Three-One–Point Pattern To move backward in a three-one–point pattern, instruct the patient to step back with the stronger lower extremity while maintaining the crutches in front of, or even with, the less functional lower extremity. The patient then steps back with the crutches and the less functional lower extremity to place them in line with the normal foot. The pattern should be repeated as necessary.

An alternative advanced technique is to instruct the patient to simultaneously move the crutches and the weaker lower extremity backward and then step backward with the stronger lower extremity until it is behind the other foot and crutches. The pattern should be repeated as necessary.

Sideward Movement

To move to the right, instruct the patient to position the left assistive device next to the outside of the left foot and the right aid approximately 6 to 8 inches away from the right foot. The patient steps sideward to the right and repositions the aids to sidestep again (Fig. 9-34).

For the four-point, two-point, and three-one–point patterns, instruct the patient to position the aids as described previously to sidestep with the right foot and then with the left foot. Reposition the aid and repeat the pattern as necessary.

For the three-point pattern, instruct the patient to position the crutches as described previously and then support the body weight on the hands and sidestep to the right. Reposition the crutches and repeat the pattern as necessary.

The patient is instructed to reverse the process to sidestep to the left.

Turning Movement

The patient should be taught to turn to the left and to the right regardless of which extremities are weakest or strongest. However, the weaker lower extremity will require more protection or support when the turn is performed, and care must be taken if the patient pivots on that lower extremity. It is suggested that the patient learn to pivot on the stronger lower extremity regardless of which lower extremity is weaker, regardless of the direction of the turn, and regardless of the type of gait pattern used. The assistive device should be used to protect the weaker lower extremity and to provide stability similar to the way the assistive devices are used during level-ground ambulation (Fig. 9-35). For example, a patient who uses bilateral assistive devices or a walker to protect the right lower extremity (RLE) can be taught to turn to the right by initially shifting weight onto the left lower extremity (LLE). The aid and RLE are moved slightly forward and toward the right as the patient pivots toward the right on the LLE. This pattern is repeated until the turn has been completed. The aid is moved in the direction of the turn to provide support and stability by maintaining the patient's COG and vertical gravity line over the BOS. To turn to the left, the aid and RLE are moved forward and to the left as the patient pivots on the LLE.

If the patient is unable to bear weight or pivot on the LLE, he or she can be taught to pivot on the RLE while elevating the LLE from the floor and moving the aid to the left.

It will be more difficult for the patient to turn (pivot) when standing on a carpeted surface. It may be necessary to teach the patient to lift the weight-bearing foot from the carpet to initiate the turn or pivot while supporting weight on the aid and on the weaker lower extremity, if it is possible to bear weight and pivot on the weaker extremity.

Encourage each patient to use caution when turning. Using caution is particularly important for elderly, poorly coordinated, or mentally confused patients. (Note: Turning by pivoting on a lower extremity on which a total hip replacement has been recently performed is absolutely contraindicated. A patient who has undergone a hip replacement must learn to pivot while bearing weight on the nonsurgical lower extremity and must avoid rotation of the pelvis or hip while bearing weight on the surgical lower extremity.)

Curbs and Stairs

Two approaches are used to ascend and descend multiple steps (stairs): (1) with the use of a handrail (banister) and (2) without the use of a handrail. It is usually desirable to initiate stair activities with the patient using a handrail to

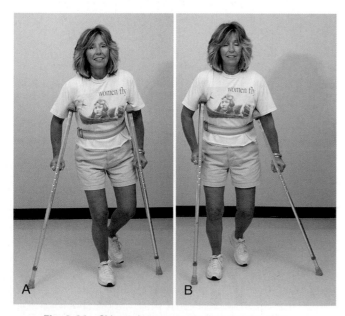

Fig. 9-34 Sideward movement to the patient's right.

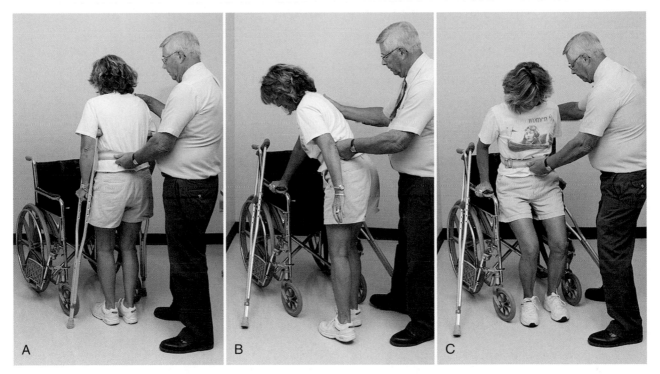

Fig. 9-35   Guarding position for turning movement.

provide maximum stability and a sense of security. However, most patients should be taught to manage stairs without using a handrail because instances are likely to occur when a handrail will not be available.

When a handrail is used, teach the patient to ascend and descend with the handrail on both the left and the right side of the stairs, because handrails may be located on only one side of the stairs in the patient's environment. For example, most stairs leading to a basement or to the second floor of a residence will have only one handrail, which could be located on either the left or right side of the stairs. If only one handrail is present and it is located on the right wall of stairs leading from the first to the second floor, it will be on the patient's right when ascending the stairs but on the left when descending. The patient may develop a preference if two handrails are available. Right-handed patients may prefer to use a handrail on the right because they can use their dominant (stronger) upper extremity on the handrail. Similarly, left-handed patients would probably prefer to use a handrail on the left. In most stair patterns in the United States, the right side of the stairway is used for ascending and descending, so teaching the patient to use the right handrail will prepare him or her for that pattern.

A patient who has only one functional upper extremity and who requires a handrail for support may experience difficulty using a unilateral handrail, depending on its location and whether the stairs are ascended or descended. A patient with a nonfunctional left upper extremity and a limited function LLE and who has functional right upper and lower extremities can be used as an example. Suppose the home has a handrail on the left wall of the stairs leading from the second floor to the first floor. To descend the stairs, the patient can be taught to reach across the body with the right upper extremity and grasp the handrail as he or she steps down first with the LLE and then steps down to the same step with the RLE. An alternative method is to have the patient descend the stairs backward so the right upper extremity will be next to the handrail. If this method is used, the patient steps down with the LLE and then steps onto the same step with the RLE. To ascend the stairs, the handrail will be on the patient's right side and the right upper extremity can be used in the conventional manner. The patient steps up with the RLE and then steps onto the same step with the LLE.

Now suppose the handrail is on the right side of the stairs. To descend the stairs, the patient uses the right upper extremity to grasp the handrail, steps down with the LLE, and then steps to the same step with the RLE. However, to ascend the stairs, the patient can be taught to face the handrail, grasp it with the right upper extremity, step up with the RLE first, and then step up onto the same step with the LLE.

These examples demonstrate the need to interrelate information about the patient and the anticipated environment as you plan and progress through the training program.

Portable, temporary curbs or stairs can be used initially, but actual curbs and stairs also should be available for instruction and practice. Demonstrate the pattern to the patient and reassure the patient that you will provide protection. The patient should not be challenged by a complete flight of stairs (approximately 10 to 12 steps) until a series of three to five steps or a single curb have been practiced. Patients who are NWB on one lower extremity and who have a cast or an orthosis that limits the movements of one lower extremity must be guarded more carefully. You must be certain the patient has sufficient strength, balance, coordination, and endurance to perform curb and stair climbing. The patient who lacks these physical qualities may find it necessary to ascend and descend stairs by sitting and advancing one step at a time using the upper extremities and one or both lower extremities to elevate the body. This method is usually the least desirable and should be used only when the patient is unable to use the other methods described.

Ascending a Curb

Bilateral Canes. To ascend a curb with bilateral canes, the patient places the stronger lower extremity onto the curb and elevates the body while simultaneously raising the weaker lower extremity and both canes onto the curb. An alternative technique is to have the patient place the canes onto the step, step up with the strongest lower extremity, then raise the weaker lower extremity onto the curb. (Note: This method decreases the amount of assistance available from the canes because the angles of the shoulders, elbows, and wrists are changed.)

Unilateral Cane. To ascend a curb with a unilateral cane, the patient places the stronger lower extremity onto the curb and elevates the body onto the curb while simultaneously raising the weaker lower extremity and cane onto the curb (Fig. 9-36). An alternative technique is to have the patient place the cane onto the curb simultaneously with the strongest lower extremity, then raise the weakest lower extremity onto the curb (Fig. 9-37).

Bilateral Crutches. *Three-One–Point Pattern.* To ascend a curb with bilateral crutches in a three-one–point pattern, the patient places the stronger lower extremity onto the curb and elevates the body while simultaneously raising the crutches and the PWB lower extremity onto the curb.

Three-Point Pattern. To ascend a curb with bilateral crutches in a three-point pattern, the patient places the weight-bearing lower extremity onto the curb with the NWB lower extremity held in hip extension and external rotation and knee extension or with the knee flexed. The patient elevates the body using the strongest lower extremity and simultaneously raises the crutches onto the curb and brings the opposite lower extremity forward.

Standard Walker. If the curb is low (4 inches or less), the patient places the walker and the stronger lower extremity onto the curb and elevates the body while simultaneously raising the weaker lower extremity onto the curb (Fig. 9-38). If the curb is of standard height (6 to 8 inches), the patient turns so the back is toward the curb and the walker

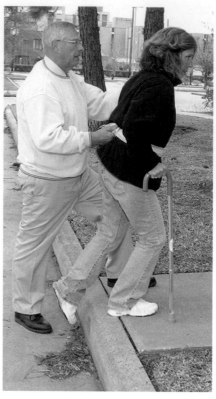

Fig. 9-36 Guarding position for ascending a curb with a unilateral cane.

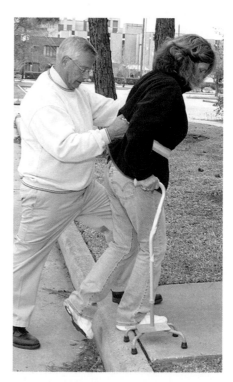

Fig. 9-37 Guarding position for ascending a curb with a unilateral four-footed cane.

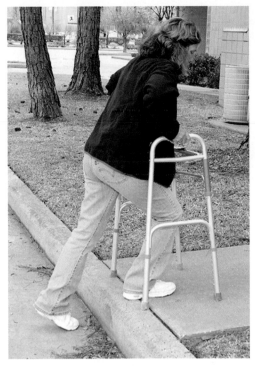

Fig. 9-38   A patient ascending a curb with a walker.

is in front of the body. The patient places the stronger lower extremity onto the curb and elevates the body while simultaneously lifting the walker and other lower extremity onto the curb. The patient backs away from the edge of the curb before turning to move forward. Some patients may be able to ascend a higher curb facing forward using the first method described, but this maneuver may be difficult because the walker may be too high for proper use of the upper extremities. For patients who are NWB, PWB, or have weak lower extremities, it may be easier to ascend the curb in the backward position; FWB patients or patients with good strength but poor balance may want to ascend the curb facing forward to avoid the turning maneuver. The patient should try both methods to determine which can be performed the most efficiently and safely.

Descending a Curb

Bilateral Canes. To descend a curb with bilateral canes, the patient simultaneously places the weaker lower extremity and both canes down onto the surface below while slightly flexing the stronger hip and knee. This latter action will help lower the patient's COG as the canes are lowered. The patient lowers the body with the strongest lower extremity and steps down after the canes and the opposite lower extremity have been placed on the lower surface.

Unilateral Cane. To descend a curb with a unilateral cane, the patient simultaneously steps down with the weaker lower extremity and cane while flexing the stronger lower extremity. The patient lowers his or her body with the strongest lower extremity and steps down after the cane and opposite lower extremity have been placed on the lower surface (Fig. 9-39).

Bilateral Crutches. *Three-One–Point Pattern.* To descend a curb using bilateral crutches with a three-one–point pattern, the same procedure described previously for use with bilateral canes can be taught.

Three-Point Pattern. To descend a curb using bilateral crutches with a three-point pattern, the patient places the crutches down onto the lower surface by slightly flexing the strongest hip and knee. The PWB lower extremity is positioned in front of the patient and over the edge of the curb. The patient steps down using the strongest lower extremity after the crutches and PWB extremity are resting on the lower surface.

Standard Walker. To descend a curb with a standard walker, the patient moves to the edge of the curb and places the walker onto the lower surface while flexing the strongest hip and knee. The weaker lower extremity is positioned in front of the patient and over the edge of the curb. The patient steps between the walker with the weaker lower extremity and then steps down with the strongest lower extremity (Fig. 9-40).

When the patient descends a curb or stairs, it is important to teach him or her to flex the hip and knee of the supporting lower extremity as the assistive device is being placed onto the step below. This technique is especially necessary for the patient using bilateral axillary crutches because it improves the patient's balance and stability. If the patient does not flex the hip and knee to lower the body, the distance between the top of the axillary rest and the axilla will increase greatly when the crutches are placed down on the next step, and the stability of the crutches will be reduced significantly. If only the trunk is inclined forward, the COG will shift forward and the vertical gravity line may not remain within the BOS. In addition, the tendency for the axillary crutches to slip forward or backward is increased when the distance between the axillary rest and the axilla is excessive; this tendency will further reduce the patient's stability. Do not overlook teaching this simple technique during the training program, because the patient's stability and safety will be improved when it is used (Procedure 9-9).

The same sequences described for the curb can be repeated to ascend and descend stairs. However, the patient should be taught initially to use a handrail when ascending or descending stairs to increase stability and safety. As has been noted previously, the patient should learn to use a handrail on the right and left to ascend and descend the stairs, regardless of which lower extremity is weaker, because it may become necessary to use a handrail on either the left or right. In addition, to enhance independence, it is important to teach the patient to ascend and descend stairs without using a handrail. Refer to Procedure 9-9 for specific instructions.

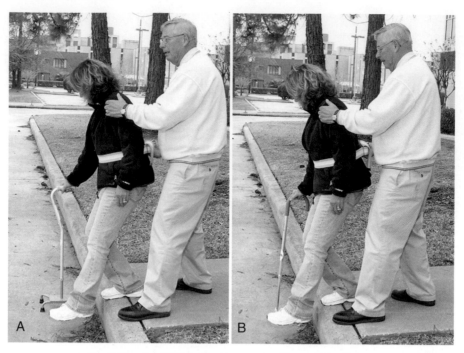

Fig. 9-39   A patient descending a curb with a unilateral cane.

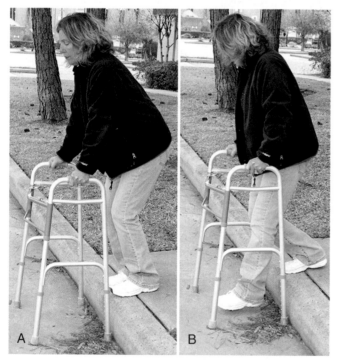

Fig. 9-40   A patient descending a curb with a walker.

Modifications of the patterns used for curbs may be necessary for stairs without handrails and can be used for any ascending or descending activity.

Ascending and Descending Stairs Using a Handrail

Bilateral Canes. To ascend or descend stairs using a handrail and bilateral canes, the patient holds both canes in one hand and uses the other on the handrail. An alternative method is to hold a cane in each hand, grasp the handrail and one cane simultaneously, and use the other cane as described for a curb. The cane held simultaneously with the handrail is held parallel to the direction of the handrail. The lower extremities are used in the same way as described for a curb.

Unilateral Cane. To ascend or descend stairs using a handrail and a unilateral cane, the patient holds the cane and the handrail simultaneously or hangs the cane on the forearm farthest from the handrail, on the belt, or in a pocket and either uses the strong hand to grasp the handrail or grasps the handrail with one hand and uses the cane in the other hand as described for ascending and descending a curb. The lower extremities are used in the same way as described for ascending and descending a curb.

Bilateral Axillary Crutches. To ascend or descend stairs using a handrail and bilateral axillary crutches, the patient places both crutches under the axilla farthest from the handrail while holding on to the handpieces, then grasps the handrail with the other hand. Guarding can be done from the side as demonstrated or from the front (downhill from the patient).

An alternative method is to have the patient place one crutch under the axilla farthest from the handrail and hold the other crutch horizontal to the crutch in the axilla; the hand without the crutch grasps the handrail (Fig. 9-41).

A third method is to have the patient place one crutch under the axilla farthest from the handrail and hold the handrail and the other crutch, which is parallel. The patient should try each of these methods to determine which is

PROCEDURE 9-9

Technique for Ascent and Descent of Stairs with Assistive Aids

For descriptive purposes, assume the right lower extremity (RLE) is the affected or weaker lower extremity when a single cane is used and when non–weight-bearing and partial–weight-bearing crutch patterns are used.

Caution: Whenever a fixed handrail is available, the person should use it for security and stability.

CANE

Ascending Pattern
- The patient faces the stairs and steps up one step with the left lower extremity (LLE).
- The LLE is used to elevate the body as the RLE and cane ascend simultaneously onto the same step.
- The patient establishes balance before ascending to the next step and then repeats the previous activities.

Descending Pattern
- The patient steps down one step with the RLE and cane simultaneously and uses the LLE to lower the body.
- The LLE descends and balance is established with both feet on the same step. These activities are repeated for the next step.

CRUTCHES: NON–WEIGHT BEARING

Ascending Pattern
- The patient faces and stands close to the stairs, uses the crutches for balance and support, and steps up with the LLE.
- The LLE is used to elevate the body as the crutches are lifted onto the same step. The patient extends and externally rotates the RLE or flexes the knee so the toes will not strike the step or become caught under the front edge of the stair tread.
- Balance is established before ascending to the next step.

Descending Pattern
- The patient stands with the LLE and crutches positioned toward the front portion of the stair tread; the RLE is held forward of the front edge of the stair tread, or the knee and hip are flexed so the heel will clear.
- The patient balances on the LLE and lowers the body by partially flexing the left hip and knee; the crutches are placed toward the front portion of the stair tread on the step below.
- The patient uses the crutches for balance and support to step down with the LLE.
- The person establishes balance before descending to the next step.

CRUTCHES: PARTIAL WEIGHT BEARING

Ascending Pattern
- The patient faces and stands close to the stairs and uses the crutches and RLE (partial weight bearing) for balance and support and steps up with the LLE.
- The LLE is used to elevate the body, stepping up with the RLE and lifting the crutches simultaneously onto the same step.
- Balance is established before ascending to the next step.

Descending Pattern
- The patient stands with the feet and crutches positioned toward the front portion of the stair tread.
- The patient balances on the LLE and lowers the body by partially flexing the left hip and knee, then lowers the RLE and crutches simultaneously to the front portion of the stair tread on the step below.
- The crutches and RLE (partial weight bearing) are used for balance and support to step down with the LLE onto the same step.
- Balance is established before descending to the next step.

Note: These same patterns can be used for ascending and descending a curb or other type of single elevation. When two-point and four-point patterns are used, the patient ascends the stairs leading with the stronger lower extremity followed by the other lower extremity and then the assistive devices are lifted simultaneously or alternately. To descend the stairs, the assistive aids are lowered to the step below simultaneously or alternately and then the patient steps down with the weaker lower extremity first, followed by the stronger lower extremity. If there is no strength difference between the lower extremities, either lower extremity may be used as the lead extremity.

most functional. The lower extremities are used in the same way as described for ascending and descending a curb. (Note: A patient who uses forearm crutches also can be taught to use these techniques.)

Standard Walker. Caution: The following techniques for ascending or descending stairs using a handrail and a standard walker are suggested only for patients who have good balance, trunk control, and extremity strength. They should be performed only when a handrail is available and when all of the feet of the walker fit on the stair treads when the walker is positioned along the patient's side. These techniques should be used for *emergency situations* rather than as routine techniques.

Ascending. To ascend stairs using a handrail and a standard walker, the patient faces the stairs and positions the walker along the side farthest from the handrail with the closed side of the walker next to the body. The front feet of the walker are placed one step above the step on which the patient stands; the rear feet remain on the step on which the patient stands (Fig. 9-42).

The patient grasps the handrail and the front hand grip or the midpoint of the horizontal bar of the walker. The

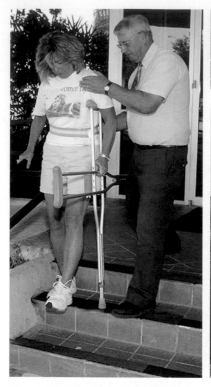

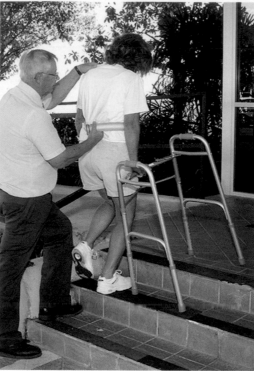

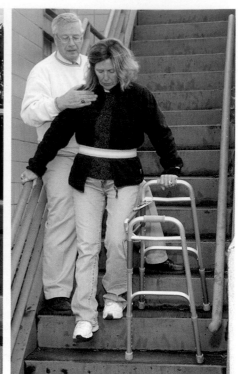

Fig. 9-41 A patient descending stairs with bilateral axillary crutches (alternative method).

Fig. 9-42 A patient ascending stairs with a walker.

Fig. 9-43 A patient descending stairs with a walker.

patient steps up with the stronger lower extremity, elevates the body, and then steps up with or lifts the weaker lower extremity. The walker is advanced up one step by the patient, and the procedure is repeated. The final step at the top of the stair is performed by placing the walker on the upper surface and using it for support as the patient steps up, similar to the way one ascends a curb.

Descending. To descend stairs using a handrail and a standard walker, the patient faces the stairs and positions the walker along the side farthest from the handrail with the closed side of the walker next to the body. The front feet of the walker are placed one step below the step on which the patient stands, and the rear feet remain on the step on which the patient is standing (Fig. 9-43).

The patient grasps the handrail and the rear hand grip or the midpoint of the horizontal bar of the walker. The weaker lower extremity descends first, which is accomplished by flexing the hip and knee of the strongest lower extremity and lowering the body; then the patient steps down with the strongest lower extremity. The walker is advanced down one step, and the procedure is repeated. The patient descends the final step using the same method described to step from a curb.

Ascending and Descending Stairs Using Axillary Crutches Caution: These procedures for ascending and descending stairs using axillary crutches are suggested only for patients who have good balance, trunk control, and strength in both upper extremities and at least one lower extremity (Figs. 9-44 and 9-45). The pattern for ascending and descending stairs is described in Procedure 9-9.

Patients with Casts or Knee Immobilizers

Below-Knee Cast. To ascend stairs or a curb, a patient with a below-knee cast has several options. Each method is designed to protect the foot and lower leg immobilized by the cast, maintain balance, and promote safety and stability for the patient.

The patient extends the hip and flexes the knee to 90 degrees so the toes will clear the curb or the stair lip. As an alternative, the patient extends and externally rotates the hip and flexes the knee.

The method selected for each patient will depend on the patient's strength, balance, coordination, and, in some instances, personal preference. The patient should try each of these methods to determine which one can be performed most effectively.

Several options are available to descend stairs or a curb. First, the patient can flex the hip and knee to 90 degrees so the heel clears the stair tread and then position the lower leg in front of the body when stepping down, or the patient can partially flex his or her hip and maintain the knee in

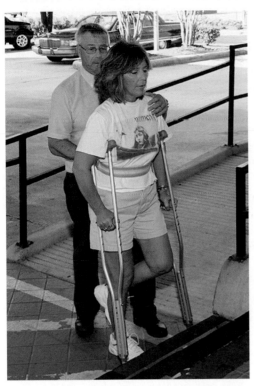

Fig. 9-44   A patient positioned to ascend stairs using bilateral axillary crutches in a non–weight-bearing pattern.

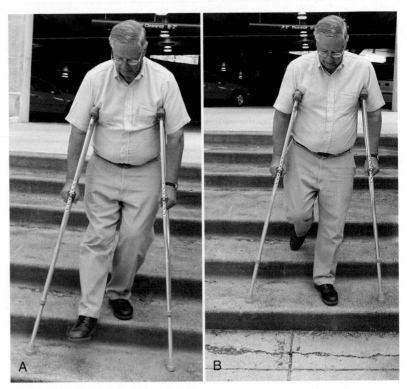

Fig. 9-45   **A,** The proper way to descend stairs independently using crutches in a non–weight-bearing pattern. **B,** The improper way to descend stairs independently using crutches in a non–weight-bearing pattern.

extension so the heel clears the stair tread (see Fig. 9-45, A). Do not teach the patient to flex the knee to 90 degrees with the hip extended because the toes are likely to contact the curb surface or stair tread when stepping down (see Fig. 9-45, B).

Full-Length Cast or Knee Immobilizer. To ascend stairs or a curb while wearing a full-length cast or knee immobilizer, the patient should extend and externally rotate the hip so the toes clear the stair lip or riser or the front of the curb when stepping up. The immobilized extremity will trail the body as the patient steps up.

To descend stairs or a curb while wearing a full-length cast or knee immobilizer, the patient partially flexes the hip so the heel clears the stair tread or curb. The immobilized lower extremity remains in front of the patient and leads the body when he or she steps down.

Doors

Patients who use assistive devices should be taught to manage opening and closing various types of doors. The patient should be familiar with several techniques to control doors with and without self-closing devices (i.e., automatic door closers). It is likely that the patient will prefer to use only one of these techniques, but independence will be enhanced if more than one method is learned and mastered.

Self-Closing Door If the door opens away from the patient, the door is approached at an angle so the patient faces the side of the door that will open (i.e., with the back to the hinges) (Fig. 9-46, A). The patient remains close to the door and the doorknob, latch, or crash bar, uses one hand to open the door, and shifts the body weight onto the opposite crutch and lower extremity, if weight bearing is permitted on that extremity. The door is opened with a quick push, and the patient returns the hand from the doorknob or crash bar to the crutch. The crutch nearest to the door is moved so the crutch tip engages the floor and the bottom of the door and serves as a doorstop (Fig. 9-46, B). The door can be opened wider by repeating this procedure as the patient moves through the doorway.

The patient moves through the doorway by pushing against the door to open it farther and by repositioning the crutch tip to keep the door open. The patient must be certain that the final step through the doorway will place the body beyond the closing arc of the door. (Note: If the door has a crash bar, the patient should open the door by pushing on the crash bar near to where it is attached to the door close to the door latch; this technique will give the patient the greatest advantage to open the door with the least expenditure of energy. A crutch tip can be used to keep the door open (Fig. 9-46, C) or, with the back to the

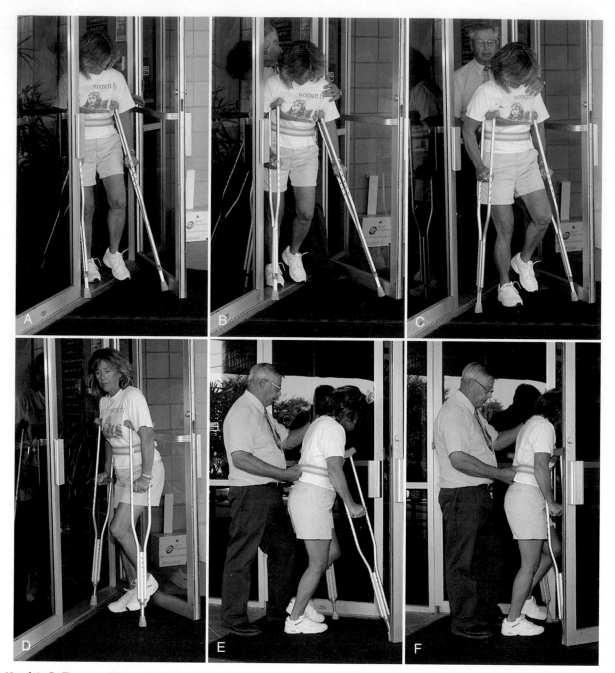

Fig. 9-46   **A** to **D,** The use of bilateral axillary crutches to negotiate a self-closing door that opens away from the patient. **E** and **F,** Use of bilateral axillary crutches to negotiate a self-closing door that opens toward the patient.

door, the body can be used to keep the door open while moving sideward (Fig. 9-46, *D*).

Some patients may prefer to place both crutches under the axilla farthest from the crash bar, holding them with the corresponding hand while grasping the crash bar with the hand nearest to the crash bar. The patient may use the crash bar as a support when stepping through the door. The patient must be instructed to push downward rather than outward on the bar while moving through the doorway to avoid opening the door too wide and affecting the BOS.

The crutches will need to be repositioned into each axilla to take the last step through the doorway.

If the door opens toward the patient, the patient approaches the opening edge of the door at an angle, facing toward the hinge side of the door. By being positioned at an angle to the door, the patient will be able to open the door a smaller amount than would be necessary if standing directly in front of it. The patient positions the body close to the door, but slightly outside the area needed to open it. The body weight is shifted onto the crutch hand grip farthest from the doorknob or latch, and the hand nearest the doorknob or latch is used to open the door by quickly pulling on the doorknob and then returning the hand from the doorknob to grip the crutch. The crutch nearest to the open edge of the door is moved so the crutch tip engages the floor and the bottom of the door to serve as a doorstop (Fig. 9-46, E). If necessary, the door can be opened wider before the patient moves through the doorway. The patient moves through the doorway by pushing against the door and repositioning the crutch tip against the bottom of the door (Fig. 9-46, F). The patient must be certain that the final step through the doorway will place the body beyond the door frame and the closing of the door.

The same procedures can be used for forearm crutches, canes, or a walker.

Standard Doors   The patient uses the same positions and techniques previously described for a door that opens away from or toward the person. However, the patient will need to open the door only wide enough for the crutches, canes, or walker and the patient to move through the doorway. The door does not need to be opened to its full width if the patient is taught to move through the doorway at an angle. The crutch or cane tip or the walker feet are not required to restrain the door. The patient will need to turn to close the door and then move sideward or backward after the door has been closed to resume the gait pattern and direction. When the door opens toward the patient, it may be necessary to back up while opening the door, especially if the door cannot be approached at an angle toward or facing the opening edge of the door.

Ascending or Descending Ramps, Inclines, or Hills

Patients can ascend a ramp, incline, or hill by using techniques similar to those used to ascend a curb or stairs. The patient should advance the aid and the stronger lower extremity before advancing the weaker lower extremity; a shorter stride may be necessary. Patients with a full-length cast or knee immobilizer will need to extend and externally rotate the hip to clear the foot when ascending the ramp, incline, or hill and will need to flex the hip when descending. With a below-knee cast, that extremity should be extended at the hip and flexed at the knee when ascending (Fig. 9-47). On a steep incline or hill, the patient may need to "zigzag" by moving diagonally when ascending or descending.

Patients can descend a ramp, incline, or hill by using techniques similar to those used to descend a curb or stairs, but the stride and placement of the assistive device(s) should be shortened (Fig. 9-48). The patient advances the weaker lower extremity and assistive device before advancing the stronger lower extremity using a short stride. Patients with a full-length cast or knee immobilizer will need to partially flex the hip to clear the foot and lead with the

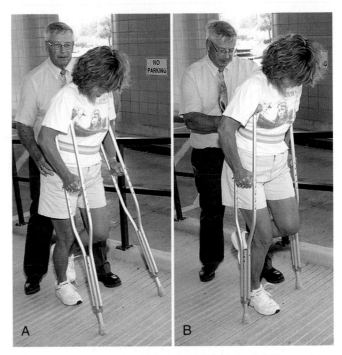

Fig. 9-47   A patient ascending a ramp with bilateral axillary crutches in a non–weight-bearing pattern.

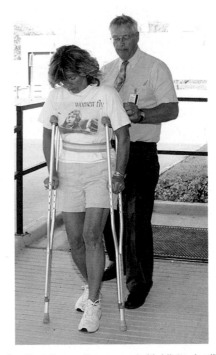

Fig. 9-48   A patient descending a ramp with bilateral axillary crutches in a partial weight-bearing pattern.

immobilized extremity. With a below-knee cast, the hip and knee should be partially flexed, with the foot positioned in front of the body to clear the foot; alternatively, the hip should be partially flexed and the knee extended to clear the foot. The affected lower extremity should not be allowed to trail the body. On a steep incline or hill, the patient may need to zigzag by moving diagonally when descending or ascending.

Elevator Access

Patients should be taught to enter and leave the elevator in a forward position whenever possible. The assistive device or the patient's hand or arm can be used to activate the device that automatically prevents the door from closing, but the patient will need to determine the type of device used to control the door (e.g., a photoelectrical beam, pressure bar, or rubber-covered flange on the edge of the door). The patient should be taught to observe the area where the floor of the elevator and the floor of the corridor meet because a space may exist between the two surfaces, and the tip of the crutch, cane, or walker must not be placed in that space. Furthermore, when some elevator cars stop, the floor may not be level with the corridor floor; patients should be alert for this potential hazard. After the patient is in the elevator, he or she will need to turn around to face forward in preparation for exiting the car and to use the control panel.

Automobile Access

Frequently, patients will find it more convenient to enter and leave a vehicle from the passenger side to avoid interference from the steering wheel. It is usually easier for patients to enter and exit automobiles that have two doors rather than four doors because in such cars the door is wider, thus providing more space in which to sit; in addition, access to the rear seat area to store the aid is more convenient (Procedure 9-10). The transfer can be performed more easily if the car seat is positioned back as far as possible to provide greater space for the lower extremities.

To enter the vehicle, the patient should approach the door at an angle so it opens away from the body (Fig. 9-49, A and B) and open it only as far as necessary to have access to the seat. The patient pivots the body to face away from the car interior and places both crutches in one hand; the other hand can be placed on the back of the seat, on the dashboard, or on the door with the window rolled down (Fig. 9-49, C and D). The patient lowers onto the seat and places the lower extremities and assistive device(s) into the vehicle (Fig. 9-49, E and F). The patient will need to slide across the seat if the car was entered on the passenger side and he or she is to drive. The patient with a full-length cast or knee immobilizer may be more comfortable in the back seat because the extremity can be placed on the seat. To drive an automobile with an automatic transmission with the RLE immobilized, that extremity can be placed on the front seat or on the floor on the passenger side of the car, or the seat can be adjusted to its most rearward position to provide more space between the front seat and the foot controls. It is not recommended that a patient drive with the RLE immobilized unless absolutely necessary. The

---

PROCEDURE 9-10

Standing Transfer Into an Automobile

TRANSFER WITH CRUTCHES

- Instruct the patient to approach the passenger door at an angle; position yourself to guard the patient by standing behind him or her and to one side.
- The patient reaches to open the door, opens it, and shifts the crutches into the hand farthest from the car.
- The free hand is positioned on a solid surface of the car (e.g., the roof, back of the seat, dashboard, door frame, or window frame with the window completely lowered), and the patient pivots so his or her back is toward the car seat.
- The body is lowered onto the car seat using the upper extremities and functional lower extremity.
- The patient pivots and places the lower extremities into the car, the crutches are placed in the car, the car door is closed, and the seat restraints are applied.

Note: For many persons, the transfer will be performed more easily if the car seat is positioned back as far as possible, and the front seat is entered. This position will make it easier to place the lower extremities and crutches in the car.

---

patient with a full-length cast or knee immobilizer on the LLE will have difficulty driving the vehicle because it will be difficult to position the LLE and still have access to the steering wheel and to the foot controls. (Caution: A person with an immobilized lower extremity should not attempt to drive an automobile with a standard transmission. A person wearing an ankle immobilizer or boot should be discouraged from driving an automobile because of the immobilizer's size and because it is difficult to maneuver.)

To leave the car, the patient opens the car door, obtains the assistive device, and adjusts the body so the lower extremities are placed outside the car. The patient grasps both crutches in one hand and places the other hand on the back of the seat, on the dashboard, or on the door frame with the window rolled down. The patient uses the upper and lower extremities to push to a standing position, places the crutches in each axilla, and steps away from the car. It may be necessary for the patient to turn to close the door and then to move backward before resuming the gait pattern and direction of travel. (Caution: The patient should never use the window glass for support.)

Transferring to the Floor from Crutches

Instances may occur when a patient wishes to sit on the floor or the ground. Several methods can be taught to allow movement from standing to sitting on the floor. This activity is not to be confused with a protective fall; transferring to the floor is an activity that the patient controls and performs independently.

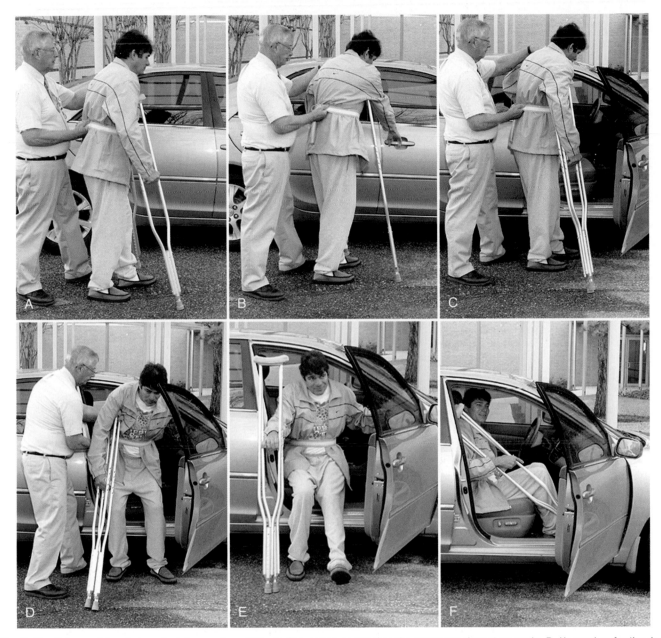

Fig. 9-49 Using crutches to transfer into a motor vehicle. **A,** The person approaches the passenger door at an angle. **B,** He reaches for the door latch. **C,** The door is opened and the crutches are placed in one hand. **D** and **E,** The person pivots, places the free hand on the dashboard, and lowers his body onto the car seat using the upper extremities and the uninvolved lower extremity. **F,** The lower extremities and crutches are placed in the car.

If the patient is NWB on one lower extremity and uses bilateral axillary crutches, both crutches are dropped to the floor and balance is maintained briefly on the strongest lower extremity. The patient then reaches forward toward the floor with the upper extremities while flexing the stronger lower extremity and extending and externally rotating the hip of the weaker lower extremity. The patient lowers the body using the strongest lower extremity until his or her hands contact the floor. The patient can kneel on the strongest knee or turn the hips and sit on the hip of the strongest lower extremity to complete the activity.

Another method would be to instruct the patient to drop both crutches and reach backward toward the floor with the upper extremities, flex the hip of the weaker lower extremity and slide the heel forward on the floor, then flex the hip and knee of the strongest lower extremity. The patient lowers his or her body using the strongest lower extremity until the hands contact the floor and then sits on the floor to complete the activity. Alternatively, you can instruct the patient to shift both crutches to the hand on the side of the weaker lower extremity and grasp both handpieces (Fig. 9-50, A and B). The body is lowered using the strongest

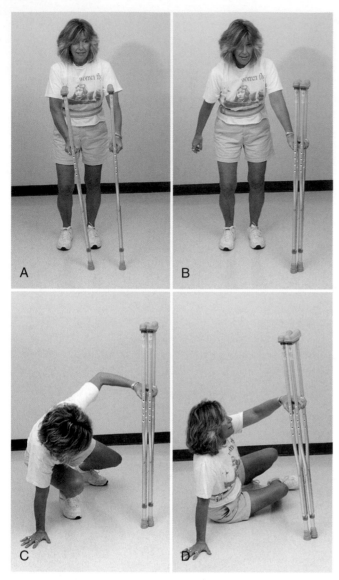

Fig. 9-50 A patient transferring to the floor using crutches.

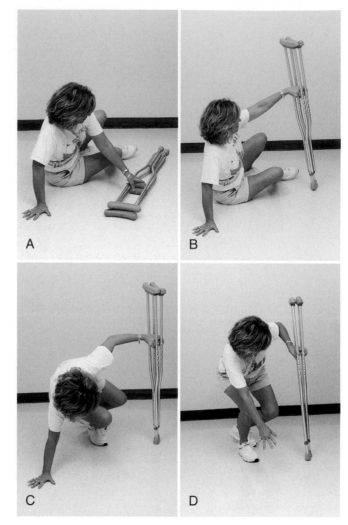

Fig. 9-51 A patient rising from the floor to a standing position using crutches.

lower extremity and the hand holding the crutches while reaching toward the floor with the opposite upper extremity (Fig. 9-50, C). The patient sits on the floor to complete the activity (Fig. 9-50, D).

Note that the patient can be taught all of these techniques or only one of them depending on his or her strength, coordination, balance, flexibility, and personal preference. The same techniques can be used for the patient who is able to partially bear weight on one lower extremity and fully bear weight on the other lower extremity.

Rising from the Floor to Standing

When rising from the floor to standing, if the patient is NWB on one lower extremity and uses bilateral axillary crutches, he or she turns so the hands and the foot of the strongest lower extremity are on the floor and assumes a

half-kneeling position with that one lower extremity. The hip of the weaker lower extremity is extended and externally rotated. The crutches are positioned within easy reach, and the patient pushes to a standing position using the strongest lower extremity and the upper extremities. The patient picks up the crutches with one hand and grasps the handpieces while still in a semistanding position. The trunk is extended, and then the patient stands erect and positions the crutches in each axilla to complete the activity.

Alternatively, the patient side sits and grasps both crutches, holding them on the same side as the weaker lower extremity (Fig. 9-51, A). The crutches are held vertically by the handpieces with the hand on the side of the weaker or more affected lower extremity (Fig. 9-51, B). The patient pushes to stand using the strongest lower extremity and both hands (Fig. 9-51, C and D); after standing, the crutches are positioned into each axilla (see Fig. 9-50, A).

In a third technique, the patient sits on the floor and flexes the strongest hip and knee so the foot is flat on the floor. The weaker lower extremity is maintained in front of the body. The patient holds both crutches by the hand-pieces, using the hand on the same side as the weaker lower extremity, or the crutches may be placed between the thighs with both hands grasping the crutch handpieces. The patient pushes to a standing position using the strongest lower extremity and the upper extremities holding the crutches; after standing, the crutches are positioned into each axilla.

Similar methods or techniques can be used for patients who use assistive devices other than axillary crutches. In some instances, the patient may prefer to use a firm object (e.g., a table, chair, sofa, tree trunk, bench, or railing) for support and stability to move to the floor or return to standing. However, the patient will be more independent when it is possible to perform these activities without the use of a firm object because such an object may not be available or accessible. Special needs or techniques may need to be resolved by problem solving with the patient. Some risks to patient safety are associated with this activity, so you must use caution. Guard the patient and use a gait belt when these techniques are practiced.

Falling Techniques

Falling Backward The patient should be taught to control his or her body if a backward fall occurs. Instruct the patient to release the crutches (or other aid), flex the trunk, and bring the chin to the chest while reaching forward (Fig. 9-52). Using this method, the force of the fall will be absorbed by the buttocks and back, and the head will be protected.

It is not recommended that the patient be taught to reach backward with the upper extremities for protection. When this method is used, the head will tend to move backward and it is more likely to strike the floor or ground. This method also can produce strains or sprains of the shoulders or elbows and fractures of the wrists. (Caution: If this activity is demonstrated or practiced, floor mats should be used to prevent injury) (Procedure 9-11).

Falling Forward When falling forward while using crutches, the patient should be taught to release the crutches so they fall to each side and reach toward the floor with the upper extremities. The patient should "break" the fall with the upper extremities and lower his or her body to the floor.

PROCEDURE 9-11

Protective Fall When Using Crutches

These procedures should be described and demonstrated by the caregiver before the patient attempts them; when the activity is practiced, the patient must be guarded closely and protective mats should be placed on the floor to prevent injury.

FORWARD FALL
- The patient releases the crutches and quickly flips them to the side; the crutches must not fall to the floor in front of the body.
- The patient reaches forward with both upper extremities and turns the head to one side.
- When the hands contact the floor, the elbows are bent to absorb some of the force of the fall.
- The body is lowered to the floor, and if no serious injury has occurred, the crutches are gathered in preparation for standing using one of the techniques presented in this chapter.

BACKWARD FALL
- The patient releases the crutches and quickly flips them to the side; the crutches must not fall to the floor behind the body.
- The patient tucks the chin toward the chest and reaches forward with both upper extremities.
- A semiflexed trunk position is maintained so the buttocks and trunk contact the floor before the back of the head.
- If no serious injury has occurred, the crutches are gathered in preparation for standing using one of the techniques presented in this chapter.

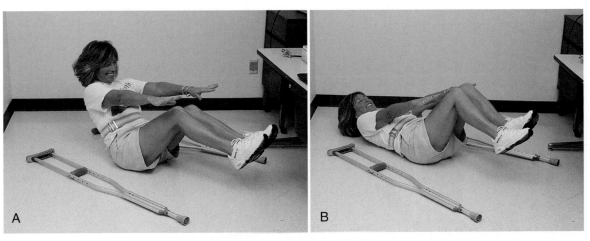

Fig. 9-52   The technique for teaching a patient how to fall backward while using crutches.

Turning the face to one side may reduce facial injuries (see Fig. 9-9).

SUMMARY

Ambulation with an aid or aids can be a potentially hazardous or dangerous activity for a patient. Therefore it is important to emphasize specific precautions to the patient and family to promote safety.

All assistive devices should be inspected and evaluated frequently for damage or disrepair. Nuts, adjustment buttons, tips, and hand grips must be secure and properly tightened or applied before the aid is used for ambulation. The patient should be instructed to examine the equipment periodically and maintain it properly. The family and the patient should be instructed to maintain the environment of the home so it will be free of hazards that could lead to patient injury. For example, small area (throw) rugs should be removed; extension cords should not lie on the floor in an area where people walk; linoleum or tile floors should not be waxed or highly polished; smooth floor surfaces should be dry and any fluids spilled should be removed immediately; wall or grab bars must be attached to wall studs, not to the wall board or plaster; one or two handrails may need to be added to stairs; and furniture should be arranged to provide adequate space for the patient to maneuver. Safety information can be provided in written form, and you should document your activities and the patient's performance according to the policies of the facility or agency with which you are employed or associated (Box 9-5).

Each patient must be instructed in the proper gait pattern and how to perform selected functional activities before initiating ambulation or attempting each functional activity. You must guide, encourage, and correct the patient until he or she is proficient and competent to perform the gait pattern safely. In addition, you must guard and protect the patient throughout the training sessions by using proper positioning and a gait belt. Demonstrations are helpful and usually necessary as part of the teaching-learning cycle. The family should be instructed how to protect or manage the patient at home, and written instructions should be provided.

The patient should be reminded to bear the body weight on the hands rather than on the axillary bars of the axillary crutch to avoid possible injury to nerves and circulatory vessels located in the floor of the axilla. The axillary bar must not be used as the primary weight-bearing surface during ambulation or when the patient is standing. Finally, inform the patient and the family how to contact you for advice or assistance after the patient has returned home. This information should be provided in writing and should include your business telephone number and the hours you are available.

self-study ACTIVITIES

- Describe the patient characteristics and abilities necessary to perform the following gait patterns: two-point, four-point, three-point (non–weight bearing), three-one–point (partial weight bearing), and modified two-point or four-point.
- Discuss the factors you would consider when selecting each of the following assistive devices: canes, axillary crutches, platform crutches, forearm crutches, walker, and parallel bars.
- Outline the assessment or evaluation techniques and procedures you would perform before initiating a gait pattern that requires assistive devices or equipment. Provide a rationale for the selection of the techniques.
- Explain how you would initially measure and confirm the fit of each assistive device; state the important principles related to the proper fit of the device.
- Explain how you would instruct a patient to use a unilateral assistive device, and provide a rationale for your instructions.
- Describe how you would guard a patient ambulating on a level surface or on stairs and when moving from a sitting to a standing position and from a standing to a sitting position.
- Describe how you would monitor a patient's response to ambulation activities and how you would use the findings to plan the patient's treatment.
- What type of assistive device would you choose for a person with Parkinson disease?

problem SOLVING

1. A 52-year-old patient with a full-length, non–weight bearing cast on the lower left extremity uses bilateral axillary crutches and is to be discharged tomorrow. He tells you that he must enter and leave his workplace through a door that has a strong self-closing device. He must pull the door to enter and push it to exit, the door has no crash bar, and a threshold must be crossed. How would you instruct him to enter and leave the building safely?

| Box **9-5** | Precautions for Ambulation in the Home |

- Remove small rugs or mats that are likely to slip or slide (e.g., area or throw rugs); be extremely cautious when using a bath mat.
- Avoid waxing floors, or use a "nonskid" wax.
- Immediately wipe fluids from noncarpeted floors.
- Check assistive devices weekly for cracks, loose nuts, or worn tips; clean dust and dirt on tips.
- Remove items stored on stair steps; be certain stair handrails are secure and strong.
- Position furniture in each room to provide a 36-inch-wide unobstructed pathway when possible; eliminate electrical cords or other loose objects from walking surfaces.
- Provide safety (grab) bars for the toilet, shower, and bathtub; be certain they are attached to wall studs or the floor.

2. A 14-year-old girl with a below-knee partial weight-bearing cast on the right lower extremity (RLE) must learn to ascend and descend steps so she can get to her bedroom at home and classrooms at school. The only handrail at either location is to her right as she ascends the stairs. What assistive device would you use and what instructions or directions will you give her to make this activity safe and effective?

3. You have been asked to give instructions for ambulation to a 45-year-old patient with a severe fracture of the RLE. He has an external fixation device and is apprehensive about ascending and descending stairs. What assistive device would you choose and what instructions or directions would you give him in teaching this necessary activity?

4. A 43-year-old woman has sustained a fracture of her right distal tibia and comes to the department directly from the emergency department. Orders are for gait training, NWB on the RLE. What questions would be appropriate to ask the patient concerning her home environment? Which assistive devices would you select for her, and what gait pattern would you choose? What activities would you teach her, and what would be your discharge goals?

5. You have a 36-year-old patient with a diagnosis of paraplegia/paresis. Both legs circumduct, and his steps are short, shuffling, and scraping; the legs scissor. What type of walking aid(s) is/are appropriate for this patient, and what gait pattern would you choose to teach?

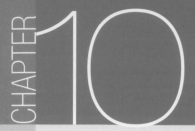

Special Equipment and Patient Care Environments

objectives *After studying this chapter, the reader will be able to:*

- Describe the use of some equipment used for special patient needs.
- Describe the precautions necessary when treating a patient using the equipment.
- Describe the progression for treating a patient in the intensive care unit.
- Understand and apply appropriate measures to resolve selected patient emergencies.
- Define acronyms used to describe special patient care units (e.g., BWICU, CCU, CSICU, CVICU, ED, ER, GICU, ICU, MICU, MSICU, NICU, OHRU, OIR, PACU, PICU, RICU, SCN, SICU, STICU, TICU, and TNCC).
- Describe treatments and special support equipment or systems that could be used with a patient in a special care unit.

key terms

Anticoagulation   The use of drugs to render the blood sufficiently unable to create a clot or mass to discourage thrombosis.

Arrhythmia   Variation from the normal rhythm, especially of the heartbeat.

Arterial monitoring line (A line)   A catheter inserted into an artery and attached to an electronic monitoring system to directly measure arterial blood pressure.

Catheter   A rubber, plastic, metal, or glass tube used to remove or inject fluids into a person.

Comminuted   Broken or crushed into small pieces.

Cyanosis   A bluish discoloration of the skin and mucous membranes caused by excessive concentration of reduced hemoglobin in the blood.

Dialysis   The diffusion of solute molecules through a semipermeable membrane passing from the side of higher concentration to the side of lower concentration; a method used in cases of defective renal function to remove elements from the blood that are normally excreted in the urine (hemodialysis).

Electrocardiogram (ECG or EKG)   A graphical record of the heart's electrical action derived by amplification of the minutely small electrical impulses normally generated by the heart.

Endotracheal tube (ETT)   A hollow tube, approximately 10 inches long, with an inflatable cuff near one end that is inserted and positioned in the trachea. After the tube has been positioned, the cuff is inflated to maintain the tube's position so the patient can breathe through the tube.

Fistula   Any abnormal, tube-like passage within body tissue, usually between two internal organs or leading from an internal organ to the body surface.

Fowler position   A position in which the head of the patient's bed is raised 18 to 20 inches above level, with the knees flexed.

Gastrointestinal (GI)   Pertaining to the stomach and intestines.

Hyperventilation   Abnormally prolonged and deep breathing.

Hypoxemia   Deficient oxygenation of the blood.

Infusion   The slow therapeutic introduction of fluid other than blood into a vein.

Infusion pump (IMED, IVAC)   An electronic device designed to automatically control the flow and rate of intravenous fluids into a patient.

International Normalized Ratio (INR)   A system established for reporting the results of blood coagulation or clotting tests.

Intravenous (IV)   Administration of fluids into a vein through the use of a steel needle or plastic catheter.

Intravenous therapy   The introduction of a fluid into a person's vein; nutrients or medications may be supplied intravenously.

Mediastinum   The mass of tissues and organs separating the sternum in front and the vertebral column behind, containing the heart and its large vessels, trachea, esophagus, thymus, lymph nodes, and other structures and tissues.

Micturition   Voiding of urine.

Monitor   An apparatus designed to observe, report, and measure a given condition or phenomenon such as blood pressure, heart rate, or respiration rate.

Myocardial infarction (MI)   Necrosis of the cells of an area of the heart muscle resulting from oxygen deprivation caused by obstruction of the blood supply.

Nasogastric (NG) tube   A plastic tube usually inserted into a nostril and ending in the stomach. It can be used to remove fluid or gas from the stomach, monitor the digestive function of the stomach, administer medications or nutrients, or obtain specimens of the stomach contents.

Oximeter   A photoelectrical device that measures oxygen saturation of the blood (also known as a pulse oximeter).

Patent   Open, unobstructed, or not closed.

Pneumothorax   Accumulation of air or gas in the pleural cavity resulting in collapse of the lung on the affected side.

Respirator   See ventilator.

Shunt   A passage or anastomosis between two natural vessels, especially between blood vessels.

Stoma   An artificial permanent opening, especially in the abdominal wall, that is made in surgical procedures.

Suprapubic   Above the pubis.

Swan-Ganz catheter   A long intravenous tube inserted into a vein (usually the basilic or subclavian vein) and terminating in the pulmonary artery. A monitor attached to the catheter measures the pulmonary artery pressure and the pulmonary capillary wedge pressure; it permits evaluation of cardiac function.

Tachypnea   Very rapid respirations.

Tract   A longitudinal assemblage of tissues or organs—especially a bundle of nerve fibers having a common origin, function, and termination—or several anatomic structures arranged in a series and serving a common function.

Traction   The exertion of a pulling or distracting force to maintain a proper position of bone ends or joints to facilitate the healing process.

Trendelenburg position   A position in which the patient lies supine with the head lower than the remainder of the body.

Turning frame   An apparatus that allows a patient's position to be changed from supine to prone and vice versa by one person by maintaining the patient's position between two frames of the apparatus; the patient may be turned horizontally or vertically depending on the apparatus used.

Ventilator   A mechanical apparatus designed to intermittently or continuously assist or control pulmonary ventilation (breathing); also referred to as a respirator.

Wedge pressure   Intravascular pressure measured by a catheter inserted into the pulmonary artery (Swan-Ganz catheter) to permit indirect measurement of mean left atrial pressure.

INTRODUCTION

Many patients who occupy hospital beds are acutely ill and require extensive nursing care. The equipment and technology available to treat and monitor these patients have improved dramatically during the past several years. Life-supporting or life-sustaining equipment is commonplace. Patients who probably would not have survived life-threatening trauma or illness several years ago are surviving now because of advances in medical treatment and equipment. Requests for treatment of these seriously ill patients by various members of the rehabilitation team have increased, in part because medical and nursing personnel have recognized the advantages of the early application of rehabilitation techniques for these patients. Consequently, occupational therapists, physical therapists, respiratory therapists, and other caregivers have become integral

---

Box 10-1 Specialized Patient Care Units

BWICU: Burn wound intensive care unit
CCU: Coronary (cardiac) care unit or critical care unit
CSICU: Cardiac surgery intensive care unit
CVICU: Cardiovascular intensive care unit
ER or ED: Emergency room or emergency department
GICU: Geriatric intensive care unit
ICU: Intensive care unit or intermediate care unit
MICU: Medical intensive care unit or mobile intensive
    care unit
MSICU: Medical surgical intensive care unit
NICU: Neurological (neuro) intensive care unit or
    neonatal intensive care unit
OHRU: Open heart recovery unit
OIR: Overnight intensive recovery
PACU: Postanesthesia care unit
PICU: Pediatric or psychiatric intensive care unit
RICU: Respiratory intensive care unit
SCN: Special care nursery
SICU: Surgical intensive care unit
STICU: Surgical trauma intensive care unit
TICU: Trauma intensive care unit
TNCC: Trauma-neuro intensive care unit

---

members of this medical management team. Many of these very ill patients initially are managed in specialized nursing units (Box 10-1).

The initial exposure to the equipment (especially mechanical ventilators) and devices used in these units can overwhelm and intimidate an inexperienced, uninformed practitioner. According to Perme and Chandrashekar (see the Bibliography), the early mobilization of a patient in the intensive care unit (ICU) who is receiving mechanical ventilation is an advanced physical and occupational therapy skill and requires specialized proficiency and instruction in specific areas that affect clinical decision making. Policies and procedures may vary by facility for all caregivers entering the ICU. The policies should be reviewed prior to provision of the initial treatment. In this book, descriptions of some of the equipment and devices frequently used to treat the seriously involved patient are presented to help the caregiver become better prepared to treat these patients in a specialized environment. However, the caregiver should be oriented specifically to the equipment and treatment protocols in each employment setting before providing patient care. If a patient emergency occurs, the caregiver should know whom to contact for assistance.

ORIENTATION TO THE SPECIAL INTENSIVE CARE UNIT

A typical patient cubicle in an ICU is likely to have several types of equipment to monitor the patient's physiological state, provide ventilation and intravenous (IV) therapy, deliver oxygen, and remove fluids from the patient (i.e., suction). The patient may have IV lines, an arterial

monitoring line (A line), a central venous catheter, a urinary catheter, drainage tubes such as an underwater sealed drain, a pulse oximeter, oxygen, or leads going from the patient to a monitor of vital signs; the patient also may be receiving respiratory support from a ventilator (respirator). Therefore it is suggested that at least two caregivers, preferably one who is familiar with the patient, be present during the initial therapy session. After you have reviewed the medical record and spoken to the patient's primary caregiver, take a few minutes to observe the unit and the patient before you initiate any treatment. Some patients will be alert, and others may be comatose or unresponsive. Most patients in specialized care units are acutely ill or seriously traumatized.

Before initiating any treatment for patients who are cognizant, it is important to obtain the patient's consent and explain the risks and advantages of treatment. Allow the patient sufficient time to ask questions.

If you are unfamiliar with the equipment being used by a patient, obtain assistance from the patient's nurse or participate in a program designed to prepare you to treat patients who are in the unit (Figs. 10-1 and 10-2, A and B). The following patient factors should be considered before and during patient treatment:

- Medical history, history of current illness, and prior level of function
- Sedation and level of alertness
- Cognition and ability to learn
- Active participation level
- Medical stability
- Activity tolerance
- Adequate proximal muscle strength to participate in active mobility training

An excellent overview of safety issues to consider before mobilizing critically ill patients has been presented in Figure 10-3.

When the patient is acutely ill, it will be necessary to reduce the intensity of the treatment that you might use with less ill patients. Shorter treatment sessions, fewer exercise repetitions, and less demand for active participation by the patient may be necessary. Careful and continuous monitoring of the patient's response to treatment will be required through observation of and communication with the patient, awareness of vital signs displayed on a monitor, and a comparison of the current responses with previous responses to treatment. It is recommended that you discuss the patient's current condition with the primary nursing person and/or the patient's physician prior to treatment, because a patient's condition may fluctuate from hour to hour and you may not be able to rely on information obtained at your previous visit or the most recent note in the medical record. Treatment guidelines and precautions for patients in the ICU are discussed in Procedures 10-1 and 10-2.

In a 2009 study presented by Phend in *Med Page Today* (see the Bibliography), researchers reported that "Exercise

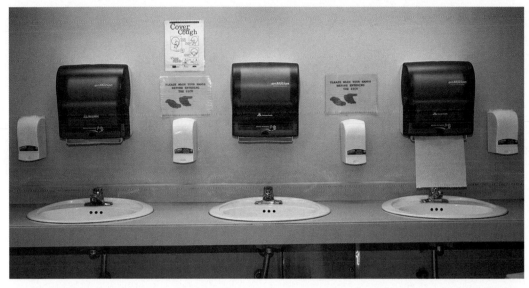

Fig. 10-1   A handwashing area at the entrance to the intensive care unit for use by visitors before entering and leaving the unit; water flow is activated when the hands are placed beneath the faucet spout. Towels automatically drop down when hands are waved in front of the sensor.

PROCEDURE 10-1

Guidelines for Treating a Patient in an Intensive Care Unit

- Review the patient's medical record before each treatment session, even when multiple sessions occur during the same day.
- Request information about the patient's current status (e.g., vital signs, physical activity level, medications, mental capacity and alertness) from nursing personnel and/or the physician.
- Wash your hands and apply protective garments as necessary.
- Observe the equipment or devices used to monitor the patient for current information about the physiological status.
- Observe the type and location of the equipment or devices being used by the patient (e.g., ventilator, intravenous line, oxygen, urinary catheter, arterial line, supplemental nutrition, and suction).
- Identify the location of all tubes, monitor lead connections, intravenous line connections and insertion sites, and patient-controlled analgesia; maintain all tubes and leads free of occlusion and tension.
- Evaluate or determine the patient's present physical and mental status before initiating treatment.
- Observe the patient and monitoring devices frequently; determine the response to the treatment; identify significant change in the condition or physiological status.
- Notify nursing personnel of significant change in the patient's condition or physiological status; document and record your activities and observations.

PROCEDURE 10-2

Precautions to Use in the Intensive Care Unit

- Avoid occlusion or excessive tension on all tubes, monitor leads, suction units, supplemental nutrition items, and oxygen lines.
- Observe and assess the patient before, during, and after treatment; determine the objective and subjective response to the treatment.
- Modify or cease treatment if the patient exhibits abnormal, unexpected, or undesired response(s) to the treatment (e.g., changes in vital signs, breathing pattern, indication of increased pain, reduced mental awareness or alertness).
- Request assistance from nursing or respiratory service personnel if you identify changes in the function or performance of the patient support systems (e.g., intravenous line, monitors, ventilation, supplemental nutrition, or drainage devices).
- Note the appearance and odor of visible wounds, wound dressings, wound drainage, and urine drainage; observe the general appearance of the patient.
- Request assistance, as necessary, to adjust or move equipment or reposition the patient.
- At the conclusion of the treatment:
  - Be certain the patient is properly positioned.
  - Elevate or replace side rails on the bed, if indicated.
  - Position the bedside table and other personal items so they are accessible to the patient.
- Inform the patient of the location of the "nurse call" device; position it to be accessible.

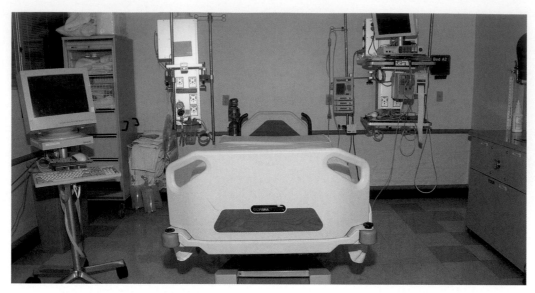

Fig. 10-2   A typical intensive care unit patient unit or cubicle prepared for patient use.

and mobilization with physical and occupational therapy within 72 hours of the start of mechanical ventilation more than doubled the rate of independent functional status at discharge, compared with the usual care. The therapy intervention included passive range of motion (PROM) exercises to the extremities every morning for unresponsive patients. Then, during interruption of sedatives, a physical and occupational therapist helped the patient with assisted and independent ROM exercises while supine in bed. As tolerated, these exercises progressed to sitting up, sitting balance activities, participation in activities of daily living (ADL), practicing sit-to-stand transfers to a chair or commode, and finally pre-gait exercises and walking." The primary outcome of this study was a return to independent functional status at discharge for 59% of the intervention group, with the ability to perform basic ADL; that is, walking independently, bathing, eating, dressing, grooming, transferring from a bed to a chair, and using the toilet. For other secondary outcomes in this study using early exercise and mobilization, see the Bibliography.

A caregiver who treats patients in an ICU will likely find that the roles will be very similar to the roles required to treat patients whose conditions are less acute or life threatening. The general, overall goals of treatment for patients in the ICU will be to minimize or prevent the adverse effects of inactivity and immobility and help each person become functionally independent.

Caregivers should be aware that several aspects of care and intervention must be considered when treating patients in the ICU. Procedure 10-3 is an example of a progression sequence for an ICU patient. One aspect of treatment is to prevent the development of contractures through the use of passive and active exercise, proper positioning, and body alignment. In addition, the use of exercise and physical activity will be important to improve the general condition of the patient. Bed mobility training will be necessary because it is a precursor to the transfer and ambulation activities that are requisites for functional independence. PROM and active range of motion (AROM) exercises help stimulate the sensory system; therefore sensory awareness and coordination may be enhanced through exercise.

Some patients may have respiratory difficulties, and they may need to be taught how to breathe more efficiently during their recovery, even when a respiratory aid is being used. Patients with respiratory deficits or who have experienced thoracic or abdominal surgery may need to be instructed how to breathe appropriately and cough effectively using their arms or a pillow to brace the incision site. For some patients, wound care management will be required, and the prevention of pressure ulcers by all caregivers is particularly important. Personal protective equipment may need to be worn by the caregiver, and compliance with the methods used to prevent the transmission of pathogens and cross-contamination of other patients may be necessary. Finally, helping the patient cope with, adjust to, or overcome painful stimuli may be accomplished through selective exercise techniques, through the use of pain-relieving electrotherapy equipment, and by being a compassionate caregiver.

TYPES OF BEDS

An electrically operated bed is the most common bed used in hospitals. This bed provides support, access to care, and the ability to alter the patient's position. However, acutely ill or traumatized patients frequently require special features that are not available on a standard hospital bed (Fig. 10-4).

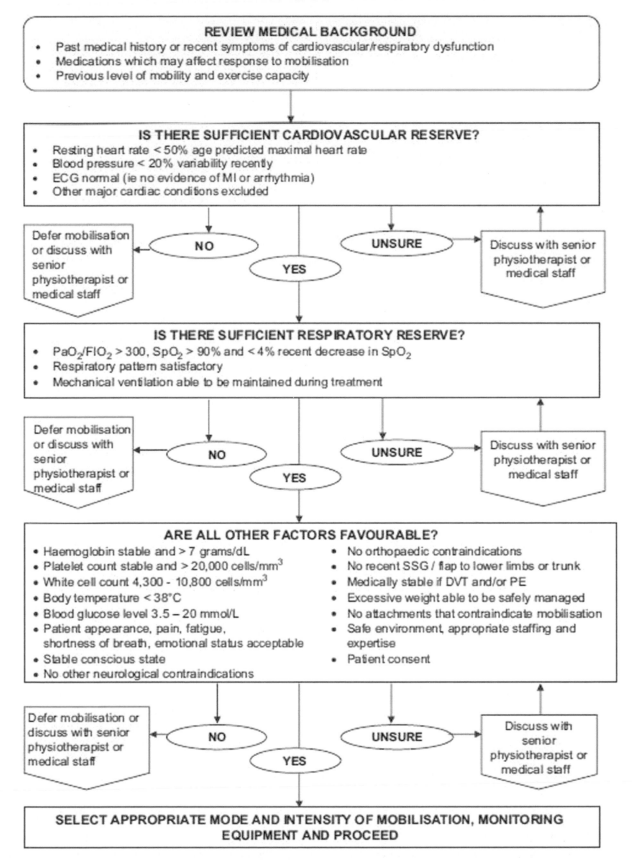

REVIEW MEDICAL BACKGROUND
- Past medical history or recent symptoms of cardiovascular/respiratory dysfunction
- Medications which may affect response to mobilisation
- Previous level of mobility and exercise capacity

IS THERE SUFFICIENT CARDIOVASCULAR RESERVE?
- Resting heart rate < 50% age predicted maximal heart rate
- Blood pressure < 20% variability recently
- ECG normal (ie no evidence of MI or arrhythmia)
- Other major cardiac conditions excluded

Defer mobilisation or discuss with senior physiotherapist or medical staff ← **NO** **UNSURE** → Discuss with senior physiotherapist or medical staff

YES

IS THERE SUFFICIENT RESPIRATORY RESERVE?
- $PaO_2/FIO_2 > 300$, $SpO_2 > 90\%$ and < 4% recent decrease in SpO_2
- Respiratory pattern satisfactory
- Mechanical ventilation able to be maintained during treatment

Defer mobilisation or discuss with senior physiotherapist or medical staff ← **NO** **UNSURE** → Discuss with senior physiotherapist or medical staff

YES

ARE ALL OTHER FACTORS FAVOURABLE?
- Haemoglobin stable and > 7 grams/dL
- Platelet count stable and > 20,000 cells/mm³
- White cell count 4,300 - 10,800 cells/mm³
- Body temperature < 38°C
- Blood glucose level 3.5 – 20 mmol/L
- Patient appearance, pain, fatigue, shortness of breath, emotional status acceptable
- Stable conscious state
- No other neurological contraindications
- No orthopaedic contraindications
- No recent SSG / flap to lower limbs or trunk
- Medically stable if DVT and/or PE
- Excessive weight able to be safely managed
- No attachments that contraindicate mobilisation
- Safe environment, appropriate staffing and expertise
- Patient consent

Defer mobilisation or discuss with senior physiotherapist or medical staff ← **NO** **UNSURE** → Discuss with senior physiotherapist or medical staff

YES

SELECT APPROPRIATE MODE AND INTENSITY OF MOBILISATION, MONITORING EQUIPMENT AND PROCEED

Fig. 10-3   An overview of safety issues prior to mobilizing critically ill patients. *DVT,* Deep venous thrombosis; *ECG,* electrocardiogram; *FIO₂,* fractional concentration of oxygen in inspired gas; *MI,* myocardial infarction; *PaO₂,* partial arterial oxygen tension; *PE,* pulmonary embolism; *SpO₂,* oxygen saturation in peripheral tissues; *SSG,* Surviving Sepsis Guidelines. From Stiller K, Phillips A. Safety aspects of mobilizing acutely ill patients. *Physiother Theory Pract* 2003;19(4):239-257, with permission of Taylor & Francis Group, LLC, http://www./taylorandfrancis.com.

PROCEDURE 10-3

Considerations for Therapy Progression of a Patient in the Intensive Care Unit

- Check vital signs and medical stability for mobilization.
- Assess the level of alertness and ability to follow commands.
- Assess bed mobility, such as rolling, scooting, and bridging:
  - How much is the patient able to assist?
  - Is the patient able to follow simple motor commands?
- Assess supine to sit transfers:
  - Is the patient able to perform the activity?
  - How much assistance is required?
- Sitting on the edge of the bed (EOB):
  - Assess trunk control and both static and dynamic sitting balance (if the patient is unable to sit on the EOB unsupported, he or she probably is not ready for transfers/ambulation)
- Establish measurable and attainable patient goals.
- Establish the treatment program:
  - The program should address functional impairments identified during the examination
  - Build on available skills to progress mobility
- EOB activities:
  - Ongoing assessments of static and dynamic sitting balance
  - Seated activities should include reaching out of base of support to determine proximal stability, which is fundamental for distal mobility of transfers/gait
- Transfer training:
  - Begin with sit to stand at EOB and progress to weight shifting with assistive devices and pregait activities (Note: If the patient does not have adequate lower extremity strength but does have independent dynamic sitting balance, transfers could be performed with a transfer board while building enough lower extremity strength for standing pivot transfers)
- Gait training:
  - Begin with weight shifting, marching in place, or short distances repeated frequently

From Wall L: Physical therapy intervention ICU: http://depts.washington.edu/pulmcc/conferences/lungday/Wall.pdf. Accessed January 23, 2011.

If the caregiver finds that the patient's position is appropriate for his or her medical condition but inappropriate for treatment, the following options are available: reschedule the treatment when the patient is positioned more appropriately, temporarily reposition the patient to permit treatment, or treat the patient as much as possible without changing his or her position. If the patient's original position needs to be changed, the caregiver should communicate with the nursing staff regarding repositioning the patient. It may be necessary to ask the nurse to reposition the patient, readjust the position of the bed, or to assist when position changes are made by the caregiver. Usually the caregiver should return the patient to his or her original position at the conclusion of the treatment session and adhere to any time schedule related to patient positioning. For example, a patient may need to follow a turning schedule and may be limited in the amount of time he or she is allowed to remain in one position. The caregiver should be aware of and comply with any special schedule the patient is expected to follow.

Standard Adjustable Bed

Most hospital beds can be adjusted using electrical controls. The controls may be located at the head or foot of the bed, on the side rail, or attached to a special cord so the patient can operate them independently. The controls should be marked according to their function and may be operated by using the hand or, in some situations, the foot. The bed can be raised and lowered in relation to the floor as a total unit, and the upper and lower components can be adjusted separately or together. On most beds, the lower portion is hinged so it can be adjusted to provide knee flexion, which in turn causes hip flexion. On some beds, the lower component will become flexed whenever the upper component is raised. This action creates hip and knee flexion, or the Fowler position, which is more comfortable for the patient and tends to prevent sliding down in the bed. Sometimes when the bed is adjusted with the upper portion raised and the lower portion flexed, the bed is considered to be "gatched."

Most beds have some type of side rails or protective devices. Some rails are lifted upward until the locking mechanism is engaged, whereas other types are adjusted by moving them toward the upper portion of the bed until the locking mechanism is engaged. When a side rail is used for patient security, it is important to be certain that the rail is locked securely before you leave. Also, check to be certain the side rail has not compressed or stretched any IV line, catheter, or other tubing. Adjust the bed into the position that will give you the best access to the patient and enable you to use proper body mechanics. The prolonged use of bed rails can be a form of patient restraint that may not be permitted legally. It may be necessary to have a physician request or order the use of all bed rails. If bed rails are used as a restraint method, it should be determined that patient safety is endangered when they are not in place. Be certain to return the patient to the original, required, or preferred position at the conclusion of the treatment.

The patient can contact nursing personnel with use of a device that is either located on the side rail of the bed or attached to an electrical cord. At the conclusion of treatment, the caregiver should be certain the patient has access to the device and is aware of its location or position. This device may be referred to as a "call button."

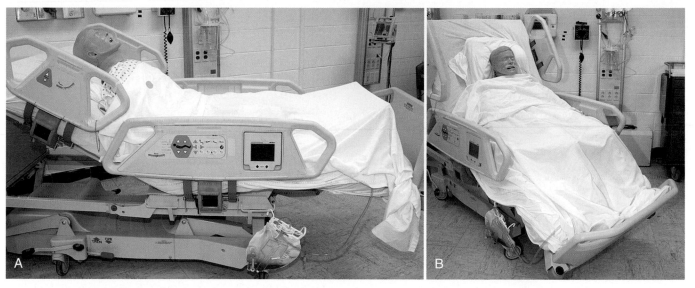

Fig. 10-4   **A,** A specialized adjustable bed. **B,** A specialized adjustable bed that allows a patient to stand when it is elevated completely.

Turning Frame (Stryker Wedge Frame)

A turning frame has an anterior and a posterior frame, each of which has a canvas cover. It has a support base that allows elevation of the head or foot ends of the frames or the entire bed. A pivot joint allows the patient to be turned in a horizontal plane from a prone to a supine position or from a supine to a prone position by one person. A similar device is the Foster frame.

A turning frame is used in the following situations: when skeletal stability and alignment are desired; to permit a patient to be turned horizontally from prone to supine or from supine to prone; when continuous maintenance of skeletal cervical traction, such as Crutchfield Tongs or a similar type of skeletal traction, is desired; and when a patient must be immobilized after a spinal fracture and safe and efficient change of position from supine to prone, or vice versa, must be performed.

This equipment has several advantages. It allows access to the patient for a variety of therapeutic interventions and nursing care; it allows one person to safely and easily turn the patient from supine to prone and back; and it allows the patient to be wheeled or transported from one location to another without being removed from the frame. Furthermore, the unit can be elevated or lowered as a unit to several heights or positions, and the height of the head or foot of the frame can be changed independently. The patient can be positioned in Trendelenburg position when supine or prone. The unit requires relatively little space, even to turn the patient, and it allows cervical traction to be applied and maintained even when the patient is turned.

The turning frame has several disadvantages. The patient can be positioned only in the supine or prone positions, and patients who weigh more than 200 lb or who are taller than approximately 6 feet will be difficult to position on the frames. Most patients who exceed these limits will not be able to tolerate this device for extended periods. Patients are at risk of experiencing skin problems as a result of shear and pressure forces related to being positioned only prone or supine, and contractures may develop unless appropriate exercise and positioning techniques are used. Furthermore, patients with complete traumatic quadriplegia have a decrease in pulmonary vital capacity when turned from the supine to prone position on the Stryker frame. In addition, occipital pressure ulcers often developed in patients who were positioned in the supine position on a Stryker frame for a long period. (Note: The development of new equipment and other technological advances in patient care have reduced the need for this piece of equipment in most hospitals in the United States, and it is now rarely used.)

Air-Fluidized Support Bed (Clinitron)

The air-fluidized bed is a rectangular or ovoid bed that contains 1600 lb of silicone-coated glass beads called microspheres. Heated, pressurized air flows through the beads to suspend a polyester cover that supports the patient. When set in motion, the microspheres develop the properties associated with fluids. The patient feels as if he or she is floating on a warm waterbed. Contact pressure of the patient's body against the polyester sheet is approximately 11 to 15 mm Hg.

This equipment is indicated for the following patients: those who have several infected lesions or require skin protection and whose position cannot be altered easily (e.g., persons with burns or spinal cord injury); those with extensive pressure ulcers or who are at risk of developing deterioration of the skin (e.g., obese persons); those with recent,

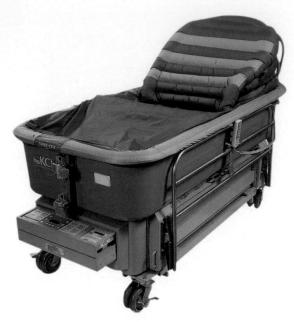

Fig. 10-5 An air fluidization bed. (Courtesy Kinetic Concepts Incorporated [KCI].)

extensive skin grafts; or those who require prolonged immobilization (Fig. 10-5).

This piece of equipment has several advantages. It reduces the need for the application of topical medications and dressings by establishing a microclimate environment favorable for the healing process. The temperature of the air in the bed can be controlled according to the needs of the patient. The bed reduces pressure on the skin, and pressure sores are less likely to develop than when a regular bed is used. Friction or shear forces to the body are reduced significantly or eliminated, and the patient can lie on the lesions or wounds for brief periods. When the unit is turned off, the polyester cover becomes a firm surface, which may be beneficial for certain therapeutic interventions or nursing care. A draw sheet can be used to assist in positioning the patient, and a two-person sliding transfer from the bed to a stretcher can be performed with the unit turned off.

The air-fluidized bed also has several disadvantages. The polyester cover (filter sheet) can be damaged (punctured) easily by a sharp object and, if the filter sheet is punctured, the microspheres will be expelled. Air flowing across the patient's skin may cause body fluids to evaporate more rapidly than normal, and thus it may be necessary to have the patient ingest small amounts of extra fluids to compensate for fluid loss. A patient may require frequent position changes because of the tendency for fluid to pool in the lobes of the lungs, and obese or tall patients are likely to be uncomfortable on this bed. The height of the bed from the floor will probably be fixed, so it may be difficult to provide care or to transfer the patient. Finally, it is a very expensive piece of equipment.

Posttrauma Mobility Beds (Keane, Roto-Rest)

Post-trauma mobility beds are designed to maintain a seriously injured patient in a stable position and maintain proper postural alignment through the use of adjustable bolsters. The bed oscillates from side to side, in a cradlelike motion, to reduce the amount of prolonged pressure on the patient's skin.

These beds are indicated for patients with restricted respiratory function or advanced or multiple pressure ulcers or for patients who require stabilization and skeletal alignment after extensive trauma or as a result of severe neurological deficits.

These beds have several advantages. The constant side-to-side motion assists in improving upper respiratory tract function and reduces the need to turn the patient to relieve pressure or prevent the development of pressure ulcers. The friction and shear forces associated with turning the patient are eliminated, and the constant motion of the bed may provide some environmental stimulation for neurologically impaired patients. Urinary stasis is reduced and bowel function is improved as a result of the constant motion of the bed (Fig. 10-6).

Several disadvantages also have been reported. Some patients may experience signs or symptoms of motion sickness, such as vertigo or nausea, and others may feel isolated from the environment as a result of a decrease in their visual orientation. Exercises and other forms of patient care may be restricted because of the bolsters and alignment supports, although some beds have ports or hatches to provide better access. Finally, sufficient space must be available to allow the bed to oscillate without interference from other objects. The bolsters and alignment supports must be maintained in position to provide proper stabilization and alignment, which is especially necessary for adequate support to the thorax.

Low Air Loss Therapy Bed

Low air loss beds have several segmented and separated air bladders that allow the limited escape of air. The amount of air pressure in each bladder is individually controlled for each patient based on the size, weight, and shape of the patient, and the bed may be adjusted to several different positions (Fig. 10-7).

This bed is indicated for patients who require prolonged immobilization, who are at high risk of developing pressure ulcers or who have existing ulcers, whose condition requires frequent elevation of the trunk to promote proper respiratory function, and who are obese.

This bed has several advantages. It can be adjusted to accommodate the need to change the patient's position to a hip and knee flexion position, a sitting position, or a semirecumbent position. The patient's position can be altered through the use of electronically operated controls.

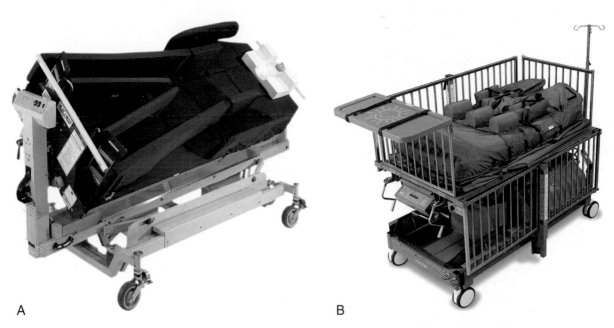

A   B

Fig. 10-6   **A,** A Roto-Rest bed. **B,** A pediatric bed. (**A,** Courtesy Kinetic Concepts Incorporated [KCI].)

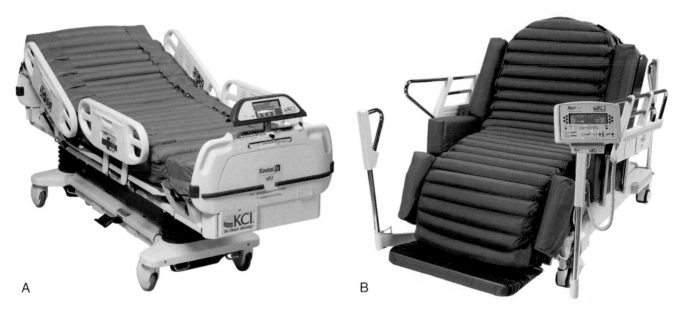

A   B

Fig. 10-7   An air suspension bed with individual air bladders. **A,** A traditional bed. **B,** A bed for a heavy patient (300 to 850 lb). (Courtesy Kinetic Concepts Incorporated [KCI].)

The patient's weight is measured by sensors in the bed, and the air bladders are inflated or deflated automatically to distribute the patient's weight.

Several disadvantages of this bed also have been reported. The air bladders can be punctured or torn by sharp objects, and frequent alterations in the patient's position must be performed to prevent pressure ulcers. (Note: To transfer a patient, you should lock the wheels, elevate the patient's trunk approximately 20 to 30 degrees, deflate the seat section, perform the transfer, and turn off the seat deflation control to reinflate the seat.)

The surfaces of the three beds described in this section may not be rigid enough to allow effective performance of the chest compressions required for cardiopulmonary resuscitation. Therefore a flat rigid wooden or plastic device must be placed beneath the patient to provide a firm solid surface before the initiation of cardiopulmonary resuscitation, or the patient may need to be transferred to the floor. It will be easier to transfer the patient when he or she is supine and is first placed on a firm support.

LIFE SUPPORT AND MONITORING EQUIPMENT

Mechanical Ventilators

Most ventilators, also known as respirators, currently use positive pressure to move or propel gas or air into the patient's lungs. The purpose of a ventilator is to maintain adequate and appropriate air exchange when normal respiration is inhibited or cannot be actively performed by the patient. A ventilator may be indicated for diseases or conditions that affect the patient's neurological or musculoskeletal control of respiration or that interfere with the exchange of gases in the lungs. A ventilator may be used when the patient experiences apnea or when the potential for respiratory distress or failure exists.

An example of respiratory distress that may develop is acute respiratory distress syndrome (ARDS); a similar syndrome affects infants. This syndrome is potentially life threatening, and its existence must be recognized soon after it affects the patient so immediate steps can be initiated to counteract the syndrome. Some of the possible causes of ARDS are systemic shock, diffuse respiratory infection, and systemic response to sepsis or extensive trauma. Clinical signs and symptoms include dyspnea, tachypnea, cyanosis, and hypoxemia. The caregiver who treats a patient with ARDS or the infant ARDS syndrome must monitor the patient's response to activity and observe the monitoring equipment frequently to be certain the vital signs and arterial blood gases (ABGs) remain within acceptable ranges or limits. A person with ARDS will have a restricted respiratory capacity and will receive respiratory assistance from a ventilator. The patient is likely to be intolerant of active exercise, especially resistive exercise, in the early stages of recovery, and complete recovery from ARDS may require several weeks. The syndrome is life threatening because it can trigger the failure of one or more major organs, such as the kidneys; therefore early detection of the syndrome and aggressive treatment are extremely important.

Types of Ventilators

Volume-Cycled Ventilators Volume-cycled ventilators are used primarily for patients who require long-term support. A predetermined volume of gas ("air"), which is dependent on the patient's needs, is delivered during the inspiratory phase of respiration, but the expiratory phase remains passive (Fig. 10-8). This type of equipment is indicated when long-term ventilation assistance is needed, for patients with severe chronic obstructive pulmonary disease (COPD), after thoracic surgery, for patients with disorders of the central nervous system, and for patients with musculoskeletal disorders that affect the respiratory system. Some musculoskeletal disorders affecting the respiratory system include a cervical spinal cord injury, a brain injury, amyotrophic lateral sclerosis, Guillain-Barré syndrome, and poliomyelitis.

Pressure-Cycled Ventilators Pressure-cycled ventilators deliver a predetermined, established maximum pressure of gas during respiration, and the inspiratory phase ends when that level is reached. The expiratory phase remains passive. The flow rate may vary from one respiration cycle to the next.

This device is indicated when only short-term ventilation is needed in the form of intermittent positive-pressure breathing and for selected patients with neuromuscular or musculoskeletal distress.

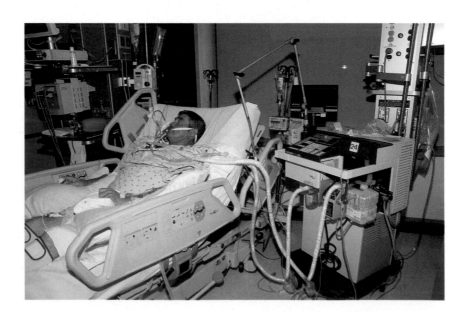

Fig. 10-8 A ventilator with computer functions.

Negative Pressure Device Currently, negative pressure ventilation is rarely used in the management of patients with respiratory problems. The primary types are the tank respirator ("iron lung") and the chest respirator ("turtle shell"). These devices create a negative pressure in the patient's chest so the environmental air pressure exceeds the internal thoracic pressure. Because of this pressure imbalance, air enters the patient's lungs passively to provide inspiration. These devices are used primarily for persons with poliomyelitis.

Modes of Ventilation

Several modes of ventilation are described in Box 10-2.

Airway Placement Usually, the gas delivered by the ventilator will be introduced into the patient through a tube in one of several possible airways. The tube is referred to as an endotracheal tube (ETT), and when it is in place, the patient is considered to be intubated. The possible locations for an ETT are in the oral pharyngeal, nasal pharyngeal, oral esophageal, nasal endotracheal, or oral endotracheal airway. Other means of insertion of the tube include a tracheostomy and laryngostomy. Each of these artificial airways provides a clear airway through the patient's nasal, oral, or other passageways to the lungs. The ETT allows suction of the bronchial tree, but insertion of the ETT restricts the patient from talking. When the ETT is removed, the patient will probably report throat discomfort, and the voice is likely to be distorted for a short period. The caregiver must avoid disturbing or accidentally disconnecting the tube of the ventilator from the ETT and bending, kinking, or occluding the connector tubing. Be certain the tubing is not obstructed by the weight of one of the patient's extremities or trapped under the bed rail.

Patients who use a ventilator can participate in various types of exercise and other bedside activities, including sitting and ambulation. The patient must be informed of the activity, and the caregiver must be certain the tubing is of a sufficient length to allow the physical activity to be performed. Because the patient will have difficulty communicating orally, questions should be asked that can be answered with head nods, a note pad and pen, or other nonverbal means. The patient's response to the activity must be monitored closely by the caregiver, and undue stress to the patient should be avoided. A patient using a ventilator probably will not tolerate exercise as well as other patients, so you should be cautious during treatment. Monitor the patient's vital signs and be alert for signs of respiratory distress such as a change in the respiration pattern, syncope, or cyanosis.

The ventilator has an auditory and visual alarm that will be activated by various stimuli such as a disconnected tube, coughing by the patient, movement of the tubing, or a change in the respiratory pattern or needs of the patient. During orientation to the special care unit, the caregiver should be instructed how to determine the cause of the alarm and how to return the system to normal function. If this education is not provided, the caregiver should obtain assistance from a nurse or respiratory therapist in the unit. Be alert for signs or symptoms of respiratory or cardiopulmonary distress exhibited by the patient, such as dyspnea, tachycardia, arrhythmia, and hyperventilation.

The caregiver should become familiar with the various types of ventilators and modes of ventilation before beginning treatment with any patient. You can attend one or more in-service orientation programs to familiarize yourself with types of ventilators and modes of ventilation.

Monitors

Patients who require special care may have their physiological status monitored by various pieces of equipment. Common monitoring parameters include cardiac and vital signs, ABGs, intracranial pressure (ICP), pulmonary artery pressure (PAP), central venous pressure (CVP), and arterial pressure (A line). Exercise can be performed by patients

---

> ### Box 10-2 Modes of Ventilation
>
> - Assist mode: The patient must develop or cause a negative pressure to "trigger" the ventilator to provide assistance to deliver gas, such as oxygen and air, to the patient.
> - Continuous positive airway pressure mode: This mode superimposes the use of positive end-expiratory pressure (PEEP) (refer to the description below) on the patient's spontaneous breathing pattern. It is particularly useful to help wean a patient from the ventilator or to help maximize the gas exchange capabilities for an immobile, inactive patient.
> - Control mode: The inspiration phase of respiration begins at timed intervals based on the patient's need for gas.
> - Assisted control mode: This mode is a combination of the previous two modes.
> - Intermittent mandatory ventilation mode: The patient's ventilation cycle is established so that ventilation occurs a minimum number of times per minute. This mode is frequently used to begin to wean the patient from the ventilator and to develop an independent respiration pattern.
> - Synchronized intermittent mandatory ventilation mode: This mode allows the ventilation cycle to be coordinated with the patient's own breathing cycle.
> - PEEP mode: This mode allows oxygen to be introduced into the patient's lungs by maintaining positive pressure at the end of expiration, which increases the alveolar surface area able to absorb the gas introduced by the ventilator and leads to maximal alveolar ventilation. The PEEP helps to expand, maintain, and keep the alveoli patent because normally they would close at the end of expiration.

who are being monitored, as long as care is taken to avoid disruption of the equipment. Many of these units have an auditory and visual signal that may be activated by a change in the patient's condition, a change in the function of the equipment, or a change in the patient's position. In some instances it will be necessary for a nurse to evaluate and correct the cause of the alarm, but in other instances the caregiver may be able to correct the cause safely. For example, you may cease exercise and allow the patient to rest until the physiological state returns to an acceptable level.

The caregiver should recognize that the patient's condition can be unstable, and caution should be used to avoid causing stress for the patient. Orientation regarding the purpose and function of the monitoring equipment and devices is recommended for persons who will treat the patient. (Caution: Be certain that you understand which parameters the various channels on the monitor are measuring or reporting at a given time and which channels are active. The channels can be changed to monitor different parameters at different times, or they can be deactivated. Therefore it is important for the caregiver to know which of the patient's physiological responses are being monitored when treatment is being provided.)

Vital Signs Monitor The patient's monitor may display current values of any of the following: blood pressure, respiration rate, temperature, blood gases, or cardiac patterns (Fig. 10-9, A and B). A portable unit can be used when a permanent, fixed monitor is not available (Fig. 10-9, C). Acceptable or safe parameters or ranges for the three physiological indicators can be set on the unit. An alarm is activated when the upper or lower limits of the ranges are exceeded or when the unit malfunctions. A graphical and

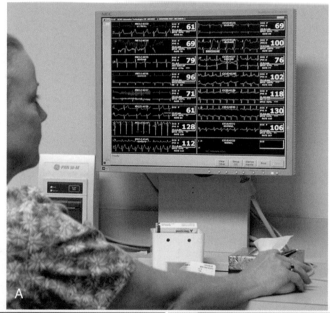

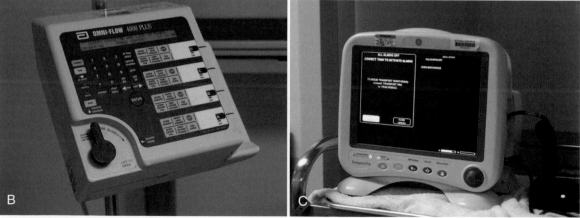

Fig. 10-9 Patient monitors. **A,** A monitor located in the nurses' unit; several patients can be monitored simultaneously. **B,** A patient monitor located in the patient's unit; heart rate, temperature, respiration rate, electrocardiogram patterns, and blood gases can be displayed separately or simultaneously. **C,** A portable monitor.

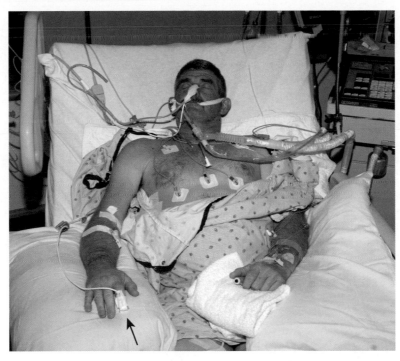

Fig. 10-10   This patient has several chest pads and leads, infusion sites, an arterial line, and an oximeter on the right index finger (*arrow*) and also receives support from a ventilator.

a digital display of the values are apparent on the monitor screen so the caregiver can observe the effects of the exercise and the patient's responses to activity.

Oximeter   An oximeter is a photoelectrical device that is used to measure the oxygen saturation (SaO_2) of the patient's blood by recording the different modulations of a transmitted beam of light affected by reduced hemoglobin (Hgb) and oxyhemoglobin. Usually, the oximeter will be positioned on or attached to a patient's finger or ear, and it measures and reports the pulse rate and the percentage of SaO_2 of the Hgb (blood) (Fig. 10-10).

Pulmonary Artery Catheter (Swan-Ganz Catheter)   The Swan-Ganz catheter is a long plastic IV tube that can be inserted into the internal jugular or the femoral vein, guided into the basilic or subclavian vein, and then passed into the pulmonary artery. This catheter is used to provide accurate and continuous measurements of PAP and detects even subtle changes in the patient's cardiovascular system, including responses to medications, stress, and exercise.

This device is indicated when measurements of right atrial pressure, PAP, and pulmonary capillary wedge pressure are desired. Readings are performed frequently; the monitor screen shows a rolling waveform and a digital reading of the various values. Normal values are right atrial pressure, 0 to 4 mm Hg; PAP, 20 to 30 mm Hg systolic and 10 to 15 mm Hg diastolic; and pulmonary capillary wedge pressure, 4 to 12 mm Hg.

Exercise can be performed with the pulmonary artery catheter in place, but it may be necessary to limit the exercise because of the location of the catheter's insertion. For example, if the catheter is inserted into the subclavian vein, shoulder flexion should be avoided and other shoulder motions should be restricted. Similar restrictions in hip flexion (i.e., not greater than 30 degrees) and abduction exist for a femoral vein insertion. Some complications associated with this catheter are pulmonary artery vascular damage, damage to intracardial structures, cardiac dysrhythmias, endocarditis, and sepsis (infection).

Intracranial Pressure Monitor   The ICP monitor measures the pressure exerted against the skull by brain tissue, blood, or cerebrospinal fluid (CSF). It is used for patients who have experienced a closed head injury, a cerebral hemorrhage, a brain tumor, or an overproduction of CSF. Normal ICP pressure is 4 to 15 mm Hg, but a fluctuation of as much as 20 mm Hg can occur as a result of a variety of routine activities.

This device is used to monitor ICP easily, to quantify the degree of abnormal pressure, to properly initiate treatment, and to evaluate the results of treatment. Some of the complications associated with this device are sepsis, hemorrhage, and seizures.

The following types of ICP monitoring devices are used:
- **Ventricular catheter.** The ventricular catheter is inserted into a lateral ventricle of the brain through a hole drilled in the skull. The ventricular catheter

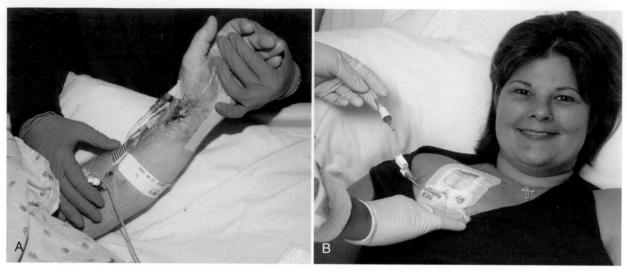

Fig. 10-11 **A,** A patient with an arterial line in the left forearm. **B,** A Hickman infusion site at the upper right chest wall.

provides a highly accurate method for monitoring the ICP and allows withdrawal of CSF.

- **Subarachnoid screw.** A screw is inserted into the subarachnoid space through a small hole drilled in the skull. This device permits accurate measurement of the ICP, but it does not permit withdrawal of CSF.
- **Epidural sensor.** A sensor plate can be placed in the epidural space, but it has proved to be a relatively inaccurate measurement device with poor reliability and therefore is rarely used.

Limited physical activities can be performed when these devices are in place; however, activities that cause a rapid increase in ICP, such as isometric exercises and the Valsalva maneuver, should be avoided. The patient should be positioned to avoid neck flexion, hip flexion greater than 90 degrees, and lying in a prone position. The patient's head should not be lowered more than 15 degrees below horizontal. As with other devices that use plastic tubing, care must be taken to avoid disruption, disconnection, or occlusion of the tube.

Central Venous Pressure Catheter The CVP catheter is a plastic IV tube used to measure pressures in the right atrium or the superior vena cava. It measures the pressure associated with the filling of the right ventricle (i.e., the diastolic pressure). Such measurement is imprecise and may be misleading regarding the function of the right ventricle. Precautions similar to those expressed previously for other catheters also apply when a CVP line is in place. Potential complications are similar to those listed for the pulmonary artery catheter.

Arterial Line (A Line) The A line is a catheter that is inserted into an artery, typically the radial, dorsal pedal, axillary, brachial, or femoral artery. The A line is used to

continuously measure blood pressure or to obtain blood samples without repeated needle punctures, and it usually provides accurate measurements. Potential complications include sepsis, hemorrhage, development of a fistula or aneurysm, ischemia, or arterial necrosis.

Exercise can be performed with an A line in place, as long as the precautions described previously are followed, especially those related to disruption of the catheter, disturbance of the inserted needle, occlusion of the line, or disconnection of the line from the inserted cannula (Fig. 10-11, A).

Indwelling Right Atrial Catheter (Hickman) The right atrial catheter is inserted through the cephalic or internal jugular vein and passes through the superior vena cava to near the tip of the right atrium (Fig. 10-11, B). This device allows administration of medications, removal of blood for testing, and measurement of CVP. When a central line catheter is used for "hyperalimentation" or total parental nutrition (TPN), it will usually be positioned into the superior vena cava for the delivery of the nutritional solution. The central line can be used with patients who will receive a bone marrow transplant, who have cancer, or who have experienced severe trauma. Potential complications associated with this device are sepsis and blood clots.

Exercise should be performed with care, and precautions similar to those described previously for other catheters should be followed.

Reference Laboratory Values

Reference laboratory values are important because they provide baseline values to which a patient's laboratory findings can be compared. Depending on the patient's diagnosis and physical and mental condition, along with institutional or physician guidelines or protocols, the approach to care and treatment will be adjusted for each individual. Persons with the same or a similar diagnosis may require very different approaches to care because of differences in their physical responses to the disease, trauma, or condition.

Cardiac status can be determined by examination of the cardiac enzyme levels in the blood after an acute myocardial infarction (MI). When an MI occurs, intercellular enzymes are released into the person's blood. The presence in the blood of the enzyme creatine kinase, and especially the enzyme found primarily in cardiac muscle—creatine kinase-myocardial bound—is an indication that an acute MI has occurred. These increased values usually return to normal levels within 2 days after the MI. The caregiver must use caution when treating a person who has had an MI and should be certain to closely observe the patient's vital signs as they appear on the cardiac monitor. The patient can receive basic care and participate in physical activities as long as the vital signs, blood chemistry, ABGs, and physical appearance remain within acceptable ranges. Adverse responses to activity, such as chest pain, fatigue, hypotension, or cardiac dysrhythmia, are indicators that the treatment may need to be modified, altered, or discontinued.

The ABG analysis provides information about the oxygenation level of the blood. A pulse oximeter, often positioned on a fingertip or an earlobe, is used to measure the pulse rate and the percentage of SaO_2 in the blood. Refer to Table 10-1 for ABG values and ranges.

During exercise or physical activity, a minimum of 90% saturation should be maintained to avoid hypoxemia and possible respiratory dysfunction. If supplemental oxygen is being provided for the patient, it should remain in place during the treatment. If the SaO_2 falls below 90% and remains there, the patient's nurse or physician should be notified and the treatment should be discontinued. Consideration should be given to altering or modifying the treatment in the future. Changes in the patient's respiration rate or pattern may occur because of a reduced SaO_2 level during exercise. If hyperventilation occurs, the patient may benefit from relaxation techniques such as abdominal-diaphragmatic or pursed-lip breathing. If hypoventilation occurs, the patient may benefit from deep-breathing techniques and an upright position with the trunk supported.

Blood chemistry analysis provides information about an individual's red blood cell (RBC) and white blood cell (WBC) count, Hgb, and hematocrit (Hct). The WBC, also known as a leukocyte, is one of the body's defense mechanisms for fighting acute or chronic disease or infection. An increased WBC count may indicate the presence of bacterial infection, leukemia, neoplasm, allergic reaction, inflammation, or tissue necrosis. A decreased WBC count may indicate bone marrow deficiency or infection with human immunodeficiency virus, or it may be attributable to radiation or chemotherapy treatments. A person with a decreased WBC count caused by an immunosuppressed condition must be monitored carefully, and the caregiver must be certain to perform thorough hand hygiene, apply protective garments, and follow precautions before treatment to reduce the possibility of cross contamination. Depending on the diagnosis and the patient's physical condition, treatment activities may need to be modified, altered, or discontinued according to the patient's response to treatment, and frequent rest periods may be necessary. Precautions for exercise activities when abnormal blood values exist are presented in Table 10-2.

Because they are bound to the Hgb contained in the cell, the RBCs transport oxygen to tissue cells throughout the body. Anemia occurs when the RBC count is decreased significantly, and polycythemia occurs when the RBC count is increased significantly. A patient with either of these conditions may participate in physical activity as long as institutional and physician guidelines or protocols are followed and the response to the activity is monitored frequently and consistently.

The Hct is used to measure the volume percentage of packed RBCs in a sample of whole blood. The Hct is particularly important in the diagnosis of polycythemia or anemia. Persons with anemia will not tolerate vigorous physical activity, and their vital signs should be monitored frequently and consistently.

The Hgb is the protein contained in the RBC that transports oxygen in the blood; it is frequently referred to as oxyhemoglobin. Anemia, trauma, surgery, or dietary iron deficiency may cause a decrease in the Hgb. A person with a low Hgb will have a reduced tolerance to physical activity and will require frequent rest periods. Persons whose Hgb is less than 8 g/dL should not receive or participate in treatment requiring physical activity.

Caregivers who provide treatment in an ICU (or coronary care unit) should become familiar with the reference values of various laboratory tests to understand the implications for treatment when abnormal values are identified. The level of activity that is appropriate or suitable for a given patient can be established by the caregiver to attain maximal function effectively without jeopardizing recovery (see Tables 10-1 and 10-2).

Anticoagulation

Anticoagulation is initiated in patients for a variety of medical reasons, the most common being to prevent clots after surgery. Anticoagulants are a class of medications used to prevent clots in high-risk patients. Several commonly prescribed anticoagulants are heparin, Coumadin (warfarin), Plavix (clopidogrel), Lovenox (enoxaparin), and Arixtra (fondaparinux sodium). Aspirin is also considered an anticoagulant. Because these drugs are in a "high-risk" category, patients must be monitored very closely. In January 2009, The Joint Commission initiated a new National Patient Safety Goal, 3 E, which requires hospitals to actively reduce the likelihood of patient harm associated with anticoagulation therapy. Anticoagulants inhibit the blood from

Table 10-1 Reference Laboratory Values

Laboratory Values	Description	Normal Values	Critical Values
Arterial blood gases			
pH	Acid-base status (<7.35 = acidosis; >7.45 = alkalosis)	7.35-7.45	pH: <7.10 or >7.59 units, first only (within past 24 hours)
$PaCO_2$	Partial pressure of carbon dioxide dissolved in arterial blood (influenced by pulmonary function)	35-45 mm Hg	$PaCO_2$: <20 or >75 mm Hg, first only (within past 24 hours)
HCO_2	Amount of alkaline substance dissolved in arterial blood (influenced by metabolic changes primarily)	22-26 mEq/L	HCO_2: <10 or >40
PaO_2	Partial pressure of oxygen dissolved in arterial blood (influenced by pulmonary function)	80-100 mm Hg	PaO_2: <40 mm Hg
O_2 saturation (SaO_2)	Oxyhemoglobin saturation or percentage of oxygen carried by hemoglobin	95%-98%	SaO_2: <60%
Selected blood chemistry values			
Red blood cells (RBCs)		4.6-6.2×10^{12}/L (male) 4.2-5.4×10^{12}/L (female)	
White blood cells (WBCs)		4.3-10.8×10^9/L	<2000 or >50,000/mm³
Hemoglobin (Hgb)		14-18 g/dL (male) 13-16 g/dL (female)	<6.5 g/dL
Hematocrit (Hct, Crit, packed cell volume)		40-54 mL/dL (male) 37-48 mL/dL (female)	<20% or >56%
Potassium (K)		3.5-5.0 mEq/L	<2.8 or >6.0 µmol/L
Bilirubin		Direct: up to 0.4 mg/dL Total: up to 1.0 mg/dL	
Creatinine		0.6-1.2 mg/dL ≥10 years of age	
Potassium		3.5-5.0 mEq/L	
Prothrombin (PTT)		25-41 seconds	
Thyroid stimulating hormone (TSH)		0.4-5.0 µU/mL	
Blood urea nitrogen (BUN)/ creatinine ratio		5-35	
"Sed rate"—erythrocyte sedimentation rate (ESR)		Female: 1-25 mm/h Male: 0-17 mm/h	
Glucose		70-115 mg/dL	<40 or >500 mg/dL
Platelet		150-450 µ 106/L	<20,000/mm³
Sodium (Na)		135-145 mEq/L	
Serum creatinine		0.6-1.5 mg/dL (male) 0.5-1.0 mg/dL (female)	
Creatine kinase (CK)—total		25-255 mL/L	
Creatine kinase-myocardial bound (CK-MB) isoenzyme	Heart related	0-5.9 mL/L	
Creatine kinase-muscle type (CK-MM) isoenzyme	Muscle related	5-70 mL/L	

Reference values may vary depending on the method used to obtain them or the source that reports them; many are gender or age dependent. The reference values (also referred to as "normal values") used for this table were obtained from the *Encyclopedia and dictionary of medicine, nursing, and allied health*, ed 7, Philadelphia, 2005, Saunders, except for the creatine kinase values. Those values were obtained from "Laboratory Values in the Intensive Care Unit," *Acute Care Perspectives, The Newsletter of Acute Care/Hospital Clinical Practice Section–APTA*, Winter 1995. Critical values were taken from the MGH *Clinical Laboratory Callback List, Pathology Service Laboratory Handbook*. Available at mghlabtest.partners.org. Accessed January 7, 2012.

Table 10-2 Precautions for Exercise with Low Blood Counts

Count	No Exercise	Light Exercise	Resistive Exercise
Hematocrit	<27%	27%-30%	>30%
Hemoglobin	8 g/dL	8-10 g/dL	>10 g/dL
Platelet	<50,000 mm^3	50,000-70,000 mm^3	>70,000 mm^3
White cells	<500 mm^3 with fever	>500 mm^3	>500 mm^3
International normalized ratio (INR)	>5.0	4.0-5.0	<4.0

clotting and adhering to the blood vessel walls and are commonly used as a preventive in patients with a history of stroke and heart attack. If not treated promptly, blood clots can be fatal.

Maintaining an acceptable range of anticoagulation can be difficult, and the therapeutic goal frequently is exceeded. When patients function in a hyperanticoagulated state, the risk of hemorrhage is increased and excessive activity and exercise should be limited. Unfortunately, no evidence-based guidelines or recommendations exist for activity limitations in patients with hyperanticoagulation. Anticoagulation with warfarin is most commonly evaluated using the International Normalized Ratio (INR), which is a system established by the World Health Organization and the International Committee on Thrombosis and Hemostasis for reporting the results of blood coagulation or clotting tests. The INR in healthy adults ranges from 0.8 to 1.2. However, a person taking the anticoagulant warfarin might optimally maintain a prothrombin time of 2 to 3 INR. If a patient exceeds an INR of 5.0, warfarin is usually withheld by the prescribing physician and vitamin K or fresh frozen plasma may be ordered to quickly lower the INR to a safer range.

In 2009, Tuzson reported in *Acute Care Perspectives* (see the Bibliography) that performing physical or occupational therapy in patients with hyperanticoagulation (i.e., an increased risk of bleeding) raises two questions: (1) Will the patient experience some minor or major trauma during therapy that will result in gross bleeding because of an increased INR? (2) Is the patient already actively bleeding externally or internally, which would make it unsafe to pursue physical activity? To address these concerns, the caregiver should monitor blood values and vital signs to ensure that the patient is medically stable and not actively bleeding prior to treatment.

Likewise, Tuzson reported the following exercise guidelines for use with patients who have an elevated INR in an acute care setting:

- If the INR is less than 4.0: The patient should be permitted to participate in a physical or occupational therapy evaluation and his or her regular exercise program. Advancement of the exercise program or greatly increasing the intensity of exercise should wait until the patient is within his or her therapeutic range.

- If the INR is between 4.0 and 5.0: Resistive exercises should not be performed and only light exercise (i.e., a rating of perceived exertion of less than or equal to 11) should be permitted. If the patient is ambulatory, any unsteadiness should be addressed with the appropriate assistive device and close supervision. All precautions to avoid a fall must be taken, especially if the patient is older than 70 years.

- If the INR is greater than 5.0: The patient should not exercise, or exercise should consist of an evaluation of the patient's current mobility in the hospital to assess the patient's safety and to assist in discharge planning. For example, if the patient is currently getting out of bed to use a bedside commode, an occupational or physical therapist should assess this level of activity to determine whether it can be safely continued. Activity should not progress until the INR has decreased. The goal of the therapy evaluation should be to evaluate the current activity level and begin the discharge planning. The role of the therapist is to determine whether the patient's current activity level is safe.

- If the INR is 6.0 or higher: Bed rest or lessening the patient's activity level until the INR is corrected should be considered. In most cases, it takes 2 days to correct the INR. If INR correction is apparent, the caregiver should discuss the case with the physician and weigh the risk of bleeding (which is significant) against the risks associated with bed rest. Patients who have normal mobility (and as a result are probably not receiving physical therapy in the acute care setting) may be allowed to mobilize on a case-by-case basis. However, even in persons with normal mobility, stairs and resistive exercises should be avoided by those who have an INR of 6.0 or higher (Table 10-3).

Feeding Devices

It may be necessary to provide nutrition for a patient who is unable to eat independently or who is unable to chew, swallow, or ingest food.

Nasogastric Tube A nasogastric (NG) tube is a plastic tube inserted through a nostril that eventually terminates in the patient's stomach. Purposes of the NG tube include removing fluid or gas from the stomach and gastrointestinal

Table 10-3	Exercise Guidelines for Patients Receiving Anticoagulation in an Acute Care Setting
International Normalized Ratio (INR)	**Activity Level**
0.8-1.2	Normal range for healthy adults; normal activity
<4.0	Physical therapy or occupational therapy evaluation and regular exercise program; no increase in intensity of exercises
4.0-5.0	Resistive exercises withheld; light exercise only; assistive devices for ambulation if unsteady
5.0-6.0	Exercise should be withheld; evaluate current activity level and assess for safety and discharge
>6.0	Bed rest should be considered by the medical team

From Tuzson A: *How high is too high? INR and acute care physical therapy.* Available at The Free Library by Farlex: http://physical-therapy.advanceweb.com/Article/Lighten-Up-on-Patients-Who-Risk-Bleeding.aspx

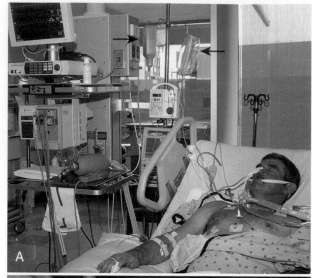

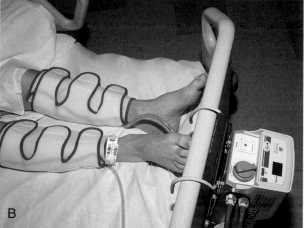

Fig. 10-12   **A,** Multiple intravenous lines with solutions for infusion. **B,** Antiembolism leg wraps (arteriovenous leg pumps).

(GI) tract, evaluating digestive function and activity in the GI tract, administering medications directly into the GI tract, providing a means to feed the patient, allowing treatment to the upper portion of the GI tract, and obtaining gastric specimens. Some patients will report having a sore throat or may have an increased gag reflex as a result of the tube. The patient will not be able to eat food or drink fluids through the mouth while the NG tube is in place. Exercise can be performed with the NG tube in place, but movement of the patient's head and neck should be avoided, especially flexion or forward bending.

Gastric Tube A gastric tube (G tube) is a plastic tube that is inserted directly into the stomach through an incision in the patient's abdomen. Many of the purposes described for the NG tube also apply to the G tube. Exercise can be performed as long as the caregiver is aware of the presence of the G tube and avoids removing the tube.

Intravenous Feeding, Total Parenteral Nutrition, and Hyperalimentation Devices IV feeding techniques permit infusion of large amounts of nutrients that are needed to promote tissue growth. They are a means to achieve an appropriate metabolic state in patients who are unable to, should not, or refuse to eat.

A catheter is inserted directly into the subclavian vein or sometimes into the jugular or another vein and then is passed into the subclavian vein. The catheter may be connected to a semipermanently fixed cannula or sutured at the point of insertion. The caregiver should carefully observe the various connections to be certain they are secure before and after exercise. A disrupted or loose connection may result in the development of an air embolus, which could be life threatening to the patient.

Usually the system will include an infusion pump, which will administer fluids and nutrients at a preselected, constant flow rate. An audible alarm will be activated if the system becomes unbalanced or when the fluid source is empty.

Exercise can be performed as long as the caregiver does not disrupt, disconnect, or occlude the tubing and cause undue stress to the infusion site. Motions of the shoulder on the side of the infusion site, especially abduction and flexion, may be restricted.

Intravenous Infusion Lines IV lines are used to infuse fluids, nutrients, electrolytes, and medications; to obtain venous blood samples; and to insert catheters into the central circulatory system to monitor the physiologic condition of the patient, especially the cardiopulmonary system (Fig. 10-12).

The components of the IV system usually consist of the solution or fluid container, which may be a bottle or plastic bag; a device to measure the number of drops of fluid administered per minute; plastic tubing; a roller clamp to control the rate of the flow of fluid; and a needle to enter the vein. Some IV systems include an infusion pump, which provides a constant, preselected fluid flow rate. Box 10-3 lists commonly used IV infusion sites.

Most IV insertions are made into superficial veins. Various sizes and types of needles or catheters are used, depending on the purpose of the IV therapy, the infusion site, the need for prolonged therapy, and site availability.

Possible complications associated with the IV administration include infiltration of fluid into the subcutaneous tissue, phlebitis, cellulitis, thrombosis, local hematoma, sepsis, pulmonary thromboembolus, air embolus, or a catheter fragment embolus. The caregiver should ensure that the IV bag is above the level of the heart when moving the patient to prevent reflux of the IV fluid. Caution must be used to avoid disruption, disconnection, or occlusion of the tubing; stress to the infusion site; or interruption of circulatory flow. The infusion site should remain dry, the needle should remain secure and immobile in the vein, and no restraint should be placed above the infusion site (for example, avoid applying a blood pressure cuff above the infusion site). The caregiver should observe the infusion site for signs of infiltration of the fluid into the subcutaneous tissue (e.g., edema, hyperemia, a report of site discomfort by the patient, reduced flow of fluid, or infection). Observe the total system to be certain it is functioning properly when you begin and end the treatment (Box 10-4).

Exercise can be performed, but disruption, disconnection, occlusion, or overstretching of the tubing must be avoided. If the infusion site is in the antecubital area, the elbow should not be flexed. The patient who ambulates with an IV line in place should be instructed to grasp the IV line support pole so the infusion site will be at the heart level. If the extremity with the infusion site remains in a dependent position, blood flow may be affected, resulting in retrograde flow of blood into the IV line tubing. Similar procedures to maintain the infusion site in a proper position should be followed when the patient is treated while in bed, on a treatment table, or on a platform mat. Activities that require the infusion site to be elevated above the level of

the heart for a prolonged period should be avoided so the proper direction of the flow of the IV fluid will be maintained.

Nursing personnel should be informed of problems related to the IV system that develop as you treat the patient. Unless the caregiver has been specifically instructed and trained to adjust, modify, alter, or otherwise correct the IV system, a qualified person should be asked to correct any problems that develop during the treatment. However, simple procedures such as straightening the tubing or removing an object that is occluding the tubing should be performed by the caregiver.

Urinary Catheters

A urinary catheter can be applied internally (i.e., an indwelling catheter) or externally. The external urinary catheter is used successfully only in male patients. A catheter inserted through the urethra and into the bladder is an internal catheter. A condom applied externally to the penis of a male patient with a drainage tube attached to it is an external catheter. No practical, acceptable, or effective external catheter has been developed for female patients.

Urinary catheters are used to remove urine from the bladder so it can drain through plastic tubing into a collection bag (Fig. 10-13), bottle, or urinal. Urinary catheters are used for a patient who has lost voluntary control of micturition. This lack of control may be attributable to a spinal cord injury, a surgical procedure, a disease such as multiple sclerosis, or the physiological changes associated with old age. Any form of trauma, disease, condition, or disorder that affects the neuromuscular control of the bladder sphincter may necessitate the use of a urinary catheter, including before and after some surgical procedures. The catheter may be used temporarily or for a prolonged period, even for the remainder of the patient's life. Common complications

---

Box **10-3** Common Intravenous Infusion Sites

- Upper extremity: metacarpal and dorsal venous plexus of the hand; basilic, cephalic, and antecubital veins
- Lower extremity: dorsal venous plexus and medial, lateral, and marginal veins of the foot; saphenous and femoral veins
- Head: superficial scalp veins (often selected for use with infants and the elderly)

Box **10-4** Complications Associated with Intravenous Therapy

- Infiltration: Cool skin or swelling around the site; swelling of the limb; sluggish flow rate
- Phlebitis: Pain in limb; erythema; edema with induration; streak formation
- Thrombophlebitis: Painful intravenous site; erythema; edema with induration; sluggish flow rate
- Air embolism: Decrease or drop in blood pressure; weak, rapid pulse; cyanosis; loss of consciousness; increase or rise in central venous pressure
- Infection of venipuncture site: Swelling and soreness at the site; foul-smelling discharge
- Systemic infection: Sudden rise in temperature and pulse rate; chills and shaking; changes in blood pressure
- Allergic reaction: Fever; swelling or generalized edema; itching or rash; respiratory distress, especially shortness of breath

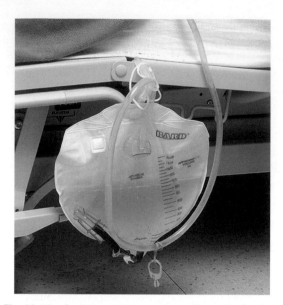

Fig. 10-13 A urinary drainage system with a collection bag.

associated with the use of a catheter are infection of the urinary tract or bladder, development of a urethral fistula, formation of bladder calculi as a result of urinary stasis, and kidney failure. Patients with a spinal cord injury above the T6 cord level may experience autonomic hyperreflexia caused by urine retention. This condition is described in Chapter 12.

Exercise of the lower extremities can be performed by a patient with a catheter as long as the caregiver avoids disruption, disconnection, stretching, or occlusion of the drainage tube. You should determine how much free tubing is available before initiating exercise to avoid causing excessive tension on the tubing. Urine drains into the collection bag as a result of the effect of gravity; therefore the bag should not be positioned above the level of the bladder for more than a few minutes. The bag should not be placed in the patient's lap when he or she is being transported by wheelchair or on the lower abdomen when he or she is lying on a wheeled stretcher. Furthermore, the bag and tubing should be positioned and secured to minimize the possibility that the bag or the tubing will be pulled or snagged. When the patient ambulates, the bag should be positioned and maintained below the level of the bladder, but it should not interfere with gait or ambulation activities.

It may be difficult to provide an adequate position to promote drainage when the patient receives hydrotherapy in an immersion tank or sit-in whirlpool. In such cases, the bag can be positioned below the level of the bladder, but the tubing will need to be elevated over the edge of the tank or whirlpool before it can be directed downward to the bag. This position of the tubing may prevent urine from draining because it will have to drain upward or against the force of gravity. You should drain any urine in the tubing into the bag before the patient is placed in the water to assist with the future drainage. The bag should not be immersed in the water. At some institutions, treatment protocols may permit clamping of the tubing or catheter before the patient is immersed so the bag can be removed for the length of the treatment. However, the flow of urine should not be occluded for an extended period and should not be occluded frequently to avoid the infection associated with the stasis of urine in the bladder.

The caregiver should observe the color of the urine and be alert for unusual odors. Foul-smelling urine, cloudy, dark urine, or urine with blood in it (hematuria) should be reported to a physician or nurse, especially if it is not mentioned in the medical record. You also should observe the flow and amount of urine in the bag. Any reduced flow or decreased production of urine should be reported. The caregiver should document and verbally report observations of abnormal urine appearance, odor, or production promptly so proper treatment can be initiated.

Infection can be a major complication for a person who uses a catheter, particularly if it is an indwelling catheter. All personnel who are involved with the patient should maintain cleanliness when treatment is provided. Precautions must be used when replacing any tubing that has been disengaged from the catheter or the collection bag, when replacing the bag, and when the catheter is inserted into the bladder. Many times it is safer to allow nursing personnel to replace or reconnect the tubing rather than reconnecting it with use of an improper technique. Treatment settings that routinely treat patients with catheters usually have specific protocols for the care of the tubing and the collection bag as well as the insertion and removal of the catheter. It is important that infection be prevented from developing in the urinary system. Therefore strict adherence to the principles of medical and surgical asepsis is necessary by all personnel, especially hand hygiene and the use of disposable gloves.

Foley Catheter The Foley type of indwelling catheter is held in place in the bladder by a small balloon that is inflated with air, water, or sterile saline solution. The catheter has two or three tubes or channels in it. The main channel allows the urine to drain, and the other channels are used to inflate the balloon and irrigate the bladder. To remove the catheter, the balloon is deflated and the catheter is withdrawn.

External Catheter The external catheter (condom) is applied over the shaft of the penis and is held in place by an adhesive applied to the skin or by a padded strap or tape encircling the proximal shaft of the penis. (Caution: The tape or strap must not be applied too tightly to avoid occlusion of the urethra or the blood supply of the penis.)

Suprapubic Catheter Another type of urinary catheter that may be encountered is a suprapubic catheter. This catheter is inserted directly into the bladder through an incision in the lower abdomen and bladder. The catheter may be held in place by adhesive tape, but care should be taken to avoid accidentally removing it.

Oxygen Therapy Systems

Administration of oxygen may be required after surgery and for patients who have a variety of conditions, including an MI and other cardiac problems, respiratory diseases, or inadequate lung function. The purpose of oxygen therapy is to provide and maintain an adequate amount of oxygen in the patient's blood in response to the patient's needs when the patient is unable to provide an adequate amount independently (Fig. 10-14). Several devices or modes can be used to deliver oxygen, and the selection of the specific device will depend on the patient's condition or illness and functional respiratory capabilities. Regardless of how it is delivered, the oxygen should be humidified to reduce its drying effect on the respiratory mucous membranes.

Modes of Oxygen Delivery

Nasal Cannula. The nasal cannula has two plastic prongs (i.e., points or tips) that are inserted into the patient's nostrils. The points are joined by a plastic connector that rests below the nose and above the patient's upper lip and is secured by tubing positioned above the ears. This mode is used most frequently for patients who require low to moderate concentrations of oxygen (e.g., patients with COPD).

Oronasal Mask. The oronasal mask is a triangular plastic device with small vent holes in it to expel exhaled air; it covers the patient's nose and mouth. It is used for short

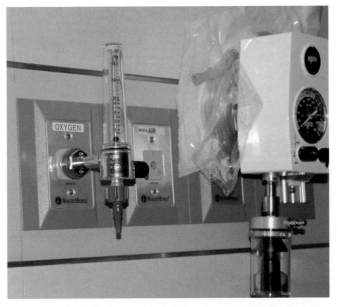

Fig. 10-14   An in-room oxygen flow meter (a wall suctioning system is to the right).

periods when moderate concentrations of oxygen are desired, such as when weaning a postsurgical patient from long-term therapy, when the need exists for higher concentrations of oxygen, or as a temporary approach until a decision is made regarding a permanent form of oxygen delivery.

Nasal Catheter. A catheter can be inserted through the nasal passage to the nasopharyngeal junction, which is located just below the level of the soft palate. The uses of this catheter are similar to those described for the nasal cannula.

Tent. Occasionally, a tent-like device that encloses the patient's trunk and head may be used, especially if the patient is restless, very young, uncooperative, or extremely ill. The edges of the tent must be sealed to prevent the loss of oxygen, and thus frequent and repeated monitoring of the system may be required by nursing personnel.

Tracheostomy Mask or Catheter. Some patients may have a temporary or permanent tracheostomy through which oxygen can be administered by a mask placed over the stoma or by a catheter inserted into the stoma.

In the hospital setting, oxygen is obtained from a wall unit when the patient is in bed or from an oxygen cylinder that accompanies the patient when he or she is out of the room. The oxygen in the cylinder or tank is compressed or pressurized, and a regulator on the tank controls the administration of the oxygen to the patient. The rate of flow, in liters per minute, is determined by a physician and is delivered and maintained by proper adjustment of the regulator valve.

Because oxygen supports combustion, care must be used to prevent a fire or an explosion. Excessive heat, such as a flame, spark, radiator, or even high room temperature, must be avoided when oxygen is administered. When the cylinder is not in use, it should be stored in a temperate, dry, and well-ventilated area and should be handled with care to avoid damage to the regulator valve or to the cylinder itself to prevent rapid release of the compressed gas. Cylinders should be transported on a wheeled carrier or on a wheeled pushcart for larger cylinders. Care should be used to avoid dropping or tipping the tank onto the floor to prevent damage to the tank or the control device. When a patient who is receiving oxygen therapy ambulates, the cylinder should accompany the patient in a wheeled carrier, be attached to a bracket on the wheelchair, or be carried by another person. Several other types of mobile oxygen supply systems can be used by persons to allow them to participate in their daily activities. The same precautions described previously should be applied to these devices (see Fig. 11-20 in Chapter 11).

Precautions to be considered when treating a patient who is receiving oxygen include avoiding disruption, disconnection, or occlusion of the tubing; maintaining the prescribed flow rate; and maintaining a free flow of oxygen. In addition, be alert for signs or symptoms of respiratory distress exhibited by the patient. If the patient reports dyspnea, shortness of breath, or cramping in the calf muscles, or if the patient exhibits cyanosis of the nail beds or lips, he or she may be experiencing respiratory or circulatory distress. Exercise or physical activity should cease, the oxygen delivery system should be evaluated for improper function, and qualified personnel may need to be contacted for assistance. The patient may obtain symptomatic relief by standing and partially flexing the trunk, while placing the upper extremities on a firm object for support. Do not place the patient in a supine position; instead, the patient should lean forward slightly when seated. The patient may rest with the forearms on the thighs, on the chair armrests, or on a firm table to relieve respiratory distress.

The prescribed flow rate must not be altered when the patient performs exercise. Complications can develop if the patient receives an overdose of oxygen, especially patients with COPD, whose usual dose is 2 L per minute. Careful monitoring of the patient's response to the exercise or activity must be performed to avoid or quickly identify an adverse response and to provide appropriate emergency care.

Chest Drainage Systems

Chest drainage tubes may be used to remove air, blood, purulent matter, or other undesirable material from the patient's chest or pleural cavity. These tubes are inserted through an incision in the chest and may be connected to a mechanical or gravity-based suction system (Fig. 10-15).

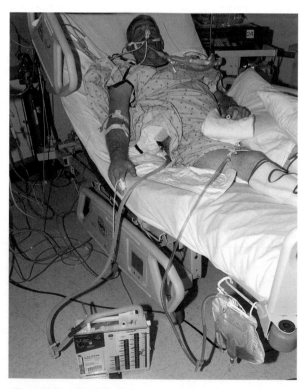

Fig. 10-15   Chest drainage system with collection reservoir.

Three types of chest tube bottle systems are used, which use one, two, or three bottles. The one- and two-bottle systems function by gravity, whereas the three-bottle system and the commercially available disposable systems use a pump to create suction.

The chest tubes are inserted in different locations depending on the type of drainage that is desired. Tubes that are placed in the anterior or lateral chest wall promote the removal of air (as in treating a pneumothorax); tubes placed inferiorly and posteriorly promote the removal of fluids and blood; and mediastinal tubes can be used to drain blood and fluid, which may be necessary after open chest or heart surgery. The drainage tubes usually are maintained securely in place with adherent dressings or sutures, but care should be used to avoid pulling on them or the connecting tubing. Additional precautions are as follows: (1) Avoid disruption of the bottles or containers located on the floor; (2) avoid disconnection or occlusion of the tubing; (3) observe the color of the drainage; (4) observe the system for proper function; and (5) monitor the patient's response to exercise or activity. For the patient who ambulates, the collection bottles should be kept below the level of the location of the inserted tube.

Other types of suction equipment used to remove pulmonary secretions are shown in Fig. 10-16.

Ostomy Devices

An ostomy is a surgically produced opening in the abdomen to allow the elimination of feces. More specifically, an enterostomy is a surgical procedure that produces an artificial stoma into the small intestine through an incision in the abdominal wall. An ileostomy and a colostomy are types of enterostomies. The stoma is covered with a plastic bag or pouch to collect waste. Most patients find it necessary to have the collection bag in place at all times, particularly if the waste is more liquid than solid. The location of the ostomy will affect the need for and the extent to which the patient will use or change the collection bag or pouch.

Three primary types of collecting devices are used for patients with an ostomy; they are designated by the way they are attached to the patient. The bag may be a two-piece pouch that attaches to a skin barrier that adheres to the patient's skin with an adhesive, a one-piece pouch attached to a skin barrier, or an adhesive-backed pouch that adheres to a separate skin barrier. The pouch may be disposable or reusable. Components of the system include an odor-proof plastic pouch, a skin barrier, a filter for gas release, and a means to attach the pouch to the skin barrier or the skin barrier to the skin, such as an adhesive seal or belt tabs.

The caregiver should be aware that the patient has an ostomy and that excessive stress to the attachment of the pouch should be avoided during treatment. Most patients can be treated with minimal concern for the development

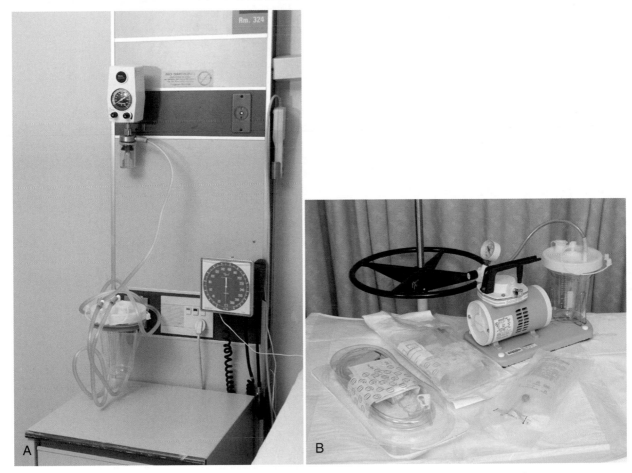

Fig. 10-16   **A,** In-room suction equipment. **B,** A mechanical suction system with a reservoir.

of complications or the need to restrict exercise or activity. The patient with a recent ostomy may be sensitive to and concerned about whether the system will function properly. The caregiver should avoid activities that may cause the patient to experience a socially embarrassing event (e.g., leakage of waste or intestinal gas). Usually, it is desirable to schedule the patient's treatment after the pouch has been emptied or to coordinate it with the patient's bowel habits.

Traction

Traction applied to an extremity can be used to align fracture segments, stretch soft tissue, reduce muscle spasm or contractures, and immobilize the patient. It may be applied to the skin or to a skeletal structure and may be applied constantly or intermittently. Skin traction must be applied with low weights because of the intolerance of the skin and soft tissue to excessive force. Skeletal traction is applied through a pin or wire inserted into bone to which traction ropes and weights are attached. Skeletal traction is used to position, immobilize, and align fracture segments to promote their proper healing.

Types of Skeletal Traction

Balanced Suspension Traction Balanced suspension traction is used primarily to treat displaced or comminuted femoral fractures. A splint under the femur (i.e., a Thomas splint) and one under the lower leg (i.e., a Pearson attachment) are used to balance and suspend the extremity. A pin or wire such as a Kirschner wire or Steinmann pin is inserted through the tibial plateau to provide traction to the distal femoral segment. Because of this arrangement, the traction will remain "balanced" even when the patient moves in bed. Exercises can be performed to the noninjured extremities, and ankle movements can be performed on the injured extremity. This type of traction requires prolonged immobilization of the patient, which can lead to secondary complications such as contractures, pressure ulcers, and sepsis. The more recent use of internal or external fixation devices, as described later in this section, has reduced the need for this type of traction and enhanced the functional recovery of the patient.

Skull Traction Skull traction is applied by tongs (e.g., Crutchfield, Gardner-Wells, Vinke, or Barton tongs) positioned into small holes drilled in the outer layer of the patient's skull. The traction is applied through a rope-weight arrangement and is used for patients with a fracture or dislocation of one or more cervical vertebrae.

Precautions to be aware of when treating the patient who has skull traction are as follows: (1) be certain the traction weights hang freely after the patient has been repositioned; (2) avoid removal or release of any traction weight during treatment, unless prescribed; (3) avoid bumping the weights, because doing so will create motion through the rope to the fracture site; and (4) note the condition of the site of the pin. Look for bleeding, skin disruption, drainage, or signs of inflammation at the site of the pin insertion. Any unusual observations should be documented and reported promptly.

A device frequently referred to as a "halo" (Fig. 10-17) can be applied to provide traction and stability to the cervical spine. The device is held in place by four pins inserted into the patient's skull and a metal ring that connects the pins, to which four vertical uprights are attached. The uprights are anchored to two over-the-shoulder plates, which are connected to a padded vest worn over the upper body. With the halo in place, the patient can be mobile and can sit, stand, and perform various activities. Exercise of the extremities can be performed, but care should be used when movement of the shoulder is attempted or when the muscles that attach to the cervical vertebrae are contracted to avoid stress to the fracture site and to the corresponding nerve roots of that area.

External Fixation External fixation is a form of stabilization and traction that uses a variety of frames applied externally to the patient's extremity (e.g., Haynes, Hoffmann, or Anderson devices). Two of these examples are shown in Fig. 10-18. These frames hold pins that have been inserted into the bone fragments of a severe fracture to maintain the fracture in alignment. This form of fixation allows earlier and greater mobility for the patient while providing excellent alignment and stabilization of the fracture segments. Ambulation on both lower extremities and exercise of the noninjured extremities or areas of the body can be performed, although weight bearing on the involved extremity may be contraindicated or limited. This form of fixation is particularly beneficial for a comminuted fracture, an extensive open fracture, or an infected open fracture or when bone grafts are involved. Be careful to avoid excess stress to the exposed frame and pins, and observe the insertion sites for evidence of adverse reactions to the pins (e.g., infection or bone deterioration). (Note: Care must be taken when the patient uses ambulation aids so the external apparatus is not struck or does not interfere with the ambulation pattern.)

Internal Fixation The internal fixation method of treatment uses hardware applied internally to or within bone to maintain its alignment and stability after fracture reduction. The hardware can include transfixation screws, bone plates, wires, nails, and intramedullary rods. The technique usually provides a shorter period of immobilization, a stable fracture site, maintenance of local circulation, and more rapid return to functional activities.

The treatment procedures selected will vary depending on the location and type of fracture, the hardware used to fixate the fracture, and the patient's general condition. Early

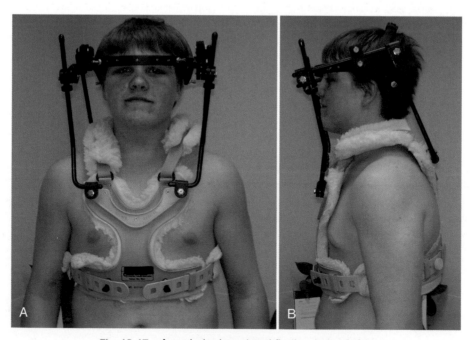

Fig. 10-17   A cervical spine external fixation device (halo).

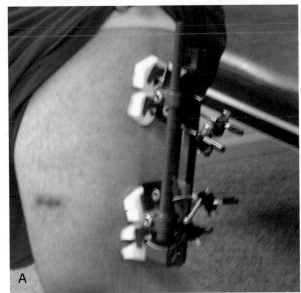

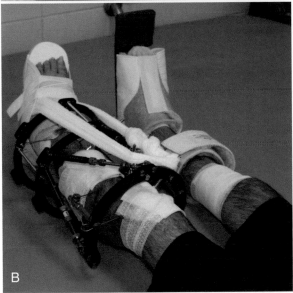

Fig. 10-18   Examples of extremity external fixation devices.

active or passive mobilization of the joints proximal and distal to the fracture should be initiated. Isometric exercise of the muscles that cross the fracture and that are immobilized (as in a cast) can be performed to maintain muscle tone, local circulation, and muscle awareness. Active and active-resistive exercise for the muscles and joints of the noninvolved extremities should be performed to maintain or improve ROM and strength.

Ambulation after a fracture in a lower extremity usually can be performed shortly after the fracture has been reduced and fixated. The amount or type of weight bearing depends on the location of the fracture, the type of fixation device, the general condition of the patient, and the orders of the surgeon.

If a surgical open reduction was performed, caution may be necessary to protect the fracture site and soft-tissue incision until healing occurs. The open reduction of the fracture has the potential for wound infection, which is a disadvantage of this procedure. In addition, the complication of the development of a venous embolus may occur after a femoral fracture. If the embolus is transported to the pulmonary artery, a life-threatening condition exists.

Patient-Controlled Analgesia

The patient-controlled analgesia system allows patients to self-administer a small predetermined dose of pain medication intravenously on demand, as frequently as every 6 minutes. A reservoir of the medication is connected by tubing to an IV line and to a small control module or pump, which the patient wears on the wrist or has at the bedside. When medication is desired, the patient presses a button on the control module; the medication moves to a small area in the control module and then passes through tubing into the IV line. The unit will not deliver more medication than the premeasured dose each time the patient activates the button. In addition, the patient cannot receive the medication more frequently than a predetermined period (e.g., every 6 minutes). The number of requests the patient has made and the number of doses the unit has delivered are recorded by the unit and are available for review. This device should not interfere with the patient's exercise program or other activities. However, the precautions outlined for IV lines should be followed.

Dialysis Treatment

Dialysis is used for patients who experience acute or end-stage renal disease. The single leading cause of end-stage renal disease is type 2 diabetes, followed by high blood pressure, glomerulonephritis, and a cystic kidney. The objectives of dialysis are to prevent infection, restore the normal level of fluids and electrolytes, control the acid-base balance, remove waste and toxic materials, and assist in or replace normal kidney function.

An important issue for patients who undergo dialysis is regular access to removal of waste products from the body. The two types of generally accepted methods of artificial kidney treatment are hemodialysis and peritoneal dialysis. Most patients who undergo dialysis receive hemodialysis, which may be provided through a prosthetic shunt or an arteriovenous fistula. Blood is pumped out of the patient's body to the dialyzer, which cleanses the blood of wastes, and the cleansed blood is returned to the body from the machine through connecting tubing. This method of dialysis is usually performed for 2- to 4-hour periods or longer and is done at least three times per week. Advantages of this method are that trained professionals are with the patient during the procedure and minimal disruption of lifestyle occurs between treatments.

Exercise and activity can be performed safely while undergoing hemodialysis, but excessive activity involving the area of the shunt and application of any occlusive item (such as a blood pressure cuff) or restraint to the upper arm of the extremity containing the shunt should be avoided.

During peritoneal dialysis, the inside lining of the abdomen acts as a natural filter. Wastes are taken out by means of the cleansing fluid called dialysate, which is washed in and out of the body in cycles. The dialysate solution is delivered into and removed from the abdomen through a catheter that has been surgically implanted in the abdominal wall. This method of dialysis is repeated several times a day or can be done automatically by a machine (cycler) during the night. Advantages of this method are that the patient can do the treatment alone and at the times and places desired.

Care should be taken to avoid pulling on the peritoneal tube or the tubing attached to it and to avoid occluding the drainage tubing.

SUMMARY

It may be necessary to treat a patient who is very ill, whose condition requires highly specialized care, or who needs a variety of devices and equipment to maintain life. These patients should be treated with caution and frequent monitoring. A patient who uses any of the devices, systems, or procedures described in this chapter should be evaluated whenever treatment is provided, and the response to treatment should be documented at the conclusion of each treatment session. Any complications or problems encountered or any deviations from the expected treatment results should be noted. Serious or unusual adverse patient responses to treatment should be discussed directly with the appropriate physician or nurse. Many of these patients are acutely ill and probably will not tolerate exercise or physical activity as easily as patients who are less ill. You are encouraged to proceed carefully by maintaining the program within the functional and physiological capacities of each patient.

self-study ACTIVITIES

- Describe how you might need to alter or modify your treatment plan and program to accommodate the types of patient conditions presented in this chapter.
- Explain the immediate and long-term actions you would perform if a patient exhibited adverse responses to the treatment received.
- Define the following: IV line, SICU, CCU, PACU, A line, NG tube, skeletal traction, external fixation, TPN or hyperalimentation, and ventilator. (Select other acronyms or terms and define them.)
- Outline the components you believe should be included in a program designed to orient or familiarize a therapist with the equipment, environment, and patient devices that are likely to be encountered in an intensive care unit.
- If a patient in an intensive care unit is unable to sit at the edge of the bed unsupported, what type of transfers would you perform to get the patient into a chair?

problem SOLVING

1. You are treating a 55-year-old patient in an intensive care unit who is on a ventilator. The treatment includes active assistive exercises to the extremities. During one of the treatment sessions, the alarm on the ventilator sounds. What are your immediate actions at this time, and what would you do if the patient exhibited signs of respiratory distress?

2. You are to treat a 63-year-old man in a surgical intensive care unit who had open heart surgery 2 days ago. He is supported by a ventilator, an IV infusion in the left forearm, and urinary and chest drainage systems. What would you do before you begin to treat him? What precautions and contraindications should you be aware of before and during the treatment?

CHAPTER 11

Basic Wound Care and Specialized Interventions

objectives *After studying this chapter, the reader will be able to:*

- Describe the functions of a dressing and a bandage.
- Describe and demonstrate the proper application and removal of a dressing.
- Describe and demonstrate the proper application and removal of a bandage that covers a dressing.
- Assess and determine the stage of a pressure ulcer.
- Describe four tests to assess peripheral venous and arterial circulation.
- Describe and demonstrate girth measurement.
- Describe a treatment approach for lymphedema.
- Describe the principles and function of compression garments and how to measure the extremities for a garment.
- Describe the functions of chest physical therapy and demonstrate postural drainage positions.
- Describe the immediate postoperative goals of a lower extremity amputation.
- Describe the uses for kinesiology taping.

key terms

Autolysis   The disintegration of cells or tissues by the enzymes of the body or cellular components in wound fluid.

Chest physical therapy (CPT)   Gravity-assisted bronchial drainage with techniques for secretion removal and breathing techniques.

Debridement   The removal of devitalized tissues from or adjacent to a traumatic or infected lesion to expose healthy tissue.

Dysvascular amputation   Denotes amputations that are caused or acquired from poor vascular status of a limb (i.e., ischemia).

Epithelialization   Healing by the growth of epithelium over a denuded surface.

Erythema   Redness of the skin caused by congestion of the capillaries in the lower layers of the skin.

Eschar   A dry scab; devitalized tissue.

Exudate   A fluid with a high composition of protein and cellular debris that has escaped from blood vessels and is deposited in tissues or on tissue surfaces.

Granulation   Any granular material on the surface of a tissue, membrane, or organ.

Induration   The quality of being hard; abnormal firmness of tissue with a definite margin.

Lymphedema   A functional overload of the lymphatic system in which lymph volume exceeds transport capabilities, resulting in obstructed lymph flow.

Maceration   The softening of a solid or tissue by soaking.

Necrosis   The morphological changes indicative of cell death.

Pressure ulcer   A localized injury to the skin and/or underlying tissue, usually over a bony prominence, as a result of pressure or pressure in combination with shear force and/or friction.

Slough   A mass of dead tissue in, or cast out from, living tissue; pronounced "sluf."

Sterile   Free from any microorganisms; aseptic.

INTRODUCTION

The care and management of wounds is an important aspect of patient treatment. The ability of the caregiver to establish and maintain a sterile or clean environment during the application of a dressing and to avoid contamination of the wound, other persons, equipment, or treatment areas is of paramount importance. The application of the principles and techniques of proper hand hygiene and the use of protective garments (see Chapter 2) are necessary activities for the caregiver when treating a wound. A wound that is contaminated or caused by pressure to the tissue overlying a bony prominence requires consistent and persistent care to enhance the healing process. The judicious use of protective positioning (see Chapter 5), nursing procedures, topical or systemic medications, appropriate nutrition and hydration supplements, and proper skin care are critical components of wound care.

The caregiver must be able to recognize the type of wound, the phase of healing it represents, and the factors that affect wound healing. Each wound should be assessed to determine its size, depth, and appearance so that subsequent assessments can be compared with the initial findings. The procedures used to assess, classify, and stage a wound are presented later in this chapter.

Information about establishing a sterile field and the application of a topical medication and its covering bandage to protect the wound from contamination are described. The caregiver must remember that prevention of wound contamination and cross-infection of others are critical elements of wound care.

Girth measurement, when performed over time, is an important process that provides objective evidence of a change in limb size as a result of edema or atrophy. These measurements also provide evidence of treatment success for a variety of disorders. Serial measurements and techniques are discussed in this chapter, as is volumetric measurement of the hand and foot.

Edema occurs when venous or lymphatic vessels (or both) are impaired. In this book, we will focus primarily on lymphedema. When impairment is so great that the lymphatic fluid exceeds the lymphatic transport capacity, the result is an abnormal collection of high-protein fluid in the interstitial spaces. Lymphedema can be primary (i.e., congenital, usually found in the lower extremities) or secondary (i.e., caused by surgical removal of lymph nodes, tumor invasion of the lymph nodes, injury or infection to the lymph drainage system, or radiation therapy, which can damage the lymph channels). Lymphedema can be found in any part of the body but is usually limited to the extremities.

Patients who have undergone an axillary or groin dissection should be informed that secondary lymphedema is a possibility, and they should be provided with instruction about preventive measures because lymphedema is a lifelong, chronic condition. Fortunately, effective treatment for both primary and secondary lymphedema is available from caregivers with specialized education. Treatment methods of complete (or complex) decongestive therapy (CDT) are presented, which includes manual lymph drainage (MLD), lymphedema care and precautions, use of a compression pump, use of compression bandages or garments, and therapeutic exercises. Two measurement techniques for upper and lower extremity compression garments also are included in this chapter.

Chest physical therapy (CPT), also known as cardiopulmonary physical therapy, is an important part of care for patients with respiratory disease (e.g., chronic obstructive pulmonary disease, cystic fibrosis, pneumonia, asthma, and carcinoma of the lung) or for patients who have undergone surgery or experienced an injury (e.g., cardiac, thoracic, or lung surgery or fractured ribs). The caregiver should be aware of specific methods of chest care used in a particular setting. In some facilities, a physical therapist will be responsible for all aspects of CPT, including postural drainage, percussion and vibration, and airway clearance (e.g., suctioning and cough techniques). In other settings, respiratory therapy or nursing personnel, or both, will have defined interventions for patients who require respiratory treatment. Suctioning techniques through the nose, mouth, or endotracheal tube are not presented in this book. However, examination and evaluation techniques and the treatment methods of postural drainage and secretion removal, as well as goals for the patient who receives CPT, are described.

Taping strategies will be addressed, with several examples of how different types of tape can be used.

WOUND MANAGEMENT

Dressings and bandages are important items associated with the care and management of wounds. The caregiver must apply the concept of the prevention of wound infection. The basic goals of wound care are listed in Box 11-1.

Phases of Healing

Three phases of wound healing are described in the literature:
- Inflammatory

Box 11-1 Basic Goals of Wound Care and Management

- Protect the wound and surrounding tissue from additional trauma
- Provide an optimal environment for wound healing
- Reduce strain on the tissues near the wound
- Protect the tissue in the area of the wound from mechanical stress or movement
- Reduce the number of pathogenic microorganisms in and around the wound
- Expedite the healing process
- Decrease or reduce the formation of scar tissue

- Proliferative
- Remodeling (maturation)

Inflammatory Phase The inflammatory process initiates wound healing. Its function is to limit tissue damage, remove injured or damaged cells, and repair the injured tissue. The inflammatory process is the body's initial local defense response to injury or trauma, and it begins immediately after injury or trauma.

The inflammatory process consists of at least three stages:
- Vascular
- Exudate
- Reparative

During the acute phase of healing, the vascular stage is characterized by hyperemia because of a change in cellular filtration pressures and an increase in the permeability of cells. These factors usually produce local edema, warmth, erythema, and discomfort, which are the cardinal signs and symptoms of inflammation.

The exudate stage can have any of several appearances: serous (typically pale yellow and transparent, as in a blister), purulent (pus), fibrinous (clotting), or hemorrhagic (bleeding). In the exudate stage, a fluid passes through the walls of vessels into adjacent tissues or spaces to help deposit fibrins and leukocytes, which are necessary to initiate wound healing.

During the reparative stage, damaged cells are replaced and true wound healing begins. Damaged cells are removed through phagocytosis, which is accomplished by polymorphonuclear cells and monocytes.

Proliferative Phase The proliferative phase overlaps the inflammatory phase with granulation, angiogenesis to reestablish capillary buds, contraction, and epithelialization of the wound site. The fibroblastic cells proliferate and collagen tissue develops to initiate scar formation. According to one theory of healing, the fibroblasts and capillary buds develop at the edges of the wound and gradually advance toward the center of the wound. A bed of granulation tissue forms gradually over the surface of the wound, and the epithelial margins begin to migrate toward the center of the wound on top of this granulation bed. This process leads to contraction of the wound and eventual formation of a scar. Epithelialization requires a moist surface, and cells travel about 3 cm from the point of origin in all directions.

Remodeling Phase The remodeling phase overlaps the proliferative phase and is characterized by the organization of the collagen tissue into a more definitive and finite pattern. Another factor associated with the remodeling phase is an increase in the tensile strength of the tissue that covers the wound (i.e., scar tissue). It is important to note that scar tissue is only 80% as strong as the original tissue.

Because the wound heals from the edges toward the center of the wound, care must be taken when removing a dressing from the wound. The dressing should be removed gently and from the edges first to avoid disrupting the healing process, particularly if exudate associated with the wound adheres to the dressing. The remodeling phase can last from 3 weeks to 2 years.

Processes of Healing

Wounds heal by first (primary) or second (secondary) intention (Fig. 11-1). First-intention healing occurs in wounds whose edges are closely related or whose edges have been approximated by sutures, staples, Steri-Strips, or other similar means. These wounds tend to heal with less likelihood of infection, in a shorter period, and with less scar formation than do other wounds. First-intention healing is the preferred and most effective method of healing.

Second-intention healing occurs in wounds with large surface areas or retracted edges or in wounds in which a large amount of tissue has been lost. These types of wounds heal by the gradual filling of the wound with granulation material. Compared with other wounds, these wounds may become infected more easily, usually require an extended healing time, and are likely to exhibit excessive scar formation. If the patient is medically sound and able to tolerate a surgical procedure, these large wounds are better able to heal with the use of skin grafts, skin flaps, or other similar surgical techniques.

Several factors can affect wound healing favorably or unfavorably. Infection or the presence of high numbers of pathogens in the wound or its surrounding tissue will delay or complicate the healing process. The size, extent, distances between the edges, location, and type of wound all can affect healing. A large, deep, irregularly shaped wound usually requires additional time to heal, as does a wound that is located where circulation is limited or impaired (e.g., the shin) (Box 11-2).

The nutritional status of the patient is also an important factor for healing. Compared with a well-nourished person, wound healing for a person with poor nutritional status and dehydration will be more difficult and require more time. A wound in an older adult may not heal as rapidly as a similar wound in a younger adult because of differences in circulation and metabolic responses to the wound. Some medications may enhance wound healing, whereas other medications may delay the healing process. A patient who has a chronic illness or who is generally debilitated will probably exhibit a delay in the healing of the wound. All patients with a wound need to maintain a full level of hydration.

Wound Classification

A burn is caused when the skin contracts in response to dry heat (fire), moist heat (steam or scalding water), chemicals, electricity, or radiation. A burn may be described according

HEALING BY PRIMARY INTENTION

HEALING BY SECONDARY INTENTION

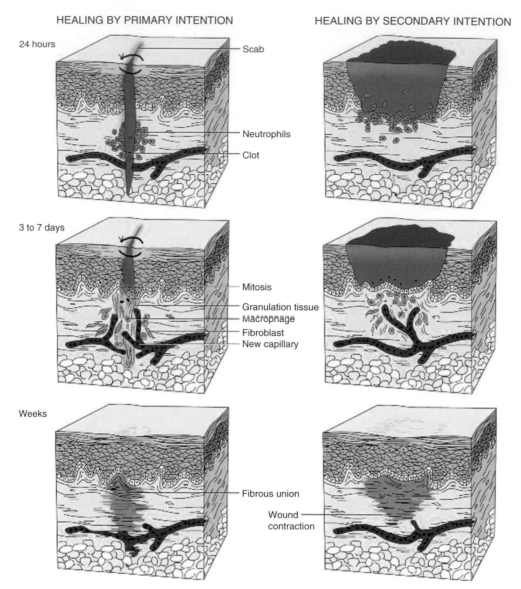

24 hours
— Scab
— Neutrophils
— Clot

3 to 7 days
— Mitosis
— Granulation tissue
— Macrophage
— Fibroblast
— New capillary

Weeks
— Fibrous union
Wound contraction

Fig. 11-1   Diagrammatic comparison of healing by primary intention (*left*) and secondary intention (*right*). (From Cameron MH: *Physical agents in rehabilitation: from research to practice,* ed 3, St Louis, 2009, Saunders.)

to the depth of the wound, for example, superficial (first degree), partial thickness/deep partial thickness (second degree), or full thickness (third degree). The skin has three major components: the epidermis, or upper layer; the dermis, or middle layer; and the subcutaneous fat, or deep layer. When the upper layer of the epidermis is affected, the burn is superficial (first degree); when the deep layer of the epidermis and the dermis are involved, the burn becomes a partial-thickness (second-degree) wound; and when the epidermis, dermis, and subcutaneous tissues (fat or bone) are involved, the burn becomes a full-thickness (third-degree) wound.

The percentage of body area involved also may be used to describe a burn, using the rule of nines or the Lund and Browder chart. The rule of nines assigns specific values to the body surface. For adults, the head and neck is 9%; each upper extremity is 9%; each lower extremity is 18%; the front trunk area is 18%; the back trunk area is 18%; and the genital area is 1%. For children, the head and neck is 18%, the lower extremities are 14%, and the remainder of the body areas have the same values as those listed for adults. The Lund and Browder chart subdivides the extremities into segments (e.g., upper arm, lower arm, and hand; thigh, leg, and foot), with specific values assigned to each area. This chart accounts for the change in body surface areas affected by growth. It is more accurate than the rule of nines when estimating the size of a burn. When more than 18% of a body surface area is involved or when the face, hands, feet, or perineum is involved, the burn is considered a major burn and usually requires admission to a burn care facility or unit.

Box 11-2   Factors That Affect Wound Healing

Depending on the presence or absence of the following factors, a positive or negative effect or influence on the healing of the wound may occur.

EXTRINSIC FACTORS
- Pressure applied to soft tissue that overlies a bony prominence
- Shear force applied to the skin, especially to the heels and sacrum
- Maceration of the skin caused by body waste, perspiration, or skin-to-skin contact (i.e., skin folds)
- Infection
- Reduced activity leading to prolonged immobility

INTRINSIC FACTORS
- General health of the patient
- Condition of the skin
- Body build and composition
- Nutritional status
- Hydration status
- Distance between the edges of the wound
- Location of the wound
- Adequacy of blood flow to the wound

Data from Morey S: *Pressure ulcer/wound care.* Presented at the Ohio Physical Therapy Association Annual Conference, April 17, 1997, Columbus, OH.

An incision is a cut or wound made by a sharp instrument such as a scalpel. An ulceration is the result of an excavation of the surface of an organ or tissue, which is produced by the sloughing or falling away of necrotic inflammatory tissue. Skin ulcers often are located on the distal lower extremities, especially in the area of the malleoli. A pressure ulcer may develop in the tissue that covers a bony prominence (e.g., the sacrum, calcaneus, or greater trochanter) when relief of pressure at the site does not occur.

The preceding information is limited in scope and comprehensiveness but provides a basic description of the process of wound healing and its relationship to wound management. Sources of additional information about the wound-healing process may be found in the Bibliography.

A case study pertaining to the treatment of burns can be found on the Evolve site accompanying this text.

Pressure Ulcers

A pressure ulcer, which sometimes is incorrectly referred to as a decubitus ulcer, pressure sore, or bedsore, is one type of wound that can complicate the care of many patients. Although a pressure ulcer may be prevented through an aggressive treatment plan of ongoing skin care, there is no assurance that these activities will prevent the development of one or more pressure ulcers. Frequent changes in the patient's position, proper and adequate nutrition, and the relief of pressure or reduction in pressure on the soft tissue that overlies bony prominences are all methods of pressure ulcer prevention. Factors that contribute to the risk of pressure ulcers are the patient's age, body condition and composition, disease state, presence of circulation or metabolic disorders, and mobility capability. Every caregiver who treats the patient should be involved in the prevention of pressure ulcers.

Causes A pressure ulcer is a wound that develops as a result of two primary factors:
- Pressure on soft tissue that exceeds the normal capillary pressure of the local circulation
- The application of friction or shear force to superficial skin

When soft tissue is compressed over bony prominences, especially the greater trochanter, sacrum, calcaneus, malleolus, and ischial tuberosity, a pressure ulcer may develop. In those areas, the capillaries that transport oxygen and nutrients to and remove waste products from the tissue become compressed between the underlying bone and the external pressure source. (Note: Table 5-1 presents the locations where pressure ulcers are most likely to develop depending on the patient's position.) When the capillaries are compressed over time, they become occluded, ischemia occurs, and the potential for tissue necrosis exists. If necrosis occurs, tissue is destroyed, and a partial-thickness or full-thickness wound will be evident.

A contributing factor to the development of a pressure ulcer is the application of shear force or friction to the patient's skin, which may occur during position changes, transfers, or exercise activities. A shear force created by the caregiver's hand or the bed linen may produce friction to the skin, which causes increased surface heat and erosion of the epidermis. The combination of prolonged pressure and episodes of shear force applied to the same area of the body causes trauma to the capillaries, skin, and underlying soft tissue, which may lead to the development of a pressure ulcer (see Box 11-2).

Patient Assessment Each patient who is admitted to a health care facility or treated at home should be assessed to determine the potential risk for development of a pressure ulcer. The person's functional abilities, such as bed mobility; activity level; wheelchair or ambulatory mobility; feeding, chewing, and swallowing capability; and transfer performance should be determined. Information about the patient's medical history and current condition, level of mental competence, nutritional status, skin condition, general physical condition, and psychosocial factors are other components of the initial assessment. Identification of specific risk factors should be one of the major outcomes of the initial assessment and examination. Caregivers who frequently treat pressure ulcers often use the Braden Scale for Predicting Pressure Sore Risk (Appendix 11) and the Pressure Ulcer Scale for Healing Tool (Appendix 12) for wound assessment. Reassessment of the wound should be performed at specific intervals and/or with changes in the patient's status.

Box **11-3**	Primary Risk Factors Associated with Pressure Ulcers

- Pressure on tissue overlying bony prominences, especially the sacrum, heels, greater trochanters, vertebral spinous processes, and ischial tuberosities
- Shear and friction forces applied to the skin
- Inadequate or improper nutrition or fluid intake
- Insensate body areas, especially those that are not sensitive to pressure
- Persistent incontinence, which leads to skin irritation, maceration, or breakdown
- Metabolic or systemic disorders or diseases, especially diabetes
- Persons with reduced mobility and contracture
- Persistent use of tobacco products

Risk Factors Some risk factors related to the development of a pressure ulcer are presented in Box 11-3. A risk assessment of a patient at the time of admission to any health care facility or when the person is treated at home by a health care practitioner is a standard of care recommended by several agencies or regulatory bodies, including the Agency for Health Care Policy and Research, the National Pressure Ulcer Advisory Panel, the Omnibus Budget Reconciliation Act, the Association for the Advancement of Wound Care, and the Wound, Ostomy, Continence Nurses Society. A patient who is at risk for the development of pressure ulcers should be identified at admission, the risk factors should be documented, and a prevention program should be initiated promptly. Every person who has contact with the patient, such as housekeeping personnel, family members, aides, technicians, and primary caregivers, should be considered members of the prevention team. These non–primary caregivers are able to observe the patient several times during the day, and their observations, comments, or suggestions can be helpful to the primary caregivers. Pressure ulcer prevention is a responsibility that should be shared by multiple individuals.

Preventive Interventions Relief of pressure on the soft tissue that overlies a bony prominence is the primary method of pressure ulcer prevention. Relief of pressure can be accomplished by elevating the area from the pressure source (e.g., using a pillow beneath the calf to elevate the heel slightly from the mattress when the person is supine), changing the patient's position frequently so an area is not in prolonged contact with a source of pressure (i.e., using a turning or positioning schedule to relieve weight bearing on a specific bony prominence), positioning the patient so an area is not in contact with a source of pressure (i.e., positioning the patient in a partial side-lying position with the use of pillows or foam wedges so he or she does not rest directly on the lowermost greater trochanter), and by separating bony prominences. If the patient is able to independently alter his or her position, instruction on how and when to do so should be provided (e.g., the patient should perform push-ups or lean to one side and then to the other while seated in a wheelchair, lift the pelvis from the mattress using the lower extremities when supine, and use a trapeze to elevate the upper body from the mattress when supine). These activities should be performed several times each hour. (Note: Because repetitive push-ups may cause trauma to the patient's wrists, this method should be alternated with other pressure relief methods.)

Pressure reduction is another preventive method that decreases but does not fully relieve the amount of pressure to an area. Examples of pressure reduction aids or approaches include air-fluidized or low-air-loss beds, "egg crate" foam, closed cell foam mattress overlays, oscillating beds, air or water mattresses, bony joint protectors (i.e., heel or elbow guards), wound protection dressings, and seat cushions (however, the ring or "donut" type of cushion should not be used because the rim of the cushion creates pressure, which occludes capillaries and deprives the local tissue of a proper blood supply and flow).

The following techniques may be used to reduce shear force and friction: using a draw sheet to position or transfer a patient; using double socks to protect the heels; elevating the head of the bed to the lowest level of comfort and function for the patient (at greater than 30 degrees of elevation the patient tends to slide down over the bed linen, creating shear to the sacrum and scapulae); instructing the patient to avoid rubbing his or her heels or elbows on the bed linen when lying supine; and not dragging the patient across the bed linen when he or she is turned, positioned, or transferred. Patients who are incontinent or have skin that is often moist should be monitored, and a moisture barrier ointment should be used frequently (Box 11-4).

According to Masspro (see the Bibliography), the rehabilitation staff can play a significant role in both the prevention and treatment of skin breakdown. Physical and occupational therapists bring a unique set of skills to a multidisciplinary pressure ulcer prevention team. Below are areas of important consideration for position changes:

- The body position of patients who are at risk for pressure sores (e.g., patients who are confused, medicated, have poor nutritional status, have fecal or urinary incontinence, are immobile, or are inactive) should be changed at least every 2 hours. Many at-risk patients will need to have their position changed more frequently.
- Most positions can be easily modified (without a full position change) at the 1-hour mark, allowing pressure relief.
- Avoid placing flaccid or weak extremities in a gravity-dependent position, which facilitates the development of dependent edema. In these cases the most distal part of the extremity should be higher than the heart.

| Box **11-4** | Guidelines for Pressure Ulcer Intervention and Management |

- Provide pressure relief or reduction to body areas susceptible to ulcer development.
- Develop and follow a schedule to alter the patient's position.
- Determine the nutritional and fluid intake needs of the patient; establish an appropriate diet and feeding schedule to meet the patient's needs.
- Initiate mobility activities that are possible, safe, and appropriate; include bed, wheelchair, and ambulation activities. Shear forces must be avoided.
- Debride necrotic tissue, as necessary, to promote healing.
- Perform wound and skin cleansing; avoid the use of toxic agents, including many types of soaps, hydrogen peroxide, and povidone-iodine (Betadine).
- Perform consistent and thorough perineal care, especially when the patient is incontinent, and use a moisture barrier ointment.
- Rinse the ulcer with a sterile saline solution with an appropriate pressure (2 to 10 psi) at the time of dressing changes.
- Develop and follow a schedule to observe, evaluate, remove, and apply dressings that is appropriate for the patient and personnel involved.
- Provide education to all caregivers involved with the patient's care, including the patient's family members; include information on prevention, care, and management.
- Plan and follow a program designed to prevent the development of pressure ulcers, especially for persons who demonstrate a high risk.
- Prevent contractures.

- The primary caregiver should use a turning schedule, and other caregivers who intervene to provide treatment should adhere to the turning schedule after treatment has been performed.
- Ideally, patients should be comfortable in whatever position they are placed. This rule may depend on the patient's problem and diagnosis. Some patient conditions (such as burns to the axilla) do not allow the patient to assume a position of comfort. In the case of burns to the axilla, the most therapeutic position is to have the patient in shoulder abduction, which usually is not a position of comfort. The position of comfort is often the position of contracture.

Table 11-1 lists body positions with suggestions for pressure reduction.

Skin Care Frequent inspection of and attention to the care of a patient's skin, particularly for patients who are incontinent, are important preventive activities. Prompt cleansing of the skin may be necessary, along with maintenance of dry, clean skin of the perineum, buttocks, and upper thighs, and the use of topical agents to provide a

moisture barrier or to moisturize dry skin. In addition, the use of lubricants, protective dressings (i.e., films, hydrocolloids, and hydrogels), and padding should help minimize shear and friction. (Caution: Massage of the tissue that overlies a bony prominence should be avoided because it may traumatize the local capillaries, which are likely to be fragile and susceptible to injury.)

Caregivers whose treatment requires handling of the extremities, especially the upper extremities, should be aware of the possibility of causing a skin tear when treating elderly patients because their skin tends to be fragile. A skin tear should be assessed and measured before it is treated. The area should be cleaned gently with sterile saline solution, and the wound edges should be dried by patting the area with gauze. Small pieces of detached epithelium that appear to be traumatized can be debrided by a qualified caregiver, and skin that appears to be viable and nontraumatized should be repositioned gently over the wound. According to a study by Solway, Consalter, and Levinson (see the Bibliography), a microbial cellulose membrane such as Dermafill can be applied and covered with a protective stockinette. This dressing is never removed but is absorbed by the wound, whereas other dressings need to be changed, can be painful, and can lead to infections.

All caregivers should avoid activities or procedures that intensify the established risk factors for a given patient. Prolonged, excessive pressure over time to bony prominences and shear and friction forces must be avoided during exercise, transfers, mobility activities, and turning or positioning of the patient. Straps used to attach splints or orthoses must not be applied too tightly, and footwear must fit properly to avoid friction or blister development. The caregiver must be aware of the potential for injury or damage to the patient's skin and must adjust the treatment program to avoid trauma (Table 11-2).

Wound Classification and Staging A pressure ulcer should be assessed and classified according to its stage or level of tissue destruction as defined by the National Pressure Ulcer Advisory Panel. The stage designation also provides a diagnosis of the amount or type of tissue insult and injury that has occurred. If the epidermis and a portion of the dermis are involved, the wound is considered to be a partial-thickness wound and the ulcer is considered to be superficial. When the entire dermis and underlying fascia, muscle, tendon, or bone are involved, the wound is considered to be a full-thickness wound and the ulcer is considered to be deep (Fig. 11-2). Table 11-3 lists and describes the four stages associated with a pressure ulcer. These stages can be described as being progressive: stage I becomes stage II and stage II becomes stage III; however, the stages cannot be described regressively. That is, as a stage III ulcer heals, it does not revert to stage II; instead, as a stage III wound heals, it continues to be classified as stage III, but the percentage of the wound that has healed is reported or a

Table 11-1 Common Body Positions and Suggestions for Reducing Pressure

Position	Suggestions for Reducing Pressure
Supine	Body is well aligned (i.e., the head is in a neutral position and is in line with the shoulders; the pillow should not be too high or too low) Heels are off the bed Elbows are supported or protected Hands are higher than the elbow, particularly if the patient has a flaccid extremity The lower extremity is in a neutral position; excessive internal or external rotation at the hips is avoided; support with towel rolls, pillows, or adjunctive devices may be needed
Side lying on the left or right side	Body is well aligned Avoid direct side lying; the patient should be about 30 degrees off a 180-degree position Carefully monitor the lowermost shoulder position The lowermost greater trochanter may need to be bridged Knees should be slightly flexed with a pillow between the legs and the legs not on top of each other, depending on patient comfort Support the lowermost foot well to avoid excess pressure on the lateral malleolus or fifth metatarsal head
Prone (Caution: This position is not well tolerated for 2 h for older adults; a change at 30 min often will need to be made; in addition, this position is not appropriate for persons with breathing problems)	Body is well aligned Have pillows and towel rolls readily available so that as the patient is rolled from a side-lying to a prone position, a pillow is under the abdomen to put the back in neutral or slight flexion, patellae are protected or bridged, the dorsum of the feet are protected or lifted, and ankles are not too far plantar flexed; the feet may hang off the end of the support surface if the patient is not in danger of injury
Sitting	Unlike when the patient is lying down, this position needs to be modified AT LEAST every 15 min Use a properly fitted wheelchair that enhances upright posture; avoid sling back and sling seat designs Use a wheelchair seat cushion (and a wedge with the wider side to the front if the patient is likely to slide forward in the chair) Educate the patient to perform pressure relief by either leaning, tipping, or doing push-ups (all are good techniques for assisting with upper extremity strength) Avoid restraints Feet should be in properly fitting shoes and well supported on properly aligned foot and leg rests

From Bergquist S, Bonnel W, Braun J, et al: CPGEC *prevention of pressure ulcers.* Available at coa.kumc.edu/gec/modules/PresUlc/PU-FramePages/ModuleContent_Main.htm.

Table 11-2 Goals of Wound Management Dependent on Wound Stage and Appearance

Stage	Appearance	Goals
I	Erythema that does not blanch when pressure is applied	Remove, relieve pressure, keep area clean; avoid friction and shear forces
II, III	Granulation/nondraining	Maintain moist wound bed; protect surrounding tissue; observe for infection
II, III	Granulation/draining	Maintain moist wound bed; protect surrounding tissue; observe for infection; absorb exudate
IV	Necrotic/nondraining	Maintain moist wound bed; protect surrounding tissue; observe for infection; soften and remove eschar, necrotic tissue
IV	Necrotic/draining	Maintain moist wound bed; protect surrounding tissue; observe for infection; soften and remove eschar, necrotic tissue
II, III, V	Infected wound	Protect the surrounding tissue; absorb exudate; contain infection

Data from Kendall K, Porter C, Carroll C et al: Evolution of Sacred Heart Hospital's wound assessment sheet. In *Acute Care Perspectives,* Newsletter of the Acute Care/Hospital Clinical Practice Section, Alexandria, Va, Summer 1995, American Physical Therapy Association.

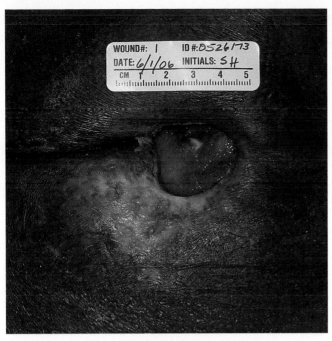

Fig. 11-2   Sacral pressure ulcer, stage III.

measurement and description of the open area of the wound are used to indicate the improvement or healing of the wound. A full-thickness wound cannot be staged if its depth cannot be measured or visualized; therefore a wound in which the base is covered with eschar or necrotic tissue or one that is covered in slough (Fig. 11-3, A) cannot be staged until the wound surface is exposed through debridement. Note that eschar (Fig. 11-3, B) on the heels, if it is dry, adherent, and intact without erythema, serves as the body's natural cover and should not be removed.

A description of a suspected deep tissue injury with intact skin cannot be classified into a stage because the extent of injury is not evident. The wound may present as a dark purple or blue hue with erythema or a blood-filled blister caused by damage of underlying soft tissue by pressure or a shear force. The deep tissue injury may be preceded by tissue that is painful, firm, or mushy, and it may be warmer or cooler than the adjacent tissue. On people with a dark complexion, the only signs may be the cardinal signs of inflammation, and thus it may be necessary to describe the affected area using objective and subjective information.

Table 11-3 Staging a Pressure Ulcer	
Stage	**Description**
Stage I	Intact skin with nonblanchable redness of a localized area, usually over a bony prominence; darkly pigmented skin may not have visible blanching—its color may differ from the surrounding area Further description: The area may be painful, firm, soft, warmer, or cooler compared with adjacent tissue; stage I may be difficult to detect in persons with dark skin tones; may indicate "at risk" persons (a heralding sign of risk)
Stage II	Partial thickness loss of dermis presenting as a shallow open ulcer with a red pink wound bed, without slough; also may present as an intact or open/ruptured serum-filled blister Further description: Presents as a shiny or dry shallow ulcer without slough or bruising (bruising indicates suspected deep tissue injury); this stage should not be used to describe skin tears, tape burns, perineal dermatitis, maceration, or excoriation
Stage III	Full-thickness tissue loss; subcutaneous fat may be visible but bone, tendon, or muscles are not exposed; slough may be present but does not obscure the depth of tissue loss; may include undermining and tunneling Further description: The depth of a stage III pressure ulcer varies by anatomic location; the bridge of the nose, ear, occiput, and malleolus do not have subcutaneous tissue and stage III ulcers can be shallow; in contrast, areas of significant adiposity can develop extremely deep stage III pressure ulcers; bone/tendon is not visible or directly palpable
Stage IV	Full-thickness tissue loss with exposed bone, tendon, or muscle; slough or eschar may be present on some parts of the wound bed; often includes undermining and tunneling Further description: The depth of a stage IV pressure ulcer varies by anatomic location; the bridge of the nose, ear, occiput, and malleolus do not have subcutaneous tissue and these ulcers can be shallow; stage IV ulcers can extend into muscle and/or supporting structures (e.g., fascia, tendon, or joint capsule), making osteomyelitis possible; exposed bone/tendon is visible or directly palpable
Unstageable	Full-thickness tissue loss in which the base of the ulcer is covered by slough (yellow, tan, gray, green, or brown) and/or eschar (tan, brown, or black) in the wound bed Further description: Until enough slough and/or eschar is removed to expose the base of the wound, the true depth, and therefore stage, cannot be determined; stable (dry, adherent, intact without erythema or fluctuation) eschar on the heels serves as "the body's natural (biological) cover" and should not be removed

Data from the National Pressure Ulcer Advisory Panel (NPUAP): *Pressure ulcer stages revised by NPUAP.* Copyright © NPUAP 2007.

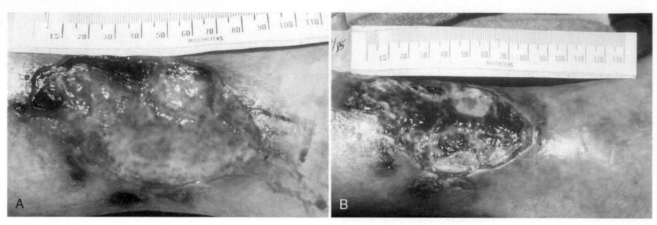

Fig. 11-3 **A,** An example of slough in a wound. **B,** An example of eschar.

- Identify the wound stage.
- Measure the wound size.
- Measure the wound depth.
- Observe and describe the tissue at the wound edges.
- Examine the wound for areas of tunneling or undermining; measure the length or depth.
- Observe and describe the characteristics of any exudate (i.e., viscosity, amount, and color).
- Observe and describe the characteristics of any necrotic tissue (i.e., color, adherence, texture, consistency, and amount).
- Describe any wound odor.
- Observe and describe the characteristics of the surrounding skin (e.g., dry, macerated, color, texture, blistered, edematous, firm, soft, or indurated [edges rolled under "epiboly"]).
- Observe and describe the characteristics of wound healing:
  - Granulation
  - Epithelialization
  - Budding
  - Wound contraction

Data from Kennedy KL: *Wound caring.* Copyright © 1997 Professional Education Systems, Inc. (800-647-8079). No further reproduction may be made without consent from the publisher.

Wound Assessment Several methods or parameters can be used to assess many characteristics of the wound (examples are provided in Box 11-5). The size is determined by measuring the longest and widest portions of the wound. The measurements are stated in centimeters, and a disposable, plastic overlay can be used to measure the wound. The overlay should be positioned on the wound so its top is directed toward the patient's head, and the measurements are made based on the configuration of the face of a clock. Length measurements are made along a line from 12 o'clock (head) to 6 o'clock (foot), and width measurements are made from 9 o'clock (left) to 3 o'clock (right).

The depth is measured by inserting a sterile cotton-tipped swab vertically into the wound until it contacts the bottom or floor of the wound. The caregiver uses a finger, thumbnail, or marker to indicate where the upper portion of the shaft of the swab exits the wound; the distance from the end of the swab to the mark on the shaft indicates the wound depth. The swab and plastic overlay must be discarded in a proper container immediately after each use. A swab can be used to determine the amount of undermining of the edge of the wound or tunneling of the wound into surrounding soft tissue. A technique similar to the one described for measuring the depth can be used to measure undermining and tunneling by inserting the swab horizontally. Again, using the clock method, the area of tunneling should be identified. Probing of these areas should be performed gently and cautiously because it will not be possible to observe the tissue that the swab contacts. The caregiver should wear clean, nonsterile gloves when performing these measurements.

Another assessment component is to observe and describe the color patterns or necrotic tissue of the wound and to estimate the percentage of content in the wound. The color red is indicative of the process of granulation, slough is yellow or grayish-brown in appearance, and eschar appears black. Epithelial tissue appears to be pink and shiny and indicates that coverage of the wound by new skin is occurring. Photographs taken periodically can be used to document the condition of the wound and the surrounding tissue (skin) and should be included in the medical record.

Wound Care Nursing personnel and rehabilitation therapists are the primary caregivers responsible for the care of a pressure ulcer. In some settings therapists are greatly involved in the measurement of wounds, the selection and application of wound dressings, and debridement. The basic elements of wound care include debridement of necrotic tissue, wound cleaning, wound dressing, and the possible use of adjunctive therapies such as electrical stimulation, a whirlpool, and pulsatile lavage. One such adjunct therapy

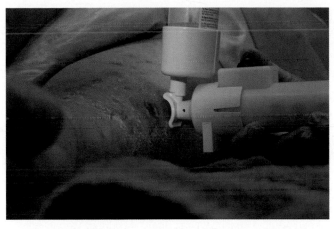

Fig. 11-4 MIST Therapy System being applied to a cellulitis wound. (Courtesy of Celleration).

| Table **11-4** | Dressing Choices and Preferred Uses |

Stage or Condition	TF	HC	HyG	AL	WD	WM	PS
I	X	X					
II	X	X	X			X	
III		X	X	X		X	X
IV				X		X	X
Necrotic/draining				X	X	X	
Necrotic/nondraining			X		X	X	
Noninfected	X	X	X	X	X	X	
Infected				X	X	X	

Data from *Acute Care Perspectives*, Newsletter of the Acute Care/ Hospital Clinical Practice Section, Alexandria, Va, Summer 1995, American Physical Therapy Association. Updated by Martiza Kennedy, RN, Clinical Manager, Northeast Wound Care Center, Humble, TX. *AL*, Alginate; *HC*, hydrocolloid; *HyG*, hydrogel; *PS*, packing strip; *TF*, transparent film; *WD*, wet to dry; *WM*, wet to moist (not the preferred treatment).

is MIST Therapy (Fig. 11-4), which produces a low-frequency ultrasound that is delivered into the wound bed via a gentle saline mist. The sound waves penetrate through the wound surface and into the wound bed to reduce bacteria, biofilm, and inflammation and accelerate the body's normal healing process. This type of noncontact delivery results in a painless treatment for the patient.

Wound healing is promoted through wound cleansing and maintenance debridement by the removal of yellow slough, fibrin, tissue exudates, and bacteria. MIST Therapy should not be used near electronic implants/prostheses (e.g., near or over the heart or over the thoracic area if the patient is using a cardiac pacemaker); on the lower back or over the uterus during pregnancy; and over areas of malignancies unless otherwise advised by a physician.

Debridement The removal of necrotic tissue from the wound allows the wound to heal more effectively. Debridement can be performed with sharp instruments (i.e., a scalpel or scissors), mechanically, chemically, or with autolysis. Sharp debridement with use of a scalpel or scissors to remove thick adherent eschar and other devitalized tissue is the most rapid method. Surgical or sharp debridement often is performed by a physician when a large amount of necrotic tissue is present (>70%). Depending on state statutes, practice acts, and the policies and procedures of the facility, a variety of persons who have the appropriate training may legally perform sharp debridement. Mechanical debridement (typically a nonselective form of debridement) can be performed through pressure irrigation (i.e., pulsed lavage), the removal of dressings (wet to dry dressings), hydrotherapy, electrical stimulation, a combination of hydrotherapy and ultrasonography, and the use of dextranomers.

Chemical debridement can be performed with the use of enzymes. Enzymatic debridement is performed with exogenous agents, such as collagenase, which are applied to the wound. The patient's self-produced (endogenous) enzymes also can be the active agent; this process is known as autolysis, or autolytic debridement, and is performed with a very occlusive dressing. Enzymatic debridement tends to be more effective for small areas of necrosis or when the patient is unable to tolerate other methods. Nutritional support may be necessary to promote improvement in skin condition, to increase the development of subcutaneous tissue, and to improve or maintain the patient's metabolism. Some patients may require supplemental enteral or parenteral feedings to ensure that sufficient nutrient levels are attained. Laboratory values such as prealbumin, albumin, and total protein levels may be helpful in deciding a course of action.

Dressings Care of the wound usually requires the selection and application of one or more types of dressings. The purposes of the dressing are to protect the wound, assist the healing process, reduce infection or contamination of the wound, and remove exudates and toxic waste when the dressing is removed. Dressings can be used to add moisture in very dry wounds or to remove and absorb moisture in wounds with large amounts of exudate. Tables 11-4 and 11-5 present information about the selection and effects of several types of dressings. Dressings that prohibit observation of the wound may need to be removed more frequently than are dressings that permit observation. Because some dressings cause maceration of the surrounding skin, a moisture barrier may need to be applied to the perimeter of the wound when those dressings are used. Dressings should be removed carefully to avoid trauma to the wound surface or surrounding tissue. The wound and its surrounding skin should be observed and assessed each time a dressing is removed, and noticeable changes from previous observations should be documented. Additives to the dressing can be utilized, such as silver products if the wound is infected

Table **11-5** Product Selection Based on Wound Severity	
Dressing	**Value/Effects**
Transparent file (e.g., Bioclusive, Tegaderm, and OpSite)	Dressing of choice for stages I and II wounds with blister formation over bony prominences; resists shear; may be applied to heels prophylactically; self-adherent and allows wound to be observed; may be used for autolytic debridement; do not use on draining or infected wounds
Hydrocolloid (e.g., DuoDerm, Restore [paste or granules], Tegasorb, Hydrocol, and DermaFilm)	Dressing of choice for stages II and III wounds with minimal drainage; provides moist wound bed; absorbs small amount of drainage; self-adherent and provides cushioning over bony prominence; do not use on infected wounds; medications cannot be used under the dressing
Hydrogel (e.g., Vigilon, ClearSite, and NU-GEL)	Recommended for stages II and III wounds with dressing covering the gel; moist wound bed is maintained; recommended for use on skin tear, cover with rolled absorbent material (Kling); may cause maceration of surrounding healthy tissue; does not protect wound from external soiling; helps clean and debride necrotic tissue
Wet to wet	Safe choice for unstaged wounds; use on stage II partial-thickness wounds and stages II and IV wounds; dressing will need to be changed every 8 h to maintain moist wound base; moisten dressing with saline solution before removal if dressing is dry to prevent bleeding and disruption of granulation bed; moisture barrier must be used on surrounding tissue to prevent maceration
Wet to dry	Use on stages II and IV wounds for debridement; slough and necrotic tissue adhere to dressing and are removed with dressing; this dressing is the most widely used and probably the most controversial, because research shows disruption of angiogenesis by dressing removal and increased risk of infection because of the need for frequent dressing changes
Calcium alginates	Use to absorb heavy drainage, but will require a secondary dressing to cover the wound (Kaltostat, Algosteril); calcium alginates may be used on infected wounds or for filling in the cavity of deep wounds
Foam dressings (e.g., Polyderm, Lyofoam, Mepilex, and Allevyn)	Used for heavily exudative wounds (especially during the inflammatory phase after debridement and desloughing when exudate is at its peak), deep cavity wounds, and weeping ulcers such as venous stasis ulcers; is very absorbent and can be left on for 3-4 days
Collagen (e.g., Collagen/Ag, BIOSTEP, and Medifil)	When added to a wound, it acts as a hemostatic agent; continued application seems to hasten healing; it absorbs 40-60 times its weight in fluid
Enzymatic debriding agents (e.g., Accuzyme, Kovia ointment, Gladase, Ethezyme, and papain-urea debriding ointment)	Particularly effective for tunneling ulcers that may be hard to see or reach; some of these debriders are selective for necrotic tissue, while others are not; by loosening necrotic debris, surgical debridement may be avoided
Hydrofiber (e.g., Aquacel and Aquacel Ag Hydrofiber)	Indicated for wounds with moderate to high exudate that are infected or at risk for infection; provides a moist wound environment and provides sustained antimicrobial activity for up to 7 days

Data from Kendall K, Porter C, Carroll C et al: Evolution of Sacred Heart Hospital's wound assessment sheet. In *Acute Care Perspectives*, Newsletter of the Acute Care/Hospital Clinical Practice Section, Alexandria, Va, Summer 1995, American Physical Therapy Association. Added to from Woundcare Information Network (see Bibliography).

or saline if hypergranulation exists. When the wound is not infected, it is desirable to minimize the need for dressing changes (i.e., every 2 or more days as opposed to every day).

Pressure Ulcer Summary Pressure ulcers are caused by pressure to the soft tissue that overlies a bony prominence. When the tissue is trapped between the bony prominence and a source of external pressure, the capillaries in the tissue are occluded, leading to local ischemia and tissue necrosis. Contributing factors are shear force and friction applied to the skin. Many risk factors predispose the patient to the

development of a pressure ulcer; therefore every patient who is admitted to a health care facility or is treated at home should be assessed for these risk factors. If risk factors are identified, a specific, aggressive prevention program should be initiated, including the use of the Braden Scale. Integral components of such a program are proper skin care, pressure relief or reduction, appropriate support surface of bed and wheelchair, proper positioning, and frequent position changes.

If a pressure ulcer occurs, it should be classified and described accurately and objectively to ensure appropriate

| Box 11-6 | Pressure Ulcer Documentation Guidelines |

- Describe the site or location of the ulcer.
- Identify the stage of the ulcer based on the classification system of the National Pressure Ulcer Advisory Panel.
- Measure and report the size of the total surface area of the ulcer.
- Measure and report the depth of the ulcer.
- Determine the evidence or extent of ulcer tunnels or undermined areas; report tissue destruction underlying intact skin along the margins of the ulcer; measure the width and length.
- Estimate and describe the percentage of color (black, red, and yellow) and the percentage of the ulcer covered with new skin; describe the composition of the ulcer (e.g., granulation, epithelialized tissue).
- Estimate and describe the type and amount of exudate (e.g., viscosity, color, and consistency).
- Describe the odor associated with the ulcer after it has been rinsed with sterile saline solution.
- Observe and report whether edema or induration exists in the tissue surrounding the periphery of the ulcer.
- Observe and report whether signs of inflammation are present in the tissue surrounding the ulcer; measure and report the area in which signs appear.
- Observe and describe the condition of the skin surrounding the ulcer (e.g., dry, moist, loose, taut, warm, or discolored).
- Observe and report any increase in pain in the area.

documentation (Box 11-6). Wound care actions such as debridement, the use of dressings, proper nutrition, and vascular/microvascular assessment are important aspects of treatment. An interdisciplinary care team should be established to maximize the care and management of the patient and the wound.

Peripheral Vascular Conditions

Wounds caused by venous or arterial insufficiency or diabetes should be differentiated from pressure ulcers. In some instances, the location and appearance of the wound will be sufficient to determine the type of wound and its cause. For example, a wound located directly over a bony prominence is suggestive of a pressure ulcer; a wound located at the medial lower leg just above the medial malleolus accompanied with edema and dark, dusky skin discoloration is suggestive of a venous insufficiency wound; and a small wound located near the ankle accompanied by localized edema is suggestive of an arterial insufficiency wound or a wound caused by diabetes. Fig. 11-5, A, depicts an ulcer on the foot of a person with diabetes and cellulitis. Fig. 11-5, B, depicts a gangrenous great toe caused by vascular insufficiency in a person with diabetes. When peripheral vascular disease problems are diagnosed early enough, they can be treated with use of a hyperbaric chamber (Fig 11-5, C).

Several assessment methods or tests are available to evaluate the status of venous and arterial circulation in the lower extremity. Peripheral venous circulation dysfunction can be caused by defective or deficient valves, occlusion of the veins, or limited function of the "calf-pumping" mechanism. Peripheral arterial circulation dysfunction usually is attributable to some form of arterial occlusion, which is associated with atherosclerosis. Both circulatory system components may exhibit acute or chronic conditions. Some tests that can be performed to determine the function of the venous and arterial peripheral circulation are presented in Tables 11-6 and 11-7. Other evaluative procedures are examination of the patient's skin, measurement of the skin temperature, palpation of the pulse at various sites, evaluation of sensation, auscultation of an artery, and measurement of blood pressure. Doppler ultrasonography and air plethysmography may be performed, but these procedures require specific training and special equipment.

Treatment procedures or activities for these types of wounds are beyond the scope of this book. However, the caregiver should be aware of his or her responsibility to notify the patient's physician when one of these conditions is identified. For most patients, prompt medical care and management of any condition that affects the peripheral venous or arterial circulation will be necessary to prevent a serious complication.

Dressings and Bandages

The composition of a dressing and its bandage varies, but in many instances several layers are involved. For example, a topical medication may be applied directly to the wound, with a nonabsorbent material (e.g., a wound contact layer of Dermanet or a Telfa pad) placed over the medication along with a second layer consisting of a cotton gauze pad; for large wounds or wounds that exhibit excessive drainage, a third layer of an absorbent material may be used, such as a foam. These three layers make up the dressing.

A fourth layer of a material such as roller gauze and a fifth layer of a material such as an elastic wrap may be used as a bandage. Depending on the purpose of or need for the dressing, the type of wound, and the purpose of or need for the bandage, various layers may be omitted or added. However, you should be able to differentiate the purposes or functions of a dressing and a bandage.

The functions of a dressing are to prevent additional wound contamination, keep microorganisms in the wound from infecting other sites, prevent further injury to the wound, apply pressure to control hemorrhage, absorb wound drainage, and assist in wound healing.

The functions of a bandage are to keep the dressing in place, maintain a barrier between the dressing and the environment, provide external pressure to control swelling, provide support or stability to an area, hold splints in place, and help the dressing accomplish its functions.

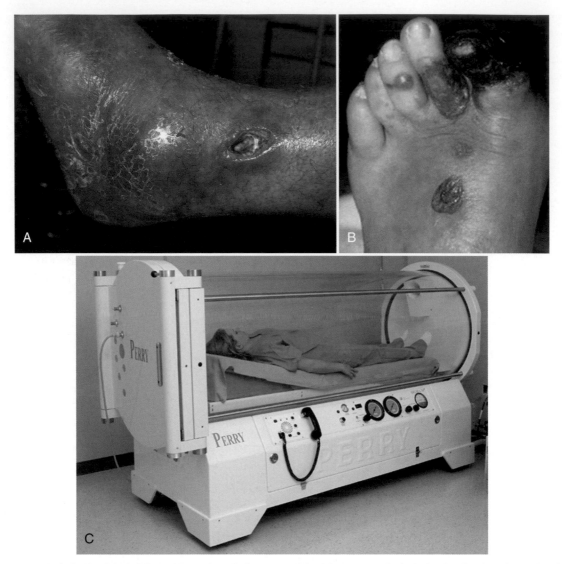

Fig. 11-5   **A,** Cellulitis of the left foot with an ulcer. **B,** Gangrene of the left great toe. **C,** A single-chamber hyperbaric chamber.

Removal of a Dressing   Before removing a dressing, the caregiver should wash his or her hands thoroughly and presume that the wound and dressing are contaminated. For self-protection, nonsterile gloves should be donned (i.e., a clean technique should be used) before the dressing is removed. Once the gloved hand has touched the dressing or the wound, it must not touch any other object, especially the skin of the patient or caregiver, the clean (sterile) dressing, or any other object in the area. Once the dressing has been removed, it and the gloves should be discarded in a closed container or nonporous bag. The caregiver should remove the gloves without touching the outside of either glove with any exposed skin, as described in Chapter 2. Immediately after the removal and disposal of the gloves, the caregiver must wash his or her hands to further reduce the possibility of cross contamination.

To remove a nonadherent dressing, the bandage may be removed independently of the dressing or with the dressing.

If you are unfamiliar with the site and shape of the wound, request information about it from the patient or other personnel who are familiar with it. The patient may be able to indicate the size and location of the wound on the corresponding extremity or on the caregiver's extremity. Bandage scissors are used to cut through the various layers of the bandage. The blunt tip of the scissors is placed under the edge of the bandage so it is next to the patient's skin. The initial cut should be made a safe distance from any edge or from the center of the wound. (Caution: Avoid cutting over bony prominences.) If you are uncertain where or how to cut the dressing, attempt to unwrap or remove the bandage without using scissors to expose the dressing; then carefully remove the dressing layers. As you remove the bandage and dressing materials, mentally note how many layers there are, the materials used, and the sequence of application of the materials, which will prepare you to reapply the dressing properly.

Table 11-6 Peripheral Venous and Arterial Circulation Tests

Test	Description
Venous sufficiency tests	
Percussion test	Used to assess the function of the valves of the saphenous vein
	With the patient standing, the caregiver palpates a proximal segment of the saphenous vein with the fingers of one hand, then uses the fingers of the other hand to tap (percuss) a distal segment of the vein
	A fluid movement will be sensed by the fingers on the proximal segment during percussion if the valves are not functioning properly
	Test both lower extremities and compare the results
Deep vein thrombo-phlebitis test	Used to assess the possible presence of a thrombus
	The caregiver grasps and lightly presses the patient's calf while passively forcing the foot into dorsiflexion; if the patient complains of pain in the calf, a positive response is reported; this is known as a positive Homans' sign
	Another method is to apply a blood pressure cuff around the patient's calf and inflate it gradually; a patient with an acute condition will not tolerate an inflation pressure higher than 40 mm Hg; once the pain threshold has been reached, do not continue to inflate the cuff; test the noninvolved lower extremity first if only one extremity is suspected of having a deep vein thrombosis
Cuff test	
Deep vein thrombo-phlebitis	Wrap a blood pressure cuff around the calf and test if the patient can tolerate a pressure of 40 mm Hg
Arterial sufficiency tests	
Rubor of dependency test	Used to evaluate the arterial circulation by observing skin color changes that occur with the lower extremity elevated and level
	When the patient is supine, observe and record the color of the plantar surface of the foot (normal = pinkish); elevate the lower extremity approximately 45 to 60 degrees for 1 minute (abnormal = rapid loss of color)
	Return the extremity to a level position; observe and record the color of the plantar surface (normal = rapid pink flush; abnormal = 30 seconds or longer for color to appear; color will be bright red)
Ankle-brachial test	Used to determine if a person has peripheral artery disease; the blood pressure is measured at the ankle and in the arm while a person is at rest; the test is often repeated after 5 min of walking on a treadmill; if the blood pressure at the ankle is the same or greater than in the arm, this is an indication of normal blood flow; if the blood pressure at the ankle is lower initially or after exercise, this is an indication of peripheral artery disease
Venous filling time test	Used to determine the length of time required for superficial veins to refill, after they have been emptied, as a result of arterial flow through the capillaries into the veins (Note: The patient must have a normal venous system)
	The patient is supine, and the lower extremities are elevated 45-60 degrees for 1 min; then the legs are dangled over the edge of the bed or table; refilling of the veins is observed and timed (normal = 10 to 15 s for refilling)
Claudication	Used to measure the length of time a patient can walk before claudication is experienced
	The patient walks on a level-grade treadmill at 1 mile/h until claudication occurs; the time elapsed is recorded when calf pain prevents continuation of walking
	The test can be repeated at specified intervals, and the time elapsed values can be compared

Data from Morey S: *Pressure ulcer/wound care.* Presented at the Ohio Physical Therapy Associated Annual Conference, Columbus, OH, April 17, 1997 and O'Sullivan SB, Schmitz TJ: *Physical rehabilitation assessment and treatment,* ed 4, Philadelphia, 2001, FA Davis.

The deepest layer of the dressing should be removed by carefully loosening and freeing the dressing from the wound edges and gently pulling it toward the center of the wound; this method provides the least disruption of the healing process. After the dressing has been removed, all dressing materials and your gloves should be discarded in a closed container as described previously, and you should wash your hands before you perform any other activity (Fig. 11-6).

When the wound has been exposed, its condition should be evaluated carefully (Box 11-7). While wearing nonsterile gloves, the caregiver should gently and carefully palpate the tissue in the area of the wound to determine the following:

- The temperature of the wound tissue in comparison with the temperature of tissue away from the wound on the same or another extremity

Table **11-7** General Assessment Activities for Peripheral Vascular Conditions

Assessment Information	Description
Objective information	
Skin examination	Observe color and compare with the opposite extremity
	Observe the condition of the skin (dry, scaly, flexible, firm, loose, taut, adherent, moist, presence of exudate)
	Palpate to sense temperature, edema, and general condition
	Observe for absence of hair
	Evaluate superficial sensation; use objects with different textures; apply light pressure; use a monofilament "feeler"
Measure skin temperature	Use a thermometer with a probe (or radiometer) to measure temperature at various sites or locations along the extremity
	Compare values with those obtained from similar sites or locations on the opposite extremity
Palpate pulses	Evaluate all major arterial pulses; refer to techniques and procedures in Chapter 3
	Evaluate the quality and rate
	Compare findings of the involved extremity with those of the noninvolved extremity
Auscultation	Use a stethoscope to listen for blood flow in the major arteries of the neck, abdomen, groin, and extremities
	Listen for a swishlike sound, which indicates fluid turbulence known as bruit; a narrowed vessel lumen will produce turbulence
Doppler ultrasound	The Doppler ultrasound looks at major blood flow in the arteries and veins in the limbs; the Doppler is passed over an area and a computer converts sound waves into a graph that indicates blood flow in the area; the sound produced when the Doppler is over a vessel can indicate the strength and quality of the pulses
Blood pressure	Perform measurement on both upper extremities; use a proper size cuff
	Follow the techniques and procedures presented in Chapter 3
Edema	Observe for and measure edema using palpation, girth, or volumetric measurements
	Compare values obtained from the involved extremity with values of the noninvolved extremity; document any pitting edema
Remeasure	Remeasure periodically to determine whether edema is regressing, progressing, or static
Subjective information	
Patient history and lifestyle	Obtain history of the current condition from the patient or a family member
	Obtain specific information about the current condition or a previous condition and the effects or result of treatments
	Determine personal habits that may affect the condition (i.e., eating habits, use of tobacco, reaction to heat or cold, sensory changes)

Data from O'Sullivan SB, Schmitz TJ: *Physical rehabilitation assessment and treatment*, ed 4, Philadelphia, 2001, FA Davis.

- The tone of the tissue
- The integrity of the wound edges or the area of healing
- The condition of the skin (e.g., dry, moist, pliable, or taut)
- The sensory response or capacity of the tissue

You should report and document your observations and findings using specific and objective terms. A nurse or physician should be notified if you observe adverse changes or a regression in the healing process or the condition of the wound since your previous observation. Remember, gloves should be worn whenever dressings are changed.

To remove a dressing that adheres to the wound, it may be necessary to soak the bandage and dressing first to reduce disruption of the healing surface of the wound when the dressing is removed. The wound bandage and dressing can be soaked in a basin, whirlpool, tub, or other similar container. An alternative method is to pour water or a saline solution over the bandage and dressing repeatedly until the hardened exudate has softened. The actual removal of the dressing should be performed as described previously. If a whirlpool is used, the turbine should not be activated until the dressing has been removed from the water. Removal of the dressing material before the turbine is turned on will prevent the dressing material from being drawn into the turbine or occluding the drain when the water is released. If edema is associated with the wound, the use of a whirlpool may increase production and decrease removal of excess interstitial fluid (edema) because of the warmth of the water and the dependent position of the extremity when it is immersed.

Application of a Sterile Dressing After the bandage and dressing are removed, the wound may require care to enhance its healing. Before a new dressing can be applied, necrotic tissue may need to be removed from the surface of the wound through the process of debridement. Debridement may be accomplished by gently rubbing the surface of the wound with a gauze pad, using pulsatile lavage with

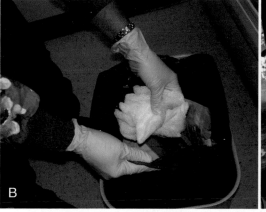
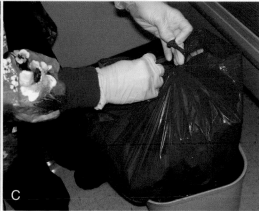

Fig. 11-6   Removal and disposal of a dressing.

Box 11-7   Wound Evaluation

- Observe and palpate the condition of the skin surrounding the wound; record your findings.
- Observe and record the color of the tissue surrounding the wound.
- Observe and record the color and appearance of the wound.
- If an exudate is present, note the type and amount.
- If an odor is present, indicate what the odor is and how pervasive it is.
- Determine whether signs of inflammation or infection are present.
- Determine whether signs of pressure or irritation are present.
- If edema or swelling is present, observe where it is located and in what amount.
- State the location of the wound and measure the size and depth of the wound.
- Whenever possible, take a photograph of the wound with the date, measure it according to facility protocol, and label it with patient's name/medical record number.
- Determine the type of wound or lesion (e.g., abrasion, puncture, laceration, burn, incision, or ulceration).

suction, running water over the surface of the wound, or using a scalpel or scissors to excise the necrotic tissue. A description of the specific methods and techniques used to debride a wound is beyond the scope of this book. The approval of a physician may or may not be required before a caregiver other than a physician can perform debridement. In many situations, only the physician is permitted to perform wound debridement. (Note: Regardless of the method used, the wound should not bleed during or after the debridement process.)

Before applying a dressing, a sterile field with the appropriate wound care materials should be established and the caregiver should wear sterile, protective clothing appropriate for the patient's condition. If it is necessary to dry the patient's skin before the dressing is applied, a sterile towel or sterile gauze should be used. The patient should be positioned comfortably so the wound is accessible. (Note: For some wounds, a clean rather than a sterile technique may be used; facility protocols and policies and procedures should always be followed in this regard.)

If debridement is to occur, an oral analgesic or an anesthetic may be applied to the wound beforehand (Fig. 11-7, A and B). Following debridement (Fig. 11-7, C),

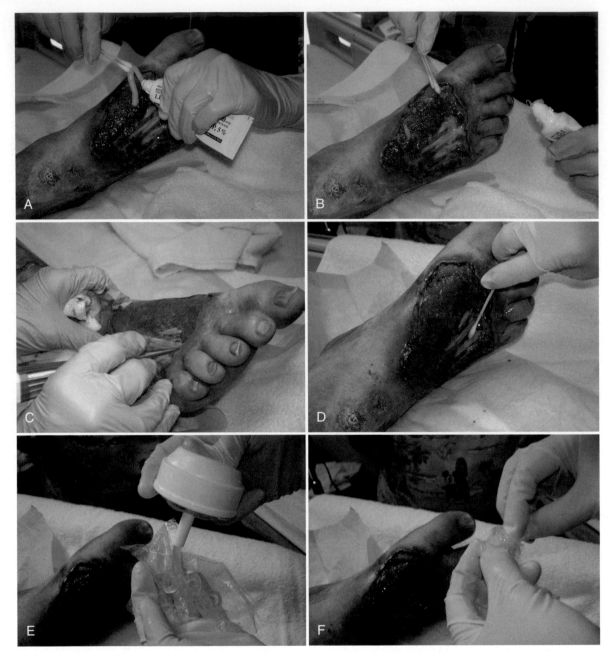

Fig. 11-7   **A** and **B,** Application of lidocaine ointment in preparation for debridement. **C,** Debridement using a rongeur. **D,** Application of Cellerate RX (activated collagen). **E** and **F,** Application of Intrasite Gel onto Dermanet.

medications can be applied directly to the wound or to the dressing material and then onto the wound. Medication or anesthetic in a tube or jar should be applied to a cotton swab, gauze pad, or other acceptable applicator and then applied to the wound (Fig. 11-7, *D* and *E*). The sterile applicator must not contact the nonsterile exterior of the tube or jar, and care must be used to avoid contaminating the contents of the tube or jar with the applicator once it has contacted the patient. Therefore a new swab or gauze pad should be used each time the medication is obtained from the tube or jar.

Select the appropriate dressing material and apply it directly to the medication base over the wound (Fig. 11-7, *F* to *I*). Be certain you maintain its sterility as it is applied by handling it with sterile gloves or sterile forceps. Once the initial layer has been applied over the wound, the upper layers of the dressing and the bandage do not need to be applied using sterile technique. Cover the dressing with the appropriate bandage materials and evaluate the tension, location, and coverage of the bandage. The bandage should have sufficient tension to secure the dressing and control edema, if edema is present or anticipated, but it must not

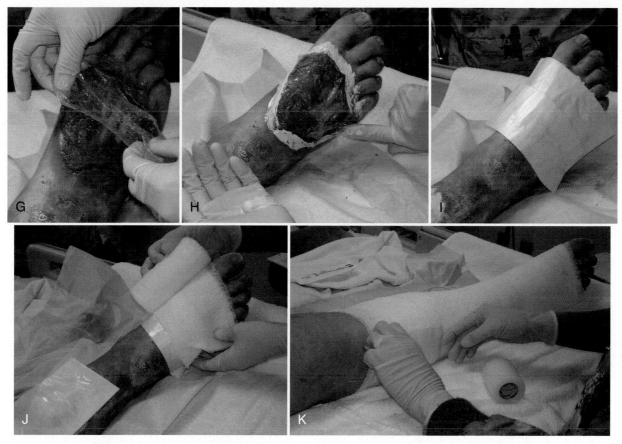

Fig. 11-7, cont'd   G, Application of Dermanet dressing. **H,** Application of Calazime protectant paste. **I,** Application of Telfa dressing. **J** and **K,** Application of a Kerlix bandage.

occlude or impede the local circulation. You may need to question the patient about the tension, or you can slide a finger under the outer edges of the bandage to determine the tension force.

The following conditions are indicators of an improperly applied bandage:

- If the color of the segment distal to the bandage becomes excessively red, blue, or pale, the bandage is usually too tight and is constricting the local circulation.
- If the patient reports pain, numbness, tingling, or a burning sensation in the segment distal to the bandage, the bandage is usually too tight and is affecting local neural receptors.
- If the exposed distal segment feels cold to the touch when compared with the similar, opposite segment, the bandage is usually too tight proximally and is constricting the flow of arterial blood to the area.
- If edema develops in the segment distal to the bandage, the bandage is usually too tight and is constricting the local lymphatic and venous circulation.
- If the bandage changes position, it is usually too loose.

When any of these conditions occurs, the bandage should be removed and reapplied. The patient should be

informed of these problems and become responsible for monitoring the bandage when he or she is not being treated or under the direct care of another person. After the bandage has been applied, the caregiver should evaluate it to determine how well it was applied. The exposed areas of tissue proximal and distal to the wound should be observed and palpated, the patient should be questioned about the sensations perceived in the extremity, and the tension of the bandage should be tested. This last activity can be accomplished by simultaneously inserting a finger beneath the deepest layer of the bandage at the proximal and distal edges of the bandage. The pressure should be essentially equal at both sites or slightly greater distally than proximally.

The patient or a family member should be instructed to evaluate the bandage periodically and to remove and reapply it when any signs or symptoms of improper application are evident. The date and time of dressing changes should be documented. The patient should be instructed about the length of time the bandage should remain in place, when it should be routinely removed (e.g., for bathing, for exercise, or if it becomes wet), and how long the wound can be free of the bandage before the bandage is reapplied. If the patient is capable of applying the bandage, instruct him or her how to remove and apply it. By observing the patient's performance, you can be certain the person understands and can perform the procedure. Written instructions may be useful for the patient and his or her family.

Bandages may be applied and used for purposes other than to cover and protect a dressing, such as to control edema or swelling, protect an injured joint, or hold a splint in place. An excellent source for wound care algorithms for step-by-step assessment, management, and treatment of wounds can be found at Hollister.com (see the Bibliography).

GIRTH MEASUREMENT

Girth measurement of an extremity to serially measure its circumference is a technique used to evaluate the presence of edema or atrophy. Possible indications for the measurement of the calf or thigh include lymphedema, anterior compartment syndrome, deep venous thrombosis, shin splints, a ruptured gastrocnemius or soleus muscle in the calf (Fig. 11-8, A), and a ruptured or strained hamstring or

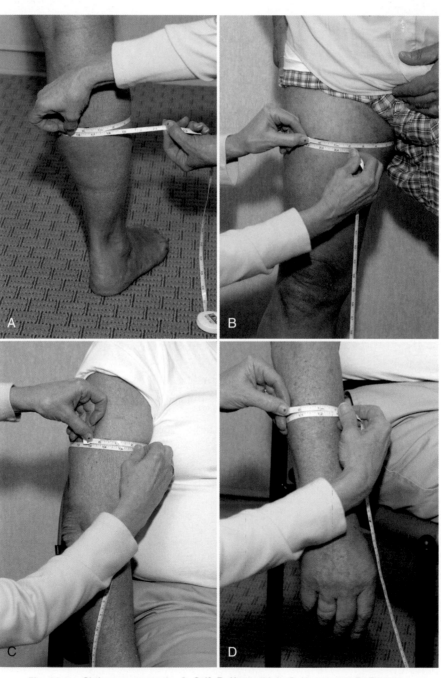

Fig. 11-8   Girth measurements. **A,** Calf. **B,** Upper thigh. **C,** Upper arm. **D,** Forearm.

quadriceps muscle in the thigh (Fig. 11-8, B). Indications for upper extremity measurement include lymphedema; fractures of the humerus (Fig. 11-8, C), radius, or ulna (Fig. 11-8, D); and severe tennis elbow. Possible causes for atrophy are use of a cast or splint for immobilization at a fracture site or certain muscle disorders such as myotonia dystrophy or amyotrophic lateral sclerosis. When measuring the upper and lower extremities, measurements should be taken bilaterally for patients with atrophy or edema in the limb(s) for a base comparison.

Use of a plastic or metal anthropometric measuring tape is recommended to obtain these measurements because it does not deteriorate, it is easy to clean, and its calibration marks can be read easily. During measurement of the lower extremity, the patient should stand on a level surface with the feet approximately 6 inches apart and the body relaxed. During measurement of the upper extremity, the extremity should be exposed in a position of relaxation. Explain the procedure to the patient for either measurement. Wrap the anthropometric measuring tape horizontally around the area where the greatest or least amount of girth appears, using sufficient pressure to maintain contact with the skin without causing an excessive indentation in the skin. When a tension gauge is available it should be used during measurement of all sites to ensure consistent pressure on the tape. Two measurements to the nearest 0.25 inch should be made at the site, and the average of the two measurements is used as the reporting value. A skin-marking pencil can be used to mark the level or location at the base of the tape of the circumferential measurement. A measurement in centimeters or inches should be taken of the distance from a bony landmark along the extremity to the mark made at the base of the tape to produce a consistent site for future values. Bony landmarks to be considered are the base of the lateral malleolus for the calf, the inferior pole of the patella for the thigh, the tip of the ulnar stylus or the base of the radial head for the forearm (Fig. 11-9), and the olecranon process for the upper arm.

Accuracy and reliability of the measurements are enhanced when the same person performs the measurements, a tension gauge is used, the patient is in the same position, measurements are made at the same time of day, and the same tape measure is used. The caregiver should apply the tape horizontally around the extremity with the same tension applied at each measuring session. Serial measurements that are performed over a specified period will provide objective evidence of the changes in the circumference of the extremity, which indirectly indicates the effect of edema or atrophy in the girth (Procedure 11-1).

Volumetric Measurement

Volumetric displacement using a volumeter is a method of measuring changes in the distal aspect of an extremity caused by edema or muscle atrophy. The technique is more

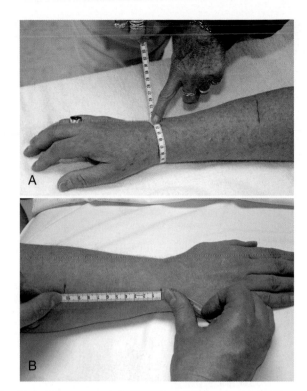

Fig. 11-9 Measurement. **A,** Circumferential measurement of the wrist. **B,** Distance measurement using the ulnar stylus as the bony landmark. Note the skin marking at the end of the tape.

accurate than girth measurements because of the irregular shape of the hand and foot, but it requires proper equipment. A volumeter (large enough to immerse a foot and ankle or a hand and wrist) with a spout and a calibrated collection container are necessary. A volumeter with a bar placed near the base is often used for hand/wrist measurement. When using a volumeter with a bar, the patient is instructed to immerse the hand so the bar falls between the third and fourth digits (Fig. 11-10).

The volumeter is filled with tepid water until it overflows, but it is not ready for use until the water ceases to drip from the spout. The calibrated cylinder is positioned so it will catch the water that overflows when the patient immerses his or her hand or foot into the water-filled volumeter. The patient should be instructed to immerse his or her hand or foot slowly and carefully into the water and to remain motionless as the displaced water flows through the spout; the two containers should rest on a firm, level surface. The calibrated container, which is usually a column, collects the expelled water. After the water is collected in the container, it should be placed on a firm, level surface and at a height that allows the caregiver to read the scale at eye level. When a series of measurements are made of the same extremity, conditions such as the water temperature, time of day, equipment, patient position, and evaluator should be replicated at each session to enhance the accuracy and reliability of the findings. Differences of several millimeters

PROCEDURE 11-1

Girth Measurements

LOWER EXTREMITY

- Explain the procedure, expose the extremity, and position the patient standing on a level surface so the extremity is relaxed.
- Use a plastic or metal anthropometric measuring tape with well-defined, easily visible calibrations.
- Palpate and mark the bony landmark (e.g., the lateral malleolus) to be used as the base for the distance measurement site on the extremity; position the free end of the tape on the mark and extend it along the extremity.
- Use a skin-marking pencil to mark the site at which the measurements are to be made (i.e., the area of greatest edema or atrophy).
- Measure and document the distance from the bony landmark to the circumferential measurement sites.
- For the circumference measurement, apply the tape around the extremity so it contacts the skin firmly and lies flat, but without causing an excessive indentation in the soft tissue; use consistent pressure and a tension gauge, if possible, as you apply the tape.
- Record the results for the circumference and the distance from the landmark to the base of the tape; document your activity and report significant findings.
- Measure the contralateral limb for comparison.

UPPER EXTREMITY

- Follow the aforementioned procedure, measuring the distance from a bony landmark (e.g., the ulnar styloid process) to the area where the circumference is to be measured (i.e., the area of greatest edema or atrophy); then measure the circumference.
- Document both the distance from the landmark and the circumference.
- If a tension gauge is used, be sure to mark the tension that was used around the circumference to permit more accurate detail for following measurements.

Note: Because girth measurements are difficult to perform on irregularly shaped areas such as the hand/wrist and foot/ankle, volumetric measurements are suggested for those areas.

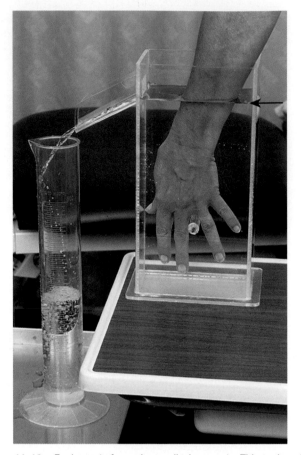

Fig. 11-10 Equipment for volume displacement. This volumeter includes a finger bar. (Note: The water level is indicated by the arrow.)

Lymphedema is the result of a functional overload of the lymphatic system in which lymph volume exceeds transport capabilities, resulting in obstructed lymph flow, swelling, pain, and susceptibility to infection. Primary lymphedema is a congenital malformation, whereas secondary lymphedema generally is acquired after surgical removal of lymph nodes, infection of the lymphatics, radiation therapy for cancer, or trauma. Lymphedema can occur in any body part but usually is seen in the limbs and is a chronic condition if it is left untreated.

Although lymphedema is not curable, several indications and contraindications for treatment exist (Box 11-8), and the condition can be managed. CDT—sometimes referred to as complete/complex decongestive physiotherapy—is one treatment protocol (Box 11-9) that can manage this chronic inflammatory condition effectively and minimize associated complications such as repeated infections, cellulitis, lymphangitis, and nonhealing ulcers. CDT includes MLD, compression bandaging, vasopneumatic compression, patient education about skin care and precautions, compression garment measurement, and remedial exercise. It is a specialized program designed to move fluid from the tissues back into the lymph drainage system to promote normal functioning and help alleviate fluid blockage.

of water displacement may occur between a person's dominant and nondominant hand. Despite these differences, it will be helpful initially to measure the displacement of water caused by the unaffected hand or foot to establish a baseline or comparison value for the affected hand or foot. Repetitive measurements can be reviewed and compared to determine the change in volume of the segment being measured (Procedure 11-2).

LYMPHEDEMA

The lymph system is a one-way drainage system designed to rid tissues of unwanted material and excess fluid.

PROCEDURE 11-2

Volumetric Measurements

- Expose the area to be assessed, seat the patient to assess the foot/ankle, and have the patient sit or stand to assess the hand/wrist. Inform the patient about the procedure and obtain the volumeter and a calibrated container.
- Fill the volumeter to overflowing with tepid water. When water no longer drips from the spout, place the calibrated container beneath the spout; be certain both containers are on a firm, level surface.
- Instruct the patient to slowly and carefully immerse the hand/wrist with the hand open and the fingers relaxed, until the fingers touch the bottom of the container. With the foot/ankle, have the patient slowly immerse the foot until it just touches the bottom of the container. Instruct the patient to leave the body part immersed, without movement, until water no longer drips from the spout. (Note: When using a volumeter with a bar, instruct the patient to immerse his or her hand so the bar separates the third and fourth digits.)
- Remove the calibrated container before the patient lifts the foot or hand from the water so any water that would drip from the body part does not drip into the calibrated container. Dry the patient's foot or hand.
- Place the calibrated container on a firm, level surface, and position yourself to read the scale at eye level.
- Record the results, document your activities, and report significant findings.
- Repeat the procedure for the uninvolved extremity for comparison.

Box 11-8 Indications and Contraindications for Lymphedema Treatment

INDICATIONS	CONTRAINDICATIONS
• Primary lymphedema	• Acute infection (the
• Secondary lymphedema	patient should be
• After a trauma, radiation	taking antibiotics at
• After a burn	least 4 days before
• After obstruction resulting	treatment)
from a tumor, scar,	• Active cancer
inflammation, or parasite	• Presence of congestive
• Idiopathic lymphedema	heart or kidney failure
• Postoperative edema	• After radiation
• Venous or arterial ulcer	treatment (requires
• Scar treatment	medical clearance)

Box 11-9 Complete (or Complex) Decongestive Therapy Objectives

- Enhance lymph drainage through the use of manual lymph drainage techniques.
- Control and reduce edema through compression bandaging.
- Use an intermittent vasopneumatic compression device as an adjunct to manual lymph drainage.
- Reduce or eliminate infections; educate the patient about techniques for meticulous skin and nail care.
- Increase function and enhance lymphatic flow through a gentle, individualized exercise program.
- Establish a maintenance program of therapy that will preserve the extremity improvements obtained from complete (or complex) decongestive therapy.
- Teach the patient to manage symptoms independently.

The use of MLD as a treatment of lymphedema has become recognized in the United States as an important therapeutic intervention. Dr. Emil Vodder developed the procedure in Cannes, France, in the 1930s. It is a superficial massage that differs from therapeutic massage in that it is gentler and is used to encourage fluid drainage from swollen areas by stimulating lymph vessels. Instead of using the kneading motion of massage, MLD involves mild stretching applied to the skin. This massage technique is systematically performed to reduce edema and move it to the main lymph drainage areas in the body. The massage increases lymphatic flow, helps break down fibrotic tissue areas, and promotes lymph system collateral development. This manual technique is specifically dependent on the location of the edema, skin tissue and integrity, and the cause of the edema.

Depending on the severity of edema, CDT may need to be performed for 2 to 8 weeks, three to five times per week, before a patient achieves normal or near-normal girth and can be fitted for a compression garment. MLD often is followed by intermittent vasopneumatic compression pumping. When lymph flow is established, a compression pump can be used to further reduce edema and, in conjunction with MLD treatment, can be applied during the control/

maintenance phase of treatment. MLD and compression pumping are followed by compression bandaging of the affected area. Short stretch bandages, with or without the use of foam padding, are applied daily to ensure that appropriate compression is maintained until the limb edema has reached a plateau in reduction. Instructions for lymphedema bandaging are provided in Procedure 11-3. The bandages are used to maximally assist compression, to provide an effective increase in lymph system flow, and to prevent reaccumulation of evacuated lymph fluid.

Short stretch bandages are made of extensible elastic material that provides high stability (support), low resting pressure, and high working pressure of the limb. The effectiveness of high working pressure is maximized by muscle and joint activity to pump the fluid proximally. Remedial exercises are performed daily while the extremity is either wrapped or has a properly fitted compression garment applied. While wearing the compression garment, patients should perform isometric and active exercises at home that focus on the affected limb, such as arm exercises for upper extremities and walking and isometric exercises for lower extremities. All exercise regimens require an individualized

Instructions for Upper Extremity Lymphedema Bandaging

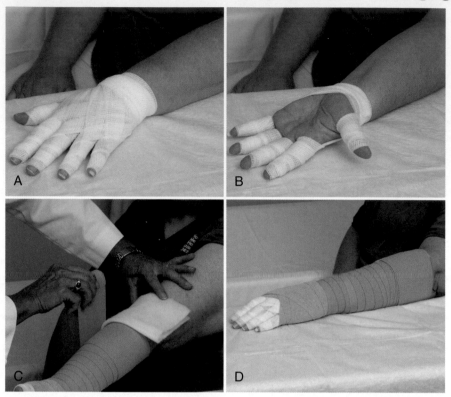

Fig. 11-11 **A** and **B,** The initial compression wrap using elasticized gauze. **C,** The third layer of the compression bandage with cotton batting to cushion the antecubital fossa; this bandage ends at the deltoid insertion. **D,** The completed compression wrap to the elbow.

All bandages start at the wrist; a minimum of three bandages (plus a finger wrap if fingers are involved) will be used for the complete wrap. It is important not to wrap above the elbow with the first two bandages. The third wrap, and fourth if needed, will cross the elbow, but do not return the bandage down across the elbow. Strive to have an even tension; the bandage should feel firm evenly up the arm when bandaging is finished. If the hand is not edematous, the finger wrap will not be used. If the wrist appears very small in comparison to the hand and forearm, a strip of foam padding may be used to fill the space before application of the wraps. Start with a finger wrap of 5 cm × 4 m, then apply a 6-cm × 5-m wrap, followed by an 8-cm × 5-m and a 10-cm × 5-m wrap, and if necessary a 12-cm × 5-m wrap.

FINGER WRAP

- Prefold in half the 5-cm × 4-m open weave soft cotton bandage, which has a high tensile strength and is available from various manufacturers.
- Anchor the white elasticized bandage at the wrist.
- Take the bandage to the tip of the thumb and wrap around the thumb to its base, overlapping by half the width. Anchor again at the wrist and take the bandage to the tip of the index finger, wrap to its base, and anchor at the wrist. Take the bandage to the third fingertip, and again wrap to its base, ending with a wrist anchor.
- Repeat this procedure for the fourth and little fingers, anchoring the final wrap at the wrist. When completed, the palmar surface should be free of bandage as shown in B, and the dorsum of the hand should be completely covered as shown in A.

6-cm BANDAGE

- This short stretch bandage is produced from 100% cotton and has long-lasting elasticity with strong to firm compression. It provides light resting pressure but high working pressure. The bandages are permeable to the air and nonirritating to the skin.
- Anchor the bandage at the wrist and wrap it around the palm of the hand three or four times to cover the palm and any areas left exposed by the finger wrap (usually at the base of the thumb).
- Continue the wrap in a spiral pattern, overlapping half of the previous bandage. Wrap to the elbow, but do not cross it.

8-cm BANDAGE

- Anchor at the wrist and wrap in a spiral pattern, overlapping each spiral by half. This bandage should cross the elbow and go to the upper arm to approximately the area of the deltoid insertion, but do not return it across the elbow. A square of soft cotton batting should be placed at the antecubital space for comfort (C) before or during application of this third bandage.

10-cm BANDAGE

- This bandage and the 12-cm bandage, if necessary, are anchored at the wrist and overlap by half of the previous bandage in a spiral pattern, crossing the elbow and ending near the deltoid insertion. These bandages will cover the previous bandages and are used for a large upper extremity.

Box 11-10	Precautions for Patients with Lymphedema

- Avoid extreme temperatures (e.g., hot baths, burns, and travel in extreme hot or cold climates).
- Avoid factors that may cause infection (e.g., insect bites, manicures, vaccinations, pet scratches, skin punctures and cuts, venography, and lymphography).
- Avoid blunt trauma (e.g., lifting heavy objects, playing tennis or golf, blood pressure cuffs, tight clothing, a heavy breast prosthesis, and tight jewelry).
- Avoid use of alcohol and nicotine.
- When traveling by air, wear a well-fitting compression garment and elevate the limb during flight.
- Maintain excellent nutrition and hydration (e.g., follow a low-salt diet; avoid fried foods and alcohol).
- Manage body weight to avoid obesity.
- Perform meticulous skin and nail care.
- Exercise daily.
- Treat infections promptly and vigorously.
- Seek treatment for even the slightest episode of lymphedema.
- Use hypoallergenic soaps and fragrances.

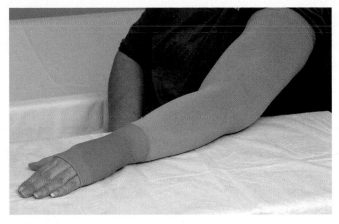

Fig. 11-12 A custom-made compression sleeve with a separate gauntlet.

approach. Proper assessment of patient strength, flexibility, functional limb mobility, and aerobic capacity should be performed before initiating treatment, and gradual progression of exercise should be expected. (Caution: Higher exertion-type exercise may damage the delicate balance of the lymph system and interstitial pressure.)

Patients with lymphedema have a high risk for the development of skin infections because of the decreased flow of high-protein lymph fluid. Precautions are listed in Box 11-10. Meticulous skin and nail care are important to prevent bacterial, viral, and other infections. Because lymphedema weakens the immune system of the affected limb, the skin must be kept moist and at an appropriate pH level. A low-pH skin lotion that contains no irritants or perfumes should be applied to the skin and nails daily. Because lymphedema is a lifelong condition, patients must be responsible for meticulous skin care and must follow precautions, perform self-massage, apply compression bandages or garments, and perform remedial exercises to ensure that CDT will have long-term success. Therefore a proficient clinician should educate the patient on all the treatment steps beginning on the first day of treatment.

Lymphedema Certification

Although CDT has been used in Europe for years with great success, it has only been recognized as the U.S. standard for lymphedema management within the past two decades. Registered nurses, physical therapists, occupational therapists, massage therapists, and other providers from several disciplines offer treatment in the United States. The technique of CDT has a strong self-care aspect, and lymphedema therapists need to be very proficient. For this reason, the Lymphology Association of North America created a national CDT certification examination, which became available in 2001.

COMPRESSION GARMENTS

Compression garments are used to control edema in an extremity, assist in the return of venous circulation in a lower extremity, and decrease the formation of extensive scar tissue resulting from a burn. The information herein, however, is limited to its use in treating lymphedema. Garments are available in both custom-made and standard prefabricated varieties (Fig. 11-12). Standard garments should not be used for patients whose circumference measurements show extreme deviations when compared with measurement tables, for patients whose length measurements vary greatly from the average, for awkwardly shaped limbs or a deformity, or when a custom-made compression garment is required. Garments may be obtained in a gradient format in which distal compression is greater than proximal compression. Standard prefabricated garments are less expensive than custom-made garments and can be obtained quickly, whereas obtaining custom-made garments can take up to 3 weeks. For this reason, most knowledgeable caregivers will measure for a custom-made garment after 10 to 15 days of treatment so the garment will be available at the end of the CDT protocol.

Theoretically, compression garments aid in reducing swelling by lessening the amount of edema formed within the involved extremity. The garments are fabricated for an individual patient from a fabric that, because of its elastic properties, produces an external, graduated compression force to the tissues. In addition to their use on the extremities, garments can be fabricated for a patient's head or trunk. These applications would be beneficial to decrease the development of scar tissue for a person who has been burned. A patient's comfort, and therefore compliance, is of importance for the maintenance of progress made during therapy. Therefore the fit is extremely important, as is the material from which the garment is made. The garment can be made from synthetic or cotton fibers, and some garments have a soft inner lining.

These garments have the following disadvantages: they can be uncomfortable (although more comfortable materials have become available), putting them on is a laborious process (often talc is used on the limb before garment application, but talc should not be used with patients who have known respiratory problems or who are allergic to it), they are unsightly, and they typically last no more than 3 to 6 months. Garments should be replaced when they begin to lose their elasticity or when they no longer fit because of a change in the patient's condition.

Measurements for a pressure-gradient garment for the upper or lower extremity can be obtained by using paper measuring tapes (Fig. 11-13) supplied by a manufacturer or by following the directions on other manufacturers' forms (Fig. 11-14; Procedure 11-4). The paper tapes allow circumferential measurements to be made approximately every 1.5 inches from the distal to the proximal aspect of the extremity. Specific landmarks on each extremity are used to properly position the tape before the application of the individual strips that are wrapped around the extremity. Complete instructions and directions, including diagrams, are provided with each measuring tape.

Other forms of measurement include use of a plastic-covered cloth tape, an anthropometric tape, or a metal tape

(see Figs. 11-8 and 11-9). For the lower extremity, the usual measurement sites are the gluteal fold, upper thigh, lower thigh, knee, calf, distal calf, ankle, instep, and metatarsal heads (see Fig. 11-14). Upper extremity measurement sites include the wrist, mid forearm, elbow, mid upper arm, upper arm at the level of the axilla, and upper arm from the axilla to the tip of the shoulder. If a strap is necessary to secure the upper extremity garment, a measurement from the tip of the shoulder to the opposite axilla must be performed. The explanation for using the measuring tape technique of an upper extremity compression garment is explained in Procedure 11-4. If the hand is edematous, it must be measured for a glove or gauntlet (i.e., a fingerless glove that may be separate from or can be attached to an upper extremity sleeve). Hand measurement sites include the circumference of the wrist, mid palm, metacarpal circumference (at the base of the fingers), the base of the thumb and each finger, and the distal interphalangeal joints of the thumb and each finger just below the nails. Distance measurements for the hand include from the wrist to the metacarpal heads, from mid palm to the metacarpal heads, and from the base of the fingers and thumb to either the nail bed for an open-fingered glove or from the base to the tip of the fingers and thumb for a closed-fingered glove (see Fig. 11-14).

Two garments should be ordered simultaneously so one garment will be available for use while the other garment is being washed. Alternate use of the two garments will extend the life of each garment. Furthermore, replacement garments should be ordered so they are available before the current garment has lost its therapeutic value. Instructions about the application, removal, and care of the garment are provided by the manufacturer.

Intermittent Vasopneumatic Compression Devices

Intermittent compression through the use of a vasopneumatic compression pump and sleeve is a method of treatment for chronic or acute edema or swelling and venous insufficiency. A variety of pumps are available. They range in cost from several hundred dollars to several thousand dollars for more advanced units. Pumps range from a single-chambered unit to up to 12 chambers (cells). Multichambered pumps inflate sequentially from the distal to to proximal position, thereby producing pressure that ascends the extremity, theoretically evacuating the edema with this wave of pressure. The use of a multichambered pump is shown in Fig. 11-15. Guidelines for pump selection, the number of chambers, the length of time of the pumping session, pumping pressure ranges, and inflation/deflation cycles vary according to the pump manufacturer and the patient's needs.

A trial is recommended so patients can compare pumping devices, if these devices are available, before a unit is obtained for home use. Multichambered, sequential pumps are used at relatively low pressures (i.e., 40 to 60 mm Hg

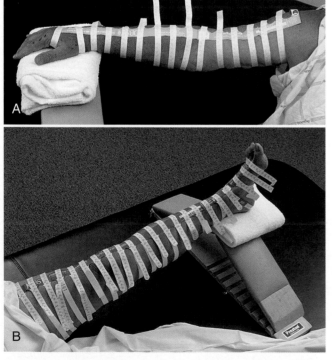

Fig. 11-13 Application of measurement tapes for a graduated compression (pressure gradient) garment. **A,** Upper extremity. **B,** Lower extremity.

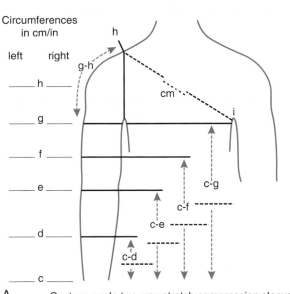

A   Custom-made two-way stretch compression sleeves

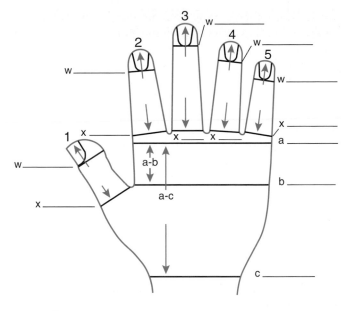

B   Custom-made two-way stretch compression hand portions

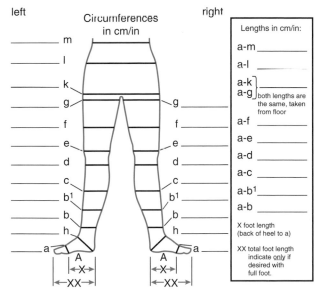

C   Custom-made medical two-way stretch compression panty hose

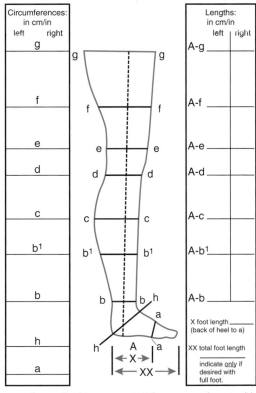

D   Custom-made medical two-way stretch compression stockings

Fig. 11-14   Measurements chart for custom-made compression garments of the upper and lower extremities. **A,** Two-way stretch compression sleeves. **B,** Two-way stretch compression hand portions. **C,** Two-way stretch compression pantyhose. **D,** Two-way stretch compression stockings. (Redrawn with permission from Julius Zorn, Juzo, 80 Chart Road, Cuyahoga Falls, OH, 2000.)

for the upper extremity and 80 to 90 mm Hg for the lower extremity) and have been advocated as part of a comprehensive lymphedema program. Compression sleeves for the upper and lower extremities are available from most compression pump manufacturers, but some must be custom-made for particular models. The sleeves are inflated and deflated by the pump (Procedure 11-5). The inflation cycle provides an external compression force to the extremity that assists in removing the edema or facilitates the return of venous blood from the extremity to the heart.

PROCEDURE 11-4

Measurement of a Pressure Gradient Garment

PAPER TAPE METHOD

Upper Extremity

- Explain the procedure, seat the patient, elevate and support the upper extremity, and expose the entire upper extremity from the top of the shoulder to the ends of the fingers.
- Apply the spine of the measuring tape along the length of the extremity; apply the paper strips at the specified landmarks (e.g., the elbow and the base of the thumb/wrist).
- Wrap each individual strip around the extremity; keep it flat, in close contact with the skin, perpendicular to the spine, and parallel to the strip above and below. Do not pull the strip so tight that it causes an indentation in the soft tissue. Attach the strip to the spine, and follow the manufacturer's instructions for pleating the spine to ensure that the garment's length will be appropriate.
- After all the strips are in place, use bandage scissors to cut each strip along the side of the spine that is scalloped (the side with round indentations); it may be helpful to use cellophane tape to reinforce the attachment of each strip to the spine.
- Label the tape with the patient's name, indicate whether it is the left or right extremity, list any specific information or instructions regarding the fabrication, fold the tape, and place it in the mailing envelope.

Lower Extremity

- Explain the procedure and position the patient supine. Support the lower extremity to elevate it from the mattress or mat and expose the lower extremity from the groin to the end of the toes. (Note: If a leotard ["panty hose"] type of garment is to be fabricated, it will be necessary to provide waist and hip measurements.)
- Apply the spine of the measuring tape along the length of the extremity; apply the paper strips at the specified landmarks (e.g., the heel/ankle).
- Wrap each individual strip around the extremity; follow the same procedure outlined for upper extremity measurements. Note that extension strips may be added to strips that are not long enough to encircle the extremity. In addition, pleats (folds) can be made on the measuring tape to adjust its length. When edema control is the goal, the extremity should be measured when the least amount of edema is present (i.e., measure early in the morning or after complete decongestive therapy if the patient is being treated). Many options and modifications are available for the garments (see Fig. 11-13).

MEASURING TAPE METHOD FOR THE UPPER EXTREMITY

- Expose the extremity, position the patient so the extremity is relaxed, supported, and elevated, and explain the procedure. If lymphedema is not bilateral, measure the unaffected contralateral extremity to obtain a baseline for comparison. Use a plastic or metal anthropometric measuring tape with well-defined, easily visible calibrations; it will be helpful if the tape can be locked at any length so it will not retract, but can be lengthened.
- Use a tension gauge, if it is available, for circumference pressure.
- To measure each of the circumferences of the extremity, apply the measuring tape around the extremity so it contacts the skin firmly and lies flat but without causing an excessive indentation in the soft tissue. Use consistent pressure as you apply the tape at each mark, and apply the tape so each measurement is parallel to the one above and below.
- Palpate and mark the ulnar stylus of the wrist to be used as the base for the series of measurement sites on the extremity. Take a circumferential measurement at the wrist.
- Use a skin-marking pencil to mark each site at which the circumferential measurements of the upper extremity are to be made; the sites should be as equidistant as possible from each other and include the mid forearm, elbow, mid–upper arm, and upper arm at the level of the axilla. If the sleeve includes the shoulder, measure from the axilla to the tip of the shoulder on the lateral aspect and from the tip of the shoulder to the opposite axilla (see Fig. 11-14, *A*).
- Measure the circumference at each site.
- Position the free end of the tape on the ulnar stylus, and extend it along the extremity to each of the premarked circumferential sites; document the distances between the ulnar stylus and each circumferential measurement site (see Fig. 11-14).
- Document your activity properly on the form provided.

(Caution: Before using compression with a lower extremity for a venous condition, arterial insufficiency and thrombophlebitis must be ruled out. If arterial insufficiency is present, the inflation phase of the intermittent compression cycle may cause additional occlusion of the arterial circulation and possibly tissue ischemia. If thrombophlebitis is present, compression has the potential to cause an embolus to enter the venous system.)

The patient is either seated or placed in a supine position for compression of the upper extremity and placed in a supine position for compression the lower extremity, the sleeve is applied, and the extremity is elevated above the level of the heart. (Note: A tubular stockinette should be applied to the person's extremity before application of the sleeve to maintain cleanliness of the inside of the sleeve.) The amount of pressure in the sleeve and the parameters of

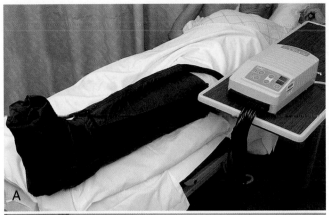

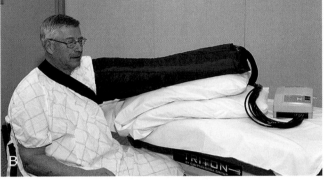

Fig. 11-15 A multichambered, sequential compression pump. **A,** Lower extremity application. **B,** Upper extremity application.

PROCEDURE 11-5

Intermittent Compression Pump

- Explain the procedure to the patient and obtain consent, measure the patient's blood pressure to ensure that pneumatic pressure does not exceed diastolic pressure, and examine the extremity.
- Position and drape the patient, expose the extremity, and apply a tubular stockinette and the sleeve to the extremity.
- The extremity should be level with or elevated above the heart.
- Adjust the controls of the unit as necessary (i.e., pressure and inflation-to-deflation ratio) and turn on the unit. The patient can be instructed to actively contract muscles during deflation cycles.
- Periodically monitor the patient during the treatment session, and provide the patient with a call device or bell that can be used during treatment. Lower the pressure or stop treatment if the patient reports tingling, numbness, or severe pain or can feel his or her pulse.
- To conclude the treatment, turn off the unit when the sleeve is deflated. (Note: If the sleeve is inflated, detach the inflation hose(s) from the sleeve and deflate it.) Remove the sleeve and discard the stockinette.
- Examine the extremity, measure the circumference (girth), and document your activities and findings.

the cycle should be established for each patient. Generally, the maximum compression force should be above the patient's systemic diastolic blood pressure but should not exceed his or her systolic pressure to avoid possible cardiovascular complications. The length of treatment time for compression pumps varies. An example of an extreme protocol would be to undergo pumping for 2 hours on and 30 minutes off during waking hours and to undergo 6 hours of continuous pumping during the night. The normal length of time for a patient to undergo compression after MLD for lymphedema would be 30 minutes.

A program of intermittent vasopneumatic compression is advantageous to reduce the edema in an extremity before measurement for a graded compression garment. When this approach is used, a more accurate measurement of the garment can be obtained and it will be more likely to control the residual edema. The application of tubular elastic gauze for a finger and hand wrap and low-stretch compression wraps to the extremity (see Fig. 11-11) after each pumping session will help minimize redevelopment of the edema and should be performed until a permanent graded compression garment is available (see Fig. 11-12).

In addition to undergoing mechanical compression, the patient may be instructed to perform active pumping exercises and to elevate the extremity two or three times per hour to assist with edema control. Finger flexion and

extension exercises for the upper extremity and active ankle pumping (i.e., repetitive dorsiflexion/plantar flexion) for the lower extremity, with the extremity elevated and supported, are two activities that are used frequently.

It is important to observe and converse with the patient periodically during each treatment session. Reports of pain, numbness, tingling, or other forms of paresthesia by the patient may indicate that the treatment should be terminated. To conclude a treatment session, the sleeve should be in the deflated mode so the sleeve can be easily removed. If the treatment is terminated with the sleeve inflated, the hose(s) attached to the control unit should be disconnected from the sleeve. Pressure to the outside of the sleeve will cause it to deflate; when the sleeve has been removed, remove and discard the stockinette. Observe and palpate the extremity and measure the circumference (girth) periodically if lymphedema is the condition being treated. Be observant for skin or circulatory changes that may have occurred as a result of the treatment, and document your activities, observations, and measurements as necessary.

These pump units may be rented or loaned for home use, and the patient should be provided with written instructions and directions about the use of the unit. Precautions to be followed should be described, and a method of communication between the patient and caregiver should be established. In addition, periodic reevaluation of the person's response to or effect of the home treatments should be performed by the caregiver. Contraindications for compression pumps include anticoagulated patients, patients with deep venous thrombosis, and patients with local cancer or malignancy, severe arterial insufficiency, lymphangitis, cellulitis, cutaneous infection, acute dermatitis, and wet dermatosis. These symptoms also may contraindicate the use of support stockings for vascular conditions.

CHEST PHYSICAL THERAPY

Also called cardiopulmonary physical therapy, CPT is an intervention process concerned with the examination, evaluation, and treatment of patients of all ages with acute and chronic lung conditions. These conditions may be attributable to primary diseases or may be secondary to other medical and surgical conditions. CPT includes the use of many examination, evaluation, and treatment techniques. The examination and evaluation of a spontaneously breathing and mechanically ventilated patient may include analysis of medical information from the patient's record (e.g., findings of a chest x-ray, arterial blood gas values, history, physical findings, and results of an exercise stress test and tolerance); chest assessment by auscultation, chest wall mobility, palpation, posture analysis, breathing pattern, and chest percussion; evaluation of cough effectiveness and productivity; joint range of motion (ROM) and muscle testing; observation of noninvasive oxygen monitoring (e.g., ear oximetry and transcutaneous oximetry) and identification of respiratory therapy appliances that might enhance CPT; assessment of any stress or tension the patient exhibits; functional evaluation of bed mobility, transfer activities, ambulation on level surfaces and stairs, and the need for assistive devices; and observation of mental status and level of acceptance of the disease, medical condition, or postoperative status.

Treatment is based on results of the initial and subsequent examination and evaluations. Most of the techniques used fall into the categories of airway clearance (secretion removal), breathing retraining/exercises, and therapeutic exercise. Airway clearance techniques facilitate loosening and removal of secretions from the tracheobronchial tree.

The following techniques may be used for airway clearance:
- Positioning for gravity drainage (Fig. 11-16)
- Chest percussion, vibration, and shaking
- Rib springing
- Cough training, stimulation, and assistance
- Forced expiratory technique (huff)
- Airway suctioning
- Oxygen, bronchodilator, and humidity therapy used in conjunction with CPT treatments

The following breathing retraining exercises often are used:

- Breathing exercises (diaphragmatic, pursed lip, segmental)
- Incentive spirometry (Fig. 11-17)
- Paced breathing techniques
- Glossopharyngeal breathing
- Sustained maximal inspiration and inspiratory hold techniques
- Respiratory muscle strength and endurance exercises

The following therapeutic exercise programs with or without oxygen support may be used:
- Relaxation training
- Posture correction
- Manual stretching of the thorax
- Chest mobilization
- Exercise techniques to improve and maintain ROM of the chest and shoulders (e.g., after a thoracotomy)
- Strength and coordination of the trunk and extremities
- Exercise endurance training
- Energy conservation techniques
- Instruction in home care programs
- Patient and family education

Goals of CPT include improvement of airway clearance, ventilation, and exercise tolerance; reduction in the work of breathing; and restoration of the patient to the fullest potential in the inpatient, outpatient, pulmonary rehabilitation, and home care settings (Fig. 11-18). Treatment settings may include medical, surgical, and cardiac intensive care units; inpatient units; preoperative and postoperative areas; labor and delivery and pediatric units; and the chronic care area. Patients may range from neonates to the very elderly. CPT home program planning, which helps the patient and family understand and participate in self-care, promotes optimal pulmonary rehabilitation in the continuum of care.

Many newer modalities are being clinically tested to determine whether they can be an adjunct to or a replacement for CPT, especially in persons with cystic fibrosis, who need daily CPT. These modalities include but are not limited to vests that vibrate the chest wall using pulses of air, airway devices that create waves of pressure through the airway as the patient exhales through the device, high-frequency chest wall compression by an oscillating thoracic cuff, and an intrapulmonary percussive ventilation device. Aerobic exercise, such as with a stationary bicycle, has been used to facilitate airway clearance.

AMPUTATIONS

Amputation is removal of a body part as a result of trauma or surgery. Surgery is performed because of pain or a disease process in the limb resulting from cancer, gangrene, infection, diabetes, or vascular insufficiencies. Because of the large amount of information needed to address each type of amputation, only above the knee (AK) and below the knee (BK) amputations in adults will be addressed in this book.

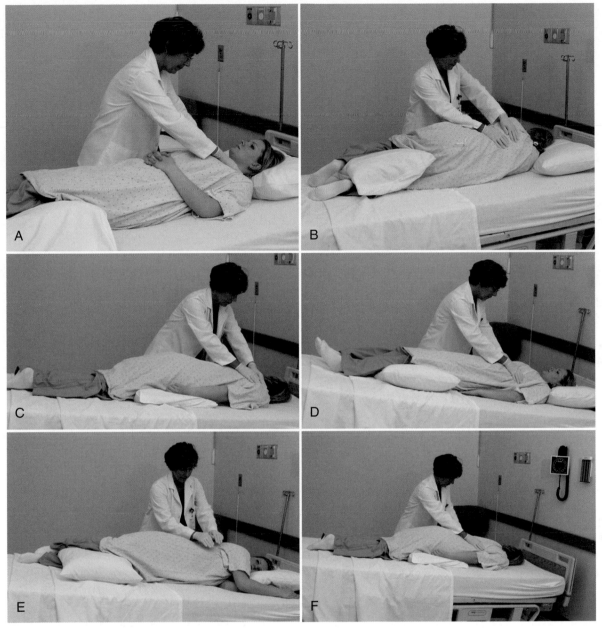

Fig. 11-16 **A,** Postural drainage position for anterior segments, upper lobes. **B,** Postural drainage position for posterior segment, left upper lobe. **C,** Postural drainage position for posterior segment, right upper lobe. **D,** Postural drainage position for anterior basal segments. **E,** Postural drainage position for left lateral basal segment. **F,** Postural drainage position for posterior basal segments.

Lower Extremity Amputations

Fig. 11-19 depicts the following types of lower extremity amputations:

- Hemicorpectomy (the entire pelvis and distal structures are removed)
- Hemipelvectomy (removal of half of the pelvis)
- Hip disarticulation (removal at the hip joint with the pelvis left intact)
- AK, also referred to as a transfemoral amputation
- Knee disarticulation (removal at the knee joint with the femur left intact)

- BK, also referred to as a transtibial amputation
- Ankle disarticulation or Syme's disarticulation (the entire ankle is removed)
- Chopart, Lisfranc, transmetatarsal
- Toe or digit (phalangeal)

The aim of rehabilitation for all lower extremity amputations is to achieve maximal independence and function. This goal can be achieved by improving the baseline musculoskeletal system, which ROM, strengthening, cardiovascular fitness, balance, mobility, coordination, and a home exercise program. The caregiver should obtain

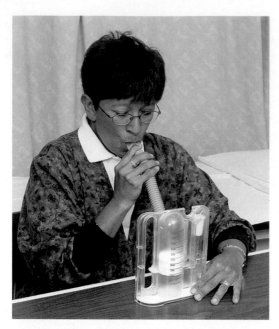

Fig. 11-17   Use of an incentive spirometer.

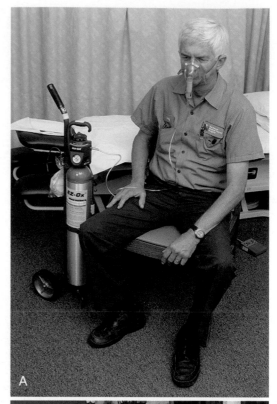

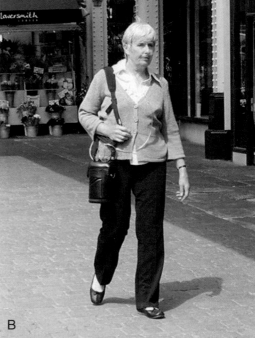

Fig. 11-18   Portable oxygen use. **A,** Use of portable oxygen cylinder with a mask. Note the trunk position and support by the forearm on the thigh. **B,** A portable oxygen tank that is carried by the patient. The patient uses a nasal cannula to receive the oxygen. (**B** from Bonewit-West K: *Clinical procedures for medical assistants,* ed 8, St Louis, 2012, Saunders Elsevier.)

knowledge about the patient's preamputation lifestyle, coping mechanisms, support system, medical limitations, comorbidities, barriers to learning, and expectations. Immediate postoperative goals are:

- Successful wound healing
- Control of edema and shaping of the residual limb
- Prevention of joint contractures (e.g., hip flexion, abduction and external rotation for the AK and BK amputations, and knee flexion for the BK amputation)
- Patient and family education concerning limb care, skin care, and residual limb and body positioning
- Control of postoperative pain (both phantom limb pain and real pain)
- Achieving independence in activities of daily living and mobility with and without a prosthesis
- Education concerning daily inspection of the residual limb, the process of fitting of a prosthetic limb, and functional outcome

After preoperative education and assessment, postoperative care begins with dressings that are applied over the amputation wound, which is usually covered by one or more of the following items: sterile gauze, nonadherent sterile gauze or colloid wound dressings, and absorbent pads. These wound dressings are worn until the wound healing is complete and the volume of the stump has stabilized.

The patient's surgeon should select the appropriate postoperative dressing used for edema control and shaping of the residual limb. The major postoperative dressing classifications are the soft dressing, the semirigid dressing, and the rigid dressing. The soft dressing could be a 4- or 6-inch Ace wrap, a compression pump, or a shrinker. The semirigid dressing would be an Unna cast or air cast, and the rigid

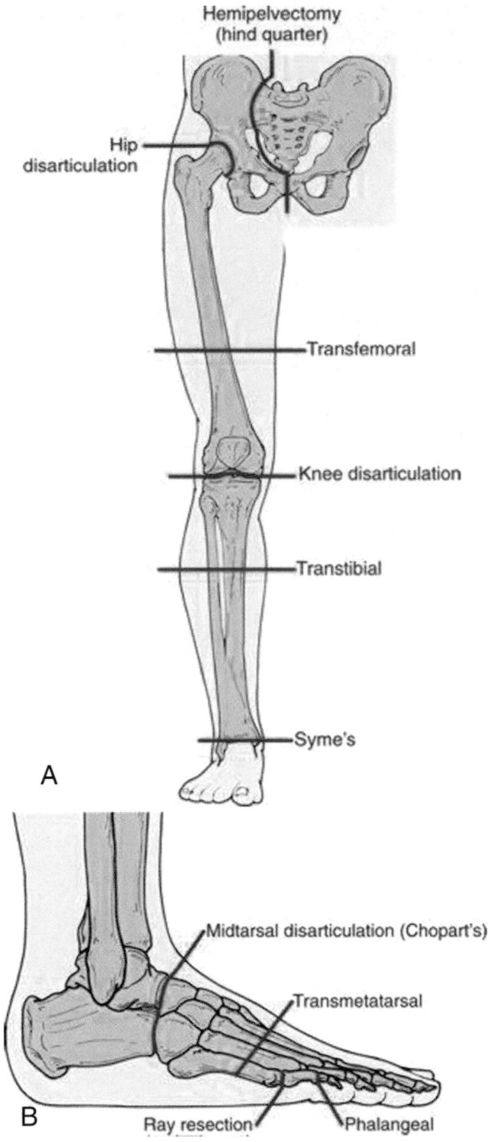

Fig. 11-19   Lower extremity amputations. **A,** Major lower extremity amputations. **B,** Minor lower extremity amputations. (From Cameron MH, Monroe LG: *Physical rehabilitation: evidence-based examination, evaluation, and intervention,* St Louis, 2008, Saunders Elsevier.)

dressing could be a non–weight bearing rigid dressing; a custom or prefabricated rigid removable dressing (RRD), an immediate postoperative prosthesis (IPOP); or a prefabricated pneumatic immediate postoperative prosthesis (airPOP).

The soft dressing is the most widely used postoperative dressing. Major advantages of soft dressings are that they are readily available and easy to apply, and they allow the wound to be checked frequently (Fig. 11-20). Disadvantages of Ace bandages are that they must be applied expertly to achieve proper tension to reduce edema without causing the tourniquet effect, they have a tendency to loosen if not wrapped properly, the limb is still at risk of injury, they must

be reapplied several times a day, and they are not the best dressing for controlling edema. Shrinker socks are more effective than bandages in controlling edema, but different sizes will be needed as the residual limb shrinks.

Wong, in an article titled "Rethinking the Standard in Preprosthetic Rehab" (see the Bibliography), is an avid supporter of the use of the semirigid dressing in postoperative amputees. He states that Unna paste has the following benefits: availability, less expense, edema reduction, wound healing, and limb shaping. Because of the self-adhering quality of Unna paste, there is no need for suspension devices that must be used with RRDs. This dressing also may be left on for up to 7 days. Wong states that some clinicians have even used the Unna dressing under a temporary prosthesis for early gait training. For a BK amputation, Wong uses one roll of Unna paste, which terminates distal to the knee. At times he needs to use two rolls for a large limb of an AK amputation that terminates at the inguinal ligament. The limb is completely covered after securing a dressing at the wound site and then covering that dressing with a thin transparent film.

The RRD has the benefit of protecting the residual limb; in addition, it is removable so that wound inspection can occur frequently, it immobilizes soft tissue to reduce pain and facilitate wound healing, and it permits progressive shrinkage of the stump by means of the addition of socks. The RRD can be made from plaster bandage, fiberglass casting, or a polymer plastic and felt. The RRD must be suspended by use of a suspension stockinette that is placed over the RRD and attached to a supracondylar plastic cuff. In a study conducted by Taylor et al. (see the Bibliography), it was found that the use of a postoperative RRD in persons with BK amputations resulted in a reduced length of acute hospital stay and a shortened time to first prosthetic casting compared with patients who had used a soft dressing.

In a study by Deutsch et al. (see the Bibliography) in which the subjects were 50 randomized, controlled dysvascular transtibial amputees who used either a soft dressing or a removable rigid dressing, no significant difference was found in the hospital stay, incidence of residual limb breakdown, time taken for limb volume to become stable, or time to prosthetic fitting. However, it was found that primary wound healing of the residual limb occurred almost 2 weeks earlier with use of the removable rigid dressing.

Postsurgical management of the amputee is carried out by the rehabilitation team and, later, by the prosthetist. A thorough, continuous rehabilitation assessment (Table 11-8) is essential to obtaining maximum independence and function. The skin on the residual limb of an amputee must be given proper care acutely, as well as before and after use of a prosthesis (if applicable). Persons with diabetes, the elderly, patients with poor nutrition, persons who smoke, and patients with dysvascular disorders must take particular care. Skin lesions and abrasions can occur from poor healing,

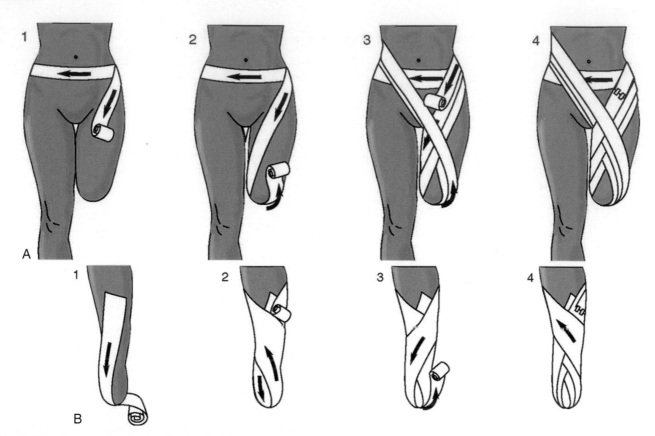

Fig. 11-20 Proper application of an Ace bandage for an amputation. **A,** Above the knee. **B,** Below the knee. (From Ignatavicius DD: *Medical-surgical nursing: patient centered collaborative care,* ed 6, Philadelphia, 2009, Saunders Elsevier.)

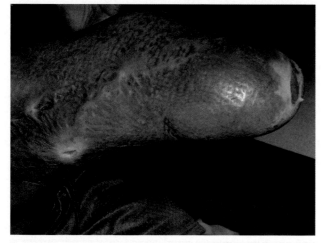

Fig. 11-21 A poor-healing skin lesion on a diabetic person caused by pressure on the skin from a prosthesis.

infections, and pressure on the skin or stump from a prosthesis (Fig. 11-21).

TAPING STRATEGIES

Many types of taping are used for particular diagnoses. Some examples of an adhesive nonstretch tape are the epicondylitis wrap (adhesive tape) and the plantar fasciitis wrap.

Epicondylitis (Tennis Elbow) Wrap

To wrap the extremity of a patient with epicondylitis, place an underwrap (i.e., a thin, porous polyurethane foam) around the wrist to prevent the tape from adhering to the underlying skin. Distract the wrist by having the patient hold the elbow at the side with the elbow bent to 90 degrees, and gently pull the wrist and hand away from the forearm. Use athletic tape that is approximately 0.5 to 0.75 inch wide. Place the tape just distal to the radial head and ulnar stylus (Fig. 11-22, A). Wrap the tape snugly over the dorsum of the wrist and then "lay on" the tape on the volar surface to avoid compression of blood vessels and the median nerve. Repeat the wrap two or three repetitions and ask the patient to extend and flex his or her wrist; motion should be limited. When treating a patient for tennis elbow, have him or her wear an adjustable tennis elbow strap approximately 1 to 2 inches distal to the olecranon process (Fig. 11-22, B).

Plantar Fasciitis Wrap

To create a plantar fasciitis wrap, first cover the entire foot with an underwrap, such as Omnifix or Cover-Roll stretch, to protect the skin. Lay the tape on as described in Fig. 11-23. This wrap is an excellent choice for acute plantar fasciitis. An orthotic should be made for a person with chronic plantar fasciitis to support the arch. Appropriate foot exercises also should be initiated.

Table **11-8**   Assessment and Interventions for Lower Extremity Amputations

	Preoperative	Postoperative
Medical history	Obtain comorbidities, surgical history, history of present incident, support system	Initiate education of comorbidities if needed
ROM	Assess active and passive ROM of all four limbs and trunk	Initiate passive ROM of residual and contralateral limb in flexion/extension and adduction and abduction; progress to active assistive ROM; advance to active ROM and stretching exercises; position to prevent contractures when sitting or in bed; use towel rolls and knee extension device if needed
Strength	Assess strength in all four limbs and trunk	Begin strengthening program for major muscle groups of upper extremity and lower extremity; progress to trunk and core stabilization exercises
Cardiovascular system	Assess fitness level and explain increase in energy level needed for prosthetic use (if applicable)	Establish cardiac precautions to exercise (heart rate, blood pressure, perceived exertion scales, shortness of breath, pallor, diaphoresis, chest pain, headache, peripheral edema); progress to antigravity exercises, isometric contractions, upper body ergometer
Balance	Assess balance and coordination and explain center of gravity changes postoperatively	Initiate sitting to sitting weight shifts, working to sit to stand, to supported standing, to single limb standing balance
Mobility	Current mobility status	Initiate and progress to independent bed mobility, rolling, positioning, transfers, and wheelchair mobility to single limb gait in parallel bars; progress to use of assistive gait device with and without prosthesis
Patient education	Safety/fall precautions, prevention of complications (residual limb care, contractures, postoperative dressings), equipment needs (wheelchair training, gait devices, residual limb socks and liners, prosthetic choices), and desensitization exercises	Positioning (bed and seated), edema control, pain control, residual limb care, wound care, application of shrinker or Ace bandages; progress to prosthetic education if applicable (donning and doffing prosthesis, care of prosthesis, sock management, skin integrity, progressive wear schedule, monitor skin integrity)
Home exercise program		Provide contact numbers, educate on limb volume management, provide home exercise program (HEP)

ROM, Range of motion.

Kinesiology Taping

Unlike many of the athletic taping procedures that are used primarily for support and/or compression of a joint during an activity, kinesiology taping is used over muscles and joints and is pulled at varying degrees of tension, or the body or body part is flexed, extended, or rotated to create the desired effect. The tape is usually worn from 2 to 5 days, and the person is able to take a shower with the tape on and pat dry.

Kinesiology tape was developed in the 1970s by Japanese chiropractor Kenzo Kase and brought to the United States in the mid 1990s. Kase's tape is called Kinesio Tex Tape, and after development it was sold only to chiropractors and physical therapists. Today several kinesiology tapes can be found on the market, and some are being sold in athletic stores for purchase by any consumer. Some of the kinesiology tape brands available are SpiderTech, which is sold in precut patterns to clinicians only; KT Tape, which is sold

in major athletic stores; Rock Tape, which is sold as an athletic enhancer; and 3B Scientific Tape.

In 2006, Yasukawa et al. performed a pilot study on the effect of using kinesiology tape in an acute pediatric rehabilitation setting. The purpose of the study was to describe the use of the kinesiology tape for the upper extremity in enhancing functional motor skills in children who were in an acute rehabilitation program. The study found statistically significant improvement from before taping to after taping. Fig. 11-24 shows a child with an obstetrical brachial plexus injury that was being treated with kinesiology tape. Jaraczewska et al., in a study on adults with hemiplegia, noted an improvement in upper extremity function with the use of kinesiology taping as an adjunct to other treatments.

Several uses for kinesiology taping have been suggested in the literature, including use of the tape for upper extremity lymphedema in patients with breast cancer, shoulder

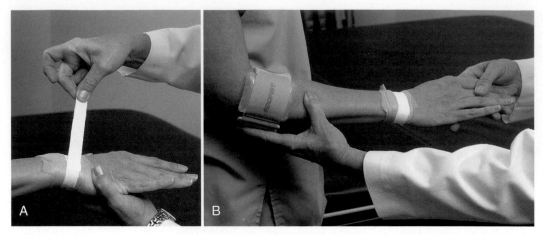

Fig. 11-22 An epicondylitis (tennis elbow) wrap. **A,** Application of underwrap, followed by 0.5-inch-wide adhesive tape. Note: The hand should be distracted from the wrist during application. **B,** A tennis elbow strap is applied.

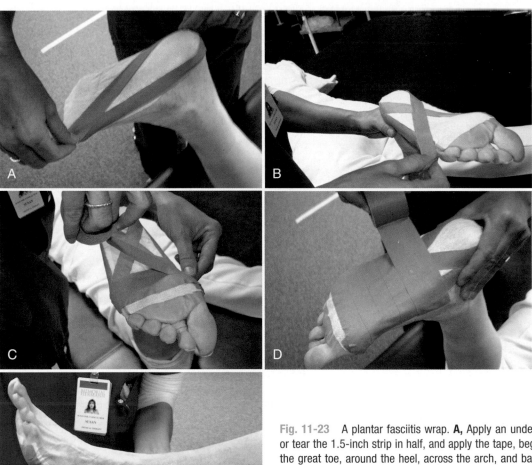

Fig. 11-23 A plantar fasciitis wrap. **A,** Apply an underwrap to protect the skin, cut or tear the 1.5-inch strip in half, and apply the tape, beginning at the lateral border of the great toe, around the heel, across the arch, and back to the lateral border of the great toe. Be sure to just lay the tape on the patient. **B,** Apply the other half of the strip, beginning at the lateral border of the fifth metatarsal head, around the heel, across the arch, and back to the lateral border of the fifth metatarsal head. **C,** With the full width, lay the tape across the metatarsals and overlap the remaining pieces by one half, moving toward the heel. **D,** The last piece of tape ends just before the calcaneus. **E,** The wrap ends on the lateral border of the foot when it is completed.

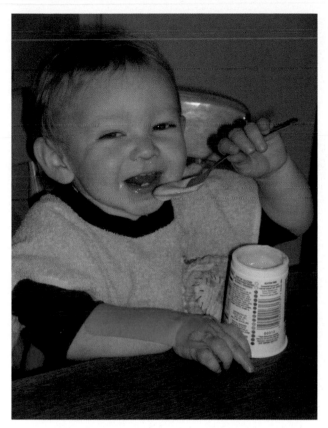

Fig. 11-24   A child taped with kinesiology tape for an obstetrical brachial plexus injury.

impingement, lateral epicondylitis, shoulder pain, low back pain, knee pain, lower extremity edema, cervical pain, strains and sprains, and for any painful joint or muscle group where support and stability are needed without compromising ROM. See Fig. 11-25 for photos demonstrating the use of SpiderTech taping.

SUMMARY

Wound care requires compliance of the caregiver with many of the principles related to infection control that are addressed in Chapter 2. When the application and removal of dressings and bandages are required for wound care, it may be necessary to develop and maintain a sterile field to protect the dressing materials and to dispose of the contaminated materials properly.

For some patients, preventing a wound from developing will be an important intervention. This intervention is particularly urgent for patients whose condition predisposes them to the development of a pressure ulcer. Assessment of the risk factors associated with a pressure ulcer and the use of measures to prevent them should be performed for all patients upon admission to a health care facility.

Patients with lymphedema should be informed about the risks and preventive measures associated with the condition. Treatment interventions to control edema include the use of specific massage and compression bandaging

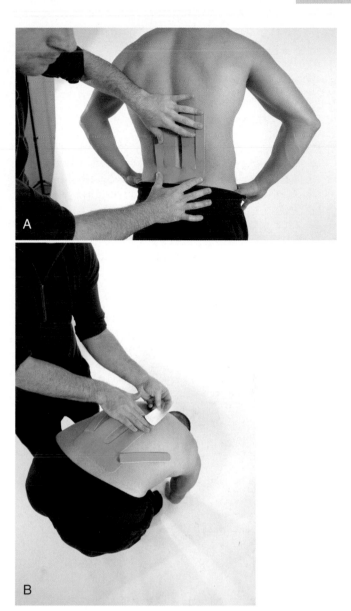

Fig. 11-25   SpiderTech low back application. (Courtesy Dr. Kevin Jardine, CEO, SpiderTech Kinesiology Tape.)

techniques, the use of an intermittent compression pump, and the measurement for and eventual application of a pressure garment for the extremity. Girth and volumetric measurements are used to evaluate the size of the extremity after each week of treatment and to provide objective data regarding the results of the interventions used.

A patient who has a respiratory infection or condition that adversely affects respiratory capacity or who is recovering from a surgical procedure affecting the chest or lungs may require chest mobility or lung secretion clearing techniques to improve respiratory status.

Postoperative goals for amputees are important for both the patients and their families. Different types of postoperative dressings are available and are dependent on the condition of the patient and the future goals for ambulation and function. The patient's surgeon is usually the person who orders the type of dressing.

self-study ACTIVITIES

- Identify persons at risk for pressure ulcers.
- Prescribe appropriate positions to assist in the prevention of pressure ulcers.
- Describe at least five signs or symptoms of an improperly applied bandage, and state a corrective action for each.
- Describe at least four instructions or precautions you should give to a patient for whom you have applied a bandage.
- Describe and demonstrate how you would evaluate the tension of the bandage.
- Describe how you would evaluate a wound at the time a dressing is changed.
- Perform girth measurements of an individual's upper and lower extremities.
- Demonstrate how to measure a person for a graded compression garment for the upper extremity.
- Describe six gravity-assisted positions for postural drainage of the lungs.
- Identify the postoperative goals for a transtibial lower extremity amputation.

problem SOLVING

1. You have been asked to give chest physical therapy to a patient who has a chest tube in the right lower lobe. What precautions would you take, and what postural drainage positions would you avoid?

2. You are treating a patient with a vasopneumatic compression device on the right upper extremity. After 10 minutes, the patient reports numbness in the right hand. What would you do to alleviate this symptom, and what precautions would you take to avoid this situation in the future?

3. You are asked to develop a plan and start a program to prevent the development of pressure ulcers in elderly patients, especially those who have limited mobility. What would you include in your plan, and how and with whom would you initiate this program?

4. If you were able to treat the patient in the case study for this chapter on the Evolve site for this text just after he was burned, what type of exercise regime and positioning would you use? Would there have been any possible contraindications to mobilization, and if so, what would they be?

CHAPTER 12

Incidents and Emergencies

objectives *After studying this chapter, the reader will be able to:*

- Explain basic, immediate, and initial treatment for selected types of patient injury or acute illnesses.
- Describe precautions to improve safety and reduce patient and employee injury in the treatment setting.
- Differentiate between heat exhaustion and heat stroke through the observation of signs and symptoms and apply appropriate treatment.
- Differentiate between an insulin reaction and acidosis through the observation of signs and symptoms and apply appropriate treatment.
- Differentiate between autonomic hyperreflexia and postural (orthostatic) hypotension through the observation and measurement of various signs and symptoms and apply appropriate treatment.
- Identify the signs and symptoms of choking and apply the Heimlich maneuver.
- Analyze patient care activities and determine the need to modify, reduce, or discontinue treatment.
- Describe at least five ways to maintain personal and patient safety.
- Identify factors to maintain a safe treatment environment.
- Describe adult cardiopulmonary resuscitation and the American Heart Association 2010 guideline changes.

key terms

Acidosis   A pathological condition resulting from the accumulation of acid or the depletion of the alkaline reserve in the blood and body tissues that is characterized by an increase in hydrogen ion concentration.

Allergen   A protein or nonprotein substance that is capable of inducing an allergy or a specific hypersensitivity.

Autonomic hyperreflexia (dysreflexia)   An uninhibited and exaggerated reflex of the autonomic nervous system as a result of a stimulus.

Cardiac arrest/death   The sudden and often unexpected stoppage of effective heart action.

Cardiopulmonary resuscitation (CPR)   The reestablishment of heart and lung action as indicated for cardiac arrest.

Convulsion   A series of involuntary contractions of the voluntary muscles.

Emergency medical technician (EMT)   A person trained to manage the emergency care of sick or injured persons during transport to a hospital or at the scene of an injury.

Hyperglycemia   An excess of glucose in the blood.

Hypoglycemia   An abnormally low level of sugar (glucose) in the blood.

Insulin   A double-chain protein hormone formed from proinsulin in the beta cells of the pancreatic islets of Langerhans.

Intubation   The insertion of a tube, as into the larynx, to maintain an open airway.

Laceration   A wound produced by the tearing of body tissue, as distinguished from a cut or an incision.

Orthostatic (postural) hypotension   A fall in blood pressure associated with dizziness, syncope, and blurred vision that occurs upon standing or when standing motionless in a fixed position.

Seizure   A convulsion or attack, as in epilepsy.

Shock   Acute peripheral circulatory failure caused by derangement of circulatory control or loss of circulating fluid.

Sternum   A plate of bone forming the middle of the anterior wall of the thorax; the breastbone.

Vasoconstriction   A decrease in the caliber of blood vessels.

INTRODUCTION

All persons who work in patient care areas have the responsibility to provide and maintain a safe environment for patient care. In freestanding service units or in a patient's home, caregivers and employees should be qualified to provide immediate emergency care. Hospital caregivers and employees should be aware of and follow departmental or institutional policies and procedures regarding emergency situations. Employees should know how to contact emergency personnel and request assistance (e.g., they should know how to use 911 or local fire, emergency medical, or police telephone numbers and should understand special emergency terms such as "code blue," "code red," and "code orange"). In addition, caregivers should observe each patient to determine whether he or she wears a medical alert bracelet or necklace. These items inform others of a patient's special conditions or needs (e.g., allergies, implants, a pacemaker, diabetes, or medication requirements).

An emergency (crash) cart is a mobile unit that contains emergency supplies such as medications, dressings and bandages, a manual resuscitation device, and intravenous infusion items (Fig. 12-1). This cart is often available in the treatment area. The contents are protected from unwarranted use by a temporary lock or seal. However, the exterior contents should be inspected daily to ensure that the defibrillator is charged properly and to determine that other equipment on the cart is ready for use. The drugs contained in the cart should be checked periodically for expiration dates, and the time and date of the check should be recorded.

All caregivers should be informed of their required legal responsibilities and limitations in providing emergency aid, especially as they relate to the "Good Samaritan" statutes of the state in which they work. In some states, an employee may be more liable when emergency care is provided by the employee in a hospital or other similar setting where medical equipment or support personnel are available. In most states, some legal protection is provided for persons who cause additional injury or trauma when emergency care is provided, particularly if the action was a lifesaving or life-sustaining measure. A review of specific professional practice acts and other state statutes may be necessary to determine one's emergency care responsibility in that state.

It should be recognized that the potential for patient and employee injuries becomes greater under certain conditions. Some examples are when too few personnel are available to manage the patients in the area, too few qualified personnel are available, personnel are excessively busy, personnel are inattentive to patient needs, equipment is poorly maintained or defective, personnel are inadequately trained, and personnel display careless behavior. The supervisor and all employees should be especially alert when personnel changes occur. Examples of such personnel changes include shift changes, times when some personnel are on vacation or ill and inexperienced workers or no replacement personnel are provided, during a holiday or weekend when fewer personnel are likely to be available, and when several acutely ill patients are being treated simultaneously.

The following patients may need close attention and care by the service unit personnel: older adults; debilitated persons; persons with decreased mental competence or cognitive deterioration; persons whose physiological status has been compromised as a result of extensive burns, a spinal cord injury, a chronic respiratory condition, an acute or chronic cardiac condition, or acute or chronic diabetes; psychologically or emotionally disturbed individuals; the

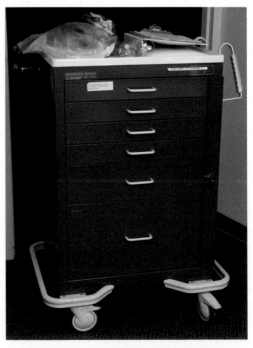

Fig. 12-1   An emergency (crash) cart.

very young; febrile patients; and patients who have been injured or involved in an unusual incident during a previous hospitalization or treatment program.

Caregivers should be aware of and be prepared to respond to an improper referral or prescription by discussing the issue with the referral source before initiating treatment. In many states a physical therapist is able to perform a physical therapy diagnosis and treat a patient without a referral or prescription (i.e., the physical therapist has direct access to the patient). It is the responsibility of the therapist to know and comply with state statutes regarding communications with a physician pertaining to the patient's response to treatment or progress as a result of the treatment provided. In addition, the therapist is responsible for recognizing when the patient's condition warrants referral to another practitioner or when the therapist lacks the competence to treat the individual. In all situations of patient care, the therapist must function within the scope of practice as defined by statutory language. It may be necessary to delay treatment until any concerns or problems with a referral have been resolved.

Precautions or contraindications associated with various treatments should be recognized and applied judiciously to reduce the incidence of injury or trauma to the patient or caregiver. In addition, the caregiver should understand and be aware of potential problems that may develop in a patient as a result of the primary diagnosis, and additional care should be used when treating patients who have a serious illness or have sustained extensive trauma. Supportive personnel should be supervised and guided to ensure that they are not asked or expected to perform any treatment activities beyond their education, training, skill, and competence.

Treatment programs or sessions may need to be modified, reduced, or terminated in response to the observed or reported changes in a patient's condition. A patient who convulses without a known cause, experiences incontinence of the bowel or bladder without a known cause, loses consciousness without a known cause, or exhibits new or different symptoms from those observed previously should be evaluated carefully before treatment is continued.

When a patient exhibits signs or symptoms of an acute illness or appears to be experiencing an adverse response to treatment (e.g., unusual vital signs, vertigo, syncope, nausea, or vomiting), the treatment should be terminated temporarily and the patient should be reevaluated by a physician before being treated again. Nursing staff, other medical personnel, and the patient's family should be informed of changes in the patient's condition. In addition, appropriate documentation must reflect the change.

Caregivers should inform mentally competent patients about the intent, anticipated or desired outcome, and potential risks associated with the planned treatment. All patients should have the opportunity to participate in the process of informed consent, presented in Chapter 1, before receiving treatment, and their autonomy regarding the

decision about whether to receive treatment should be respected. The patient should be given the opportunity to ask questions or seek additional information about the treatment. If the treatment is refused, the decision should be accepted, and nursing and other medical personnel should be notified. The caregiver may find it helpful or necessary to confer with a physician, nurse, or other practitioner who is involved in the care of the patient to assist with the resolution of a dilemma related to a patient's lack of consent. The decision should be documented in the patient's medical record by the caregiver.

Injuries or trauma that may be sustained by a patient who receives treatment include burns, lacerations, muscle strains, ligamentous sprains, heat stress, hematomas, fractures, respiratory distress, and cardiovascular distress.

The physical environment in which the patient is treated and the equipment used to treat patients should be maintained to meet the standards established by various agencies. These agencies include the Occupational Safety and Health Administration, The Joint Commission, the Department of Public Health, the Commission on Accreditation of Rehabilitation Facilities, the Comprehensive Out-patient Rehabilitation Facility, and the National Institute of Occupational Safety and Health. The policies and procedures established by the hospital or treatment facility also should be followed.

PRINCIPLES AND CONCEPTS

Health care providers must be aware of the need to maintain a safe environment for treatment. The service unit director or department manager is responsible for developing safety education and awareness programs for all of the employees in the department. Staff meetings and orientation programs regarding environmental, employee, and patient safety should be developed, implemented, and repeated periodically. General guidelines to reduce and avoid patient or employee injury should be included in the unit's policy/procedures or safety manual. Employees should be required to read this material periodically, and their comprehension of this material should be evaluated. Failure to provide information and training sessions on safety could create increased organizational or personnel liability and reduce the level of the quality of care.

Written policies and procedures should identify and explain the following elements:

- Patient scheduling patterns, the least acceptable ratio of personnel to patients, and what is to be done when unacceptable ratios occur
- The maintenance and monitoring of records such as referrals, patient status documentation (i.e., progress reports), treatment protocols, and incident reports
- Plans for the evacuation and care of patients and the expected function of all personnel at the time of an emergency, such as a fire or other disaster
- First-aid or immediate emergency care plans

- Restriction or access of visitors to the treatment areas
- Security measures for patient and employee valuables and procedures for items that are lost or found
- The establishment of equipment inspection, repair, and maintenance records
- The process and procedures for general infection control and handling of toxic materials (i.e., the Medical Safety Data Sheet manual)
- The application and use of protective clothing, handling of body fluids, management of patients who are placed in isolation, and changing the dressings of infected wounds
- Employee job duties, descriptions, and responsibilities
- Supervisory relationships, lines of communication, a table of organization, the span of control, and the chain of command of the facility and the service area

The physical environment and equipment should be prepared, inspected, and maintained to ensure the following conditions:

- Proper levels of ventilation, temperature, humidity, light, and noise
- Routine janitorial and housekeeping services
- Equipment functions according to the manufacturer's standards
- Structural hazards are minimized or eliminated
- Equipment is properly attached or fixed to structurally sound areas (i.e., it should be attached to wall studs, bolted to the floor, or attached to ceiling joists or rafters)
- Equipment and supplies not in use are stored, line cords and electrical outlets are protected by a built-in ground (i.e., they are ground fault interrupted), and wheels on movable equipment have locks
- Emergency exits and evacuation routes are clearly marked and displayed for patients, visitors, and employees
- Emergency equipment (e.g., fire extinguishers or hoses, first aid kits, intubation airways, and an automated external defibrillator) is available, accessible, and ready for use
- A metabolic cart or "crash cart" is available with its components clearly marked and ready to use; drugs are not expired
- Floor surfaces are clean and dry, and loose or torn carpeting and other similar hazards (e.g., line cords on the floor) are eliminated

Safety related to patient care is the responsibility of the service unit personnel. It is imperative that all personnel understand and comply with safe personal and patient care practices. Regardless of the goal of treatment, the primary responsibility of any practitioner is to "do no harm" to the patient.

Employee injuries are frequently associated with activities that require lifting, carrying, pushing, pulling, and reaching. The development, use, and application of proper body mechanics are presented in Chapter 4. It may be helpful to review that information for suggestions to prevent injury to yourself and to the patient. You should always be alert to the possibility that patient injury can occur, and you should anticipate that unusual events might occur (i.e., "expect the unexpected"). The supervisor or department manager has several specific responsibilities, as listed in Box 12-1.

Prevention is an important aspect of patient and employee safety. Care should be taken during an assisted transfer, lifting activities, ambulation activities, and when using equipment. Certain patient conditions, such as wound management, require special attention to avoid infection of the wound and cross contamination of other persons. Personal cleanliness in the form of proper hand washing or use

---

Box 12-1 Responsibilities of Managers/Directors

- Be certain that each employee is qualified and competent for all assigned duties and responsibilities. The manager should observe and evaluate each employee's performance at least once a year.
- Be certain that each employee understands the duties, responsibilities, and expectations of the job. This understanding can be ascertained during the orientation of a new employee, at staff meetings, and at performance evaluation sessions.
- Develop and implement an ongoing safety training and awareness program for unit personnel.
- Instruct and teach personnel how to establish appropriate professional interpersonal relations with each patient. Each patient must receive individualized care and should be considered as an entire person rather than as a patient with a specific impairment.
- Instruct and teach personnel how to obtain informed consent from each patient before initiating or extensively altering treatment.
- Instruct personnel to explain all treatment procedures to each patient and to monitor, guide, instruct, or direct the patient during treatment.
- Instruct personnel to refer the patient to another caregiver when they do not have the appropriate skills or are not competent to treat the patient.
- Instruct personnel to contact the referral source to clarify a referral or prescription that is considered to be inaccurate or incomplete or that contains a contraindicated procedure before initiating treatment.
- Instruct personnel to clarify any referral or prescription if they are unsure of its intent or expected outcome before initiating treatment. A verbal referral or prescription should be transferred to written form within 24 hours of its receipt, and the written form must be signed by the person who originally provided it.
- Be certain that personnel report malfunctioning equipment or other forms of breaches of safety are corrected promptly.

of hand rubs before and after each patient treatment, after eating, and after toileting is essential for successful infection control. The best way to maintain your personal safety is through the use of proper body mechanics, proper personal hygiene, familiarity with the operation of equipment, familiarity with the methods of infection control, and by performing the safety techniques or procedures for which you have been educated and trained.

An injury to a patient can occur even though safety measures are applied diligently and consistently. However, an injury is less likely to occur when safe practices are used. The primary caregiver of the patient who sustains an injury should follow the steps provided in Procedure 12-1. These procedures may vary slightly from facility to facility, but they are necessary to protect the employee, facility, and patient.

Each employee must be aware of the need for the consistent application of preventive measures to maintain a safe environment and the safe care of each patient. The

---

PROCEDURE 12-1

Responses to Patient Injuries

- Immediately provide or obtain emergency care for the patient according to established organizational policies and procedures and the competence of the caregiver. Do not leave the patient unattended (except to summon assistance), but attempt to prevent any further injury and act to stabilize the patient's physiological status. When it is apparent that assistance from trained personnel (e.g., emergency medical technicians, a rapid response team, a trauma team, or a cardiopulmonary resuscitation team) is needed, they should be contacted before on-the-scene emergency care is initiated in order to reduce response time. If two or more persons are at the scene, one person should contact the support team while the other begins to provide emergency care.
- After the emergency phase is concluded, document the incident with objective and factual information. Indicate the type of emergency care that was provided and by whom. List the persons who witnessed or observed the incident, who was notified about the incident, the time the incident occurred, and any events leading up to the incident. Do not confer with the patient or relatives about the incident, and do not express information to anyone that would indicate you were negligent or at fault.
- Notify your immediate superior, the department manager/director, or the risk manager of the incident.
- File an incident report with the appropriate person within the organization; it may be necessary to document the incident in the patient's medical record.
- Notify the insurance carrier of the incident (in a large facility, this notification may be performed by the risk manager).

---

employee's thoughts and behavior should be directed to promote safety for the patient, visitors, other employees, and himself or herself. Each employee should be prepared to react to emergency situations quickly, decisively, and calmly. Any emergency or first aid treatment provided by departmental personnel should be performed according to institutional policies and procedures and the training of the employee. All such incidents should be documented completely after the incident. Institutional and community agency emergency telephone numbers should be posted by each telephone, and employees must use these numbers when assistance is required or desired.

EMERGENCY CARE

Although the role of the caregiver may be to provide immediate initial aid, the caregiver should make an effort to obtain immediate assistance from the most qualified individual available, such as a physician, a nurse, an emergency medical technician, a rapid response team, or other medical personnel. Obtaining such assistance in the hospital may be relatively easy, and trained personnel who will react quickly when called are likely to be readily available. However, in the patient's home, outpatient clinic, a school, an athletic facility, or even an extended care facility, assistance may be difficult to obtain and may require time. The caregiver should be aware of sources of assistance within the setting and external to the setting, and the most appropriate source should be contacted promptly. Judgment on the part of the caregiver will be required to determine whether assistance should be obtained before or after initiating emergency care or first aid. (In most situations, it is best if assistance is requested before emergency care is initiated unless the delay of immediate aid is life-threatening to the patient [e.g., in the case of excessive arterial bleeding].) Any care that has been provided before assistance arrives will need to be described to the persons who provide additional care, including objective information about the patient's condition and previous events associated with the incident.

SUPPORT DEVICES

A bandage, adhesive tape, or an external support (orthosis) may be used when an emergency situation occurs and some form of support or control for the area is needed. In general, these items can be used to stabilize a segment, restrict motion of a joint, or control edema or joint effusion. An orthosis (e.g., a splint) provides the greatest amount of control but may not be as available as adhesive tape or a bandage. The most common injury that would require use of a bandage for any of these purposes is a sprain or strain. Examples of bandage materials are shown in Fig. 12-2.

Bandage Materials

Materials often used for a bandage are muslin (i.e., nonelastic unbleached cotton), woven elastic porous cotton (i.e., an Ace bandage), rolled gauze, a stockinette (i.e., a tube formed of loosely knit cotton), low-stretch bandages (e.g., Comprilan, Rosidal K, and KompriBAND), and adhesive tape. Low-stretch bandages offer more support than Ace bandages and are usually used for edema control. An elastic bandage can be used multiple times until the elasticity is lost; it should then be discarded. An elastic bandage can be washed with soap in warm water and dried while lying on a flat surface on an absorbent towel. (The bandage will stretch excessively if it is dried while hanging, as from a clothesline.) Once it is dry, the bandage should be rolled so it is ready for use. An elastic bandage provides limited support and protection to a joint but can be an effective temporary method to control or reduce edema. This type of bandage usually is available in widths of 2, 3, 4, and 6 inches.

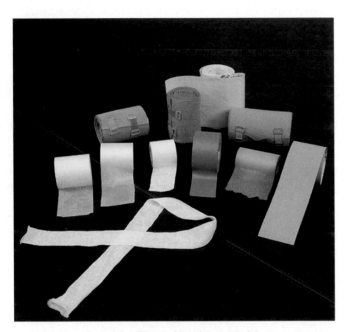

Fig. 12-2 Types of bandage materials.

Adhesive or athletic tape is used when more support or protection of a joint is needed than can be provided by any of the bandage material(s) described previously. A common use for this tape is for first- and second-degree sprains of the ankle when an air cast or gel-filled splint is not available. This tape also is used as a preventive bandage for athletes to reduce the possibility of a sprain to various joints, especially the ankle and knee. The usual width of the tape is 1.5 to 2 inches. The tape may be rigid or have some capacity to "stretch" and usually requires an underwrap to protect the skin.

Types of Bandages

Triangular A triangular bandage is a large piece of cloth cut or formed into a triangle (e.g., a square piece of cloth folded diagonally becomes a triangle). It is most often used as a temporary sling to support the weight of a patient's upper extremity. When it is used for this purpose, the cloth triangle must be large enough to contain the patient's forearm and hand. To apply the sling, use the following procedure:

- Flex the elbow of the injured extremity to slightly more than 90 degrees with the palm facing the chest.
- Place the apex of the sling at the elbow, and bring the outer end over the forearm and shoulder of the injured upper extremity (Fig. 12-3, A).
- Bring the other end of the sling under the forearm and over the shoulder of the uninjured upper extremity (Fig. 12-3, B).
- Tie the ends in a square knot positioned to one side of the spinous processes of the patient's neck.
- Have the patient relax the shoulder, and be certain the sling trough supports the forearm and hand.
- Pull the free apex end of the sling over the elbow, and pin or tape it to the front of the sling; the hand and forearm should be horizontal or elevated slightly above horizontal (Fig. 12-3, C).

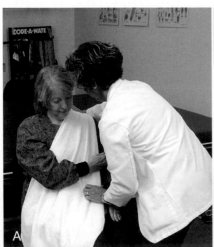
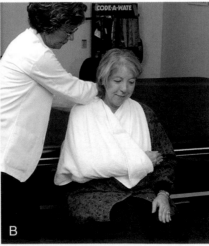
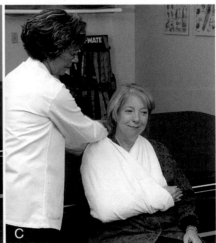

Fig. 12-3 Application of a triangular bandage.

Cravat A cravat also can be used to support the upper extremity, but it will not support the patient's upper extremity as well as a triangular sling.

- To form the cravat, fold a square or rectangular cloth into a series of overlapping layers to the width desired. A belt, necktie, or scarf can be used to form a cravat.
- Loop the cravat over the forearm of the injured upper extremity.
- Tie the two free ends behind and to one side of the patient's neck using a square knot, or if a belt is used, use the belt buckle to make the loose ends secure.

Ankle Wrap An ankle wrap can be used to support and contain swelling of the ankle after a sprain has occurred. An elastic bandage (such as an Ace wrap), a low-stretch bandage, or adhesive tape can be used. The foot should be wrapped while in dorsiflexion and either eversion or inversion, depending on which ligaments have been sprained. The forefoot should be wrapped in a circular pattern with "figure of eights" around the ankle and back to a circular pattern above the ankle (Fig. 12-4).

Protective Splints, Sleeves, or Slings Some patients may find it necessary to use a splint, sleeve, or sling to immobilize, stabilize, and protect a joint or extremity or to control edema. Fig. 12-5 shows an adjustable sling. The joints affected most frequently are the elbow, wrist, thumb, knee, and ankle. When the knee is involved, a knee immobilizer orthosis is often used. Fig. 12-6 depicts the application of a knee immobilizer orthosis. (Note: The knee immobilizer is usually donned in the long sitting or sitting position if the patient is not full weight bearing). Ambulation while wearing a knee immobilizer may require that the patient elevate the hip of the lower extremity with the immobilizer or plantar flex the opposite foot so the foot clears the floor and allows the leg to complete the swing phase. Stairs and steps must be managed one step at a time.

Other examples of protective devices are presented in Fig. 12-7. Some of these items are available over the counter at a drugstore, pharmacy, sporting goods store, or department store, whereas others must be custom-fabricated and fit for the individual. Uses vary and include protection during athletic competition, prevention of contractures, or immobilization of a joint during the healing of an injury. (Note: Ambulation while wearing a protective boot (see Fig. 12-7, *E*) may result in discomfort in the person's contralateral hip and lower back because the thick sole of the boot creates a leg length discrepancy of the two lower

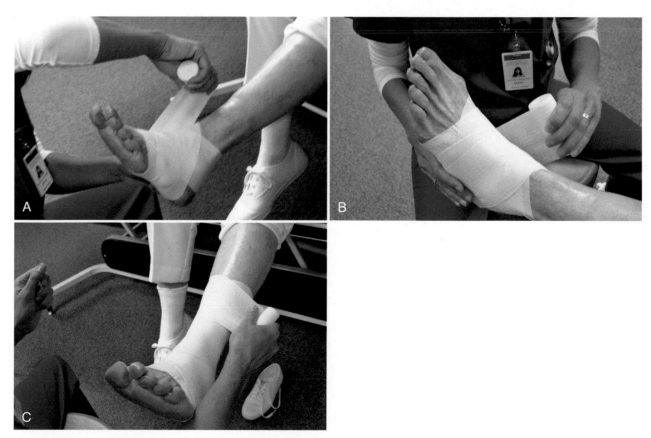

Fig. 12-4   An ankle wrap. **A** and **B,** The forefoot is wrapped in a circular pattern, and the ankle is wrapped in a figure of eight pattern. The foot should be in dorsiflexion during the wrap. **C,** The area above the ankle is wrapped in a nonocclusive circular pattern and secured with tape or a bandage clasp.

extremities. This discrepancy causes abnormal stress to the opposite hip and lumbar structures.)

EMERGENCY CARE FOR SPECIFIC CONDITIONS

When an injury or change in the patient's condition requires first aid or emergency care, you should be aware of some of

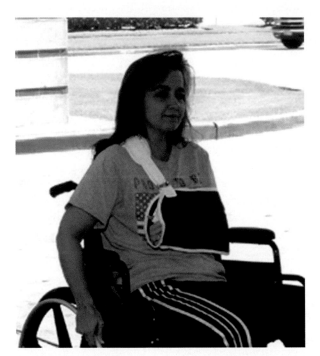

Fig. 12-5 An adjustable sling designed to support the forearm and shoulder.

the emergency aid that can be provided. The best way to be prepared to provide emergency care is to participate in an educational program or course provided by a qualified instructor or agency.

Allergic Reactions

An allergic reaction occurs when one's immune system overreacts to a specific substance, known as an allergen. A person may demonstrate sensitivity to an allergen when exposed to pollen; dust; various foods such as eggs, shellfish, milk, wheat, soy, and nuts (especially peanuts); insect stings; chemicals (e.g., dyes, cleansers, and pesticides); or medications, especially antibiotics. A caregiver may experience a reaction to the latex in gloves or the chemicals in hand cleansers. A patient may experience similar reactions to these items and also may exhibit an allergic reaction to specific medications or dyes used in some imaging procedures.

You should differentiate between an allergic reaction and an adverse effect of a medication. An allergic reaction can be identified when one or more of the signs or symptoms listed in Box 12-2 appear. An adverse effect is a consequence other than the one for which the medication was intended and which frequently has an adverse effect on another organ. Some examples of adverse effects are nausea, muscle ache, vomiting, visual disturbance, drowsiness, abdominal discomfort, intestinal cramping, diarrhea, and headache. When any of these adverse effects severely affect the person's physical, cognitive, or emotional status, the prescribing physician should be contacted.

Allergic reactions can be classified as mild, moderate, or severe. In most instances, a person with a mild or moderate

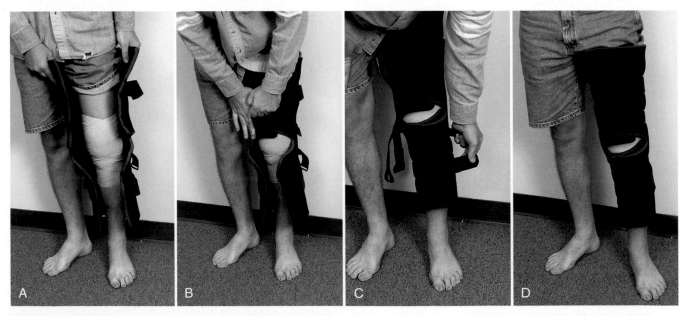

Fig. 12-6 Application of a knee immobilizer while standing. (Note: This person is weight bearing as tolerated and as such prefers to apply his knee immobilizer while standing. Most people apply it in a sitting position.)

| Box **12-2** | Signs and Symptoms of an Allergic Reaction |

MILD/MODERATE REACTION	**SEVERE REACTION**
Itchy skin	Swelling of the face or mouth
Skin redness, rash, areas of swelling	Difficulty swallowing, speaking
Itchy, watery eyes	Wheezing, difficulty breathing
Sneezing	Abdominal pain, nausea, vomiting
Hives at several body sites	Dizziness or syncope

reaction exhibits several signs and symptoms that usually are not life threatening (see Box 12-2). However, a severe reaction can be life threatening and requires prompt medical attention. When an allergen attacks the immune system, an excessive amount of histamine is released into the body. Therefore an initial treatment is the use of an antihistamine (e.g., diphenhydramine), which is contained in many over-the-counter medications used to control nasal and sinus congestion. The antihistamine may be administered orally, or in the case of moderate or severe reactions, it may be infused. Follow-up treatment may include a regimen of an oral corticosteroid (e.g., prednisone) until the symptoms diminish. Topical anti-itch medications usually are of little value in these situations; however, the application of calamine lotion or cool compresses may reduce the itching sensation temporarily. First-aid procedures for allergic reactions are presented in Procedure 12-2. The caregiver and patient should be aware of the signs and symptoms of a severe reaction, such as difficulty swallowing or breathing, and obtain immediate medical attention.

When treating a person with an allergic reaction, the objectives are to identify and reduce or remove the cause of the allergy, if possible, and to prevent or reduce the extent of the allergic reaction.

Lacerations

When treating a person with a laceration, the objectives are to prevent contamination of the wound and control the bleeding. Treatment for a laceration is described in Procedure 12-3.

Shock

When treating a person who is in shock, the objectives are to identify and reduce or remove the cause, when possible, and to prevent or reduce the extent of the physiological state of shock. Signs and symptoms of shock include pale, moist, cool skin; shallow and irregular breathing; dilated pupils; a weak, rapid pulse; diaphoresis; dizziness or nausea; and syncope. Treatment is described in Procedure 12-4.

PROCEDURE **12-2**

Initial Treatment for an Allergic Reaction

MILD/MODERATE REACTION
- Calm and reassure the person.
- Identify the allergen and help the person avoid further contact with it or remove it (in the case of an insect stinger).
- Apply cool compresses or calamine to itchy areas.
- Observe the person for signs/symptoms of increased distress.
- Obtain medical assistance or refer the person for such assistance.

SEVERE REACTION
- Check the person's airway; if it is compromised, seek medical assistance and begin rescue breathing and cardiopulmonary resuscitation.
- Calm and reassure the person.
- Help the person ingest or inject emergency allergy medication if it is available; do not use an oral medication if the person has breathing difficulty.
- Position the person to prevent shock.

PROCEDURE **12-3**

Initial Treatment of Lacerations

- Wash your hands, apply protective gloves, and apply a clean or sterile, nonabsorbent towel or similar object to the wound. Continue to wear protective gloves during the treatment of the wound. Obtain additional assistance and contact emergency services personnel as necessary.
- If the blood flow is excessive, elevate the wound above the level of the heart to reduce blood flow to the area.
- In some instances, the wound can be cleansed with an antiseptic or by rinsing it with water.
- Place a clean towel or sterile dressing over the wound, and apply direct pressure to a bleeding wound.
- Encourage the patient to remain quiet and to avoid using the extremity.
- If arterial bleeding occurs (demonstrated by spurting blood), it may be necessary to apply intermittent, direct pressure to the artery above the level of the wound or directly over the wound. Such pressure is applied most frequently to the brachial and femoral arteries to restrict blood flow to the distal wound site. However, prolonged pressure with the use of a tourniquet should be avoided. The person should be transported to a site where appropriate medical care can be provided unless assistance can be brought to the patient.

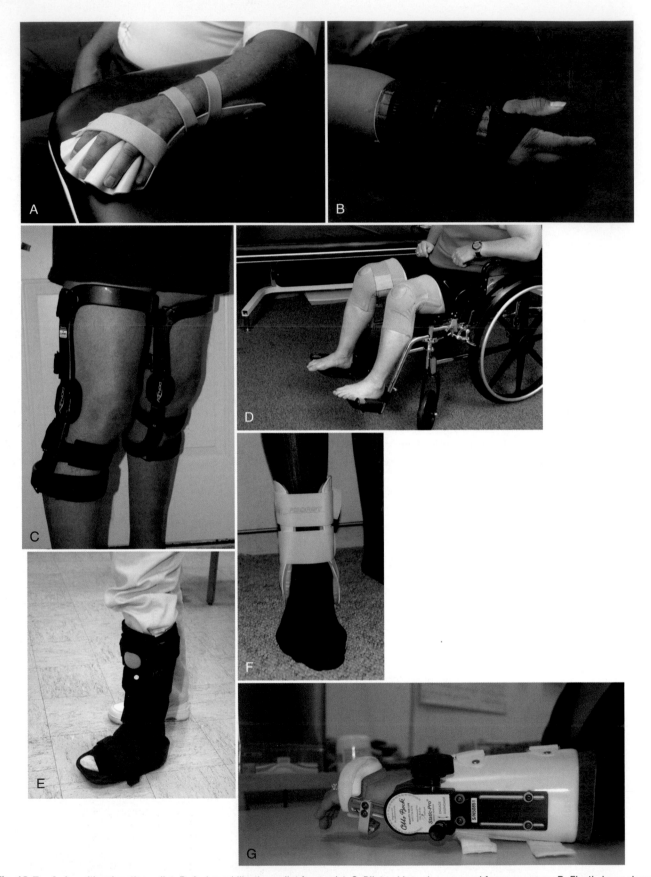

Fig. 12-7 **A,** A positional resting splint. **B,** An immobilization splint for a wrist. **C,** Bilateral knee braces used for genu varum. **D,** Elastic knee sleeves. **E,** An immobilization splint ("rocker boot") for the ankle. **F,** A gel-filled ankle splint. **G,** A dynamic wrist orthosis splint.

PROCEDURE 12-4

Initial Treatment of Shock

- Determine the cause of the shock (e.g., excessive bleeding, the inability to adjust to moving from a supine to a sitting or standing position, or a response to excessive heat), and remedy it if possible. Monitor the person's blood pressure and pulse rate. Obtain additional assistance and contact emergency support personnel as necessary.
- Place the person in a supine position with the head slightly lower than the lower extremities. If head and chest injuries are present or if respiration is impaired, it may be necessary to place the person supine with the body flat or with the head and chest elevated slightly. If bleeding is the apparent cause of the shock and the wound is visible, attempt to control the bleeding as described for a laceration.
- A cool compress may be applied to the person's forehead for comfort, and a light blanket may be used to prevent loss of body heat.
- Have the person remain quiet and avoid exertion.
- After the symptoms have been relieved, gradually return the person to an upright position and monitor him or her to ensure regression of the condition.
- Request transportation so the patient can be taken to a facility where proper care and treatment can be provided.

Orthostatic (Postural) Hypotension

Some patients may experience orthostatic (postural) hypotension. Usually this condition is accompanied by signs and symptoms similar to those described for shock. Orthostatic hypotension occurs most frequently when the person attempts to stand rapidly from a stooped, kneeling, recumbent, or sitting position. Older adults, persons who use anti-hypertension medication, persons with a decreased ability to return venous blood from the periphery to the heart (e.g., patients with spinal cord injury), persons with hypotension, and persons who have been immobilized in a recumbent position for an extended period are most likely to demonstrate orthostatic hypotension. The reduced venous return from the lower extremities results in decreased filling of the left ventricle, which leads to decreased cardiac output and, eventually, decreased cerebral perfusion. As a result, the person experiences dizziness and possibly syncope when rising to stand.

The initial measures used to resolve hypotension are the same as those listed in Procedure 12-4. Some measures that can be taken to prevent this condition are to wrap the patient's lower extremities from the feet to the groin with elastic bandages; apply an abdominal binder or corset; apply elastic hose (half or full length); instruct the patient to perform active ankle dorsiflexion-plantar flexion exercises ("ankle pumps") and alternate knee-to-chest exercises

frequently while supine or sitting; allow the patient to accommodate to the upright position gradually by slowly elevating the head of the bed to various levels; or use a tilt table to elevate the patient by increments.

In a severe case, it may be necessary to apply a full-body pressurized garment (i.e., a G suit) to stabilize the patient's venous circulation. The abdominal binder, elastic lower extremity wraps, elastic hose, and G suit provide external pressure to the veins of the extremities and trunk, which helps return venous blood to the heart and reduces the pooling or collection of venous blood in the lower extremities and abdomen. The active use of the lower extremity muscles will assist in "pumping" or moving the blood. The gradual elevation of the patient from a recumbent to a sitting or standing position allows the vascular system to accommodate physiologically to the changes in position.

Falls

Falls are common occurrences in the daily lives of many adults and children. Some falls result from risk-related occupations or activities or sports, whereas other falls occur because of carelessness, ill health, or the process of aging. Prevention of falls is an important component of patient safety, and one of the National Patient Safety Goals of The Joint Commission is to "Reduce the risk of patient harm resulting from falls." Some attention is being given to informing and teaching older adults how to prevent or at least reduce the possibility of falling, but more education is needed. Some of the human and environmental factors related to falls are presented in Box 12-3. A conscientious caregiver will offer suggestions and instruct patients how to prevent a fall and how to protect themselves if a fall occurs. This instruction is especially important for persons who use ambulation aids, who are older, who have decreased proprioception or balance, or who are visually impaired. The Tinetti Assessment for balance and gait, the Berg Balance test, the Timed Up and Go Test, the Timed One-Legged Standing Test, and Czuka's Sit-to-Stand Test are a few tools that can assist in testing a patient for risk of falls.

Fractures

When treating a person with a fracture, the objectives are to protect the fracture site and avoid further injury to it, prevent shock, reduce pain, and prevent wound contamination if the bone ends have penetrated the skin. Emergency care should not include any attempt to align the fracture segments or "set" the fracture. Treatment is described in Procedure 12-5.

Burns

When treating a person with a burn, the objectives are to prevent wound contamination, relieve or reduce pain, and prevent shock. Treatment is described in Procedure 12-6.

Box **12-3** Risk Factors Related to Falls

HUMAN FACTORS	ENVIRONMENTAL FACTORS
Persons older than 65 years	Uneven or irregular walking surface
Impaired vision or hearing	Doorway thresholds
Use of assistive devices for ambulation or support	Area rugs, throw rugs, scatter rugs
Decreased strength, flexibility, proprioception, balance, or coordination	Obstacles in the area (e.g., furniture, electrical cords, toys, or miscellaneous objects)
A previous history of falling	Insufficient lighting
Episodes of vertigo, seizures, or syncope	Wet, icy, snow covered, or waxed surfaces
Use of medications such as antihypertensives, sedatives, or pain modifiers	Steps, especially those with a tread that overhangs the riser
Inattentiveness while walking	Absence of nonskid strips or mat in the bathtub
	No handrail on either side of the stairs or steps
	Chairs with an unstable base or without armrests
	No handrails in the shower or bathtub

Convulsions/Seizures

When a person has a convulsion or seizure, the objectives are to protect the patient from injury should a fall or excessive involuntary movements of the extremities occur and to protect his or her modesty or privacy. Treatment is described in Procedure 12-7.

Choking

When a person is choking, the objectives are to restore and maintain a patent airway and normal breathing. Treatment is described in Procedure 12-8 and Fig. 12-8.

Heat-Related Illnesses

When treating a person with a heat-related illness, the objectives are to remove or reduce the cause of the illness and return the individual to a state of normal homeostasis.

The two primary forms of heat-related illness are heat exhaustion and heat stroke (Table 12-1). Of the two, heat exhaustion poses the least threat to life, whereas heat stroke is considered a medical emergency because it can be life threatening. Both illnesses can result from a hot, humid environment, vigorous physical activity, dehydration, and depleted body electrolytes. Persons who are treated with hydrotherapy and persons who participate in vigorous aerobic exercise in a warm, humid environment should be observed periodically for signs or symptoms of heat

PROCEDURE **12-5**

Initial Treatment of Fractures

- Obtain information about the injury from the patient if he or she is conscious (e.g., its cause, location, the extent of discomfort, and any restriction of motion). Obtain additional assistance and contact emergency services personnel as necessary.
- Observe the site of the injury or the position of the extremity; examine and evaluate the patient's general appearance and condition. Monitor the patient's blood pressure and pulse rate.
- Gently palpate the area and surrounding tissue to evaluate swelling or edema and tenderness. Deformity and soft-tissue bruising may indicate that a fracture has occurred.
- Avoid movement or activity that has the potential to cause additional damage to the site.
- Apply support to the site to stabilize it, but do not attempt to align the bone ends. Use a firm object to stabilize the fracture before transporting the patient. A pillow folded around the site, canes or crutches applied on either side of a lower extremity fracture, or a flat piece of wood applied to either side of the fracture site can be used. On small extremities, a large magazine can be wrapped around the site.
- Cover an open fracture site with a sterile towel or dressing, but do not attempt to reinsert the bone ends beneath the skin.
- If a spinal fracture is suspected, do not move the patient. Call 911 or the emergency response system if you are in an outpatient setting, or obtain immediate assistance from appropriate emergency personnel if you are working in an inpatient environment.

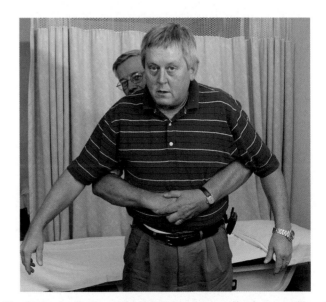

Fig. 12-8 Application of the Heimlich maneuver. Hands are positioned above the umbilicus and below the diaphragm, and pressure is exerted in and up.

PROCEDURE 12-6

Initial Treatment of Burns

- Remove or eliminate the agent causing the burn or remove the patient from the agent and contact skilled personnel when the burn wounds are extensive or involve the face, hands, perineum, or feet. Obtain additional assistance and contact emergency services personnel as necessary.
- Cut away or remove clothing near the site of the burn, but do not attempt to remove clothing that lies over or is part of the wound. Remove jewelry from the patient if edema has not developed and if the jewelry can be removed without causing additional trauma.
- A clean or sterile dressing or towel can be loosely laid over the wound. In some instances a moist dressing will be more comfortable for the patient. Do not apply any cream, salve, ointment, or a similar substance (such as butter or lard) to the wound, because these substances will mask the appearance of the wound and may lead to infection or a delay in healing.
- If the wound has been caused by a toxic chemical, use a copious amount of water to wash the wound site to dilute the substance. However, avoid washing the chemical onto an unaffected portion of the skin to prevent causing a burn to that area.
- Observe the patient for shock, respiratory distress, and other symptoms or injuries. Prepare the patient for transportation or transport to a facility that is prepared to manage this type of injury.

PROCEDURE 12-7

Initial Treatment of Seizures

- Place the person in a safe location and position; do not attempt to restrain or restrict the convulsions. Obtain additional assistance and contact emergency services personnel as necessary.
- Monitor the rate and quality of respiration. A period of tonic contraction of all body muscles may occur, which will cause respiration to cease for up to 50 to 70 seconds, after which respirations may be slower and deeper than normal for a brief period.
- Assist in keeping the patient's airway patent, but do not attempt to open the mouth by placing any object between the teeth. Never place your finger or a wooden or metal object in the patient's mouth, and do not attempt to grasp or position the tongue.
- When the convulsions subside, turn the person's head to one side in case vomiting occurs.
- Allow the patient to rest after the convulsions cease and protect his or her modesty and privacy. It may be helpful to cover the person with a blanket or screen him or her from view. Sphincter control may be lost during or at the conclusion of the seizure, resulting in the involuntary discharge of bladder or bowel contents.
- The patient should be evaluated by a physician to determine the cause of the seizure if the cause is not known.

Table 12-1	Signs and Symptoms of Heat-Related Illnesses	
Observations	**Heat Exhaustion**	**Heat Stroke**
Skin	Profuse diaphoresis	Dry; no diaphoresis
Nausea	Present	Present
Headache	Present	Present
Breathing	Shallow, rapid	Labored
Pulse	Weak, rapid	Strong, rapid
Color	Pale	Flushed or changes to gray
Temperature	Normal or slightly elevated	Very elevated (106° F-110° F)
Behavior	Exhaustion, collapse	Exhaustion, collapse, convulsions
Consciousness	Unconscious	Unconscious
Eyes	Pupils normal	Pupils contract, then dilate

exhaustion or heat stroke. Heat stroke may follow heat exhaustion if the person is not treated properly when the signs of heat exhaustion appear. Muscle cramps in the legs and abdomen may be the initial indicators of a heat-related illness. Rest, increased fluid intake, and gentle stretching

and massage to the affected areas are methods used to relieve these symptoms.

Heat Exhaustion When the signs and symptoms of heat exhaustion are observed, it is important to cool the person and counteract the effects of dehydration. Emergency initial treatment procedures are presented in Procedure 12-9. You may need to treat the person for shock, and you should be alert for signs or symptoms of heat stroke. The person should not be given salt tablets by mouth as part of the treatment, because the ingestion of excess salt may interfere with the person's ability to readjust the electrolyte balance to a normal state. Fluids containing selected electrolytes can be administered frequently to help the person compensate for the loss of electrolytes from excessive exercise.

Heat Stroke Heat stroke is life threatening, and its signs and symptoms must be recognized quickly so that emergency first-aid treatment can be initiated promptly. Emergency first-aid treatment procedures are presented in Procedure 12-10. A person with heat stroke will require care and treatment by qualified medical personnel and must be transported to a medical facility as quickly as possible.

Insulin-Related Illnesses

When treating a person with an insulin-related illness, the objectives are to restore him or her to a normal

PROCEDURE 12-8

Initial Treatment for Choking

When assisting a conscious adult or a child who is older than 1 year:
- Ask the person if he or she is choking. If the person can speak, cough, or breathe, do not attempt to provide further assistance but remain close by until it appears that he or she is no longer in distress.
- If the person is unable to speak, cough, or breathe, check his or her mouth and remove any visible foreign object.
- If the person cannot speak, cough, or breathe, position yourself behind him or her. Clasp your hands over the person's abdomen slightly above the umbilicus but below the diaphragm.
- Make a closed fist of one hand, and cover it by your other hand; give three or four forceful abrupt thrusts against the person's abdomen to forcefully compress the abdomen in and up (called the Heimlich maneuver; see Fig. 12-8). Continue to apply the thrusts until the obstruction becomes dislodged or is otherwise relieved or the person becomes unconscious.
- Obtain advanced medical assistance.

When assisting an unconscious adult or child who is older than 8 years:
- Place the person in a supine position and ask others to contact advanced medical assistance.
- Open the person's mouth and use your finger to attempt to locate and remove the foreign object (i.e., perform a finger sweep).
- Open the airway by tilting the head back and lifting the chin forward (i.e., a head tilt–chin lift) and attempt to provide ventilation using the mouth-to-mouth technique.
- If respiration does not occur, administer 6 to 10 subdiaphragmatic abdominal thrusts using the heel of one hand reinforced by the other hand (i.e., the Heimlich maneuver).
- If this approach is unsuccessful in initiating respiration, repeat the finger sweep, open the airway, attempt to provide ventilation, and perform the abdominal thrusts. Be persistent and continue these procedures until the object is removed or advanced medical assistance arrives. (Note: Avoid performing a blind finger sweep in children who are younger than 8 years. Instead, lift the

chin to expose the oral cavity and remove a foreign body if you see it.)
- After the object has been removed, it may be necessary to initiate cardiopulmonary resuscitation techniques to stabilize the person's cardiopulmonary functions.

When assisting a conscious infant (younger than 1 year):
- Support the head and neck with one hand and place the child in a prone position over your forearm, with the head lower than the trunk and your forearm supported on your thigh.
- Perform four gentle but forceful interscapular blows with the heel of your free hand.
- Immediately after applying the blows to the upper back, turn the infant supine with the head lower than the trunk, and perform four thrusts to the lower sternum with two fingers.
- Repeat the back blows and sternal thrusts until the object is expelled.

When assisting an unconscious infant:
- Place the infant supine and ask others to contact advanced medical assistance.
- Perform a tongue-jaw lift and remove any foreign object if it is visible.
- Open the airway using a slight head tilt–chin lift technique described previously and attempt to ventilate the infant.
- Perform four back blows and four sternal thrusts if respiration has not been started.
- If the foreign body has not been removed, repeat the sequence until the foreign object is extracted.
- If the foreign body has been removed and the infant is not breathing, initiate basic cardiopulmonary resuscitation techniques (i.e., open the airway, use mouth-to-mouth and nose ventilation, and perform chest compressions with two fingers to initiate a heart rate).

Note: All persons who have experienced a choking incident should be examined by a physician as soon as possible. This information is based on the recommendations of the American Heart Association (AHA). A pamphlet containing diagrams and this information can be obtained from most affiliate offices of the AHA.

---

insulin-glucose state and to remove, correct, or compensate for the cause of the condition.

It is important to differentiate between the conditions of hypoglycemia (i.e., hyperinsulinemia, or an insulin reaction) and hyperglycemia (i.e., acidosis), as outlined in Table 12-2. An insulin reaction can be caused by too much systemic insulin, too little food intake, or excessive exercise in relation to the metabolic state of the person. Acidosis can be caused by too little systemic insulin, the intake of too much food or improper food (i.e., excessive sugar), or insufficient physical activity in relation to the metabolic state of the person. Treatment should be scheduled accordingly.

Insulin Reaction (Hypoglycemia) If the person is conscious, have him or her ingest some form of sugar (e.g., candy or orange juice). If the person is unconscious, glucose may need to be provided intravenously. The person should rest, and all physical activity should be stopped. Hypoglycemia is not as serious as acidosis, but the person should be given the opportunity to return to a balanced metabolic state as quickly as possible. It may be necessary to provide counseling about how to balance food intake and exercise or how to monitor blood glucose levels and the insulin dosage regularly and with greater care.

PROCEDURE 12-9

Initial Treatment for Heat Exhaustion

- Place the person in a comfortable position in a shady or covered area or in a room that is well ventilated. Loosen or remove the person's outer clothing and monitor his or her vital signs. Obtain additional assistance and contact emergency service personnel as necessary.
- Sponge the person's forehead and neck with a cold compress or ice bag. Cool wet towels or sheets can be used to cool the person, and water or a solution containing electrolytes may be given by mouth if the person is conscious.
- Observe the person for shock or other physiological changes and treat the symptoms as appropriate. Vomiting, refusal of fluids, or loss of consciousness indicates that the condition is becoming worse.
- Request transportation so the person can be taken to a facility where proper care and treatment can be provided if no relief of signs and symptoms occurs within a short time or if further progression of the signs or symptoms occurs.

PROCEDURE 12-10

Initial Treatment for Heat Stroke

- Place the person in a semireclining position in a shady or well-ventilated covered area or room. Remove his or her outer clothing and monitor pulse and respiration rates. Obtain additional assistance and contact emergency services personnel immediately.
- Cool the person quickly with large amounts of cool or cold water or apply cold, wet compresses, towels, or sheets to the body. Ice bags can be applied to the wrists, ankles, each groin area, each axilla, and the lateral neck areas to cool the large blood vessels.
- Heat stroke is a life-threatening condition, and prompt emergency care must be provided. The person should be transported to a medical facility as quickly as possible.

Table 12-2   Warning Signs and Symptoms of Insulin-Related Illnesses

Observation	Insulin Reaction (Hypoglycemia)	Acidosis (Hyperglycemia)
Onset	Sudden	Gradual
Skin	Pale, moist	Flushed, dry
Behavior	Excited, agitated	Drowsy
Breath odor	Normal	Fruity odor
Breathing	Normal to shallow	Deep, labored
Vomiting	Absent	Present
Tongue	Moist	Dry
Hunger	Present	Absent
Thirst	Absent	Present
Glucose in urine	Absent or slight	Large amounts

PROCEDURE 12-11

Initial Treatment of Autonomic Hyperreflexia

- Initially place the person in a sitting or semirecumbent position to reduce the hypertension. Do not place the person in a supine position.
- If the noxious stimulus can be identified, it should be removed or relieved. Common stimuli are an occluded catheter, restricted straps or clothing, or a completely filled urine retention bag that prevents further drainage of urine from the bladder.
- Monitor the person's vital signs frequently, provide reassurance, and obtain qualified medical assistance.
- Be aware that this condition could occur at any time, and be prepared to assist the patient.

Acidosis (Hyperglycemia) Acidosis can lead to a diabetic coma, and death can occur if this state is allowed to persist. It should be considered a medical emergency that requires prompt action, including assistance from qualified personnel. The patient should not be given any form of sugar. Usually an injection of insulin is needed, and a nurse or physician should provide care as quickly as possible.

Autonomic Hyperreflexia (Dysreflexia)

When treating a person with autonomic hyperreflexia, the objectives are to determine and remove the noxious stimulus causing the condition and return the person to a level of normal homeostasis.

Autonomic hyperreflexia occurs in persons with a relatively recent complete injury to the cervical and upper thoracic portions of the spinal cord down to the T6 cord level. Signs and symptoms include severe hypertension, bradycardia, profuse diaphoresis above the level of the cord lesion, a pounding headache, a general feeling of discomfort, red skin blotches, and piloerection ("goose bumps"). The person may convulse, respiration may become difficult, and the person may become unconscious.

Various noxious stimuli below the level of the spinal cord lesion (e.g., bladder distention caused by urine retention, fecal impaction, open pressure ulcers, tight straps from an orthosis or urine retention bag, localized pressure, or exercise) may cause a massive sympathetic system response that cannot be controlled or counteracted by higher centers in the brain because of the location of the spinal cord injury. The result is uncontrolled, widespread peripheral arterial vasoconstriction, which causes severe hypertension. This condition should be considered a medical emergency, and a physician should be contacted for immediate assistance. Treatment is described in Procedure 12-11.

Cardiac Arrest/Death

When treating a person who is undergoing cardiac arrest, the objective is to maintain the cardiopulmonary system at a level sufficient to sustain life until the person can be transported to a medical facility.

All health care practitioners should be trained and certified to perform cardiopulmonary resuscitation (CPR). The information presented in this section is a summary of the CPR techniques developed by the American Heart Association (AHA) in 2010 for an adult undergoing cardiac arrest.

The AHA has changed the guidelines for the first time since their inception in 1962 and now instructs bystanders (those not trained in basic life support techniques) to compress the person's chest at a rate of 100 times per minute to a depth of 2 inches until paramedics arrive or the bystander is unable to continue compressions. Untrained lay rescuers are no longer advised to stop the compressions to administer breaths to a person undergoing cardiac arrest who is found out in the community. The AHA guidelines also have been revised in that the acronym A-B-C (Airway, Breathing, and Circulation) has been changed to C-A-B or Circulation (chest compressions), Airway, and Breathing for those trained in CPR.

The AHA guidelines state that persons with training in CPR should check to see if the patient is unconscious. If he or she doesn't respond and two people are available, one should seek qualified medical assistance by calling the 911 emergency telephone service or a community emergency medical technical support unit (e.g., an emergency medical service, local fire department, police department, or hospital) and locate an automated external defibrillator (AED) if possible. The other responder with training in CPR should immediately begin CPR with 30 chest compressions (which should take approximately 18 seconds) before checking the airway and giving two rescue breaths. Early recognition of a sudden cardiac arrest is based on responsiveness and abnormal breathing. Persons experiencing a cardiac arrest may present with no respirations, gasping respirations, or even what may appear to be a seizure.

If the responder is alone and trained and has immediate access to a phone, 911 should be called unless it is known that the victim has become unresponsive as a result of suffocation (i.e., drowning). In this case, CPR with compressions followed by two breaths should be provided first for 2 minutes before calling 911 or an emergency service (Procedure 12-12). If wireless communication is used (e.g., a cellular phone or a citizens' band [CB] radio), the exact location of the victim must be provided so that other rescuers can find the site. CPR should be administered until qualified medical personnel arrive, until the patient is revived and exhibits the ability to maintain vital signs independently, or until the initial rescuer is unable to continue providing support. CPR in itself usually is not sufficient to revive or maintain life for a person who experiences a sudden cardiac arrest/death ("heart attack"), but it is one link in a chain of events designed to provide the best opportunity for survival. The sequence of the chain of events is

---

PROCEDURE 12-12

Cardiopulmonary Resuscitation for Adults

- Establish unresponsiveness by shaking the person's shoulder while asking in a loud voice, "Are you all right?" If he or she is unresponsive and is not breathing or is only gasping, activate the emergency response system by calling 911 or a similar emergency service and obtain an automated external defibrillator (AED) (if available). (Note: If you suspect that the victim has become unresponsive as a result of asphyxiation [drowning], begin cardiopulmonary resuscitation [CPR] for 2 minutes before calling 911.)

- If you have not been trained in CPR, begin and continue chest compressions at a rate of 100 per minute and a depth of at least 2 inches. To do so, place the heel of one hand on the chest midway between the nipples, place your other hand over the first hand, keep your elbows straight and your shoulders directly over your hands, and press down firmly. Continue to compress the chest until you see signs of movement or until emergency medical personnel take over.

- If you are trained in CPR, begin with 30 chest compressions as previously described and then open the airway by using the head-tilt, chin-lift maneuver.

- Check for normal breathing; if breathing is absent or abnormal, seal the person's mouth with yours, pinch the nose closed, give one breath lasting one second into the mouth, and see if the chest rises. If it does rise, give the second breath; if it does not rise, reposition the head and give two rescue breaths.

- Check for any response in less than 10 seconds (e.g., independent breathing, a groan, a facial expression, or a carotid pulse).

- If no response occurs, start chest compressions again; 30 compressions in 18 seconds with 2 deep, slow breaths constitute one cycle.

- If an AED is available, apply it after five cycles of CPR (about 2 minutes), follow prompts from the AED, and continue with CPR (refer to Procedure 12-13 for use of an AED).

- Continue CPR until medical assistance arrives or the person shows signs of recovery.

- These procedures are appropriate to use for adults and for children 8 years and older.

- All health care personnel should be certified in CPR and recertified every 2 years. The American Heart Association (AHA) recommends a review yearly or sooner.

Note: If the cardiac arrest was witnessed by a trained health care worker, after establishing responsiveness and breathing, activate the emergency response system, obtain and use an AED, begin CPR, and follow the AED directions until assistance arrives. Information about CPR is available from the AHA.

Box 12-4 Chain of Events: Cardiac Arrest/Death

- Call 911 or a similar emergency service if two or more responders are present; for a lone responder, begin with 30 chest compressions and then call 911. If the person is known to be a victim of asphyxiation or drowning, complete five cycles of cardiopulmonary resuscitation (CPR) (about 2 minutes) before calling 911.
- Initiate CPR starting with 30 chest compressions at a depth of 2 inches; obtain an automated external defibrillator (AED) unit (if available).
- Apply the AED after 2 minutes of CPR; follow the AED prompts.
- Continue CPR and use of the AED (following prompts) until an emergency medical technician service arrives.
- Transport the person to the emergency department for evaluation and treatment.
- Admit the person to the cardiac care unit.

PROCEDURE 12-13

Use of an Automated External Defibrillator

- Call 911 or a similar emergency service, obtain and turn on the automated external defibrillator (AED), and position it near the person.
- Initiate cardiopulmonary resuscitation (CPR); perform five cycles, and then position yourself at the side of the person near the AED.
- Expose the person's chest from the shoulders to the waist; apply the AED pads to the chest where indicated by the AED.
- Allow the AED to "analyze" (it may be necessary to press an "analyze" button on the unit).
- Follow the prompts from the AED. If a "shock" is indicated by the AED, move away from the person, clear the immediate area, and press the "shock" button on the unit.
- Follow additional prompts from the AED and continue CPR until medical assistance arrives or the person shows signs of recovery.

listed in Box 12-4, and the activities should be performed in the shortest possible time.

An AED may not be available until emergency medical technicians arrive; however, if it is available, it should be used after five cycles of CPR are administered when breathing and pulse are absent. Procedures for use of an AED are listed in Procedure 12-13. The AED is programmed by an internal computer that instructs the user how to apply the unit (Fig. 12-9). AED units have become more accessible to the general public, especially on commercial aircraft and cruise ships; in office buildings, public schools, public service vehicles, and colleges; and at facilities or events where large numbers of persons gather. Likewise, oronasal or "pocket" masks may be placed in easy-to-see areas in case CPR needs to be administered (Fig. 12-10). At some locations, a resuscitation unit (i.e., an Ambu bag) may even be available to provide respiration for the patient. To use this unit, the caregiver squeezes and releases the flexible canister ("bag") at the rate of normal breathing (i.e., every 5 seconds in an adult and every 2 seconds in a child), producing a cycle of inspiration and expiration (Fig. 12-11).

SUMMARY

The guidelines presented in this book regarding patient care and the treatment environment, general patient safety considerations, and the employment of qualified, competent, and properly trained personnel should be reviewed. The patient must be informed of the intent and desired outcome of treatment. The caregiver should be prepared to provide emergency care or obtain assistance if an adverse reaction to treatment occurs.

Emergency equipment (e.g., an emergency or "crash" cart) and supplies should be accessible in the treatment area, and the telephone numbers of qualified advanced medical assistance personnel should be posted near all

telephones (e.g., 911 and internal emergency numbers or codes [e.g., "Doctor Blue," "Doctor Heart," and "Code Orange"]). Periodic reviews of emergency procedures should be included in staff education programs, and CPR retraining of personnel should be performed by qualified instructors at least every 2 years.

Special care and attention should be provided to any patient whose condition has the potential to develop into a more serious problem. For instance, patients who require full-body immersion or who use a therapeutic pool should be provided with fluids before, during, and after treatment to avoid heat exhaustion. Patients injured at or above the T6 cord level should be monitored for noxious stimuli, especially retention of urine, to avoid autonomic hyperreflexia. Treatment for patients with diabetes should be scheduled so patients will not be adversely affected by an insulin injection or food intake before receiving treatment. These persons should be counseled to adjust their food or insulin intake according to the type of treatment or amount of physical activity required. Patients with a history of convulsions should be reminded to use anticonvulsive medications consistently and according to the prescriptive instructions.

Each patient's vital signs should be monitored frequently, especially patients whose conditions have the potential to lead to an emergency. The Valsalva maneuver should be avoided by instructing patients not to hold their breath and to breathe regularly during exercise. A patient who has been recumbent for extended periods or who has a reduced ability to return peripheral venous blood to the heart should be observed and monitored when moving from a recumbent or sitting position to a more upright position. This patient should be given the opportunity to accommodate gradually

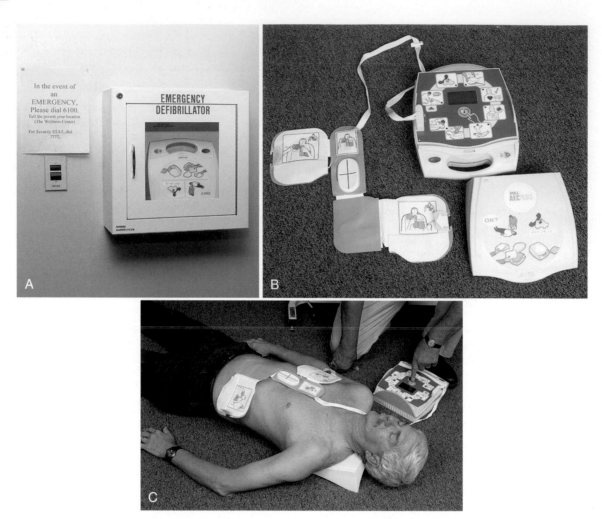

Fig. 12-9 **A,** A wall-mounted automated external defibrillator (AED) unit. **B,** An AED training unit. **C,** Demonstration of the application of an AED unit.

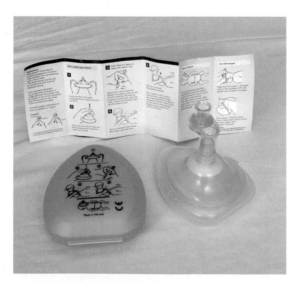

Fig. 12-10 An oronasal mask.

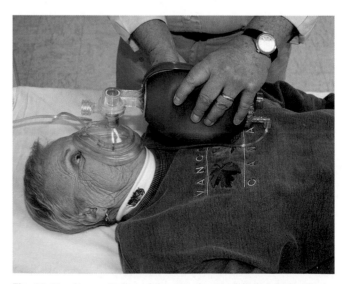

Fig. 12-11 Demonstration of the use of a resuscitation device (Ambu bag).

to an upright position, and measures should be used to relieve symptoms of hypotension. The patient should be protected until it is determined that he or she has accommodated sufficiently to sit or stand safely without experiencing the symptoms of orthostatic hypotension.

Finally, the caregiver should observe each patient for signs or symptoms of an abnormal physiological response to treatment and should be prepared to act when an emergency occurs.

self-study ACTIVITIES

- Describe your responsibilities, obligations, and actions for a patient who experiences an injury during or as a result of treatment.
- Explain how you would treat a person who has experienced heat stroke, heat exhaustion, an insulin reaction, acidosis, or autonomic hyperreflexia.
- Differentiate the signs and symptoms of heat exhaustion and heat stroke.
- Differentiate the signs and symptoms of orthostatic hypotension and autonomic hyperreflexia.
- Outline the content you believe should be included in a safety orientation and prevention program for caregivers in both inpatient and outpatient facilities.
- Describe the activities you would perform to monitor a patient's response to treatment.

problem SOLVING

1. You are in your first special clinical education experience where you assist the athletic trainer at a rural high school in Texas. During the early fall, football practice is in progress and the temperature is 88°F with a relative humidity of 85%. What preparatory actions would you take? What possible medical emergency should you anticipate occurring? What actions would you perform if an emergency occurred?

2. You are treating an 85-year-old woman with a fractured right femur. She has a long leg cast on her right lower extremity, and you are at the bedside to get her up and help her ambulate with a walker. As she stands, she reports dizziness and becomes diaphoretic. What is your initial action? What would you do to assist in determining the possible causes for this patient's reaction?

3. A 28-year-old woman is at a baby shower and has eaten some peanuts. Immediately, she indicates that she cannot swallow. What should you do, and what type of reaction do you think she is having?

4. A 68-year-old man is playing golf with three other persons and suddenly collapses while putting. You are in the group and are the first person to reach him. He is not breathing, and you are unable to palpate a pulse. What would you do from that point forward to provide emergency care for him?

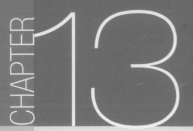

CHAPTER 13

Americans with Disabilities Act and Environmental Assessments

objectives *After studying this chapter, the reader will be able to:*

- Explain the purpose of the Americans with Disabilities Act (ADA).
- Describe the emphasis of the four primary titles of the ADA.
- Define the terms associated with the ADA.
- Discuss the roles a consultant could perform related to the ADA.
- Describe the major environmental assessments to be performed for a residence, workplace, and community.
- Describe actions an employer or businessperson can perform to respond to the employment and accessibility requirements of the ADA.
- Describe the basic components for the assessment of a home, workplace, and community.
- Describe the specifications and features for a wheelchair-accessible home.

key terms

Accessible housing A residence built or modified to meet specific requirements for accessibility and that enables an individual to function at his or her optimal level of independence.

Adaptable housing A residence designed so that some of its features can be altered to enable a person to function as independently as possible.

Universal design housing A residence designed to be used by all persons to their greatest level of independence without the need for adaptation.

INTRODUCTION

Persons with disabilities have faced discrimination with regard to employment and limited access to workplaces, businesses, and transportation for many years. Groups and organizations such as the Equal Employment Commission, the President's Committee on Employment of People with Disabilities, the National Easter Seals Society, Paralyzed Veterans of America, the Multiple Sclerosis Society, the Arthritis Foundation, and the American Physical Therapy Association have advocated improvement in mobility, access, and employment opportunities for persons with health conditions and disabilities. Previous federal legislation was designed to protect persons with disabilities from discrimination through the use of certain requirements or incentives. The Civil Rights Act of 1964, the Fair Housing and Architectural Barriers Act of 1968 and its amendments in 1988, Section 504 of the Rehabilitation Act of 1973, and Education for All Handicapped Children Act of 1975 are examples of legislation that pertains to persons with impairments. However, the Americans with Disabilities Act (ADA), which was signed on July 26, 1990, and amended in 2008, provided enforceable prohibitions and standards that ban discrimination based on disability. The ADA was designed to extend the civil rights for people with disabilities to improve their opportunity for employment by private sector employers; to provide access to public bus and train service, including Amtrak; to provide access to public accommodations and services; and to provide access to certain types of telecommunications. The ADA is federal antidiscrimination legislation designed to remove employment and access barriers for persons with disabilities.

According the Department of Justice (DOJ), the purpose of the Amendments Act of 2008, which became effective on January 1, 2009, is to carry out the ADA's objectives of providing "a clear and comprehensive national mandate for the elimination of discrimination" and "clear, strong,

Table 13-1 Definition of Disability

Phrase	Definition
Physical or mental impairment	Any physiological disorder or condition, cosmetic disfigurement, or anatomic loss affecting one or more of the following body systems: neurological, musculoskeletal, special sense organs, respiratory (including speech organs), cardiovascular, reproductive, digestive, genitourinary, hemic and lymphatic, skin, and endocrine
	Any mental or psychological disorder such as mental retardation, organic brain syndrome, emotional or mental illness, and specific learning disabilities
	Includes but is not limited to such contagious and noncontagious diseases and conditions as orthopedic, visual, speech, and hearing impairments; cerebral palsy; epilepsy; muscular dystrophy; multiple sclerosis; cancer; heart disease; diabetes; mental retardation; emotional illness; specific learning disabilities; human immunodeficiency virus disease (whether symptomatic or asymptomatic); tuberculosis; drug addiction; and alcoholism
	Does not include homosexuality or bisexuality
Major life activities	Functions such as caring for one's self, performing manual tasks, walking, seeing, hearing, speaking, breathing, learning, and working
A record of such an impairment is regarded as having such an impairment	A history of, or has been misclassified as having, a mental or physical impairment that substantially limits one or more major life activities
	Has a physical or mental impairment:
	• That does not substantially limit major life activities but that is treated by a private entity as constituting such a limitation;
	• Has a physical or mental impairment that substantially limits major life activities only as a result of the attitudes of others toward such impairment; or
	• Has none of the impairments of this definition but is treated by a private entity as having such an impairment

The term "disability" means, with respect to an individual, a physical or mental impairment that substantially limits one or more major life activities of such individual; a record of such an impairment; or being regarded as having such an impairment.
From the Americans with Disabilities Act Title II Regulations, Part 35 Nondiscrimination on the Basis of Disability in State and Local Government Services (as amended by the final rule published on September 15, 2010).

consistent, enforceable standards addressing discrimination" by reinstating a broad scope of protection and to reject the requirement enunciated by the Supreme Court in several court cases. Revisions were made in 2010 to the Title II Rule and the Title III Rule.

One of the biggest changes in the ADA Amendments Act of 2008 and the 2010 Revisions is the definition of the term "disability" (Table 13-1).

The ADA has five titles: Title I, Employment; Title II, Public Service (including public transportation); Title III, Public Accommodations; Title IV, Telecommunications; and Title V, Miscellaneous Provisions. As of March 15, 2012, all deadlines for compliance with all regulations have expired, and the legislation is in full effect. It is important to understand that the ADA interfaces with or is related to other state and federal laws, such as the Family and Medical Leave Act, the Occupational Safety and Health Act, and workers' compensation laws that are in effect in each state. Employers, owners, managers, administrators, and persons who are involved with the employment of workers should become familiar with these acts and laws to understand how they may interact with the ADA. Information and assistance with these relationships can be obtained from state and federal departments of labor and local or federal Equal Employment Opportunity Commission offices.

According to American Community Survey figures released in 2006 and published by the United States Census Bureau, 38 million persons who were older than 16 years and were of the noninstitutional population had some type of disability, and approximately 25.6% of them were employed. (Disability data are not available from the 2005-2009 American Community Survey data set because of changes in the disability questions in 2008.) The 2011 statistics from the U.S. Department of Labor Statistics found that within the same parameters of disabled people, the employment rate was 17.7% and the disabled population was 27.6 million.

DEFINITIONS

- **Disability:** A person who has a physical or mental impairment that substantially limits one or more of the major life activities of such individual; a record of such an impairment; or being regarded as having such an impairment. Communicating, working, walking, standing, lifting, bending, caring for oneself, breathing, learning, seeing, hearing, speaking, reading, thinking, sleeping, concentrating, eating, and performing manual tasks are considered major life activities.
- **Physical or mental impairment:** An individual must have a physical or mental impairment. As explained in

paragraph (1)(i) of the definition, "impairment" means any physiological disorder or condition, cosmetic disfigurement, or anatomic loss affecting one or more of the following body systems: neurological; musculoskeletal; special sense organs (which would include speech organs that are not respiratory such as vocal cords, the soft palate, the tongue, etc.); respiratory, including speech organs; cardiovascular; reproductive; digestive; genitourinary; hemic and lymphatic; skin; and endocrine. It also means any mental or psychological disorder, such as mental retardation, organic brain syndrome, emotional or mental illness, and specific learning disabilities (as taken from the DOJ's 2010 Title II ADA regulation).

- **Reasonable accommodation:** Making modifications at the job site or workplace that will enable persons with disabilities to easily perform a specific job. Some examples of reasonable accommodations are having a physically accessible workplace, restructuring a job, or adjusting a work schedule or hours of work to meet an individual's needs.
- **Undue burden:** An action necessary to provide a reasonable accommodation that would cause the employer or owner significant difficulty or expense. Several factors are considered to determine whether a hardship would occur for the employer or owner; these factors include the size of the business, number of employees, type of operation of the business, nature and cost of the needed accommodation, and whether the accommodation would have an adverse effect or pose a risk to other employees.
- **Qualified individual with a disability:** A person who can perform the essential functions of a given job or activity, with or without the benefit of reasonable accommodation. In other words, the person must have the knowledge, skills, and mental and physical capabilities to perform the essential elements of a particular job.
- **Covered entity:** An employer, an employment agency, a labor organization or joint labor management organization, and state and local governments are examples of covered entities.
- **Handicap:** A physical or attitudinal constraint that is imposed on a person, regardless of whether that person has an impairment, that places the person at a disadvantage.

Many of the terms in these definitions are not specific and therefore are subject to interpretation. The person with a disability, the employer, an attorney, and state or federal agency personnel may differ in their interpretation of the language contained in the ADA. At the time the act became effective, it was anticipated that a great amount of litigation would occur in relation to the meaning and interpretation of ADA language; however, the anticipated level of litigation has not occurred.

GENERAL ASPECTS OF THE AMERICANS WITH DISABILITIES ACT

As previously outlined, the ADA contains four primary Titles, each of which addresses a specific protected category and has separate compliance requirements. Persons in the private sector who own, manage, or lease a business or are employers and who are involved with any type of business, public service, housing, or workplace regulated by Titles I and III should become familiar with the provisions of those titles. The amended ADA states that all private sector employers who employ 15 or more persons for at least 20 weeks in a calendar year and an industry affecting commerce with 25 or more employees for the same amount of time are required to comply with Title I. In addition, because of the requirements of Title III related to accessibility to public accommodations and most commercial facilities, employers and business owners and their agents are affected even if they employ fewer than 15 persons.

Title I prohibits an employer from discriminating against a qualified individual with a disability on the basis of that disability alone. This prohibition affects job application and hiring procedures, opportunities for advancement, compensation and salary matters, and job training activities. An employer could be considered to have discriminated against a qualified person with a disability if the employer does not make reasonable accommodations for the individual or denies employment based on the need to make reasonable accommodations unless the employer can demonstrate that the needed accommodations would cause an undue hardship on the operation of the business (Box 13-1).

When a qualified individual with a disability is hired, the employer is required to make accommodations for a known impairment that would enable that employee to achieve the same level of performance and to enjoy benefits equal to those of an average, similarly situated person without an impairment. However, the accommodation does not have to ensure equal results or provide exactly the same benefits. The employee must request the accommodation and may suggest an appropriate accommodation. The employer is allowed to review and propose more than one type of

Box **13-1**	**Examples of Workplace Accommodations**

- Modification of work schedule
- Modification of job activities or requirements
- Employee reassignment or relocation
- Modifications to the physical plant
- Assistive devices such as teletypewriter, a telecommunications device for the deaf, a telephone amplifier, and large-print manuals
- Modification of existing furniture or equipment for wheelchair users
- Accessible restrooms, entrances, hallways, doorways, and parking area

accommodation and to select the one that is most appropriate or reasonable without leading to undue hardship, providing that it effectively allows the person with an impairment to perform the job. Accommodations must be determined on the basis of each individual's needs because the nature and extent of the impairment and the requirements of a job will vary. Examples of reasonable accommodations, depending on the impairment and job requirements, are adjusting the height or changing the cutout area of a desk, adjusting the height and location of shelves, relocating file cabinets, repositioning telephones and other pieces of office equipment, modifying standard office or telecommunications equipment, modifying testing and training activities or procedures, and providing readers or interpreters for persons with a vision or language impairment.

Title III is designed to protect persons with disabilities on the basis of their disability from discrimination related to full and equal access to services, facilities, accommodations, goals, privileges, and advantages of any place of public accommodation by the person who owns, leases, or operates a site, place, or facility classified as public accommodation. Virtually every type of private entity or business whose operation affects commerce is considered to be a public accommodation (Box 13-2).

For existing facilities and those to be constructed, structural physical barriers must be removed or not included. Title III usually requires removal, modification, or alteration of structural barriers when the changes can be made reasonably and accomplished without significant difficulty or expense.

The following adjustments typically can be made to provide greater access for persons with disabilities:
- Installation of ramps
- Widening of doorways
- Use of door hardware that is more functional than a knob that must be turned (Fig. 13-1, A and B)

Box **13-2** Examples of Public Accommodations

- Hotels or motels
- Restaurants or bars
- Theaters or auditoriums
- Convention centers or lecture halls
- Grocery stores, shopping centers, or sales or retail establishments
- Laundromats, gas stations, or professional offices
- Public transportation buildings
- Museums or libraries
- Parks or zoos
- Amusement parks
- Places of education
- Day care centers or senior centers
- Gymnasiums, spas, or bowling alleys

- Provision of an alternative pathway with a firm surface to buildings, parking areas, or areas within a building
- Installation of support (grab) bars or rails (Fig. 13-1, C and D)
- Increased space in restrooms to accommodate a wheelchair
- Creation of accessible parking spaces
- Use of telephones and water fountains accessible from a wheelchair
- Curb cutouts

In addition, auxiliary services and aids must be provided to individuals with a vision or hearing impairment (Fig. 13-2). Auxiliary services could be as simple as having the server in a restaurant read the menu selections to persons who are visually impaired or having the server be prepared to use a pad and pencil to communicate with persons who are hearing impaired. An aid that may be required is a telephone or an outlet for a portable device that will serve the needs of persons with hearing impairments, such as a telecommunication display device. The provisions of Title III do not apply to exempted entities, including private clubs and establishments that are exempt from Title II of the Civil Rights Act of 1964, religious organizations or entities controlled by religious organizations, Native American tribes, and entities operated by governments that are exempt from Titles I and II. Appendix 13 provides examples of Title III requirements or accommodations.

COMPLIANCE AND IMPLEMENTATION OF REGULATIONS

Employers, managers, administrators, and persons with disabilities should become educated about the employment of persons with disabilities. Consultation with human resources personnel, legal counsel, external qualified consultants, current employees with disabilities, and department supervisors is a recommended initial step. Review of the application form, process, and procedures; selection and hiring procedures; and evaluation, advancement, and training opportunities and activities will help determine the current and necessary level of compliance with Title I. Time should be spent to determine the essential functions of a job, prepare a comprehensive job description written in functional terms (e.g., able to lift 50 lb or able to stand for 2 hours at a time), observe the workplace layout and environment, and prepare an on-site job analysis for each job of the business. The physical and mental requirements of the job should be identified, as should any special skills or abilities that are needed. Specific education and training qualifications and any certification or licensure credentials that are required should be listed.

The employer and any agents involved with the hiring process must be aware of restrictions associated with the limits imposed on preemployment inquiries of applicants. Before making an offer or during the application phase of the employment process, impairment-related questions,

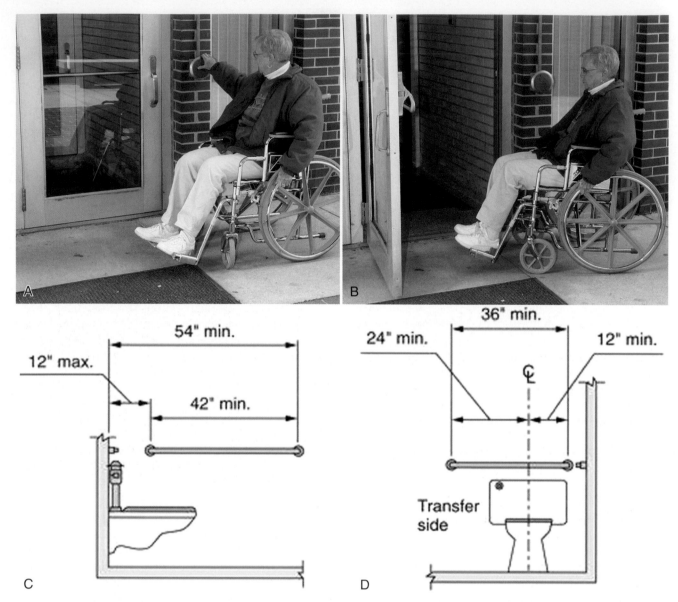

Fig. 13-1 **A,** Electrically operated doors for a public building. Pressing the control disk opens the outer and inner doors. **B,** A person approaches the door to enter; the doors close after a preset period has elapsed. (Note: Wheeling over a raised threshold at the outer door may be difficult for some wheelchair users.) **C,** Recommended placement of grab bars on the side walls of a public bathroom. **D,** Recommended placement of grab bars on the back wall of a public bathroom. (Redrawn from Department of Justice, Americans with Disabilities Act Accessibility Guidelines for Buildings and Facilities, 2002, in Cameron MH, Monroe LG: *Physical rehabilitation: evidence-based examination, evaluation, and intervention,* St. Louis, 2008, Saunders Elsevier.)

medical history information, and medical examinations are prohibited by the ADA unless they are specifically job related. An applicant can be asked whether he or she can perform specific essential job functions such as lift and carry objects, stand for prolonged periods, climb a ladder, or use specific pieces of office equipment. When an interview is conducted, the questions asked and the discussion should relate to the information requested on the application and the functional requirements of the job. The interviewer is

permitted to ask the applicant about the duties that were performed in a previous job. Questions about any visible physical characteristics of the applicant, present health status, and psychiatric history or previous addiction to drugs are prohibited (Box 13-3).

Medical examinations or evaluations are permitted if they are performed after an offer of employment has been made, providing all employees in a specific job category receive the same type of examination. The medical

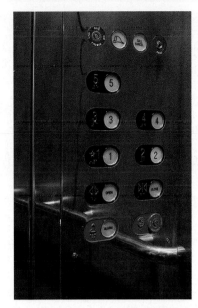

Fig. 13-2   Elevator controls with Braille symbols.

Box 13-3   **Suggestions for Employers to Facilitate Hiring Persons with Disabilities**

- Learn where to locate and how to recruit people with disabilities.
- Learn how to communicate and interact with people who have disabilities.
- Be certain that company applications and employment forms do not ask for disability-related information and are formatted to be accessible to all persons with disabilities.
- Prepare written job descriptions that clearly and specifically identify the essential functions of a job.
- Be certain that company medical examinations, evaluations, or tests comply with the Americans with Disabilities Act (ADA).
- Be prepared to provide reasonable accommodations needed by a qualified applicant to compete for the job.
- Treat persons who have a disability with dignity and respect.
- Know that persons protected by the ADA include those with acquired immunodeficiency syndrome, cancer, mental retardation, deafness, blindness, learning impairment, or brain injury as a result of trauma.
- Train supervisors and other employees about making reasonable accommodations.
- Use procedures to maintain and protect medical records as confidential; follow Health Insurance Portability and Accountability Act guidelines.
- Prepare and train all employees to communicate, interact, and work with people with disabilities.

information that is obtained must be placed in a file or separated from the person's personnel file. Preemployment tests for illegal drug use are permitted because such testing is not considered to be part of a medical examination by the ADA. However, employers and their agents should understand that a person who has successfully completed a drug or alcohol abuse rehabilitation program or is enrolled in such a program and is drug-free is protected from discrimination by the ADA.

When a person with an impairment is hired and the impairment is made known, the employer should be prepared to address the need for reasonable accommodation to provide a better opportunity for the employee to perform the job, as described previously. An ADA catalog has been produced by the National Easter Seals Society that lists videocassettes and audiocassettes, books, and posters that address the ADA, attitude awareness, training, and issues related to employment, transportation, and housing. One item listed in the catalog is *The Workplace Workbook: An Illustrated Guide to Job Accommodations and Assistive Technology* by James Mueller, which was published by the Dole Foundation in 1992. It is designed to be a resource for businesses with regard to accommodating people with disabilities and the types of problems that may be caused by inappropriate workspace design.

The employer must consider the requirements for accessibility contained in Title II that are different from the reasonable accommodation requirements of Title I. Consultation with a knowledgeable architect, qualified design professional, or health care professional (e.g., a physical therapist, occupational therapist, or industrial health specialist) or current employees with disabilities may help the employer reach decisions necessary to comply with Title

III. The 2010 Standards for Accessible Design took effect March 15, 2010, and employers must be in compliance with these standards by March 15, 2011. The 2010 Standards are basically the combination of the 1990 ADA and the Architectural Barriers Act of 1968. More information on the revised ADA Regulations that implement Title II and Title III can be found at ada.gov on the Internet.

Existing facilities classified as public accommodations are required to remove structural architectural barriers when removal is readily achievable. Access into a facility or an establishment for persons with impairments, freedom of movement, and access to goods and services once inside the facility should be given immediate attention. Suggestions and examples of how this goal can be accomplished have been presented previously. If the removal of existing architectural barriers is not readily achievable, the facility, establishment, or entity must provide its goods, services, facilities, privileges, advantages, or accommodations through alternative methods if such methods are readily achievable. For example, to comply with these requirements, a business may need to provide a "drive-through" window, offer home deliveries, or provide catalog sales. (Note: "Readily achievable" is defined as being able to be accomplished easily and

Box **13-4**	Examples of Title III Removal of Barriers Categories

- Providing curb cuts in sidewalks and entrances
- Repositioning shelves
- Rearranging tables, chairs, vending machines, display racks, and other furniture
- Repositioning telephones
- Adding raised markings on elevator control buttons
- Installing grab bars in toilet stalls
- Rearranging toilet partitions to increase maneuvering space
- Installing a raised toilet seat
- Widening doors
- Removing high-pile, low-density carpeting
- Creating designated accessible parking spaces
- Eliminating a turnstile or providing an alternative accessible path

Box **13-5**	Accessibility Audit Requirement Categories

- Ramps and slopes
- Doors and hallways
- Signage
- Steps, stairs, and elevators
- Flooring
- Obstacles and protrusions
- Reach range and clear space
- Seating
- Equipment (e.g., telephones, drinking fountains, controls and receptacles, and toilet rooms)
- Accessible path and walkway
- Parking and loading zone
- Alarms, signs, and warnings
- Area for emergency refuge

Box **13-6**	Activities for an Americans with Disabilities Act Consultant

- Educate employers, managers, supervisors, employees, and persons with disabilities about the Americans with Disabilities Act (ADA), particularly Titles I and III.
- Perform an on-site job analysis and identify essential job functions.
- Perform an on-site environmental evaluation.
- Help develop function-based job descriptions.
- Advise on job-related accommodation needs.
- Advise on the removal of physical barriers and the improvement of access internally and externally.
- Perform physical capacity and functional ability testing of current and prospective employees based on essential job functions.
- Help develop policies and procedures related to compliance with the ADA.

performed without difficulty or expense.) The DOJ's ADA Standards for Accessible Design (2010) can be found at access-board.gov on the Internet. These standards are consistent with the updated ADA guidelines issued by the Board in 2004. However, the DOJ's revised Title II regulation and Title III regulation implement additional provisions in certain facilities, as found at access-board.gov and listed below:

- Social service center establishments
- Housing at places of education
- Assembly areas
- Medical care facilities
- Residential dwelling units
- Detention and correctional facilities
- Places of lodging

Some examples of "Removal of Barriers" in Title III of the 2010 ADA Standards are provided in Box 13-4. On or after March 15, 2012, elements in existing facilities that do not comply with the specifications for elements in the 1991 Standards must be modified to the extent readily achievable in order to comply with the requirements in the 2010 Standards. The categories of the accessibility audit requirements for public accommodations are listed in Box 13-5. Specific requirements, specifications, and guidelines for each of these categories are contained in the Code of Federal Regulations, DOJ, Civil Rights Division, 28 CFR, Part 36, March 15, 2011. According to data available from the President's Committee on Employment of People with Disabilities, approximately 80% of the costs to make existing facilities accessible have been less than $1000, and 50% of the changes have cost less than $50. Extensive remodeling of a facility usually is not required, but creative and innovative ways of thinking are important elements to be used to resolve the majority of accommodation or accessibility problems.

A qualified and knowledgeable health care professional consultant (i.e., a physical or occupational therapist) is a valuable resource for an employer. Activities or roles that could be expected of such a consultant are presented in Box 13-6. The employer should review and evaluate the consultant's credentials, qualifications, and past consultation experiences to determine his or her level of expertise or competence before contracting for services. The desired and expected outcome or product of the consultation, the time frame for the consultation, costs and expenses that are anticipated, and the method of payment for the services should be clearly identified to the satisfaction of the persons involved with the consultation.

The ADA also provides some tax incentives to encourage employers and business owners to comply with the act. The Internal Revenue Service allows a deduction of up to $15,000 per year for expenses associated with the removal of qualified architectural and transportation barriers. In addition, small businesses are eligible to receive a tax credit of up to $5000 for certain costs that are incurred to comply with the ADA. When the two incentives are added, a small business owner could accrue $20,000 in tax incentives in 1 year. However, an employer should be aware that financial penalties exist if the employer does not comply with the requirements of the ADA. For all tax-related matters, consultation with a tax advisor is recommended to review and assist with the preparation and filing of the appropriate documents.

ASSESSING THE ENVIRONMENT

Many persons whose physical abilities have been compromised or reduced because of injury, illness, or disease will need to adapt to their environment, or the environment may need to be modified to permit mobility and functional activities that are safe and energy conserving. Therefore a health care professional may be asked to perform an assessment of the person's current and future environments. The assessment process should incorporate the concepts and recommendations contained in the ADA, especially when the person's workplace and use of community services and buildings are assessed. Three primary environments to be evaluated are the person's residence, place of employment, and the community. Persons who use a wheelchair or ambulation aids for mobility often encounter environmental barriers that adversely affect their mobility or functional capacity. These persons frequently require accommodations to enable them to gain greater mobility or improved functional capacity. Furthermore, persons with a visual or hearing deficit also may require modifications to their residences, workplaces, and community to enhance their functional abilities.

The application of universal design concepts for the living areas of persons with an impairment or who are elderly should be considered during the environmental assessment process. Some examples of universal design features for the home include wider doors and halls; the use of lever-type doorknobs and faucet handles; relocation of lighting controls and electrical outlets; recessed areas under sinks, cabinets, and work counters; varied heights of countertops; and relocation of cabinets for easier access. The use of these and other similar building accommodations in an original structure would classify it as accessible housing and would provide a more functional environment for the elderly, persons with various disabilities and mobility limitations, or a wheelchair user without requiring extensive remodeling or cost. Adaptable housing is defined as when an existing home is modified to include the features presented previously. Persons who are building a new home or remodeling an existing one may find it beneficial to incorporate suggestions associated with the universal design approach in case there is a need for the home to be as accessible as possible in the future.

Assessment Process

Several activities are necessary to perform an assessment of the environment, including the following: at least one interview with the patient, family, and employer; at least one site visit to the residence (Box 13-7), workplace (Box 13-8), and most frequently used community sites (Box 13-9); completion of an assessment form or record; and a final written document containing recommendations, diagrams, photographs, or plans of proposed residence and workplace modifications designed to improve mobility, access, or functional abilities. The process may require several interview sessions or site visits and should be performed using interprofessional collaboration. Persons who may be involved include a physical therapist, an occupational therapist, a social worker, a nurse, a public health practitioner, an architect, a contractor, and an employer.

Box **13-7** **Basic Assessment of the Residence**

EXTERNAL FEATURES
- Sidewalk/driveway: condition, type of surface, width, length, and slope
- Garage/carport: attached or detached, size, and access
- Approach to entry: steps, porch, landing, and illumination
- Entry: door width, threshold height, and space for access into a room
- Access to grounds

INTERNAL FEATURES
- General considerations: door widths; threshold heights; hall widths; presence of stairs; location, height, and access to electrical outlets/switches; size and space available in rooms; type of and access to lighting; location of and access to communication units (e.g., telephone and computer); location of and access to safety devices (e.g., smoke/carbon monoxide detectors, circuit breaker panel, surveillance/security controls, and emergency exit); location of and access to heating/cooling controls; access to and operation of windows; floor surfaces/coverings
- Living/family room: furniture configuration and ability to reposition furniture; type of and access to furniture; access to entertainment equipment
- Kitchen: access; location, layout, and position of sink, counter surfaces, and cabinets; location of, type of, and access to appliances and their controls; location of plumbing; space for wheelchair mobility
- Bathroom: access to sink, commode, tub/shower, mirror, and medicine cabinet; location of plumbing; safety features present or needed (e.g., grab bars, a raised toilet seat, a shower chair, and protection from hot water pipes)
- Bedroom: location, height, and access to the bed; access to other furniture, closets, and clothes

Box **13-8** Basic Assessment of the Workplace

EXTERNAL FEATURES
- Location of parking area: size, condition, and type of surface
- Location and availability of designated parking spaces
- Approach to entry: steps, illumination, and platform
- Entry: door width, size, means of opening/closing, and threshold height
- Location of sidewalk: type of surface, condition, and width

INTERNAL FEATURES
- Access to work station/office
- Door and hall widths
- Floor surfaces and coverings
- Access to job equipment, supplies, cabinets, desk, work surface, and space
- Access to rest room and its facilities
- Access to eating area and its facilities
- Access to elevator and escalator
- Access to water fountain and refreshment machines

Note: Compliance with requirements for reasonable accommodations stipulated by the Americans with Disabilities Act should be determined.

Box **13-9** Basic Assessment of the Community

- Location and type of public transportation and access to such transportation
- Location, type, and condition of sidewalks, curb cuts, and crosswalk indicators
- Location of and access to designated parking spaces at restaurants, shopping centers, grocery stores, theaters, banks, and other public buildings
- Entry to buildings: steps, door widths, means of door opening/closing, and thresholds heights
- Access to facilities in public buildings: telephone, restroom, counter surfaces, checkout areas, aisles, emergency exits, water fountain, elevator, and escalator
- Access to recreation areas and facilities

Note: Compliance with requirements for reasonable accommodations stipulated by the Americans with Disabilities Act should be determined.

When possible, the patient and a family member should be present during at least one site visit.

Periodic, short, predischarge home visits from a health care facility by the patient can help identify the patient's abilities and limitations and the barriers to mobility and function in the residence. Such visits also may make it possible to determine the modifications that are needed and whether they can be accomplished to sufficiently meet the patient's needs. It may be helpful to perform one visit in the evening or after dark and during inclement weather.

Planning for the patient's return to community life must be initiated well in advance of the anticipated date of discharge, especially the assessment process, to permit sufficient time to perform any needed modifications or obtain any needed special equipment for the residence or workplace. Materials and items to be used for the site visits are a tape measure (at least 6 feet long), a flashlight, graph paper to plot changes, a camera, a voice recorder, an assessment form, and a laptop computer.

Accessible Housing A residence is considered to be accessible if a person with a disability is able to function in it as independently as possible. One way to accomplish this goal is to construct the house with universal design features. Another approach is to modify or adapt an existing structure to make it accessible. If the latter solution is used, it may only be necessary to make minor modifications such as adding an entry ramp to compensate for steps, installing wall- or floor-mounted safety ("grab") bars, or purchasing an elevated toilet seat. However, other structures may require extensive interior remodeling or even the construction of new space to make the home accessible.

The optimal configuration for an accessible home is a single-story house with an open floor plan that has minimal walls, doors, and hallways. A second option is a multistory house with an accessible bedroom and bathroom on the first level. An attached garage and entries without steps would be desirable features for either structure. A person's type of disability will determine which modifications or features are needed to make the residence accessible. Some specifications and features for accessible housing for persons with hearing, vision, and physical impairments are presented in Table 13-2 and Box 13-10. This type of information can be obtained through many sources; some are listed in the Bibliography, and others can be located by searching the Internet.

The amount and type of remodeling or structural changes that can be accomplished may depend on factors such as whether the person owns or rents the residence, the present structure and grounds can accommodate the remodeling or construction desired, the modifications will comply with building code requirements, the costs of the modifications are reasonable and affordable, a qualified contractor is available, the residence is single or multiple level, and what effect the modifications may have on the subsequent sale or rental of the residence. Despite these factors, fulfilling the needs of the patient is the most important consideration. It should be recognized that not all modifications may be able to be completed at the same time, and priorities may need to be established to complete the entire project. The assessor(s) should identify the modifications necessary to improve the disabled person's mobility or function and provide recommendations about how to complete them. This activity should be done through consultation with the disabled person and his or her family members and employer.

Table 13-2 Specifications and Features for a Wheelchair-Accessible Home

Feature	Specifications
GENERAL CONSIDERATIONS	
Sidewalk width	36 inches minimum; slope no greater than for ramp (see below); smooth, firm surface
Door width	32 inches minimum, 36 inches preferable; clearance and space needed for chair to open door and enter; pocket doors conserve space and make access easier during an emergency
Hall width	32 inches minimum, 40 inches preferable
Threshold height	Absent or 0.5-inch maximum
Electrical outlets	18 inches from the floor; ground fault interrupting
Electrical controls	48 inches maximum from the floor, 40 inches optimal; rocker-type switch
Telephone access	18 inches from the floor; jacks in every room
Floor surface	Firm (wood, tile, linoleum); slip resistant; 0.5-inch or less pile carpet; firm underlay
Door handles	36 inches maximum from the floor, lever type
Window height	36 inches from the floor; vertical sliding or crank operation
Ramp	36 to 48 inches wide; no more than 1-inch rise for each foot of vertical rise (length); firm, slip-resistant surface; ramps longer then 30 feet will need to change direction and may need a landing area
Access	30 × 48–inch clearance in front of fixtures, work areas, and appliances
Reach zone	Comfortable reach for seated person is 20 to 44 inches
KITCHEN	
Floor plan	U- or L-shaped is best
Turning radius	5 × 5 feet optimal
Counter tops, work surfaces	30 to 34 inches from the floor; adjustable or varied heights are beneficial; 29 inches for knee clearance minimum
Sink height	32 to 34 inches from the floor; open front with insulated or shielded plumbing; 5- to 8-inch depth
Range	32 to 34 inches from the floor; smooth cook top, front controls; side-hinged oven door beneficial
Cabinets	Positioned within access and reach zone as much as possible; toe kick area on base cabinets should be recessed more than the normal 4 inches
Outlets	Located within the access and reach zone
Microwave and small appliances	Located within the access and reach zone
BATHROOM	
Toilet	16 inches or less from the floor if wheeled commode/shower chair is used; 18 inches from the floor for sitting transfer; 3-foot space needed in front and to one side for wheelchair clearance
Roll-in shower	30 × 60 inches minimum; 5 × 4 feet preferable
Regular shower	36 × 36 inches with fixed seat; handheld shower head; single lever water control
Sink	34 inches maximum from the floor; bowl depth slopes from front to back
Bathtub	With integral seat, waterproof floor, and floor drain, 30 × 60 inches minimum, 18 inches deep; adequate space needed for wheelchair clearance
Safety ("grab") bars	24 to 30 inches long; height and position according to individual needs; must be attached to floor, wall stud, or reinforced underlay (three-quarter-inch plywood attached to studs)
BEDROOM	
Bed height	18 to 22 inches from the floor; firm mattress; adequate space for wheelchair for transfer on one side
Closet	Sliding entry doors; rods adjustable or 48 inches maximum from the floor; "roll-in" closet is beneficial
Dressers	Height and width fall within the access and reach zone; D-shaped handles beneficial
Room size	Provides free space for wheelchair access and clearance for transfers, obtaining clothing
GARAGE	
Height	10-foot minimum if a raised roof van is used; 8 feet for a wheelchair lift; 5 feet for a wheelchair transfer; should have direct entrance into the house

Adapted with permission from Lema A: *Simplified disabled housing solution (system 1 and system 2)*. Copyright 2006 Lema, Brady and Lema LLC. No further reproduction can be made without written permission from the author.

Consultation with an architect and contractor is recommended for major remodeling or construction projects. Awareness by the health care professional of the requirements for access and reasonable accommodations in the workplace that are contained in the ADA will assist in providing meaningful suggestions and recommendations. A variety of environmental assessment forms can be found in the literature or through Internet sources. Many treatment facilities have developed forms that specifically meet their needs and those of the patient-related community environment.

Box 13-10	Features for Hearing and Vision Deficits/Loss

HEARING DEFICIT/LOSS
- A text telephone, teletypewriter, telecommunications device for the deaf, or an amplified handset
- Visual signals for alarms, a security system, telephone ringers, and doorbells/knockers
- Closed caption for television

VISION DEFICIT/LOSS
- Tactile sensors or labels for switches, thermostats, lamps, and other controls
- Warning strips for step edges, changes in elevation, and thresholds
- Computer or voice-command technology to activate various systems or household appliances
- An audible cue for activation of alarms, appliances, controls, and lights
- Furniture placement to provide an unobstructed travel path
- Lighting intensity appropriate for the extent of visual loss

Basic areas or items to be considered during the assessment of a person's residence, workplace, and community are presented in Boxes 13-7 through 13-9.

SUMMARY

On July 26, 1990, the ADA was signed, and most requirements contained in this Act became effective on July 26, 1992. The Act was amended by the ADA Amendments Act of 2008, which became effective January 1, 2009. The ADA requires the DOJ to publish ADA design standards that are consistent with the guidelines published by the U.S. Architectural and Transportation Barriers Compliance Board (Access Board). These rules address recreation facilities, play areas, State and local government facilities (i.e., detention facilities and courthouses), and, finally, the revision of the Access Board's 1991 guidelines. The new standards took effect on March 15, 2012, and replace the DOJ's original ADA standards. These changes have been adopted, with some modifications, as the 2010 Standards for Accessible Design.

Each of the four ADA primary Titles contains regulations, guidelines, and prohibitions specific to that title. The purpose of the ADA is to provide a clear, rational mandate for the elimination of discrimination against persons with disabilities, based on the disability, through comprehensive and enforceable prohibitions. The act was designed to extend the civil rights for people with disabilities in the areas of employment (Title I); access to certain types of public transportation, including Amtrak, and access to government employment, facilities, and services (Title II); access to goods, services, and facilities classified as public accommodations (Title III); and access to auxiliary devices and aids such as telecommunications (Title IV) (Table 13-3).

Table 13-3	Summary of Americans with Disabilities Act Titles I through IV

Title No.	Summary
Title I: Employment	Employers may not discriminate against a person with a disability in hiring or promoting if the person is otherwise qualified for the job; employers will need to provide "reasonable accommodations" to persons with disabilities, including job restructuring and equipment modification, but they need not provide accommodations that impose an "undue hardship" on business operations; regulated by the Equal Employment Opportunity Commission
Title II: Public Service	State and local governments may not discriminate against qualified individuals with disabilities; all government facilities, including public transportation and communication, must be accessible; regulated by the Secretary of Transportation
Title III: Public Accommodations	Public accommodations operated by private entities such as restaurants, hotels, retail stores, and theaters may not discriminate against individuals with disabilities; auxiliary aids and services must be provided to individuals with vision or hearing impairments or other individuals with disabilities, unless an undue burden would result; physical barriers in existing facilities must be removed if removal is readily achievable; if not readily achievable, alternative methods to provide service or access, if they are readily achievable, must be provided; all new construction and alterations to public accommodations must be accessible; regulated by the Attorney General
Title IV: Telecommunications	Companies or businesses offering telephone service to the general public must offer telephone relay services to individuals who use telecommunication devices for the deaf or similar devices; regulated by the Federal Communications Commission

The ADA is complex legislation that requires careful study before an individual can become reasonably familiar with it. Many terms and concepts are not defined specifically and at times may appear to be ambiguous and subject to interpretation; therefore assistance or consultation with a variety of persons, including an architect, an attorney, an industrial health specialist, or a health care professional, may be necessary to gain information and suggestions about compliance with the act. Many resources are available that provide specific information about the many requirements of the ADA; several of them are located in the Bibliography.

Although most of the requirements of the ADA have been in effect since July 1992, increased education is needed for employers, persons with disabilities, members of many professions, students enrolled in health care education programs, and society in general about the purpose and extent of the ADA. Many health care professionals profess themselves to be advocates for persons with disabilities, but they have not been active in promoting or providing information about the ADA. Graduates of many professional education programs have limited knowledge of the ADA, which limits their ability to educate others or serve as advocates for persons with disabilities. Minimal research has been performed and published related to the effect or outcomes of the act for employers, persons with disabilities, or society; therefore continued investigation of the values, limitations, costs, enforcement, and awareness of the effects of the ADA on society seems warranted.

self-study ACTIVITIES

- State the purpose of the Americans with Disabilities Act (ADA).
- List and describe the major themes of Titles I through IV of the ADA.
- Describe how you could serve as a consultant to an employer to assist with compliance for Titles I and III of the ADA.
- Visit several workplaces or businesses and identify structural architectural barriers; explain how they could be eliminated or modified to comply with Title III of the ADA.
- Outline activities an employer could perform to become prepared to employ persons with disabilities.
- Propose three or four topics related to the ADA that would be appropriate for investigation and research.

problem SOLVING

1. You and an occupational therapist are scheduled to perform an assessment of a patient's home. The patient will use a wheelchair for mobility indefinitely. What preparatory activities would you perform, and with whom would you perform them? What areas should be assessed during the site visit?

2. You have been delegated to assess the workspace at the reception desk for a new employee who uses a wheelchair. What aspects of the office and areas of the facility should be evaluated?

3. You have been asked to perform an assessment of a two-story home for a person who needs to use a wheelchair for mobility because of a stroke. The house has two front steps, four rear steps, and a detached garage with a manual door. A den is located on the first floor, all bedrooms and bathrooms are on the second level, and a laundry room is located on the first floor. What procedures would you use to assess the home? What are some early recommendations for exterior and interior modifications you would provide to make the house more accessible?

4. You have been asked to evaluate the living quarters of a person who is blind. What specific exterior and interior features and specifications would you recommend for this person?

Bibliography

ABC 7 News, TheDenverChannel.com: *Hospital survival guide, updated December 15, 2010* (website): http://www.thedenverchannel.com/health/26146492/detail.html. Accessed December 1, 2011.

AbleData: *AbleData informed consumer guide to accessible housing* (website):. http://www.abledata.com/abledata.cfm?pageid=191907&filename=Accessible_Housing_ICG.htm. Accessed December 1, 2011.

Access 4911: *The President's Committee on Employment of People with Disabilities* (website): http://www.access4911.org/president's_committee.htm. Accessed December 1, 2011.

The accessible housing design file, Florence, KY, 1991, Barrier Free Environments.

Adaptable housing, Washington, DC, 1989, U.S. Department of Housing and Urban Development.

Adaptive Access: *Home changes* (website): Adaptiveaccess.com. Accessed May 29, 2011.

Agency for Health Care Policy and Research: *Clinical practice guideline: treatment of pressure ulcers*, Silver Spring, MD, 1994, Agency for Health Care Policy and Research.

Agency for Health Care Policy and Research: *Quick reference guide*, Silver Spring, MD, 1994, Agency for Health Care Policy and Research.

Agency for Healthcare Research and Quality: *Medical errors and patient safety* (website): ahrq.gov. Accessed May 5, 2011.

Alexander GJ: Time for a new law on health care advance directives, *Hastings Center Law J* 42(3):755-778, 1991.

American Academy of Family Physicians: *Blood pressure monitoring at home* (website): http://familydoctor.org/familydoctor/en/diseases-conditions/high-blood-pressure/diagnosis-tests/blood-pressure-monitoring-at-home.html. Accessed December 1, 2011.

American Academy of Orthopedic Surgeons: *Atlas of orthotics*, St Louis, 1975, Mosby.

American Academy of Physician Assistants: *Final regulations allow PAs to order patient restraint or seclusion* (website): http://www.hospitalmedicine.org/AM/Template.cfm?Section=Reference_Material&Template=/CM/ContentDisplay.cfm&ContentID=17070. Accessed December 1, 2011.

American Association of Retired Persons: *Product report: wheelchair*, Washington, DC, 1990, American Association of Retired Persons.

American Association of Retired Persons: *Resources: navigating the world of caregiving* (website): http://assets.aarp.org/external_sites/caregiving/options/viewall_resources.html. Accessed December 6, 2011.

American Heart Association: *American Heart Association 2005 guidelines for CPR and ECC* (website): Americanheart.org. Accessed March 11, 2007.

American Heart Association: *Cardiopulmonary resuscitation*, Dallas, 1987, American Heart Association.

American Heart Association: *First aid for choking*, Dallas, 1988, American Heart Association.

American Heart Association: *High blood pressure*, New York, 1969, American Heart Association.

American Heart Association: *Hypertension* (website): Hyper.ahajournals.org. Accessed December 1, 2011.

American Heart Association: *Recommendations for human blood pressure determination by sphygmomanometers*, Dallas, 1984, American Heart Association.

American Medical Association: *HIPPA privacy standards* (website): Ama-assn.org. Accessed November 11, 2010.

American Heart Association Emergency Cardiac Care Committee and Subcommittees: Guidelines for cardiopulmonary resuscitation and emergency cardiac care, part II, adult basic life support, *JAMA* 268:2184-2198, 1992.

American Medical Association: *Informed consent* (website): http://www.ama-assn.org/ama/pub/physician-resources/legal-topics/patient-physician-relationship-topics/informed-consent.page. Accessed December 1, 2011.

American Medical Association Council on Ethical and Judicial Affairs: *Principles of medical ethics—E-8.08, informed consent* (website): http://www.ama-assn.org/ama/pub/physician-resources/medical-ethics/code-medical-ethics/opinion808.page. Accessed December 1, 2011.

American Occupational Therapy Association: Enforcement procedures for Occupational Therapy Code of Ethics, *Am J Occup Ther* 58(6):1085-1086, 2004.

American Physical Therapy Association: *APTA guide for professional conduct, principle 2.4, patient autonomy and consent* (website): Apta.org. Accessed October 8, 2010.

American Physical Therapy Association: *Defensible documentation for patient/client management* (website): http://www.apta.org/Documentation/DefensibleDocumentation/. Accessed December 1, 2011.

American Physical Therapy Association: *Guide for professional conduct* (website): http://www.apta.org/uploadedFiles/APTAorg/Practice_and_Patient_Care/Ethics/GuideforProfessionalConduct.pdf#search=%22Guide%20for%20Professional%20Conduct%22. Accessed December 1, 2011.

American Physical Therapy Association: *Guide to physical therapist practice*, ed 2, Alexandria, VA, 2001, American Physical Therapy Association.

American Physical Therapy Association: *Guidelines, physical therapy documentation of patient/client management* (website): http://www.apta.org/uploadedFiles/APTAorg/About_Us/Policies/BOD/Practice/DocumentationPatientClientMgmt.pdf#search=%22Guidelines%20Physical%20Therapy%20Documentation%20of%20Patient%2fClient%20Management%22. Accessed December 1, 2011.

American Physical Therapy Association: *Liability awareness, informed consent* (website): Apta.org. Accessed November 11, 2010.

American Physical Therapy Association: *Research, hooked on evidence* (website): Hookedonevidence.org. Accessed January 15, 2011.

American Physical Therapy Association: *Vision 2020* (website): http://www.apta.org/Vision2020/. Accessed December 1, 2011.

American Physical Therapy Association, Agency for Healthcare Research and Quality: *Informed consent* (website): www.apta.org. Accessed August 5, 2010.

American Red Cross: *Community first aid and safety*, St Louis, 1993, Mosby.

Americans with Disabilities Act: *Accessibility guidelines checklist for buildings and facilities, October 1992* (website): http://access-board.gov/adaag/checklist/a16text.html. Accessed December 1, 2011.

Americans with Disabilities Act: *Accessibility requirements*, Washington, DC, December 1991, U.S. Architectural and Transportation Barriers Compliance Board.

Americans with Disabilities Act: *Tax incentives packet on the Americans with Disabilities Act* (website). http://www.ada.gov/archive/taxpack.htm. Accessed December 1, 2011.

Americans with Disabilities Act: *Title II regulations: part 35 nondiscrimination on the basis of disability in state and local government services (as amended by the final rule published on September 15, 2010)* (website). http://www.ada.gov/regs2010/titleII_2010/titleII_2010_regulations.htm. Accessed December 1, 2011.

Amundsen LR: Assessing exercise tolerance: a review, *Phys Ther* 59:534-537, 1979.

Anderson JC, Towell ER: Health publications: perspectives on assessment of physical therapy error in the new millennium, *J Phys Ther Educ* Winter 2002.

Apparelyzed: *Custom wheelchairs: the trend from functionality to individuality* (website): http://apparelyzed.com/wheelchair/custom-wheelchairs.html. Accessed December 1, 2011.

Apts D, Blankenship K: *The American back school manual*, Ashland, KY, 1980, American Back School.

Armstrong DG, Holtz-Neider K, Wendel C et al: Skin temperature monitoring reduces the risk for diabetic foot ulceration in high-risk patients, *Am J Med* 120:1042-1046, 2007.

ArmstrongMH,PriceP:*Wet-to-drygauzedressings:factandfiction*(website):http://www.woundsresearch.com/article/2284.AccessedDecember1,2011.

Arnold MJ, Hill D, Shephard J: Everyday ethics: state licensure, the law and ethics. *OT Practice* 6(11), 2001.

Association for Practitioners in Infection Control: *Guidelines for exposure determination and prevention,* Cincinnati-Dayton, OH, 1992, Association for Practitioners in Infection Control.

Auscultation 1 (website): http://www.medicanalife.com/video/6d71 fed1079d34a/Auscultation-1. Accessed December 5, 2011.

The Auscultation Assistant: *Breath sounds* (website): http://www.med.ucla.edu/wilkes/lungintro.htm. Accessed December 6, 2011.

Back owner's manual, Daly City, CA, 1991, Physicians Art Service.

Back pain, San Bruno, CA, 1986, Krames Communications.

Back tips for health care providers, San Bruno, CA, 1987, Krames Communications.

Barclay L. *Rates of invasive healthcare-associated MRSA infections may be declining* (website): http://www.medscape.com/viewarticle/726883. Accessed December 1, 2011.

Barrier-free house plans, Des Plaines, IL, 1995, Professional Builder.

Beaumont J-L: *Basics of pulmonary auscultation* (website): http://infiresources.ca/fer/Depotdocument_anglais/Pulmonary_Auscultation.pdf. Accessed December 6, 2011.

Bennett JE, Dolin R, editors: *Principles and practice of infectious diseases,* ed 7, Philadelphia, 2009, Churchill Livingstone Elsevier.

Bergen A, Colongelo C: *Evaluating the environment: problem solving worksheet,* Camarillo, CA, 1984, Everest and Jennings.

Bergquist S, Bonnel W, Braun J et al: *CPGEC prevention of pressure ulcers* (website). http://coa.kumc.edu/gec/modules/PresUlc/PU-FramePages/ModuleContent_Main.htm. Accessed December 1, 2011.

Bergstrom N, Braden B, Boynton P, et al: Using a research-based assessment scale in clinical practice, *Nurs Clin North Am* 30:539-551, 1995.

Berkley Bionics: *Introducing eLegs* (website): http://www.youtube.com/watch?feature=player_embedded&v=WcM0ruq28dc. Accessed December 1, 2011.

Bemis-Dougherty A: What is ICF? *PT Magazine,* February 2009.

Beyer JE, Denyes MJ, Villarruel AM: The creation, validation and continuing development of the oucher: a measure of pain intensity in children, *J Pediatr Nurs* 7:335-346, 1992.

Blackmer J: Rehabilitation Medicine: 1. Autonomic dysreflexia. *Canadian Medical Association Journal* (serial online): http://canadianmedicaljournal.ca/content/169/9/931.full?sid=9d309995-b4d1-4d05-9e18-a91d90e5bb4d. Accessed December 1, 2011.

BloodBook.com: *Blood test results—normal ranges* (website): http://www.bloodbook.com/ranges.html. Accessed December 1, 2011.

Blood-borne infections: a practical guide to OSHA compliance. Arlington, TX, 1992, Johnson & Johnson Medical.

Body substance precautions in schools: recommendations, Columbus, OH, 1991, The Ohio Department of Health.

Bogey R: *Gait analysis* (website): http://emedicine.medscape.com/article/320160-overview. Accessed December 1, 2011.

Bolognia JL, Jorizzo JL, Rapini RP: *Dermatology,* ed 2, St Louis, 2007, Mosby Elsevier.

Bonewit K: *Clinical procedures for medical assistants,* ed 3, Philadelphia, 1990, WB Saunders.

Boulton AJM, Armstrong DG, Albert SF, et al: Comprehensive foot examination and risk assessment, *Diabet Care* 31:1679-1685, 2008.

Brian Mac Sports Coach: *Core stability* (website): http://brianmac.co.uk/corestab.htm. Accessed December 1, 2011.

Brown V, Graf S: *Lecture notes and handouts,* Columbus, OH, 1985, Physical Therapy Division, School of Allied Medical Professions, The Ohio State University.

Brookside Associates Multimedia Edition. *Closed cuff surgical gloving* (website): brooksidepress.org. Accessed December 21, 2010.

Brookside Associates Multimedia Edition. *Surgical gown solo dress* (website): brooksidepress.org. Accessed December 21, 2010.

Buerhaus PI: Lucien Leape on the causes and prevention of errors and adverse events in health care, *Image J Nurs Sch* 31:281-292, 1999.

Burkhauser RV, Houtenville AJ: *A guide to disability statistics from the current population survey—annual social and economic supplement (March CPS).* Ithaca, NY: 2006, Cornell University.

Burn Center at Westchester Medical Center: *A guide to burn management in the emergency department* (website): wcmc.com. Accessed March 11, 2007.

Cailliet R: The shoulder in the hemiplegic patient. In *Shoulder pain,* ed 3, Philadelphia, 1991, FA Davis.

Caring Connections: *Advanced directives* (website): www.caringinfo.org/i4a/pages/index.cfm?pageid=3284. Accessed December 1, 2011.

Caring Connections: *Download your state's advance directives* (website). http://www.caringinfo.org/i4a/pages/index.cfm?pageid=3289. Accessed December 1, 2011.

Carr J, Shepherd R: *A motor relearning program for stroke,* ed 2, Rockville, MD, 1987, Aspen.

Carroll K, Edelstein JE: *Prosthetics and patient management: a comprehensive clinical approach,* Thorofare, NJ, 2006, Slack.

Case-Smith J: *Practical aspects of using outcomes measures. model program for linking allied health education, research and practice,* Columbus, OH, 1996, School of Allied Medical Professions.

Center for Universal Design, College of Design, North Carolina State University: *Gold, silver, and bronze universal design features in houses* (website): http://www.ncsu.edu/www/ncsu/design/sod5/cud/pubs_p/docs/GBS.pdf. Accessed December 6, 2011.

Centers for Disease Control and Prevention: *2007 Guideline for isolation precautions: preventing transmission of infectious agents in healthcare settings* (website): http://www.cdc.gov/hicpac/2007IP/2007isolationPrecautions.html. Accessed December 5, 2011.

Centers for Disease Control and Prevention: *Diabetes public health resource* (website): www.cdc.gov/diabetes/. Accessed December 6, 2011.

Centers for Disease Control and Prevention: *Economics of preventing hospital-acquired infection* (website): http://wwwnc.cdc.gov/eid/article/10/4/02-0754_article.htm. Accessed December 1, 2011.

Centers for Disease Control and Prevention: Increase in adult *Clostridium difficile*–related hospitalizations and case-fatality rate, United States, 2000-2005, *Emerg Infect Dis J* (serial online): http://wwwnc.cdc.gov/eid/article/14/6/07-1447_article.htm. Accessed December 5, 2011.

Centers for Disease Control and Prevention, National Center on Birth Defects and Developmental Disabilities: *Joint range of motion video* (website): www.cdc.gov/NCBDDD/video/JointROM/intro/index.html. Accessed December 1, 2011.

Centers for Medicare and Medicaid Services: *PT, OT, and SLP services and the mapping of international classification of functioning, disability and health (ICF): mapping therapy goals to the ICF* (website): https://www.cms.gov/TherapyServices/downloads/Mapping_Therapy_Goals_ICF.pdf. Accessed December 6, 2011.

Chandrasekhar AJ: *Screening physical exam self evaluation lung auscultation* (website): http://www.meddean.luc.edu/lumen/MedEd/medicine/pulmonar/pd/step29e.htm. Accessed December 5, 2011.

Cholewicki J, Juluru K, Radebold A, et al: Lumbar spine stability can be augmented with an abdominal belt and/or increased intra-abdominal pressure, *Eur Spine J* 8(5):388-395, 1999.

Choosing a wheelchair system. *J Rehabil Res Dev Clin* Suppl(2):1-116, 1990.

Circulation: *2010 American Heart Association guidelines for cardiopulmonary resuscitation and emergency cardiovascular care science* (website): circ.ahajournals.org. Accessed April 11, 2011.

Circulation: *2010 International consensus on cardiopulmonary resuscitation and emergency cardiovascular care science with treatment recommendations* (website): circ.ahajournals.org. Accessed April 11, 2011.

Clarkson HM, Gilewich GB: *Musculoskeletal assessment*, Baltimore, 1989, Williams & Wilkins.

Code of Federal Regulations: *28 CFR Part 36: Nondiscrimination on the basis of disability by public accommodations and in commercial facilities* (website): http://www.ada.gov/reg3a.html. Accessed December 5, 2011.

College of Occupational Therapists of Manitoba: *Practice guideline, October 2006: informed consent in occupational therapy practice* (website): http://www.cotm.ca/upload/InformedConsent.pdf. Accessed December 6, 2011.

Connolly JB: A new breed of consultant, *Clin Manage* 12:72-80, 1992.

Contract Laboratory.com: *Normal blood values for lab blood testing* (website): http://www.contractlaboratory.com/labclass/normalbloodvalues.cfm. Accessed December 6, 2011.

Coruth F, Thompson F: *Transfer and lifting techniques for extended care*, Vancouver, BC, 1983, Evergreen Press.

Craig JV, Lancaster GA, Taylor S, et al: Infrared ear thermometry compared with rectal thermometry in children: a systematic review, *Lancet* 360:306-309, 2002.

Cress ME, Kinne S, Patrick DL, et al: Physical functional performance in persons using a manual wheelchair, *J Orthop Sports Phys Ther* 32:104-113, 2002.

Custom seamed measuring manual, Charlotte, NC, 2005, Jobst.

Cutson TM, Bongiorni D, Michael JW et al: Early management of elderly dysvascular below-knee amputees, *J Prosthet Orthot* 6(3):62-66, 1994.

Danger signs and symptoms: clinical skillbuilders, Springhouse, PA, 1990, Springhouse Corporation.

Daniels L, Worthingham C: *Muscle testing: techniques of manual examination*, ed 5, Philadelphia, 1986, WB Saunders.

Deutsch A, English RD, Vermeer TC, et al: Removable rigid dressings versus soft dressings: a randomized, controlled study with dysvascular, trans-tibial amputees, *Prosthet Orthot Int* 30(1):102-103, 2006.

Disabled and Productive: *Automated transport and retrieval system for wheelchairs enables driver independence* (website): http://www.disabledandproductive.com/blog-posts/automated-transport-and-retrieval-system-for-wheelchairs-enables-driver-independence/. Accessed December 6, 2011.

Disabled and Productive: *Hiding a wheelchair chest strap* (website): http://www.disabledandproductive.com/index.php?s=Hiding+a+Wheelchair+Chest+Strap+. Accessed December 5, 2011.

Disabled World: *Life in a wheelchair* (website): http://videos.disabled-world.com/video/19/life-in-a-wheelchair. Accessed December 5, 2011.

Disabled World: *Wheelchair transfer by rope swing* (website): http://videos.disabled-world.com/video/154/wheelchair-transfer-by-rope-swing. Accessed December 5, 2011.

Domenico RL, Ziegler WZ: *Practical rehabilitation techniques for geriatric aides*, Rockville, MD, 1989, Aspen.

Dr. Greene.com: *Droplet transmission* (website): http://www.drgreene.com/azguide/droplet-transmission. Accessed December 5, 2011.

Duff JF: *Youth sports injuries*, New York, 1992, Macmillan.

Easter Seals: *Disability etiquette* (website): http://www.easterseals.com/site/PageServer?pagename=ntl_etiquette. Accessed December 5, 2011.

Easter Seals: *Easter Seals resources for employers* (website): easterseals.com. Accessed March 13, 2007.

Easter Seals: *Easy access housing for easier living* (website): http://www.easterseals.com/site/DocServer/Easy_Access_Housing.pdf?docID=11023. Accessed December 5, 2011.

Easter Seals: *Project ACTION* (website): http://projectaction.easterseals.com/site/PageServer?pagename=ESPA_homepage. Accessed December 5, 2011.

Eberhardt K: *Wheelchair accessible housing, Rehabilitation Institute of Chicago* (website): lifecenter ric.org. Accessed March 11, 2007.

Edelstein JE: Preprosthetic management of patients with lower- or upper-limb amputation, *Phys Med Rehabil Clin North Am* 2(2):285-297, 1991.

eHow: *How to charge wheelchair batteries* (website): http://www.ehow.com/how_6949833_charge-wheelchair-batteries.html. Accessed December 5, 2011.

eHow: *How to make your home handicap accessible* (website): http://www.ehow.com/how_12076386_make-home-handicap-accessible.html. Accessed December 5, 2010.

Eichenfield LF, Frieden LJ, Esterly NB: *Neonatal dermatology*, ed 2, Philadelphia, 2008, Saunders.

Emergency procedures: clinical skillbuilders. Springhouse, PA, 1991, Springhouse Corporation.

Engle H: *Back to basics with skin and wound care (slide presentation)*, Humble, TX, June 2006, Memorial Hermann Northeast.

Erdos EE, Jared M, Steinheiser JM: *Basic intravenous therapy (seminar proceedings)*, Beachwood, OH, 1992, NCS Healthcare.

Eric Martin and Associates Architects: *Draft information sheet* (website): http://www.emaa.com.au/documents/accessdocs/Draft_Information_Sheet_for_Adaptable_Housing.pdf. Accessed December 5, 2011.

Evans N, Robertson L: *Reducing medical errors for Florida physical therapists and physical therapy assistants* (website): http://www.therapyceu.com/courses/261/index_pt.html. Accessed December 5, 2011.

Feldt KS: The checklist of nonverbal pain indicators (CNPI), *Pain Manag Nurs* 1(1):13-21, 2000: https://www.healthcare.uiowa.edu/igec/tools/pain/nonverbalPain.pdf. Accessed December 5, 2011.

Field JM, Hazinski MF, Sayre MR, et al: Part 1: executive summary: 2010 American Heart Association guidelines for cardiopulmonary resuscitation and emergency cardiovascular care, *Circulation* 122(18 Suppl 3):S640-S656, 2010.

Fish DJ, Nielsen JP: Clinical assessment of human gait, *J Prosthet Orthot* 5:39-48, 1993.

Fit back workout, San Bruno, CA, 1990, Krames Communications.

Flint PW, Haughey BH, Lund VJ, et al: *Cummings otolaryngology: head and neck surgery*, ed 5, Philadelphia, 2010, Mosby Elsevier.

Freed M, Hofkosh J, Kaplan L, et al: Choosing ambulatory aids, *Patient Care* 15:20-35, 1987.

Freed M, Hofkosh J, Kaplan L, et al: Using ambulatory aids, *Patient Care* 21:36-46, 1987.

Frontera WR: *DeLisa's physical medicine and rehabilitation: principles and practice*, ed 5, Philadelphia, 2011, Lippincott Williams & Wilkins.

Furlan JC, Fehlings MG: Cardiovascular complications after acute spinal cord injury: pathophysiology, diagnosis, and management, *Neurosurg Focus* 25(5):E13, 2008.

Gailey RS, Clark CR: Physical therapy management of adult lower-limb amputees. In *Atlas of limb prosthetics: surgical, prosthetic, and rehabilitation principles*, ed 2, Rosemont, IL, 1992, American Academy of Orthopedic Surgeons.

Garritan S, Jones P, Kornberg T, et al: Laboratory values in the intensive care unit, *Acute Care Perspect* Winter 1995.

Ghasemi Z, Martin T: The role of the physical therapist in the intensive care unit, *Acute Care Perspect* Winter 1995.

Giannangelo K, Bowman S, Dougherty M, et al: *ICF: Representing the patient beyond a medical classification of diagnoses* (website): http://perspectives.ahima.org/index.php?option=com_content&view=article&id=86:icf-representing-the-patient-beyond-a-medical-classification-of-diagnoses&catid=39:clinical-terms-a-vocabularies&Itemid=85. Accessed December 5, 2011.

Global Medical Sales: *Bariatric wheelchair 1000 lb capacity* (website): http://www.globalmedicalsales.com/Bariatric-I-1000Chair.html. Accessed December 1, 2011.

Gomella LG, editor: *Clinician's pocket reference*, ed 6, Norwalk, CT, 1989, Appleton & Lange.

González-Iglesias J, Huijbregts P, César Fernández-de-las-Peñas C, et al: Differential diagnosis and physical therapy management of a patient with radial wrist pain of 6 months' duration: a case report, *J Orthop Sports Phys Ther* 40(6):361-368, 2010.

Goodman CC, Snyder TK: *Differential diagnosis in physical therapy*, ed 3, Philadelphia, 1999, Saunders.

Gordon College: *Range of motion, body mechanics transfers & positioning* (website): http://www.gdn.edu/Faculty/jprue/RangeofMotion.ppt#324,69, Turning a Patient. Accessed December 6, 2011.

Gould R, Barnes SS: *Shoulder pain in hemiplegia* (website): http://emedicine.medscape.com/article/328793-overview. Accessed December 5, 2011.

GPO Access: *Electronic Code of Federal Regulations (e-CFR), Title 28, Judicial Administration* (website): http://ecfr.gpoaccess.gov/cgi/t/text/text-idx?sid=777770cd1100d678b551edad47fce271&c=ecfr&tpl=/ecfrbrowse/Title28/28tab_02.tpl. Accessed December 5, 2011.

Greene L, Goggin R: *Save your hands! The complete guide to injury prevention and ergonomics for manual therapists*, ed 2, Coconut Creek, FL, 2008, Body of Work Books.

Guidelines for documentation, Presented at: Rosegate Convalescent Center, 1991, Columbus, Ohio.

Hamilton HK, editor: *Nursing procedures*, Springhouse, PA, 1983, Intermed Communications.

Hammill RR, Beazell JR, Hart JM: Neuromuscular consequences of low back pain and core dysfunction, *Clin Sports Med* 27(3):449-462, 2008.

Hazinski MF, Nolan JP, Billi JE, et al: Part 1: executive summary: 2010 international consensus on cardiopulmonary resuscitation and emergency cardiovascular care science with treatment recommendations, *Circulation* 122(16 Suppl 2):S250-S275, 2010.

Helpguide.org: *Advance health care directives and living wills: make your end-of-life choices now to ensure your wishes are met* (website): http://www.helpguide.org/elder/advance_directive_end_of_life_care.htm. Accessed December 5, 2011.

Hettiaratchy S, Papini R: Initial management of a major burn: II—assessment and resuscitation, *BMJ* 329(7457):101-103, 2004.

Hill PH: *Making decisions*, Reading, MA, 1979, Addison-Wesley.

Hill WM: When a lawyer gets a hold of the chart: what to include, *Acute Care Perspect* 15(2), 2006.

Hillegass E: Exercise assessment: an important outcome tool in the acute care setting, *Acute Care Perspect* 16(1), Spring 2007.

Hollis M: *Safe lifting for patient care*, ed 2, Oxford, UK, 1985, Blackwell Scientific.

Hollister Global: *Wound care algorithms* (website): hollister.com. Accessed April 10, 2011.

Hoppenfeld S: *Physical examination of the spine and extremities*, New York, 1976, Appleton-Century-Crofts.

Hosford D: *Hosford differential diagnosis tables* (website): http://www.ptcentral.com/site/1/docs/diagnose-10day-trial.pdf. Accessed December 5, 2011.

Hospital infection control. In: *Employee orientation notebook*, Columbus, OH, 1992, Riverside Methodist Hospital.

How to transfer a patient from bed to wheelchair using a Hoyer lift (website): http://www.videojug.com/film/how-to-transfer-a-patient-from-bed-to-wheelchair-using-a-hoyer-lift. Accessed December 5, 2011.

Howell D: *Core strength—core stability: controversy regarding definition—does it ensure enhanced athletic performance?* (website): http://damienhowellpt.com/pdf/core%20strength.pdf. Accessed December 5, 2011.

Hughes RG, Blegen MA: *Chapter 37: medication administration safety* (website): http://www.ahrq.gov/qual/nurseshdbk/docs/HughesR_MAS.pdf. Accessed December 5, 2011.

Infection control for nursing students: prevention and control of infection (website): faculty.ccc.edu. Accessed April 15, 2011.

Institute of Medicine: *To err is human: building a safer health system* (website): http://www.iom.edu/Reports/1999/To-Err-is-Human-Building-A-Safer-Health-System.aspx. Accessed December 5, 2011.

Intravenous therapy, Deerfield, MA, 1995, Channing Bete.

James R, Hart JM: Neuromuscular consequences of low back pain and core dysfunction, *Clin Sports Med* 27(3):449-462, 2008.

The Janda Approach to Chronic Pain Syndromes: *Janda syndromes* (website): http://www.jandaapproach.com/the-janda-approach/jandas-syndromes/. Accessed December 6, 2011.

Jette AM: Toward a common language for function, disability, and health, *Phys Ther* 86(5):726-734, 2006.

Johannes L: *Putting on the stripes to ease pain* (website): http://www.theratape.com/education-center/kinesiology-taping-news/45-putting-on-the-stripes-to-ease-pain/. Accessed December 5, 2011.

The Joint Commission: *2011 Hospital national patient safety goals* (website): http://www.jointcommission.org/assets/1/6/2011_HAP_NPSG_EASYTOREAD_docs_112-29.pdf. Accessed December 6, 2011.

The Joint Commission: *Accreditation program: hospital chapter: national patient safety goals* (website): www.jointcommission.org. Accessed February 18, 2011.

The Joint Commission: *Facts about Joint Commission accreditation standards* (website): http://www.jointcommission.org/assets/1/18/Standards1.PDF. Accessed December 6, 2011.

The Joint Commission: *National patient safety goals* (website): www.jointcommission.org/patientsafety/nationalpatientsafetygoals/. Accessed December 9, 2011.

Jordan-Marsh M, Yoder L, Hall D, et al: Alternate Oucher Form testing: gender, ethnicity, and age variations, *Res Nurs Health* 17:111-118, 1994.

The Journal of the American Medical Association: *Pressure ulcers* (website): http://jama.ama-assn.org/content/296/8/1020.full.pdf. Accessed December 6, 2011.

Karnath B, Boyars MC: *Pulmonary auscultation* (website): http://turner-white.com/memberfile.php?PubCode=hp_jan02_pulmonary.pdf. Accessed December 5, 2011.

Keep yourself healthy at home: a guide for adults with diabetes, Deerfield, MA, 2000, Channing Bete.

Kendall FP, McCreary EK: *Muscle testing and function*, ed 3, Baltimore, 1983, Williams & Wilkins.

Kendall K: Evolution of Sacred Heart Hospital's wound assessment sheet, *Acute Care Perspect* Summer 1995.

Keenan JM: *Review of SOAP note charting* (website): 06_Keenan_Review_SOAP_Note_Charting.pdf. Accessed December 5, 2011.

Kennedy KL: *Wound caring*, Eau Claire, WI, 1997, Professional Education Systems.

Kennedy KL: *Wound caring (seminar)*. Presented at: Annual Meeting of the Ohio Chapter of the American Physical Therapy Association, March 17, 1997, Columbus, OH.

Kenney WL: *ASCM's guidelines for exercise testing and prescription*, ed 5, Baltimore, 1995, Williams & Wilkins.

Kettenbach G: *Writing S.O.A.P. notes*, Philadelphia, 1990, FA Davis.

Kibler WB, Press J, Sciascia A: The role of core stability in athletic function, *Sports Med* 36(3):189-198, 2006.

Kirby RL, Swuste J, Dupuis DJ, et al: The wheelchair skills test: a pilot study of a new outcome measure, *Arch Phys Med Rehabil* 83:10-18, 2002.

Kirsch NR: Bringing us up to code, *PT in Motion* 1(1):64-66, 2009.

Kirch NR: Matter of vitals concern, *PT in Motion* 44-46, 2010.

Kirsch NR: New and improved, *PT in Motion* 1(2):50-55, 2009.

Kisner C, Colby LA: *Therapeutic exercise: foundations and techniques*, ed 3, Philadelphia, 1996, FA Davis.

Koblenzer L, Gyuricza B: *Nursing concepts and procedures relevant to physical therapy*, Cleveland, OH, 1982, Physical Therapy Department, Department of Health Sciences, Cleveland State University.

Kohn LT, Corrigan JM, Donaldson MS, editors, Committee on Quality of Health Care in America, Institute of Medicine: *To err is human: building a safer health system*, Washington, DC, 2000, National Academy Press.

Kumar V, Cotran RS, Robbin SL: *Basic pathology*, ed 5, Philadelphia, 1992, Saunders.

Kutner L: The living will: a proposal, *Indiana Law J* 44(1):539-554, 1969.

Kyler-Hutchison P: Ethical reasoning and informed consent in occupational therapy, *Am J Occup Ther* 42(5):283-287, 1988.

LaRusso L: *Are ear thermometers accurate?* (website): http://www.vnacare-newengland.org/body.cfm?id=103&chunkiid=24766. Accessed December 5, 2011.

Leape LL: Error in medicine, *JAMA* 272:1851-1857, 1994.

Leetun DT, Ireland ML, Willson JD, et al: Core stability measures as risk factors for lower extremity injury in athletes, *Med Sci Sports Exerc* 36(6):926-934, 2004.

Lehmkuhl LD, Smith LK, Weiss EL: *Brunnstrom's clinical kinesiology*, ed 5, Philadelphia, 1996, FA Davis.

Lema A: *Simplified disabled housing solution: a quality of life tool for caring new home developers* (website): simplifieddisabledhousing.com. Accessed March 11, 2007.

Lewis C: Wheelchair use for the older patient, *Phys Ther Forum* 11:4-7, 1992.

Lewis LV: *Fundamental skills in patient care*, Philadelphia, 1976, JB Lippincott.

Living your life with diabetes: a self-care handbook, Deerfield, MA, 2006, Channing Bete Company.

Magee DJ: *Orthopedic physical assessment*, ed 3, Philadelphia, 1996, WB Saunders.

Marshall PW, Murphy BA: Core stability exercises on and off a Swiss ball, *Arch Phys Med Rehabil* 86(2):242-249, 2005.

Massachusetts General Hospital: *Pathology service laboratory handbook: MGH critical values callback list* (website): http://mghlabtest.partners.org/CriticalValues.htm. Accessed December 5, 2011.

Masspro: *Taking the pressure off, recommendation #8: therapy's role in skin protection* (website): http://www.masspro.org/NH/PS/docs/educationtraining/Taking%20the%20Pressure%20Off.8.09.pdf. Accessed December 5, 2011.

Mayo Clinic Staff: *Cardiopulmonary resuscitation (CPR): first aid* (website): http://www.mayoclinic.com/health/first-aid-cpr/FA00061. Accessed December 5, 2011.

McArdle WD, Katch FI, Katch VL: *Essentials of exercise physiology*, ed 4, Philadelphia, 1994, Lea & Febiger.

McCash T: *Procedures for the ADA*, Dublin, OH, 1991, Meacham and Apel Architects.

McCulloch JM, Kloth LC: Decision point: wound dressings, *PT Magazine* 4:52-62, 1996.

McCulloch JM, Kloth LC, Feddar JA: *Wound healing: alternatives in management*, ed 2, Philadelphia, 1995, FA Davis.

Medicare and Medicaid Programs: Hospitals conditions of participation: patients' rights (42 CFR Part 482), *Fed Regist* 71(236):71378-71428, 2006.

Medicare.gov: *Make adjustments to schedule and routine; planning for your discharge* (caregiver information videos) (website): Medicare.gov. Accessed January 17, 2011.

MedlinePlus: *Leg amputation-discharge* (website): w.nlm.nih.gov/medlineplus/ency/patientinstructions/000014.htm. Accessed December 5, 2011.

Medline Plus: *Temperature measurement* (website): http://www.nlm.nih.gov/medlineplus/ency/article/003400.htm. Accessed December 5, 2011.

Medline Plus: *Vital signs* (website): http://www.nlm.nih.gov/medlineplus/ency/article/002341.htm. Accessed December 5, 2011.

Medscapetoday: *The alternate forms reliability of the Oucher Pain Scale: history of the Oucher* (website): http://www.medscape.com/viewarticle/505826_2. Accessed December 5, 2011.

The Merck Manual Home Health Handbook: *Pressure sores* (website): http://www.merckmanuals.com/home/sec18/ch205/ch205a.html. Accessed December 6, 2011.

Meta-ot: *OT assessments and outcome measures* (website): http://metaot.com/ot-assessments-outcome-measures. Accessed December 6, 2011.

Meyer K: *Ten commandments for communicating with persons with disabilities*, Columbus, OH, 1992, Axis Center for Public Awareness of People with Disabilities.

Minnesota Department of Health: *Airborne precautions* (website): http://www.health.state.mn.us/divs/idepc/dtopics/infectioncontrol/pre/airborne.html. Accessed December 6, 2011.

Minor SD, Minor MA: *Patient care skills*, ed 2, Norwalk, CT, 1990, Appleton & Lange.

Mirone JA: Understanding the Americans with Disabilities Act. *Healthcare Trends Trans* 4:36-38, 1993.

Mitchell T: *Posture matters* (website): http://www.aquafit.com/PostureMattersArticle.pdf. Accessed May 20, 2007.

Mobility-Advisor.com: *Wheel chair information and mobility resource guide* (website): http://www.mobility-advisor.com/. Accessed December 6, 2011.

MoonDragon's Health & Wellness: *Positioning the patient, care giver information* (website): http://www.moondragon.org/health/disorders/patientpositions.html. Accessed December 6, 2011.

Morey S: *Pressure ulcer wound care*. Presented at: Meeting of the Ohio Physical Therapy Association, April 17, 1997, Columbus, OH.

Mosby's Medical Dictionary, ed 8: *Medical asepsis* (website): http://medical-dictionary.thefreedictionary.com/aseptic+technique. Accessed December 6, 2011.

Mowder-Tinney JJ: *Wound care management and therapeutic positioning: using evidence practice* (seminar) (website): http://www.jjmowder.com/wound_care_management_and%20therapeutic_positioning_info.htm. Accessed December 6, 2011.

Mueller J: *The workplace workbook 2.0, an illustrated guide to workplace accommodation and technology*, Washington, DC, 1992, Dole Foundation.

Murdock KR: ICU paraphernalia: physical therapy implications, *Acute Care Perspect* Winter 1995.

MVS *pulmonary auscultation* (website): http://sprojects.mmi.mcgill.ca/mvs/RESP01.HTM. Accessed December 6, 2011.

Najdeski P: Crutch measurement from the sitting position, *Phys Ther* 57:826-827, 1977.

Natale A, Taylor S, LaBarbera J et al: SCIRehab project series: the physical therapy taxonomy, *The Journal of Spinal Cord Medicine* (serial online): http://www.ncbi.nlm.nih.gov/pmc/articles/PMC2718813/. Accessed December 6, 2011.

National Archives: *Teaching with documents:the Civil Rights Act of 1964 and the Equal Employment Opportunity Commission* (website): http://www.archives.gov/education/lessons/civil-rights-act/. Accessed December 6, 2011.

National Council for Community Behavioral Healthcare, Policy Action Center: *Policy resources: restraints and seclusion—rules chart* (website): http://www.thenationalcouncil.org/cs/public_policy/restraints_seclusion_rules_chart. Accessed December 6, 2011.

National Pressure Ulcer Advisory Panel: *A selected bibliography: pressure ulcer assessment, prevention and treatment*, Buffalo, NY, 1995, National Pressure Ulcer Advisory Panel.

National Pressure Ulcer Advisory Panel: *Pressure Ulcer Scale for Healing (PUSH), PUSH tool 3.0* (website): http://www.npuap.org/PDF/push3.pdf. Accessed December 6, 2011.

National Pressure Ulcer Advisory Panel: *Pressure ulcer stages revised by NPUAP* (website): http://www.npuap.org/pr2.htm. Accessed December 6, 2011.

National Pressure Ulcer Advisory Panel: *Statement on pressure ulcer prevention* (website): http://www.npuap.org/positn1.htm. Accessed December 6, 2011.

NC State University: *Center for Universal Design, publications* (website):. http://www.ncsu.edu/project/design-projects/udi/publications/. Accessed December 6, 2011.

Noftz JB: *Differential diagnosis for the healthcare professional*. Presented at: Meeting of the Ohio Physical Therapy Association, October 2005, Columbus, OH.

Norkin C, Levangie P: *Joint structure and function: a comprehensive analysis*, ed 2, Philadelphia, 1990, FA Davis.

NorthWest Arkansas Community College: *Body mechanics and transfer techniques* (website): http://faculty.nwacc.edu/rcrider/Transfers.pdf. Accessed December 1, 2011.

Northwest Regional Spinal Cord Injury System: *Choosing a wheelchair* (website): http://sci.washington.edu/info/newsletters/articles/03sum_wheelchair.asp. Accessed December 6, 2011.

Nursing Crib: *Principles of surgical asepsis* (website): http://nursingcrib.com/nursing-notes-reviewer/principles-of-surgical-asepsis/. Accessed December 6, 2011.

Nursing photobook annual, Springhouse, PA, 1987, Springhouse.

Occupational Safety and Health Administration, Department of Labor: Occupational exposure to bloodborne pathogens; final rule, *Fed Regist* 56:64003-64182, 1991.

Office of the Attorney General: *Consumers advance health care directive: what's important to you* (website): http://ag.ca.gov/consumers/general/adv_hc_dir.htm. Accessed December 6, 2011.

Ohio Hospital Association: Occupational exposure to bloodborne pathogens: OSHA's final rule, *OHA Bull* December 20, 1991.

The Ohio State University Medical Center: *Patient education home* (website): https://patienteducation.osumc.edu/Pages/Home.aspx. Accessed December 6, 2011.

Okamoto GA, Phillips TJ, editors: *Physical medicine and rehabilitation*, Philadelphia, 1984, WB Saunders.

Oregon Association of Hospitals and Health Systems: *Standardization of emergency code calls* (website): http://www.oahhs.org/quality/initiatives/ercodes.html. Accessed December 6, 2011.

OrthoNet: *Amputations II-3* (website): http://www.orthonet.on.ca/amputations-ii-3. Accessed December 6, 2011.

Orthopedics International–Spine: *Lifting without hurting your back* (website): http://www.oispine.com/subject.php?pn=correct-lifting-056. Accessed December 6, 2011.

Orthopedics International–Spine: *Spine care at the office* (website): http://www.oispine.com/subject.php?pn=spine-care-057. Accessed December 6, 2011.

O'Sullivan SB, Schmitz TJ: *Physical rehabilitation: assessment and treatment*, ed 4, Philadelphia, 2001, FA Davis.

O'Sullivan SB, Schmitz TJ: *Physical rehabilitation*, ed 5, Philadelphia, 2006, FA Davis Co.

O'Toole M, editor: *Encyclopedia and dictionary of medicine, nursing and allied health*, Philadelphia, 1992, Saunders.

O'Toole M, editor: *Miller-Keane encyclopedia and dictionary of medicine, nursing, and allied health*, ed 5, Philadelphia, 1992, Saunders.

Page C, Swisher L: *Professionalism in physical therapy history, practice, and development*, Philadelphia, 2005, Saunders.

Page P, Frank CC, Lardner R: *Assessment and treatment of muscle imbalance: the Janda approach*, Champaign, IL, 2010, Human Kinetics.

Palmer ML: Gross muscle testing, *Clin Manage* 5:18-24, 1985.

Palmer ML, Toms J: *Manual for functional training*, ed 3, Philadelphia, 1992, FA Davis.

Paralyzed Veterans of America/Consortium for Spinal Cord Medicine: *Acute management of autonomic dysreflexia: individuals with spinal cord injury presenting to health-care facilities*, ed 2, Washington, DC, 2001, Paralyzed Veterans of America.

Paramedicine.com: *Patient positioning* (website): http://www.paramedicine.com/pmc/Patient_Positions.html. Accessed December 6, 2011.

PartnersAgainstPain.com: *Pain management tools* (website): http://www.partnersagainstpain.com/hcp/pain-assessment/tools.aspx. Accessed December 6, 2011.

Paz JC, Panik M: *Acute care handbook for physical therapists*, Burlington, MA, 1997, Butterworth-Heinemann.

Pellecchia GL, Lugo-Larcheveque N, DeLuca PA: Differential diagnosis in physical therapy evaluation of thigh pain in an adolescent boy, *J Orthop Sports Phys Ther* 23(1):51-55, 1996.

Perme C, Chandrashekar R: Early mobility and walking program for patients in ICU: creating a standard of care, *Am J Crit Care* 8(3):212-220, 2009.

Perry AG, Potter PA: *Clinical nursing skills and techniques*, ed 2, St Louis, 1990, Mosby.

Perry J: *Gait analysis: normal and pathological function*, Thorofare, NJ, 1992, Slack.

Perry J: Kinesiology of lower extremity bracing, *Clin Orthop Relat Res* 102:18-31, 1974.

Person first, Columbus, OH, 1995, AXIS Center for Public Awareness of People with Disabilities.

Phend C: *Early PT in ICU may prevent disability after discharge* (website): http://www.medpagetoday.com/CriticalCare/GeneralCriticalCare/14179. Accessed December 6, 2011.

Phillips AM: Uniform performance of patient care processes: what does it mean and how can we succeed? *Acute Care Perspect* 8(4):2-4, 10-11, 2000.

Polich S, Faynoor SM: Interpreting lab test values, *PT Magazine* 4:76-88, 1996.

Poor posture hurts, San Bruno, CA, 1986, Kramer Communications.

Powell KR. Fever. In Kliegman RM, Behrman RE, Jenson HB, editors: *Nelson textbook of pediatrics*, ed 18, Philadelphia, 2007, Saunders Elsevier.

Preferred Health Choice Mobility and Patient Aid Center: *Measure for wheelchair: how to take simple wheelchair measurements* (website): http://www.phc-online.com/Measure-for-wheelchair_a/6.htm. Accessed December 5, 2011.

Procedures, Springhouse, PA, 1983, Intermed Communications.

PulseOximeterHelp.Com: *How to use a pulse oximeter* (website): http://www.pulseoximeterhelp.com/category/how-to-use-a-pulse-oximeter/. Accessed December 6, 2011.

PulseOximeterHelp.com: *Why you need a pulse oximeter* (website): http://www.pulseoximeterhelp.com/pulse-oximeter-articles/why-you-need-a-pulse-oximeter/. Accessed December 6, 2011.

Purtilo R: *Health professional and patient interaction*, ed 4, Philadelphia, 1990, WB Saunders.

Pyrek KM: *Breaking the chain of infection* (website): http://www.infection-controltoday.com/articles/2002/07/breaking-the-chain-of-infection.aspx. Accessed December 5, 2011.

The Quality Interagency Coordination Task Force: *Patient's rights and responsibilities* (website): www.consumer.gov/qualityhealth/rights.htm. Accessed March 20, 2007.

Quinn E: *Core training is more than just ab exercise* (website): http://sportsmedicine.about.com/od/abdominalcorestrength1/a/NewCore.htm. Accessed December 6, 2011.

Quizlet: *Vital signs flash card sets* (website): http://quizlet.com/subject/vital-signs/. Accessed December 6, 2011.

Ragnarsson KT: *Clinical perspectives on wheelchair selection: prescription considerations and a comparison of conventional and lightweight wheelchairs* (website): http://www.rehab.research.va.gov/mono/wheelchair/ragnarsson.pdf. Accessed December 6, 2011.

Rantz MF, Courtial D: *Lifting, moving and transferring patients*, ed 2, St Louis, 1981, Mosby.

Rasul AT Jr, Wright J: Total joint replacement *rehabilitation* (website): http://emedicine.medscape.com/article/320061-overview. Accessed December 6, 2011.

Rea: *13 Steps to a basic seating posture* (website): www.invacare-rea.com. Accessed December 6, 2011.

Resha D: *Wound care* (website): http://www.vuburncenter.com/downloads/WoundCare.pdf. Accessed December 6, 2011.

Richardson CA, Snijders CJ, Hides JA, et al: The relation between the transversus abdominis muscles, sacroiliac joint mechanics, and low back pain, *Spine* 27(4):399-405, 2002.

Richardson T: *Physical therapy diagnosis, what is a SOAP note?* (website): http://physicaltherapydiagnosis.blogspot.com/2008/01/what-is-soap-note.html. Accessed December 6, 2011.

Romani-Ruby C: *Corrective exercises: swayback posture* (website): http://www.ideafit.com/fitness-library/corrective-exercises-swayback-posture. Accessed December 6, 2011.

Rosenfeld J: *An injury occurring during physical therapy may be the result of the malpractice of the physical therapist* (website): http://www.nursinghomesabuseblog.com/physical-therapy-malpractice/. Accessed December 1, 2011.

Rules and Regulations Occupational Safety and Health Act. *Fed Regist* 56:64, 175, 182, December 1991.

Russek LN: Examination and treatment of a patient with hypermobility syndrome, *Journal of the American Physical Therapy Association* (serial online): http://ptjournal.apta.org/content/80/4/386.full. Accessed December 6, 2011.

Saunders HD: *For your back: a self-help manual*, Minneapolis, MN, 1985, Viking.

Saunders JB, Inman VT, Eberhart HD: The major determinants of gait in normal and pathological gait, *J Bone Joint Surg Am* 35A:543-558, 1953.

Scott R, Cooperman J: *Legal and ethical practice issues in physical therapy*. Presented at: Ohio Physical Therapy Association Meeting, April 16, 1997, Columbus, OH.

Scott RW: Promoting legal awareness in physical and occupational therapy, St Louis, 1997, Mosby.

Scully RM, Barnes MR, editors: *Physical therapy*, Philadelphia, 1989, JB Lippincott.

Shumway-Cook A, Brauer S, Woollacott M: Predicting the probability for falls in community-dwelling older adults using the Timed Up & Go Test, *Phys Ther* 80:896-903, 2000.

Simmers L: *Diversified health occupations*, ed 6, Albany, NY, 2004, Thomson Delmar Learning.

Skaar JR: *Kinesio-taping for the arthritic hip & knee* (website): http://www.orthopaediced.com/theater.php?title=Kinesio-taping%20for%20the%20Arthritic%20Hip%20and%20Knee&loc=videos/Kinesiotaping&name=Janet%20Robinson-Skaar,%20PT&vidtype=Presentation. Accessed December 6, 2011.

Skirven TM, Osterman AL, Fedorczyk, JM, et al: *Rehabilitation of the hand and upper extremity*, ed 6, St Louis, 2011, Mosby.

Slabaugh PB, Nickel VL: Complications with use of the Stryker frame, *J Bone Joint Surg Am* 60A(8):1111-1112, 1978.

Smith EB, Rasmussen AA, Lechner DE, et al: The effects of lumbosacral support belts and abdominal muscle strength on functional lifting ability in healthy women, *Spine (Phila Pa 1976)* 21(3):356-366, 1996.

Smith LK, Weiss EL, Lehmkuhl D: *Brunnstrom's clinical kinesiology*, ed 5, Philadelphia, 1996, FA Davis.

Snyder AR, Parsons JT, Valovich McLeod TC, et al: Using disablement models and clinical outcomes assessment to enable evidence-based athletic training practice, part I: disablement models, *J Athl Train* 43(4):428-436, 2008.

Solway DR, Consalter M, Levinson DJ: Microbial cellulose wound dressing in the treatment of skin tears in the frail elderly. *Wounds* (serial online): http://www.woundsresearch.com/content/microbial-cellulose-wound-dressing-treatment-skin-tears-frail-elderly. Accessed December 6, 2011.

SpiderTech: *How does SpiderTech work?* (website): http://www.nucapmedical.com/explained.html. Accessed December 6, 2011.

Sports Injury Clinic: *Introduction to core stability* (website): http://www.sportsinjuryclinic.net/cybertherapist/corestability.php. Accessed December 6, 2011.

Squidoo: *Plantar fasciitis physical therapy exercises* (website): http://www.squidoo.com/plantar-fasciitis-physical-therapy-exercises. Accessed December 6, 2011.

Steffen TM, Hacker TA, Mollinger L: Age- and gender-related test performance in community dwelling elderly people: Six-Minute Walk Test, Berg Balance Scale, Timed Up & Go Test, and gait speeds, *Phys Ther* 8:128-137, 2002.

Steffen TM, Mollinger LA: Age- and gender-related test performance in community-dwelling adults, *J Neurol Phys Ther* 29:181-188, 2005.

Stiller K: Safety issues that should be considered when mobilizing critically ill patients, *Crit Care Clin* 23:35-53, 2007.

Stucki G: International Classification of Functioning, Disability, and Health (ICF): a promising framework and classification for rehabilitation medicine, *Am J Phys Med Rehabil* 84:733-740, 2005.

Study Stack: *Physical therapy study stacks* (website): http://www.studystack.com/PhysicalTherapy. Accessed December 6, 2011.

Supporting Safer Healthcare: Restraint and seclusion—a hot topic for hospitals (website): http://www.supportingsaferhealthcare.com/2009/02/restraint-and-seclusion-a-hot-topic-for-hospitals-html/. Accessed December 6, 2011.

Swanson MA: *Crutches on the go*, Bellevue, WA, 1974, Medic.

Tate RL: *A compendium of tests, scales and questionnaires: the practitioner's guide to measuring outcomes after acquired brain impairment* (website): http://www.psypress.com/common/sample-chapters/9781841695617.pdf. Accessed December 6, 2011.

Taylor L, Cavenett S, Stepien JM, et al: Removable rigid dressings: a retrospective case-note audit to determine the validity of post-amputation application, *Prosthet Orthot Int* 32(2):223-230, 2008.

Taylor PM, Taylor DK, editors: *Conquering athletic injuries*, Champaign, IL, 1988, Leisure.

Techniques for moving patients, Deerfield, MA, 1989-1990, Dray Publications.

Thomas DR, Rodeheaver GT, Bartolucci AA, et al: Pressure ulcer scale for healing: derivation and validation of the PUSH tool, *Adv Wound Care* 10:96-101, 1997.

Thomas SS, Supan TJ: A comparison of current biomechanical terms, *J Prosthet Orthot* 2(2):107-114, 1990.

Thompson SR: *DeLee, Drez, and Miller's orthopaedic sports medicine*, ed 3, Philadelphia, 2009, Saunders Elsevier.

Transport Accident Commission: *Occupational therapy resources* (website): http://www.tac.vic.gov.au/jsp/content/NavigationController.do?areaID=22&tierID=1&navID=9D709A5E7F000001013259CA41FC8C59&navLink=null&pageID=1420. Accessed December 6, 2011.

Tuzson A: *How high is too high? INR and acute care physical therapy* (website): http://www.thefreelibrary.com/How+high+is+too+high%3F+INR+and+acute+care+physical+therapy.-a0200343149. Accessed December 6, 2011.

TVclip.BIZ: *Maintaining a sterile field* (website): http://www.tvclip.biz/video/aPl2XdGF4JM/maintaining-a-sterile-field.html. Accessed December 6, 2011.

TVclip.BIZ: *Sterile dressing sutured wound* (website): http://www.tvclip.biz/video/1FEf_HH-tWE/sterile-dressing-sutured-wound-courtesy-of-ati.html. Accessed December 6, 2011.

TVclip.BIZ: *Wound irrigation and culture and wet-to-dry dressing change* (website): http://www.tvclip.biz/video/dnh2gTifyo4/wound-irrigation-and-culture-and-wet-to-dry-dressing-change.html. Accessed December 6, 2011.

Umiker W: *Management skills for the new health care supervisor*, Rockville, MD, 1988, Aspen.

Umphred DA, editor: *Neurological rehabilitation*, ed 2, St Louis, 1990, Mosby.

Universal Design Alliance: *FAQs on universal design* (website): http://www.universaldesign.org/faqs_universaldesign.htm. Accessed December 6, 2011.

Universal Design Living Laboratory: *Resources: links to third party sites* (website): http://www.udll.com/resources/index.cfm. Accessed December 6, 2011.

University of California Office of the President: *Legal Medical Record Standards, Policy No. 9420* (website): http://www.ucop.edu/ucophome/coordrev/policy/legal-medical-record-policy.pdf. Accessed December 5, 2011.

University of Iowa Carver College of Medicine: *Pain assessment in advanced dementia scale (PAINAD)* (website): http://www.healthcare.uiowa.edu/igec/tools/pain/PAINAD.pdf. Accessed December 6, 2011.

University of Kansas Medical Center: *Proper patient positioning* (website): http://coa.kumc.edu/gec/modules/presulc/physicaltherapy/proper_patient_positioning.htm#Prone. Accessed December 6, 2011.

University of Missouri, School of Health Professions, Department of Physical Therapy: *Lab values* (website): http://web.missouri.edu/~proste/lab/. Accessed December 6, 2011.

University of Oklahoma Health Sciences Center: *Body mechanics and patient transfers* (website): http://moon.ouhsc.edu/belledge/ptcare/bodmech.pdf. Accessed December 1, 2011.

U.S. Census Bureau: *S1802, Selected economic characteristics for the civilian noninstitutionalized population by disability status, data set: 2006, American Community Survey* (website): http://factfinder.census.gov/servlet/STTable?_bm=y&-state=st&-qr_name=ACS_2006_EST_G00_S1802&-ds_name=ACS_2006_EST_G00_&-CONTEXT=st&-redoLog=true&-_caller=geoselect&-geo_id=01000US&-format=&-lang=en. Accessed December 6, 2011.

U.S. Census Bureau: *S1810, Disability characteristics, data set: 2009, American Community Survey 1-year estimates*, (website): http://factfinder.census.gov/servlet/STTable?ds_name=ACS_2009_1YR_G00_&qr_name=ACS_2009_1YR_G00_S1810&_lang=en. Accessed December 6, 2011.

U.S. Department of Health and Human Services: *Health information privacy, all case examples* (website):. http://www.hhs.gov/ocr/privacy/hipaa/enforcement/examples/allcases.html#case11. Accessed December 6, 2011.

U.S. Department of Health and Human Services: *OCR privacy brief: summary of the HIPAA privacy rule* (website): http://www.hhs.gov/ocr/privacy/hipaa/understanding/summary/privacysummary.pdf. Accessed December 6, 2011.

U.S. Department of Health and Human Services: *Office for Civil Rights—HIPAA* (website): www.hhs.gov/ocr/hipaa. Accessed March 15, 2007.

U.S. Department of Health & Human Services: *Summary of the HIPAA privacy rule* (website): http://www.hhs.gov/ocr/privacy/hipaa/understanding/summary/index.html. Accessed December 6, 2011.

U.S. Department of Health & Human Services: *Understanding health information privacy* (website): http://www.hhs.gov/ocr/privacy/hipaa/understanding/index.html. Accessed December 6, 2011.

U.S. Department of Health and Human Services, Agency for Healthcare Research and Quality: *Patient safety and medical errors* (website): http://www.ahrq.gov/qual/errorsix.htm. Accessed December 6, 2011.

U.S. Department of Health and Human Services, Agency for Healthcare Research and Quality: *Prehypertension is a considerable health risk, particularly for people age 45 and over* (website): http://www.ahrq.gov/news/press/pr2004/prehyppr.htm. Accessed March 11, 2007.

U.S. Department of Health & Human Services, Agency for Healthcare Research and Quality: *PSNet, Patient Safety Network, glossary* (website): http://www.psnet.ahrq.gov/glossary.aspx#S. Accessed December 6, 2011.

U.S. Department of Health and Human Services, Agency for Policy and Research: *Pressure ulcers in adults: prediction and prevention (clinical guideline 3, AHCPR 92-0047)*, Washington, DC, 1992, U.S. Department of Health and Human Services, Agency for Policy and Research.

U.S. Department of Health and Human Services, Centers for Medicare & Medicaid Services: *42 CFR Parts 410, 416, and 419 Medicare program: changes to the ospital Outpatient Prospective Payment System and CY 2011 payment rates; changes to the Ambulatory Surgical Center Payment System and CY 2011 payment rates; changes to payments to hospitals for graduate medical education costs; corrections* (website): http://edocket.access.gpo.gov/2011/pdf/2011-5674.pdf. Accessed December 5, 2011.

U.S. Department of Health and Human Services, Centers for Medicare & Medicaid Services: *Medicare and Medicaid programs; hospital conditions of participation: patients' rights* (website): cms.gov. Accessed January 9, 2011.

U.S. Department of Health and Human Services, National Institutes of Health: *NHLBI issues new high blood pressure clinical practice guidelines* (website): www.nhlbi.nih.gov/new/press/03-05-14.htm. Accessed December 6, 2011.

U.S. Department of Health and Human Services, Office of Minority Health: *National standards on culturally and linguistically appropriate services (CLAS)* (website): http://minorityhealth.hhs.gov/templates/browse.aspx?lvl=2&lvlID=15. Accessed December 6, 2011.

U.S. Department of Justice: *1991 ADA Standards for Accessible Design* (website): http://www.usdoj.gov/crt/ada/stdspdf.htm. Accessed December 6, 2011.

U.S. Department of Justice: *2010 ADA standards for accessible design* (website): http://www.ada.gov/2010ADAstandards_index.htm. Accessed December 5, 2011.

U.S. Department of Justice: *28 CFR, Part 35, Nondiscrimination on the basis of disability in state and local government services* (website): http://www.ada.gov/archive/curbrule.txt. Accessed December 5, 2011.

U.S. Department of Justice: *A guide to disability rights laws* (website): http://www.ada.gov/cguide.htm. Accessed December 6, 2011.

U.S. Department of Justice: *ADA home page* (website): http://www.ada.gov/index.html. Accessed December 6, 2011.

U.S. Department of Justice: *Americans With Disabilities Act of 1990, as amended* (website): http://www.ada.gov/pubs/ada.htm. Accessed December 5, 2011.

U.S. Department of Justice: *Fact sheet: adoption of the 2010 standards for accessible design* (website): http://www.ada.gov/regs2010/factsheets/2010_Standards_factsheet.html. Accessed December 5, 2011.

U.S. Department of Justice: *Revised ADA regulations implementing Title II and Title III* (website): http://www.ada.gov/regs2010/ADAregs2010.htm. Accessed December 5, 2011.

U.S. Department of Labor, Occupational Safety and Health Administration: *Ergonomics* (website): http://www.osha.gov/SLTC/ergonomics/index.html. Accessed December 6, 2011.

U.S. Department of Labor, Occupational Safety and Health Administration: *Guidelines for nursing homes: ergonomics for the prevention of musculoskeletal disorders* (website): http://www.osha.gov/ergonomics/guidelines/nursinghome/final_nh_guidelines.html. Accessed December 6, 2011.

U.S. Department of Labor, Occupational Safety and Health Administration: *Healthcare wide hazards: ergonomics* (website): www.osha.gov/SLTC/etools/hospital/hazards/ergo/ergo.html. Accessed December 6, 2011.

U.S. Department of Veterans Affairs, Department of Defense: *VA/DOD clinical practice guideline for management for rehabilitation of lower limb amputation, January 2008* (website): http://www.healthquality.va.gov/amputation/amp_sum_508.pdf. Accessed December 5, 2011.

U.S. Equal Employment Opportunity Commission: *Americans with Disabilities Act Title I technical assistance manual*, Washington, DC, January 1992, U.S. Equal Employment Opportunity Commission.

U.S. Equal Employment Opportunity Commission: *Section 902 definition of the term disability, notice concerning the Americans With Disabilities Act Amendments Act of 2008* (website): http://www.eeoc.gov/policy/docs/902cm.html. Accessed December 6, 2011.

Van Hook FW, Demonbreun D, Weiss BD: Ambulatory devices for chronic gait disorders in the elderly, *Am Fam Physician* 67(8):1717-1724, 2003.

van Velzen AD, Nederhand MJ, Emmelot CH, et al: Early treatment of trans-tibial amputees: retrospective analysis of early fitting and elastic bandaging. *Prosthetics and Orthotics International* (serial online): http://poi.sagepub.com/content/29/1/3.abstract. Accessed December 6, 2011.

Vaughn H: *Flexion rotation test (FRT), description of how to perform flexion rotation test (FRT) with CROM device* (website): http://www.youtube.com/watch?v=HlbDCw5tMX4&NR=1. Accessed December 6, 2011.

Victoria University: *Critical care nursing at Victoria University: burn injuries and management* (website): staff.vu.edu.au. Accessed March 11, 2007.

Videosurf: *The new nursing assistant: measuring vital signs* (website): http://www.videosurf.com/video/the-new-nursing-assistant-measuring-vital-signs-140961946. Accessed December 6, 2011.

Videosurf: *The new nursing assistant: positioning* (website): http://www.videosurf.com/video/the-new-nursing-assistant-positioning-1246772322?vlt=kosmix. Accessed December 6, 2011.

Villarruel A, Denyes M: Pain assessment in children: theoretical and empirical validity. *ANS Adv Nurs Sci* 14:31-39, 1991.

Voss DE, Ionta MK, Myers BJ: *Proprioceptive neuromuscular facilitation*, ed 3, Philadelphia, 1985, Harper & Row.

Wall L: *Physical therapy intervention ICU* (website): http://depts.washington.edu/pulmcc/conferences/lungday/Wall.pdf. Accessed December 6, 2011.

Warden V, Hurley AC, Volicer L: Development and psychometric evaluation of the Pain Assessment in Advanced Dementia (PAINAD) scale, *J Am Med Dir Assoc* 4(1):9-15, 2003.

Watkinson A: *End feel—normal and abnormal* (website): http://www.watkinson.co.nz/end_feel.htm. Accessed January 4, 2011.

WebMD: *Diabetes Health Center: diabetes overview* (website): diabetes.webmd.com/default.htm. Accessed December 6, 2011.

WebMD: *Fitness: increasing core stability* (website): http://www.webmd.com/fitness-exercise/core-stabilization-76. Accessed December 6, 2011.

Weiss M: *Class notes and handouts*, Canton, OH, 1982, Stark Technical College.

Weiss M: *Class notes and handouts*, Columbus, OH, 1875, Physical Therapy Division, School of Allied Medical Professions, The Ohio State University.

West K: *The CDC's new hand washing guidelines* (website): http://grayless.com/firstresponder/The%20CDCs%20New%20Hand%20Washing%20Guidelines.pdf. Accessed December 6, 2011.

Wilner LS, Arnold R: *#126 Pain assessment in the cognitively impaired* (website): http://www.eperc.mcw.edu/display/router.aspx?docid=72630&. Accessed December 6, 2011.

Wilson AB Jr: *Wheelchairs: a prescription guide*, Charlottesville, VA, 1986, Rehabilitation.

Wintz MN: Variations in current manual muscle testing, *Phys Ther Rev* 39:466-475, 1959.

Wolf L: *Clinical decision making in physical therapy*, Philadelphia, 1985, FA Davis.

Wong CK, Edelstein JE: Effect of Unna postoperative dressings on timing of prosthetic fitting and functional outcome [abstract], *J Orthop Sports Phys Ther* 27(1):69, 1998.

Wong DL, Baker C: Pain in children: comparison of assessment scales, *Pediatr Nurs* 14:9-17, 1988.

Wong DL, Baker C: *Reference manual for the Wong-Baker FACES Pain Rating Scale*, Duarte GA, 2000, City of Hope Pain/Palliative Care Resource Center.

Wong K: *Rethinking the standard in preprosthetic rehab* (website): http://physical-therapy.advanceweb.com/Article/Rethinking-the-Standard-in–Preprosthetic-Rehab.aspx. Accessed December 6, 2011.

Wood EC, Becker PD: *Beard's massage*, ed 4, Philadelphia, 1990, WB Saunders.

Wood LA, editor: *Nursing skills for allied health services*, Philadelphia, 1975, WB Saunders.

World Confederation for Physical Therapy: *Declaration of principle—informed consent* (website): www.wcpt.org/policies/principles/consent.php. Accessed October 8, 2010.

World Health Organization: *Towards a common language for functioning, disability and health: ICF* (website):. http://www.who.int/classifications/icf/training/icfbeginnersguide.pdf. Accessed December 6, 2011.

Wound Care Information Network: *Wound care product and category index* (website): http://www.medicaledu.com/prodindx.htm. Accessed December 6, 2011.

Youdas JW, Kotajarvi BJ, Padgett DJ, et al: Partial weight-bearing gait using conventional assistive devices, *Arch Phys Med Rehabil* 86(3):394-398, 2005.

YouTube: *Lite gait training* (website): http://www.youtube.com/watch?v=LBvFUdfvWS0&feature=related. Accessed December 6, 2011.

YouTube: Measurement of the patient for a wheelchair seating system (website): http://www.youtube.com/watch?v=-SF-CYWRGww. Accessed December 6, 2011.

Zeller JL, Lynm C, Glass RM: *Pressure ulcers* (website): http://jama.ama-assn.org/content/296/8/1020.full. Accessed December 6, 2011.

OUTPATIENT PHYSICAL THERAPY
Initial Evaluation Page 1

Identification

Diagnosis:_____ Date of Onset/Surg _____

Learning Needs Assessment: How do you learn easiest?

☐ Visual/written ☐ Auditory ☐ Demonstration ☐ Other_____

Educational Assessment & Motivational Level: ☐ Asks questions ☐ Eager to learn

☐ Anxious ☐ Uncooperative ☐ Unable to answer ☐ Seems uninterested ☐ Denies need for education

Barriers to Treatment: (cognitive/emotional, physical/developmental, cultural):

Resolution to Identified Barriers:

Do you feel safe at home? ☐ Yes ☐ No   If no, does pt want to see a social worker? ☐ Yes ☐ No

Present History/Reason for Referral:

☐ X-ray ☐ MRI ☐ CT Scan ☐ Bone Scan ☐ EMG ☐ Precautions:
Results:

Pain Assessment:

Constant/Intermittent

Location/Quality:

None   Worst
0 1 2 3 4 5 6 7 8 9 10

Symptoms ↑with:

Best _____ Worst _____

Symptoms ↓ with:

Hand Dominance ☐ Right ☐ Left

Functional Status: (* denotes pain)	Pre-onset:	Current:	Occupation:
Self-care			
Transitional Mobility			Status:
Driving			
Walking			Recreation:
Stairs			
			Other:

PMH:

☐ Heart ☐ Diabetes
☐ HBP ☐ COPD
☐ Pregnancy ☐ Cancer
☐ VNA

Medication: Allergies:

Signature: _____ Date: _____ Time: _____am/pm

Appendix 1   Outpatient physical therapy initial evaluation form. (From Roberto MD: *Outpatient initial evaluation forms,* Melrose, MA, 2009, Hallmark Health System.)

Continued

OUTPATIENT PHYSICAL THERAPY
Initial Evaluation   Page 2

Identification

NEUROLOGICAL:

Sensation:

☐ WNL   ☐ Altered   ☐ Sharp   ☐ Dull

Location: _____

Dermatomes:	**Myotomes:**
☐ WNL	☐ WNL
☐ Affected: _____	☐ Affected: _____

OTHER:

Reflexes: ✓ WNL   -- Hypo   + Hyper

	Left	Right
Biceps (C5, C6)	_____	_____
Triceps (C7)	_____	_____
Brachioradialis (C5, C6)	_____	_____
Patella Tendon (L4)	_____	_____
Achilles Tendon (S1)	_____	_____

POSTURE: ☐ WNL   ☐ NA

GAIT ☐ WNL ☐ NA

ACTIVE MOVEMENTS: ☐ N/A   ☐ WNL

Key: ● End ROM   ✕ Pain Limiting   ↬ Deviation

Cervical: FB   SBL   SBR   RL   BB   RR

Lumbar: FB   SBL   SBR   RL   BB   RR

PASSIVE INTERVERTEBRAL MOVEMENT: ☐ N/A   ☐ WNL

Segment	Motion	Grade

Key:
0 Ankylosed
1 Mod Restriction
2 Min Restriction
3 Normal
4 Min Increase
5 Mod Increase
6 Unstable

MCKENZIE: ☐ NA	PDM	ERP		PDM	ERP
Pretest pain standing			Pretest pain sitting		
FIS			PRO		
Rep FIS			Rep PRO		
EIS			RET		
Rep EIS			Rep RET		
Pretest pain lying			RET EXT		
FIL			Rep RET EXT		
Rep FIL			Pretest pain lying		
EIL			RET		
Rep EIL			Rep RET		
SGIS (R)			RET EXT		
Rep SGIS (R)			Rep RET EXT		
SGIS (L)					
Rep SGIS (L)					

Signature: _____   Date: _____   Time: _____am/pm

Appendix 1, cont'd

H OUTPATIENT REHABILITATION SERVICES
Patient-Specific Functional Scale

Identification

The Patient-Specific Functional Scale

This useful questionnaire can be used to quantify activity limitation and measure functional outcome for patients with any orthopedic condition.

Clinician to read and fill in below: Complete at the end of the history and prior to physical examination.

Initial Assessment:

I am going to ask you to identify up to three important activities that you are unable to do or are having difficulty with as a result of your _____ problem. Today, are there any activities that you are unable to do or having difficulty with because of your _____ problem? (Clinician: show scale to patient and have the patient rate each activity).

Follow-up Assessments:

When I assessed you on (state previous assessment date), you told me that you had difficulty with (read all activities from list at a time). Today, do you still have difficulty with: (read and have patient score each item in the list)?

Patient-specific activity scoring scheme (Point to one number):

0	1	2	3	4	5	6	7	8	9	10

Unable to perform activity

Able to perform at the same level as before injury or problem

(Date and Score)

Activity	Initials	Time				
1.						
2.						
3.						
4.						
5.						
Additional						

Total score = sum of the activity scores/number of activities
Minimum detectable change (90%CI) for average score = 2 points
Minimum detectable change (90%CI) for single activity score = 3 points

Appendix 2 Patient-specific functional scale. (PSFS developed by: Stratford, P., Gill, C., Westaway, M., & Binkley, J. (1995). Assessing disabillity and change on individual patients: a report of a patient specific measure. Physiotherapy Canada, 47, 258-263. Reproduced with the permission of the authors.)

⌘ OUTPATIENT PHYSICAL THERAPY

□ **Malden** □ **Medford** □ **Melrose** □ **Reading**

Identification

□ **INITIAL PLAN OF CARE**

CURRENT PROBLEM LIST: Initial Pain ____/10	STG'S (2 WEEKS):	LTG'S 4 WEEKS:
□ 1. Current Pain ____/10	↓'d pain _____ to_____/10	↓'d pain _____ to _____/10
□ 2. Decreased Strength		
□ 3. Decreased ROM		
□ 4.		
□ 5.		
□ 6.		
□ 7.		
□ 8. No HEP	Independent w/ current HEP	Independent w/ current HEP

CURRENT TREATMENT   PLAN: (Check All That Apply)

□ Hot /Cold Pack   □ Electrical Stimulation   □ Bike/UBE/Treadmill   □ Iontophoresis _____

□ Therapeutic Exercise   □ Biofeedback/NMR   □ Balance/Gait Training   □ Ultrasound/ Phonophoresis

□ Functional Activities   □ Paraffin   □ Body Mechanics   □ Traction (Mechanical/Manual)

□ Joint Mobilization   □ Whirlpool   □ Bracing/Taping   □ Soft Tissue Mobilization

□ Home Exercise Program   □ Isokinetic   □ Home ES   □ Stretching/AROM/PROM

□ Patient/Family Education

Frequency: _____ times/week   **Duration:** _____ weeks

PATIENT GOALS/PERCEPTION OF TREATMENT:

REHABILITATION POTENTIAL: □ Excellent   □ Good   □ Fair   □ Poor

_____   _____   _____am/pm

Therapist's Signature   Date   Time

I have received the attendance policy, pain management literature and my intended treatment plan and I agree to participate accordingly.

I certify that the outpatient services outlined above are required and are authorized by me with a written plan of treatment to be reviewed by me every 30 days. This patient is under my care and is in need of Physical Therapy.

_____

Patient/Guardian Signature

_____

_____

MD Signature   **Date**

Medicare mandates that the MD sign & date all Plans of Care within a timely manner.

Appendix 3   Initial plan of care form. (From Roberto MD: *Outpatient rehabilitation forms,* Melrose, MA, 2009, Hallmark Health System.)

OUTPATIENT THERAPY

Identification

INTERIM NOTE
❑ SportsAid ❑ 101 Main ❑ MWH ❑ Reading

Note #_____ Please refer to treatment flow sheet & Plan of Care for specifics of patient treatment.

Pain/Subjective: /10 **Pain Meds:** ❑ No ❑ Yes _____

Objective:
ROM

Strength

Function

Other

Treatment Goals:
❑ Progressing as anticipated ❑ Progressing slowly ❑ Not progressing ❑ Revised ❑ Met

Assessment:

Plan:
❑ Continue Treatment Per POC

Therapist Signature: _____ **Date:** _____ **Time:** _____ am/pm

Note #_____ Please refer to treatment flow sheet & Plan of Care for specifics of patient treatment.

Pain/Subjective: /10 **Pain Meds:** ❑ No ❑ Yes _____

Objective:
ROM

Strength

Function

Other

Treatment Goals:
❑ Progressing as anticipated ❑ Progressing slowly ❑ Not progressing ❑ Revised ❑ Met

Assessment:

Plan:
❑ Continue Treatment Per POC

Therapist Signature: _____ **Date:** _____ **Time:** _____ am/pm

Appendix 4 Interim note form. (From Roberto MD: *Outpatient rehabilitation forms,* Melrose, MA, 2009, Hallmark Health System.)

OUTPATIENT PHYSICAL THERAPY
Patient Education & Home Exercise Flowsheet

Identification

DATE	TIME	PATIENT EDUCATION	HOME EXERCISE PROGRAM	COMMENTS
		❑ Demo ❑ Handout ❑ Verbal	❑ See Handout	
		❑ Demo ❑ Handout ❑ Verbal	❑ See Handout	
		❑ Demo ❑ Handout ❑ Verbal	❑ See Handout	
		❑ Demo ❑ Handout ❑ Verbal	❑ See Handout	
		❑ Demo ❑ Handout ❑ Verbal	❑ See Handout	
		❑ Demo ❑ Handout ❑ Verbal	❑ See Handout	
		❑ Demo ❑ Handout ❑ Verbal	❑ See Handout	
		❑ Demo ❑ Handout ❑ Verbal	❑ See Handout	

KEY:
1. Pain Management
2. Transitional Mobility
3. Static Postural Education
4. Dynamic Postural Education
5. Ergonomics
6. Body Mechanics
7. Knowledge of Injury/Diagnosis
8. Splint Education
9. Family Education
10. Adaptive Equipment Education

Appendix 5   Patient education and home exercise flow sheet. (From Roberto MD: *Outpatient rehabilitation forms,* Melrose, MA, 2009, Hallmark Health System.)

H OUTPATIENT OCCUPATIONAL THERAPY
SPLINT EVALUATION

Identification

Diagnosis:_____ Date of Onset/Surg _____

Learning Needs Assessment: How do you learn easiest?

☐ Visual/written ☐ Auditory ☐ Demonstration ☐ Other_____

Educational Assessment & Motivational Level: ☐ Asks questions ☐ Eager to learn

☐ Anxious ☐ Uncooperative ☐ Unable to answer ☐ Seems uninterested ☐ Denies need for education

Barriers to Treatment: (cognitive/emotional, physical/developmental, cultural):

Resolution to Identified Barriers:

Do you feel safe at home? ☐ Yes ☐ No If no, does pt want to see a social worker? ☐ Yes ☐ No

PMH:	**Medications/Allergies:**	**Precautions:**

Present History/Reason for Referral: Vocation:

Hand Dominance ☐ R ☐ L

Results: ☐ X-ray ☐ MRI ☐ CT scan ☐ Bone Scan ☐ EMG ☐ VNA ☐ Other

Pain Assessment: Location/Quality: Constant/Intermittent None Worst 0 1 2 3 4 5 6 7 8 9 10 Symptoms ↑with: Symptoms ↓ with:	**Sensation:** ☐ NT ☐ WFL **Edema:** ☐ NT ☐ WFL
ROM: ☐ NT ☐ WFL	**Strength:** ☐ NT ☐ WFL

Treatment Summary:

Type of Splint fabricated: _____

☐ Patient instructed in wear, care & skin precautions

☐ Patient/other is independent in splint donning/doffing

☐ Patient provided with written information re: wear/care/precautions for home

☐ Patient educated re: diagnosis, work modifications as appropriate _____

☐ Other

Signature: _____ Date: _____ Time:_____ ☐ am ☐ pm

I certify that the outpatient services outlined above are required and are authorized by me. The above custom-made /fitted splint was medically necessary for this patient who is under my care and is in need of Occupational Therapy.

_____   _____
MD Signature   **Date**

Appendix 6   Splint evaluation form. (From Roberto MD: Outpatient Initial Evaluation Forms, OT. Melrose, MA, 2009, Hallmark Health System.)

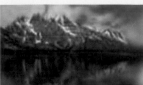

Lakeside Rehab
123 Lakeside Drive
Colorado Springs, Co   80917

(888) 401-4400

Fax (615) 259-3605

Physical Therapy	# Initial Evaluation / Examination	Page 1 of 2

Patient Name: Willow, William	**Date:** 06/12/07	
Medical Record #: HK- 987654	**DOB:** 02/20/51	
Account #: HWC - 8765	**Treating Clinician:** Thomas Hook, DPT, OCS	
Provider: Rehab Clinic of Colorado Springs		
Provider #: 25489631		

Patient Information

Address: 956 Hamleton Street	**Physician:** John Nutting, MD	
B-89	**Physician #:** 1235	
Colorado Springs, Colorado 80923		
Occupation: Carpenter	**# of Approved Visits:** 10	
Gender: Male	**Medicare #:** n/a	
Contact Person: Mary Willow	**Medicaid #:** n/a	

Rehabilitation Information / History

	Onset Date	Code	Description
Primary Diagnosis:	03/06/07	892.1	Open Wound Of Foot Except Toe(S) Alone, Complicated
Other Diagnosis:	01/01/99	357.2	Polyneuropathy In Diabetes

Preferred Practice Pattern:	Integumentary D: Impaired integumentary integrity associated w/full-thickness skin involvement/scar formation
Recent Physical Therapy:	Outpatient rehab clinic - within the last sixty days
Prior Functional Status:	Straight cane - Mild pain or limitation in ambulation, work, IADL's or recreation
Required Equipment:	Debridement supplies
Weight Bearing Status:	Right lower extremity - 33% partial weight bearing
Safety Measures:	Instruct patient and/or family in safety precautions Protect against falls and injury
Rehabilitative Prognosis:	Good rehab potential to reach and maintain prior level of function
Mental Status:	Alert - slightly confused - able to follow 3 or more step directions
Concerns that led to PT:	Decreased functional ability secondary to progression of diagnosis
System Review, History:	Mr. Willow has a history of insulin dependent diabetes for over 8 years. He step on a nail and received a puncture wound to his right foot early March. The wound has significantly deteriorated over the past 3 months.

Patient has a history of behavioral health risks: **Yes**

Patient has been a smoker for years and inconsistent with insulin routine.

Patient / Caregiver concur with established goals: **Yes**

Emotional response to health status: Fair	**Reported Eating Habits:** Fair	
Patient's communication skills: Good	**Reported Sleeping Patterns:** Good	
Knowledge of Exercise and Fitness: Fair	**Reported Energy Level:** Fair	
Frequency of Exercise sessions per week: 3		

Patient is aware of and understands his/her diagnosis and prognosis: **Yes**

Functional Measures

Ambulation: Even Terrain	**Distance**
Current Level: Straight cane - Independent with difficulty	200 Feet
Goal: Straight cane - Independent	>1,000'

Appendix 7   Electronic example of an initial evaluation/examination form for a patient with a wound. (Courtesy The Rehab Documentation Company, Inc.)

Physical Therapy ## Initial Evaluation / Examination

Patient Name: Willow, William	**Date:** 06/12/07	
Medical Record #: HK- 987654	**DOB:** 02/20/51	
Account #: HWC - 8765	**Treating Clinician:** Thomas Hook, DPT, OCS	
Provider: Rehab Clinic of Colorado Springs		
Provider #: 25489631		

Ambulation: Uneven Terrain	**Distance**
Current Level: Straight cane - Limited - Minimal assistance	40 Feet
Goal: Straight cane - Independent	100 Feet

Stair Climbing	**Steps**
Current Level: Straight cane - Independent with railing with difficulty	3 Steps
Goal: Straight cane - Independent with railing	10 Steps

Functional characteristics and analysis: Secondary to the ulcer on the lateral side of patient's right foot, he is unable to wear a shoe and is only 50% partial weight bearing. As a result he has much difficulty in ambulating and in climbing up and down stairs.

Impairment Goals; Short Term: Pain is decreased by 50% in 2 weeks
Weight-bearing status is improved by 50% in 2 weeks

Functional Goals; Long Term: Ambulation is improved to prior level of function
Stair climbing is improved to prior level of function

Physical Findings

Wound Care

Wound Care Site #: 1	Location: Foot - right - malleolus (lateral) Stage: III

Measurements: (cm) Length: 24	Width: 30	Depth: 15

Drainage: Moderate, Dark yellow

Infection: Pseudomonas

Characterstics: Foul Odor; Eschar; Inflammation; Associated Pain; Necrotic Tissue

Risk Factors: Nutritionally Compromised

Anticipated Goals:

Gait, locomotion, and balance are improved
Performance of and independence in ADL's and IADL's are increased
Wound and soft tissue healing is enhanced

Additional Comments: The circulation in both lower extremities is significantly impaired secondary to diabetes. The puncture wound has deteriorated to the above dimensions and the wound is now infected. Patient is taking an oral antibiotic and applying antibiotic ointment to the affected area BID. The necrotic tissue is tightly packed with some eschar. The patient will benefit greatly from selective debridement.

Interventions (CPT Code)

Physical Therapy Evaluation 97001

Wound Care Selective > 20 Sq CM 97598

Frequency of PT: Three times weekly

Duration of PT: 4 weeks

Thomas Hook, PT	06/14/07
Thomas Hook, DPT, OCS	Date
State License #: TN #76565	

Appendix 7, cont'd

Lakeside Rehab

123 Lakeside Drive
Colorado Springs, Co 80917

(888) 401-4400

Fax (615) 259-3605

Physical Therapy   # Initial Evaluation / Examination   Page 1 of 3

Patient Name:	Flintstone, Frederick	**Date:** 01/15/07
Medical Record #:	123	**DOB:** 08/02/61
Account #:	1234567892	**Treating Clinician:** Thomas Hook, PT
Provider:	Lakeside Rehabilitation	
Provider #:	25489631	

Patient Information

Address:	123 Opry Way	**Physician:**	James L. Smith, MD
		Physician #:	123
	Nashville, Tennessee 37203		
Occupation:	Engineer	**# of Approved Visits:**	12
Gender:	Male	**Medicare #:**	111-22-2333A
Contact Person:	Wilma Flintstone	**Medicaid #:**	

Rehabilitation Information / History

	Onset Date	Code	Description
Primary Diagnosis:	12/25/06	844.2	Sprain Of Cruciate Ligament Of Knee
Other Diagnosis:	07/11/07	781.2	Abnormality Of Gait

Preferred Practice Pattern: Musculoskeletal E: Impaired joint mobility, motor function, muscle performance, ROM associated w/localized inflammation

Recent Physical Therapy: Outpatient rehab clinic - within the last sixty days

Prior Functional Status: Independent with no pain or limitation in ambulation, IADL's, work or recreation

Required Equipment: Ace wrap for knee; Crutches

Weight Bearing Status: Right lower extremity - 25% partial weight bearing

Safety Measures: Ambulate with an assistive device & assistance of another person
Instruct patient and/or family in safety precautions
Progressive activity as tolerated

Rehabilitative Prognosis: Excellent rehab potential to reach and maintain prior level of function

Mental Status: Alert and oriented in all spheres - cooperative and motivated

Concerns that led to PT: Decreased functional ability secondary to pain or increased pain

System Review, History: This 45 y. o. male presents with a diagnosis of right anterior cruciate ligament sprain with an onset date of 12/25/06 when he fell down the porch steps while carrying packages. He is seen initially on this date for evaluation and treatment by this therapist due to persistent pain and limited ambulation. Previous medical history of insignificance. The patient is motivated to participate in treatment to achieve his functional goal of propelling his car and returning to work in rock quarry.

Patient has a history of behavioral health risks:	**No**
Patient / Caregiver concur with established goals:	**Yes**
Patient is aware of and understands his/her diagnosis and prognosis:	**Yes**

Functional Measures

Ambulation: Even Terrain	**Distance**
Current Level: Crutches - Supervision - Standby assistance	100 Feet
Goal: No assistive device - Independent with difficulty	>1,000'

Appendix 8   Electronic example of an adult physical therapy initial evaluation/examination form. (Courtesy The Rehab Documentation Company, Inc.)

Physical Therapy   # Initial Evaluation / Examination   Page 2 of 3

Patient Name: Flintstone, Frederick		**Date:** 01/15/07	
Medical Record #: 123		**DOB:** 08/02/61	
Account #: 1234567892		**Treating Clinician:** Thomas Hook, PT	
Provider: Lakeside Rehabilitation			
Provider #: 25489631			

Ambulation: Uneven Terrain	**Distance**
Current Level: Crutches - Extensive - Moderate assistance	35 Feet
Goal: Straight cane - Independent	100 Feet

Stair Climbing	**Steps**
Current Level: Crutches - Extensive - Moderate assistance	4 Steps
Goal: Straight cane - Independent	15 Steps

Tolerance to IADLs

Current Level: Moderate - Severe pain and limitation during and/or after a specific IADL affecting performance

Goal: No pain nor limitation during and/or after a specific IADL affecting performance

Tolerance to Work Activities

Current Level: Moderate - Severe pain and limitation in a specific work activity affecting performance

Goal: No pain and limitation in a specific work activity affecting performance

Functional characteristics and analysis: Mr. Flintstone is having difficulty in ambulation and requires moderate assistance with crutches on uneven terrain to maintain 25% weight bearing status for the right lower extremity. Due to this limitation, he is not able to propel his car, or climb into the crane for work at the quarry.

Impairment Goals; Short Term: Joint inflammation, or restriction & pain are reduced by 50% in 2 weeks
Pain is decreased by 50% in 2 weeks

Functional Goals; Long Term: Ambulation/stair climbing are improved to prior level of function
Work performance in related activities is improved to prior level of function

Physical Findings

Pain

Site: Joint Pain - Knee - Right; At Rest 5/10; With Activity 8/10; Dull; Cramping; Radiating

Exacerbating Factors: At rest interrupting sleep; Weight bearing beyond recommendations; Extended periods of time without joint elevation

Relieving Factors: Ice to the affected area; Elevation of effected extremity

Goals for Pain: Decrease pain at rest and during weight bearing activities to 0/10.

Pain Medication: Non-Prescription

Additional Comments: Mr. Flintstone is taking Advil 3 times daily for pain.

Dynamic Balance

Current Level: 1/5 Berg Balance Scale -Scored 0-12 High risk of falls

Goal: 5/5 Berg Balance Scale -Scored 50-56 Low risk of falls

Special Orthopedic Tests of Extremities	
Knee - Anterior drawer test - Indicates a tear of the anterior cruciate ligament	Positive
Knee - Apley compression test - Indicates a meniscus tear	Negative

Palpation

Location: Joint - knee - Right
Finding: Edema - generalized and moderate
Location: Joint - knee - Right
Finding: Joint restriction - moderate
Location: Joint - knee - Right
Finding: Pain - moderate with palpation

Continued

Initial Evaluation / Examination

Patient Name:	Flintstone, Frederick	**Date:**	01/15/07
Medical Record #:	123	**DOB:**	08/02/61
Account #:	1234567892	**Treating Clinician:**	Thomas Hook, PT
Provider:	Lakeside Rehabilitation		
Provider #:	25489631		

Girth

Location:	Knee Joint Line		
Right Side:	52 cm	**Left Side:**	44 cm
Location:	Knee Joint Line + 16 cm proximal		
Right Side:	48 cm	**Left Side:**	38 cm

Initial Eval Level

Knee		Strength Right	Strength Left	Active ROM Right	Active ROM Left	Passive ROM Right	Passive ROM Left
	Flexion	3/5	5/5	71°	145°	85°	145°
	Extension	2+/5	5/5	-20°	0°	-15°	0°

Goal

Knee		Strength Right	Strength Left	Active ROM Right	Active ROM Left	Passive ROM Right	Passive ROM Left
	Flexion	5/5	5/5	135°	145°	140°	145°
	Extension	5/5	5/5	0°	0°	0°	0°

Knee Comments: Joint play is moderate-severely limited in posterior and forward movements of tibia on femur, and medial and lateral translation of tibia on femur.

Impairment Observations

The right knee is swollen and painful with palpation, movement and weight bearing >25% on the right lower extremity. Strength and range of motion in right knee is impaired and will be assessed with each treatment.

Interventions (CPT Code)

Physical Therapy Evaluation 97001

Gait Training &/or Stair Climbing - Therapeutic Procedure - 1+ Areas 97116

Therapeutic Exercises - Therapeutic Procedure - 1+ Areas 97110

Ultrasound - Modality to 1+ Areas - Each 15 Min 97035

Frequency of PT:	Three times weekly
Duration of PT:	6 weeks

Thomas Hook, PT

01/15/07

Thomas Hook, PT

Date

State License #: 310

Appendix 8, cont'd

Lakeside Rehab
123 Lakeside Drive
Colorado Springs, Co 80917

(888) 401-4400
Fax (615) 259-3605

| Occupational Therapy | **Plan Of Care** (Initial Evaluation) | Page 1 |

Patient: **Rubble, Barney**

MR #: **1234**   DOB: **01/01/1981**

OT: **Cynthia Morris-Hosking OTR**

Plan of Care Date: **Friday, April 14, 2006**

Provider: **Lakeside Rehabilitation**

Onset Date of Medical Diagnosis with ICD9:   02/25/2006   Wrist - Fracture (Closed) - Colles' 813.41

Occupational Therapy Diagnosis: Muscle - Weakness 728.87
Pain - Wrist 719.43

Problems	**Goals**
Grooming and Oral Hygiene: Independent with difficulty	Grooming and Oral Hygiene: Independent
Donning Orthosis/Prothesis/Splint Fasteners/Buttons: Independent with difficulty	Donning Orthosis/Prothesis/Splint Fasteners/Buttons: Independent
Tolerance to Community Activities: Moderate limitation in a specific IADL affecting performance	Tolerance to Community Activities: No limitation in a specific IADL
Tolerance to Work Activities: Moderate - Severe limitation in a specific work activity affecting performance	Tolerance to Work Activities: No limitation in a specific work activity
Pain#1: Joint Pain - Radio-carpal - Right; At Rest 2/10; With Activity 6/10; Dull; Localized	Goals for Pain: Client to have 0/10 pain in right upper extremity at rest and with activity.

Skills and Components - Short Term Goals

Short Term Goal(s): Joint inflammation, or restriction & pain are reduced by 50% - 2 weeks

Areas of Occupation - Long Term Goals

Long Term Goal(s): Functional use of right upper extremity as dominant extremity for all tasks. in 4 weeks

Skilled Analysis of Safety Deficits or Problems: Barney is right hand dominant and has difficulty with ADL's as he is doing most tasks with his left hand. He is unable to carry food or trays at work, and is unable to operate a mouse or keyboard with his right hand. Handwriting is legible with difficulty. Difficulty with coin manipulation for in hand skills.

Specific Joints
(Note: Blank indicates Strength / Range of Motion are within functional limits or not tested)

Forearm	**Initial Eval Level**						**Forearm**	**Goal**					
	Strength		Active ROM		Passive ROM			Strength		Active ROM		Passive ROM	
	Right	Left	Right	Left	Right	Left		Right	Left	Right	Left	Right	Left
Supination	3-/5		40°		45°		Supination	5/5		75°		75°	
Pronation	3-/5		60°		65°		Pronation	5/5		75°		75°	

Wrist	**Initial Eval Level**						**Wrist**	**Goal**					
	Strength		Active ROM		Passive ROM			Strength		Active ROM		Passive ROM	
	Right	Left	Right	Left	Right	Left		Right	Left	Right	Left	Right	Left
Flexion	3-/5		15°		20°		Flexion	5/5		70°		70°	
Extension	3-/5		15°		20°		Extension	5/5		70°		70°	
Ulnar Deviation	2/5		5°		8°		Ulnar Deviation	5/5		25°		25°	
Radial Deviation	2/5		3°		5°		Radial Deviation	5/5		15°		15°	

Lakeside Rehabilitation

Appendix 9   Electronic example of an occupational therapy plan of care form. (Courtesy The Rehab Documentation Company, Inc.)

Continued

Occupational Therapy

Plan Of Care   (Initial Evaluation)

Page 2

Patient: **Rubble, Barney**

MR #: **1234**   DOB: **01/01/1981**

OT: **Cynthia Morris-Hosking OTR**

Plan of Care Date: **Friday, April 14, 2006**

Provider: **Lakeside Rehabilitation**

Initial Eval Level				Goal		
Grip Strength	Right	Left		**Grip Strength**	Right	Left
Gross Grasp:	20	85		Gross Grasp:	85	85
3 Point Pinch:	5	15		3 Point Pinch:	12	15
2 Point Pinch:	3	10		2 Point Pinch:	10	10
Lateral Pinch:	5	12		Lateral Pinch:	12	12

Assessment: Moderate edema in right wrist and hand. Guarding with active range of motion due to pain. Soft tissue limitations for passive range of motion. Able to use a gross grasp and pinch with right hand with limited strength.

Interventions (CPT Code)

Occupational Therapy Evaluation 97003

Self Care/Home Management Training - Direct contact 97535

Therapeutic Activities - Direct patient contact 97530

Manual Therapy Techniques - 1+ Regions 97140

Frequency of OT: Three times weekly

Duration of OT: 4 weeks

Date	James L. Smith MD		Date	Cynthia Morris-Hosking OTR
				State Lic #: 309

Software Reg #: Q0R88-0R0R0-RAMKZ-WU7ZL

Lakeside Rehabilitation

Appendix 10 Wheelchair Features/Components

Feature/Component	Value	Advantage	Disadvantage
Aluminum or titanium frame	Lighter weight than a standard chair (ultralight)	Compared with a standard chair, less exertion is required to propel it; it causes less stress to upper extremities; and it reduces cumulative trauma to upper extremities in long-term users	More expensive than a standard chair
Rigid frame	Stronger and usually lighter than a standard chair	Compared with a standard chair, it requires less maintenance and has a smaller turning radius; used for ultralight and sport-style chairs	More difficult than a standard chair to store or transport; feet cannot be used for propulsion; difficult to stand up from
Folding frame	Allows chair to be folded	Can fold for storage or transport; removable front rigging allows feet to propel; can swing away or remove front rigging for standing transfer or better approach to objects in front of chair	Requires more maintenance than other chairs; cross frame may wear or loosen over time; not as strong as a chair with a rigid frame; weighs more than the rigid frame chair
Cushion	Helps distribute pressure to reduce skin breakdown; provides support for pelvis	Adds comfort; helps position pelvis and support body weight	Requires maintenance; must be removed before chair can be folded; may interfere with sitting transfers; does not eliminate pressure to ischial tuberosities
Solid or molded backrest	Supports trunk	May help accommodate or correct some postural deviations; improves sitting balance and posture for better use of upper extremities	Increases chair weight; must be removed to fold chair; requires maintenance
Headrest with lateral supports	Prevents lateral or forward flexion of head and neck	Improves posture; provides cues for neutral head alignment	Requires periodic adjustment; restricts head movement; adds weight and expense
Lateral trunk supports	Provide support to trunk	Improve trunk posture; promote hands-free sitting balance	Require periodic adjustment; may cause skin irritation or breakdown over ribs or upper arm; add weight and expense
Lateral or medial thigh supports	Prevent excessive hip adduction or abduction	Improve lower extremity alignment	Interfere with transfers; may cause skin irritation or breakdown; add weight and expense
Hip guides	Prevent or may correct pelvic obliquity	Improve pelvic alignment and sitting balance	Increase risk of skin breakdown over the greater trochanters; add weight and expense
Side guards on armrest	Contain and position cushion; help maintain neutral pelvis	Prevent clothing from contacting drive wheels	May interfere with sitting transfer; may cause pressure to greater trochanters or lateral thigh
Removable/ reversible cutout (desk type) armrest	Allows position changes for armrest	With cutout portion forward, allows chair to get close to table or desk; with armrest forward, provides surface to push from for standing transfer	Can disengage if used to lift chair; lock mechanism requires ability to manipulate
Solid tires	Eliminate flat tires	Least expensive; minimal maintenance	Less comfort and less traction than other tires; may be difficult to propel on some surfaces

Continued

Feature/Component	Value	Advantage	Disadvantage
Semipneumatic or pneumatic tires	Greater comfort	Provide some shock absorption and a smoother ride than other tires	Pneumatic tires require maintenance and may deflate; semipneumatic tires have flat inserts and provide a smoother ride without tire maintenance; both are more expensive than solid tires
Magnesium ("mag") wheels	Stronger than spoke wheels	Maintain wheel shape better	Bearings tend to wear and may require replacement
Plastic-coated hand rims	Provide a better grip on hand rims	Improve friction for better propulsion, especially when hand grip is diminished	Plastic coating may crack or chip; coating may need to be replaced
Drive wheel camber	Increases lateral stability	Makes it easier to propel and turn the chair	Increases overall chair width
Adjustable rear axle	Allows adjustment of center of gravity of the chair	With the axle forward, it is easier to propel and turn the chair and perform a "wheelie"	With the axle forward, the chair is more likely to tip backward; requires more maintenance
Quick-release axles	Chair wheels can be removed	Make it easier to transport the chair; allow wheels to be interchanged	Require maintenance; provide a risk that the wheel may disengage when in use
Rigid front rigging	Stabilizes the front of the chair	Provides a solid footrest, especially for sport-type chairs	Makes it more difficult to stand; feet cannot be used for propulsion; limits front approach to objects or furniture
Swing-away front rigging	Able to alter position of front rigging	Removable; feet can be used for propulsion; allows better access to objects in front of chair when removed or swung away	Requires maintenance; requires ability to manipulate the control mechanism; can disengage if used to lift the chair
High-mount wheel locks	Provide better access to wheel locks	Make it easier to reach and engage the locks	May interfere with sitting transfer; may interfere with hand propulsion
Scissor wheel locks	Lock drive wheels	Do not protrude from chair; less likely to interfere with functional activities	Are more difficult to reach and operate
Lap belt	Prevents pelvis from sliding forward; helps position pelvis	Allows upper trunk movements for functional activities	Can become tangled in wheels when not fastened; upper trunk can fall forward
Chest strap	Prevents upper trunk from falling forward; compensates for poor trunk control or sitting balance	Prevents forward movement (flexion) of the upper trunk	Can become tangled in wheels when not fastened; limits trunk movements
Chest harness	Compensates for poor trunk control and sitting balance	Decreases forward shoulder or kyphotic postures; prevents forward movement (flexion) of upper trunk	Can be a choking hazard; limits trunk movements

Modified from Meehan R, Skolsky RJ: Navigating the options, *Rehab Management* 18:34-37, 2005.

Appendix **11**

BRADEN SCALE FOR PREDICTING PRESSURE SORE RISK

Patient's Name _____ Evaluator Name _____ Date of Assessment

SENSORY PERCEPTION Ability to respond meaning-fully to pressure-related discomfort	**1. Completely Limited** Unresponsive (does not moan, flinch, or grasp) to painful stimuli, due to diminished level of consciousness or sedation OR limited ability to feel pain over most of body	**2. Very Limited** Responds only to painful stimuli. Cannot communicate discomfort except by moaning or restlessness OR has a sensory impairment which limits the ability to feel pain or discomfort over 1/2 of body.	**3. Slightly Limited** Responds to verbal com-mands, but cannot always communicate discomfort or the need to be turned OR has some sensory impairment which limits ability to feel pain or discomfort in 1 or 2 extremities.	**4. No Impairment** Responds to verbal commands. Has no sensory deficit which would limit ability to feel or voice pain or discomfort.				
MOISTURE Degree to which skin is exposed to moisture	**1. Constantly Moist** Skin is kept moist almost constantly by perspiration, urine, etc. Dampness is detected every time patient is moved or turned.	**2. Very Moist** Skin is often, but not always moist. Linen must be changed at least once a shift.	**3. Occasionally Moist** Skin is occasionally moist, requiring an extra linen change approximately once a day.	**4. Rarely Moist** Skin is usually dry, linen only requires changing at routine intervals.				
ACTIVITY Degree of physical activity	**1. Bedfast** Confined to bed.	**2. Chairfast** Ability to walk severely limited or nonexistent. Cannot bear own weight and/or must be assisted into chair or wheelchair.	**3. Walks Occasionally** Walks occasionally during day, but for very short distances, with or without assistance. Spends majority of each shift in bed or chair.	**4. Walks Frequently** Walks outside room at least twice a day and inside room at least once every two hours during waking hours.				
MOBILITY Ability to change and control body position	**1. Completely Immobile** Does not make even slight changes in body or extremity position without assistance.	**2. Very Limited** Makes occasional slight changes in body or extremity position but unable to make frequent or significant changes independently.	**3. Slightly Limited** Makes frequent though slight changes in body or extremity position independently.	**4. No Limitation** Makes major and frequent changes in position without assistance.				
NUTRITION Usual food intake pattern	**1. Very Poor** Never eats a complete meal. Rarely eats more than 1/3 of any food offered. Eats 2 servings or less of protein (meat or dairy products) per day. Takes fluids poorly. Does not take a liquid dietary supplement OR is NPO and/or maintained on clear liquids or IV for more than 5 days.	**2. Probably Inadequate** Rarely eats a complete meal and generally eats only about 1/2 of any food offered. Protein intake includes only 3 servings of meat or dairy products per day. Occasionally will take a dietary supplement OR receives less than optimum amount of liquid diet or tube feeding.	**3. Adequate** Eats over half of most meals. Eats a total of 4 servings of protein (meat, dairy products) per day. Occasionally will refuse a meal, but will usually take a supplement when offered OR is on a tube feeding or TPN regimen which probably meets most of nutritional needs.	**4. Excellent** Eats most of every meal. Never refuses a meal. Usually eats a total of 4 or more servings of meat and dairy products. Occasionally eats between meals. Does not require supplementation.				
FRICTION & SHEAR	**1. Problem** Requires moderate to maximum assistance in moving. Complete lifting without sliding against sheets is impossible. Frequently slides down in bed or chair, requiring frequent repositioning with maximum assistance. Spasticity, contractures or agitation leads to almost constant friction.	**2. Potential Problem** Moves feebly or requires minimum assistance. During a move, skin probably slides to some extent against sheets, chair, restraints or other devices. Maintains relatively good position in chair or bed most of the time but occasionally slides down.	**3. No Apparent Problem** Moves in bed and in chair independently and has sufficient muscle strength to lift up completely during move. Maintains good position in bed or chair.					
				Total Score				

NATIONAL
PRESSURE
ULCER
ADVISORY
PANEL

Pressure Ulcer Scale for Healing (PUSH)
PUSH Tool 3.0

Patient Name_____ Patient ID# _____

Ulcer Location _____ Date _____

Directions:

Observe and measure the pressure ulcer. Categorize the ulcer with respect to surface area, exudate, and type of wound tissue. Record a sub-score for each of these ulcer characteristics. Add the sub-scores to obtain the total score. A comparison of total scores measured over time provides an indication of the improvement or deterioration in pressure ulcer healing.

LENGTH X WIDTH (in cm²)	0	1	2	3	4	5	Sub-score
	0	< 0.3	0.3 – 0.6	0.7 – 1.0	1.1 – 2.0	2.1 – 3.0	
		6	7	8	9	10	
		3.1 – 4.0	4.1 – 8.0	8.1 – 12.0	12.1 – 24.0	> 24.0	
EXUDATE AMOUNT	0	1	2	3			Sub-score
	None	Light	Moderate	Heavy			
TISSUE TYPE	0	1	2	3	4		Sub-score
	Closed	Epithelial Tissue	Granulation Tissue	Slough	Necrotic Tissue		
							TOTAL SCORE

Length x Width: Measure the greatest length (head to toe) and the greatest width (side to side) using a centimeter ruler. Multiply these two measurements (length x width) to obtain an estimate of surface area in square centimeters (cm²). Caveat: Do not guess! Always use a centimeter ruler and always use the same method each time the ulcer is measured.

Exudate Amount: Estimate the amount of exudate (drainage) present after removal of the dressing and before applying any topical agent to the ulcer. Estimate the exudate (drainage) as none, light, moderate, or heavy.

Tissue Type: This refers to the types of tissue that are present in the wound (ulcer) bed. Score as a 4 if there is any necrotic tissue present. Score as a 3 if there is any amount of slough present and necrotic tissue is absent. Score as a 2 if the wound is clean and contains granulation tissue. A superficial wound that is reepithelializing is scored as a 1. When the wound is closed, score as a 0.

- 4 – **Necrotic Tissue (Eschar):** black, brown, or tan tissue that adheres firmly to the wound bed or ulcer edges and may be either firmer or softer than surrounding skin.
- 3 – **Slough:** yellow or white tissue that adheres to the ulcer bed in strings or thick clumps, or is mucinous.
- 2 – **Granulation Tissue:** pink or beefy-red tissue with a shiny, moist, granular appearance.
- 1 – **Epithelial Tissue:** for superficial ulcers, new pink or shiny tissue (skin) that grows in from the edges or as islands on the ulcer surface.
- 0 – **Closed/Resurfaced:** the wound is completely covered with epithelium (new skin).

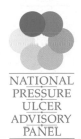

NATIONAL
PRESSURE
ULCER
ADVISORY
PANEL

Pressure Ulcer Healing Chart
To monitor trends in PUSH Scores over time
(Use a separate page for each pressure ulcer)

Patient Name_____ Patient ID# _____

Ulcer Location _____ Date _____

Directions:
Observe and measure pressure ulcers at regular intervals using the PUSH Tool.
Date and record PUSH Sub-scores and Total Scores on the Pressure Ulcer Healing Record below.

Pressure Ulcer Healing **Record**

Date													
Length x Width													
Exudate Amount													
Tissue Type													
PUSH Total Score													

Graph the PUSH Total Scores on the Pressure Ulcer Healing Graph below.

Pressure Ulcer Healing **Graph**

PUSH Total Score													
17													
16													
15													
14													
13													
12													
11													
10													
9													
8													
7													
6													
5													
4													
3													
2													
1													
Healed = 0													
Date													

Appendix **13** Examples of Title III Requirements and Accommodations

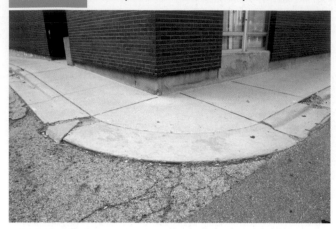

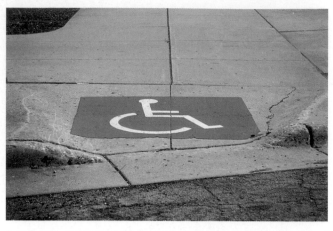

A curb cutout showing uneven surfaces and lack of crosswalk markings; some cutouts may not be in good repair or be functional for wheelchair access.

A curb cutout showing smooth, gradual elevation from the street level to the sidewalk, a wide cutout, and a large turning area on the sidewalk in all directions.

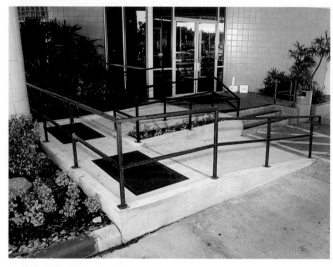

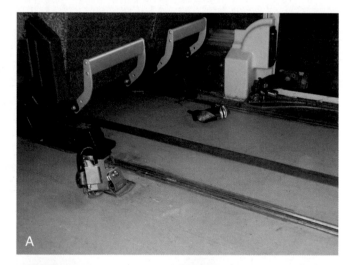

A ramp to a public building showing the ramp width, an even surface, and adequate space to turn the wheelchair where the direction and slope of the ramp change.

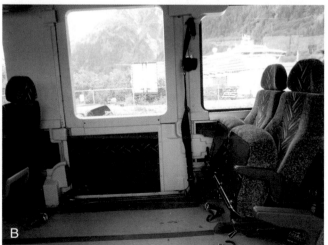

A public bus with wheelchair accommodations at the side entrance.

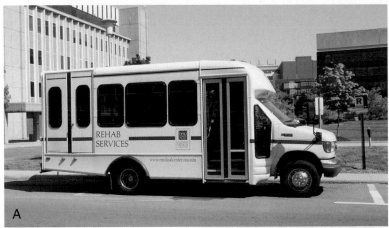

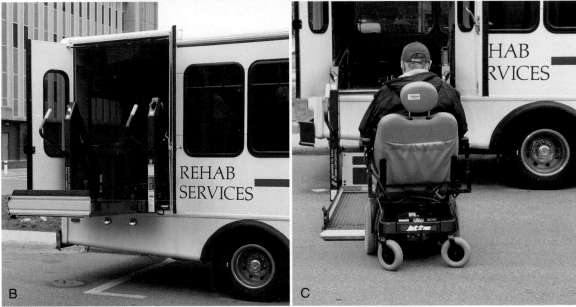

A public bus converted to accommodate a wheelchair. The bus has space and restraints for wheelchairs.

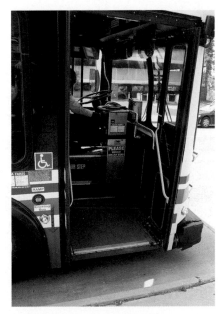

A kneeling bus in the lowered position (operated by the Central Ohio Transit Authority).

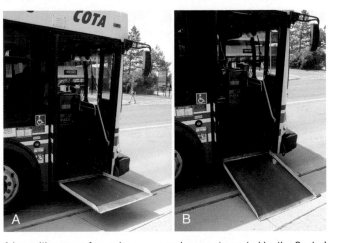

A bus with a ramp for easier access and egress (operated by the Central Ohio Transit Authority).

Index

Page numbers followed by "f" indicate figures, "t" indicate tables, and "b" indicate boxes.